Polit & Beck

Canadian 🍁

Essentials

of Nursing

Research

Fourth Edition

2019

Kevin Woo, PhD, RN, FAPWCA

Associate Professor
Queen's University
Kingston, Ontario, Canada

⬛. Wolters Kluwer

Philadelphia • Baltimore • New York • London
Buenos Aires • Hong Kong • Sydney • Tokyo

Acquisitions Editor: Christina C. Burns
Development Editor: Dan Reilly
Editorial Coordinator: Lindsay Ries
Marketing Manager: Sarah Schuessler
Production Product Manager: David Saltzberg
Design Coordinator: Joan Wendt
Manufacturing Coordinator: Karin Duffield
Prepress Vendor: Aptara, Inc.

9 8 7 6 5 4 3 2 1

Printed in China

Library of Congress Cataloging-in-Publication Data
ISBN-13: 978-1-4963-0146-8
ISBN-10: 1-4963-0146-3
Cataloging-in-Publication data available on request from the Publisher.

LWW.com

To students, clinicians, educators, researchers and all levels
of knowledge users in nursing.

Kevin Woo, PhD, RN, FAPWCA is an Associate Professor at Queen's University, School of Nursing and School of Rehabilitation in Kingston, Canada. His clinical and research interests focus on chronic disease management, gerontological nursing, wound healing, knowledge translation, and patient safety using a variety of research methods.

Canadian Essentials of Nursing Research, Fourth Edition, helps students learn how to read and critique research reports, and to develop an appreciation of research as a path to enhancing nursing practice.

This edition is designed to help students become true consumers of nursing research, with concepts being introduced carefully and difficult ideas presented thoughtfully, so that students can easily learn how to read and critique research reports. With a clear and non-intimidating writing style, the text highlights Canadian-specific research set in a Canadian context. The book also features Canadian references to engage students and foster an appreciation of research as a path to enhancing nursing practice. The fourth edition of this book and its online resources will make it easier and more satisfying for nurses to pursue a professional pathway that incorporates thoughtful appraisals of evidence.

LEGACY OF *ESSENTIALS OF NURSING RESEARCH*

This edition is focused on the art—and science—of research critique. The text offers guidance to students who are learning to appraise research reports and use research findings in practice.

The basic principles that helped to shape this edition of the book are:

1. An assumption that competence in doing and appraising research is critical to the nursing profession
2. A conviction that research inquiry is intellectually and professionally rewarding to nurses
3. An unswerving belief that learning about research methods need be neither intimidating nor dull

Consistent with these principles, the text presents research fundamentals in a way that both facilitates understanding and arouses curiosity and interest.

NEW TO THIS EDITION

New Organization

In this edition, the parts are organized by methodologic content. So, for example, Part 3 in this edition covers designs and methods for quantitative, qualitative, and mixed methods research, and Part 4 is devoted to analysis and interpretation in quantitative and qualitative studies. (Please see "Organization of the Text" later in this preface for more information.) This new organization offers greater continuity of methodologic concepts and will facilitate better understanding of key methodologic differences between quantitative and qualitative research. This new organization will better meet the needs of students and faculty.

Manageable Text for One-Semester Course

The text has been streamlined to make it more manageable for use in a one-semester course. The length has been reduced by organizing content differently and by keeping essential information in the text while moving background/advanced content online.

Enhanced Accessibility

To make this edition even more user-friendly than in the past, a concerted effort has been made to simplify the presentation of complex topics. Most importantly, the coverage of statistical information has been reduced and simplified. The chapter on measurement has been eliminated in favour of presenting a shorter, more digestible section on this topic in the chapter on quantitative data collection, which is supplemented by information in the chapter on statistical analysis. In addition, throughout the book, more straightforward, concise language has been used.

New Content

In addition to updating the book with new information on conventional research methods, content has been added on the following topics:

- Quality improvement projects, describing how they are distinct from research studies and evidence-based practice (EBP) projects. This new content is found in Chapter 13.

- Clinical significance, a seldom mentioned but important topic among researchers in other health care fields that has only recently gained traction among nurse researchers. This new content is found in Chapter 15.

THE TEXT

The content of this edition is as follows:

- **Part 1, Overview of Nursing Research and Evidence-Based Practice,** introduces fundamental concepts in nursing research. Chapter 1 summarizes the background of nursing research, discusses the philosophical underpinnings of qualitative research versus quantitative research, and describes major purposes of nursing research. Chapter 2 offers guidance on using research to build an evidence-based practice. Chapter 3 introduces readers to key research terms and presents an overview of steps in the research process for both quantitative and qualitative studies. Chapter 4 focuses on research journal articles, explaining what they are and how to read them. Chapter 5 discusses ethics in nursing studies.

- **Part 2, Preliminary Steps in Quantitative and Qualitative Research,** further sets the stage for learning about the research process by considering aspects of a study's conceptualization. Chapter 6 focuses on the development of research questions and the formulation of research hypotheses. Chapter 7 discusses how to retrieve research evidence (especially in electronic bibliographic databases) and the role of research literature reviews. Chapter 8 presents information about theoretical and conceptual frameworks.

- **Part 3, Designs and Methods for Quantitative and Qualitative Nursing Research,** presents material on the design and conduct of all types of nursing studies. Chapter 9 describes fundamental design principles and discusses many specific aspects of quantitative research design, including efforts to enhance rigor. Chapter 10 introduces the topics of sampling and data collection in quantitative studies. Concepts relating to quality in measurements—reliability and validity—are introduced in this chapter. Chapter 11 describes the various qualitative research traditions that have contributed to the growth of constructivist inquiry and presents the basics of qualitative design. Chapter 12 covers sampling and data collection methods used in qualitative research, describing how these differ from approaches used in quantitative studies. Chapter 13 emphasizes mixed methods research, but the chapter also discusses other special types of research such as surveys, outcomes research, and quality improvement projects.

- **Part 4, Analysis and Interpretation in Quantitative and Qualitative Research**, presents tools for making sense of research data. Chapter 14 reviews methods of statistical analysis. The chapter assumes no prior instruction in statistics and focuses primarily on helping readers to understand why statistics are useful, what test might be appropriate in a given situation, and what statistical information in a research article means. Chapter 15 discusses approaches to interpreting statistical results, including interpretations linked to assessments of clinical significance. Chapter 16 discusses qualitative analysis, with an emphasis on ethnographic, phenomenologic, and grounded theory studies. Chapter 17 elaborates on criteria for appraising trustworthiness and integrity in qualitative studies. Finally, Chapter 18 describes systematic reviews, including how to understand and appraise both meta-analyses and metasyntheses.

- At the end of the book, students are offered additional critiquing support. **In the appendices, full-length Research Articles** appear—two quantitative, one qualitative, and one mixed methods—that students can read, analyze, and critique. Students can model their critiques on the **full critiques of two of those studies provided or compare their work to the ones provided**. A glossary at the end of the book provides additional support for those needing to look up the meaning of a methodologic term.

FEATURES OF THE TEXT

Many of the classic features that were successfully used in previous editions have been retained to assist those learning to read and apply evidence from nursing research:

- **New! Canadian Research Examples** make research real and interesting to nursing students, as well as appropriate to the Canadian health care environment. These examples illustrate key chapter concepts, while the accompanying Critical Thinking Exercises help build students' critical thinking skills.

- **Tips!** The text offers practical tips on how to apply the abstract notions of research methods in a real-world context, and makes abstract nursing research concepts easily understandable.

- **Critiquing Guidelines** help students learn to really *read* nursing research reports, helping them to learn to focus on the portions of a study that will help students use research in practice. Electronic versions of these guidelines are also on the Point.

- **Chapter Objectives, Key Terms, and Bulleted Summary Points** help students new to this critical subject matter hone in on what's most important.

- **Full-length Research Articles** in the text's appendices provide opportunities for nursing students to read, analyze, and critique recent research.

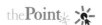
the**Point**

Canadian Essentials of Nursing Research, Fourth Edition, has ancillary resources designed with both students and instructors in mind, available on the**Point** website.

Student Resources Available on the**Point**

- **Supplements for Each Chapter** further students' exploration of specific topics. A full list of the supplements appears on page xv. These supplements can be assigned to provide additional background or to offer advanced material to meet students' specific needs.

- **Interactive Critical Thinking Activity** brings the Critical Thinking Exercises from the textbook (except those focused on studies in the appendices) to an easy-to-use interactive tool that enables students to apply new skills that they learn in each chapter. Students are guided through appraisals of real research examples and then ushered through a series of questions that challenge them to think about the quality of evidence from the study. Responses can be printed or e-mailed directly to instructors for homework or testing.

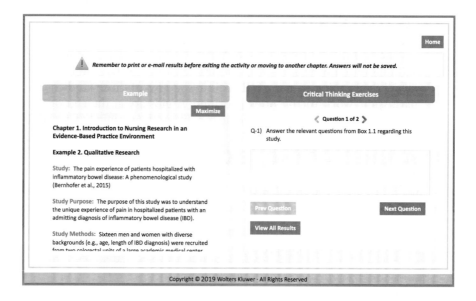

- **Answers to Critical Thinking Exercises** are provided for questions related to the studies in Appendices A and B of the textbook.

- **Journal Articles** from Wolters Kluwer journals are provided for additional critiquing opportunities. Many of these are the full journal articles for studies used at the end-of-chapter Research Examples. All journal articles that appear on the**Point** are identified in the text with ⚡ and are called out in the References lists for appropriate chapters with a double asterisk (**).

- **Internet Resources with relevant and useful websites** related to chapter content can be clicked on directly without having to retype the URL and risk a typographical error. This edition also includes **links to all open-access articles cited in the textbook; these articles** are called out in the References lists for appropriate chapters with a single asterisk (*).

- **Critiquing Guidelines** and **Learning Objectives** from the textbook are available in Microsoft Word for your convenience.

- **Nursing Professionals' Roles and Responsibilities.**

Instructor's Resources Available on thePoint

- In addition to all of the student resources noted above, instructors will also have access to the following ancillaries:
  - NEW! **Test Generator Questions** are completely new and written by the book's authors for the fourth edition, offering hundreds of multiple-choice questions to aid instructors in assessing their students' understanding of the chapter content.

- **An Instructor's Manual** includes a preface that offers guidance to improve the teaching experience. We have recognized the need for strong support for instructors in teaching a course that can be quite challenging. Part of the difficulty stems from students' anxiety about the course content and their concern that research methods might not be relevant to their nursing practice. We offer numerous suggestions on how to make learning about—and teaching—research methods more rewarding. The contents of the Instructor's Manual include the following for each chapter:
  - **Statement of Intent.** Discover the authors' goals for each chapter.
  - **Special Class Projects.** Find numerous ideas for interesting and meaningful class projects. Check out the Icebreakers and activities relating to the Great Cookie Experiment with accompanying SPSS files.
  - **Test Questions and Answers.** True/false questions, plus important application questions that test students' comprehension and their ability to put their new critiquing skills to use. The application questions focus on a brief summary of a study and include several short-answer questions (with our answers), plus essay questions. These application questions are intended to assess students' knowledge about methodologic concepts and their critiquing skills.

- **Answers to the Interactive Critical Thinking Activity.** Suggested answers to the questions in the Interactive Critical Thinking Activity are available to instructors. Students can either print or e-mail their responses directly to the instructor for testing or as a homework assignment.

- **PowerPoint Presentations** offer summaries of key points in each chapter for use in class presentations. These slides are available in a format that permits easy adaptation and include questions that can be used on their own or are compatible with audience response programs and devices to assess students' grasp of important concepts.

- **An Image Bank** includes figures from the text.

- **Strategies for Effective Teaching** offer creative approaches for engaging students.

CLOSING NOTE

It is my hope and expectation that the content, style, and organization of this fourth edition of *Canadian Essentials of Nursing Research* will be helpful to those students who want to become skilful, thoughtful readers of nursing studies in the Canadian health care environment and to those wishing to enhance their clinical performance based on research findings. Many examples are drawn from our vibrant nursing research community in Canada to inspire, inculcate, and instil the passion for nursing scholarship.

KEVIN WOO, PhD, RN, FAPWCA

Learning Objectives
focus students' attention
on critical content ⟶

Learning Objectives

On completing this chapter, you will be able to:

- Understand why research is important in nursing
- Discuss the need for evidence-based practice
- Describe broad historical trends and future directions in nursing research
- Identify alternative sources of evidence for nursing practice
- Describe major characteristics of the positivist and constructivist paradigm
- Compare the traditional scientific method (quantitative research) with constructivist methods (qualitative research)
- Identify several purposes of quantitative and qualitative research
- Define new terms in the chapter

Key Terms alert
students to important
terminology ⟶

Key Terms

- Assumption
- Cause-probing research
- Clinical nursing research
- Clinical significance
- Constructivist paradigm
- Empirical evidence
- Evidence-based practice
- Generalizability
- Journal club
- Nursing research
- Paradigm
- Positivist paradigm
- Qualitative research
- Quantitative research
- Research
- Research methods
- Scientific method
- Systematic review

Examples help students
apply content to real-
life research ⟶

Example of inclusion and exclusion criteria • • • • • • • • • • •
Stinson et al. (2016) studied the effectiveness of online peer mentoring programmes for adolescents with arthritis. To be eligible, adolescents had to be diagnosed with juvenile idiopathic arthritis, has access to Skype, and between the ages of 12 and 18 years. Children were excluded if they had cognitive impairment or psychiatric conditions, such as schizophrenia or bipolar disorder.

Tip boxes describe
what is found in actual
research articles ⟶

☞ **TIP** If attrition is random (i.e., those dropping out of a study are similar to those remaining in it), then there would not be bias. However, attrition is rarely random. In general, the higher the rate of attrition, the greater the risk of bias. Biases are usually of concern if the rate exceeds 10% to 15%.

How-to-tell Tip boxes
explain confusing issues
in actual research
articles ⟶

☞ **HOW-TO-TELL TIP** How can you tell a problem statement? Problem statements are rarely explicitly labeled. The first sentence of a research report is often the starting point of a problem statement. The problem statement is usually interwoven with findings from the research literature. Prior findings provide a rationale to support the problem statement and highlight gaps in knowledge. In many articles, it is difficult to disentangle the problem statement from the literature review, unless there is a subsection specifically labeled "Literature Review" or something similar.

Critiquing Guidelines boxes lead students through key issues in a research article ⟶

Box 7.1 Guidelines for Critiquing Literature Reviews

1. Does the review seem thorough and up-to-date? Did it include major studies on the topic? Did it include recent research?
2. Did the review rely mainly on research reports, using primary sources?
3. Did the review critically appraise and compare key studies? Did it identify important gaps in the literature?
4. Was the review well organized? Is the development of ideas clear?
5. Did the review use appropriate language, suggesting the tentativeness of prior findings? Is the review objective?
6. If the review was in the introduction for a new study, did the review support the need for the study?
7. If the review was designed to summarize evidence for clinical practice, did it draw appropriate conclusions about practice implications?

Research Examples highlight critical points made in the chapter and sharpen critical thinking skills ⟶

RESEARCH EXAMPLES WITH CRITICAL THINKING EXERCISES

In this section, we describe the sampling and data collection plan of a quantitative nursing study. Read the summary and then answer the critical thinking questions that follow, referring to the full research report if necessary. Example 1 is featured on the interactive *Critical Thinking Activity* on thePoint website. The critical thinking questions for Example 2 are based on the study that appears in its entirety in Appendix A of this book. Our comments for these exercises are in the Student Resources section on thePoint.

EXAMPLE 1: SAMPLING AND DATA COLLECTION IN A QUANTITATIVE STUDY

Study: Insomnia symptoms are associated with abnormal endothelial function (Routledge et al., 2015) (Some information about the study was provided in Rask, Brigham, and Johns (2011).)

Purpose: The purpose of this study was to test the hypothesis that insomnia symptoms are associated with reduced endothelial function in working adults.

Critical Thinking Exercises provide opportunities to practice critiquing actual research articles ⟶

Critical Thinking Exercises

1. Answer the relevant questions from Box 10.1 regarding this study.
2. Answer the relevant questions from Box 10.2 regarding this study.
3. Are there variables in this study that could have been measured through observation but were not?
4. If the results of this study are valid and reliable, what might be some of the uses to which the findings could be put in clinical practice?

Summary Points review chapter content to ensure success ⟶

Summary Points

- The **research design** is the overall plan for answering research questions. In quantitative studies, the design designates whether there is an intervention, the nature of any comparisons, methods for controlling confounding variables, whether there will be blinding, and the timing and location of data collection.
- Therapy, Prognosis, and Etiology questions are cause-probing, and there is a hierarchy of designs for yielding best evidence for these questions.
- Key criteria for inferring causality include (1) a **cause** (independent variable) must precede an **effect** (outcome), (2) there must be a detectable relationship between a cause and an effect, and (3) the relationship between the two does not reflect the influence of a third (confounding) variable.
- A *counterfactual* is what would have happened to the same people simultaneously

- Crossover designs are inappropriate if there is a risk of *carryover effects*.
- The control group can undergo various conditions, including an alternative treatment, a **placebo** or pseudointervention, standard treatment ("usual care"), or a *wait-list* (*delayed treatment*) condition.
- **Quasiexperiments** (*trials without randomization*) involve an intervention but lack a comparison group or randomization. Strong quasiexperimental designs introduce controls to compensate for these missing components.
- The **nonequivalent control-group, pretest–posttest design** involves a **comparison group** that was not created through randomization and the collection of pretreatment data from both groups to assess initial group equivalence.
- In a **time-series design**, outcome data are collected over a period of time before and after the intervention, usually for a single group.
- **Nonexperimental** (*observational*) **studies** include **descriptive research**—studies that

Special Icons alert students to important content found on thePoint

Angela Gillis, PhD
Professor Emeritus
St. Francis Xavier University, Rankin School
  of Nursing
Antigonish, Nova Scotia, Canada

Lyn Merryfeather, PhD, RN
University of Victoria
Lake Cowichan, British Columbia, Canada

Kim Mitchell, MN, RN
Instructor
Red River College
Winnipeg, Manitoba, Canada

Joyce O'Mahony, PhD, RN
Assistant Professor
Thompson Rivers University
Kamloops, British Columbia, Canada

Cheryl Pollard, PhD, RN
Associate Professor
Faculty of Nursing
MacEwan University
Edmonton, Alberta, Canada

ACKNOWLEDGMENTS

This book could not have happened without the dedication and hard work of many people, not least of all the staff at Wolters Kluwer. In particular, I want to express my appreciation for the support and encouragement of Senior Acquisitions Editor Christina Burns and Editorial Coordinator Lindsay Ries, and thank them for their exemplary efforts.

With nursing care becoming increasingly more complex within an ever-changing practice environment, there is a need to constantly inquire, appraise, and translate evidence to inform clinical decision making, improve patient-oriented outcomes, and effect system changes to bring about a comprehensive, cost-effective care delivery model. I want to acknowledge Dr. Polit and Dr. Beck for their vision and endeavour to advance nursing science, as well as their original book that continues to be highly regarded as a seminal text in Nursing Research. I am grateful for the opportunity to work on this edition of *Canadian Essentials of Nursing Research*.

Finally, I also want to acknowledge Canadian nursing researchers and their candescent scholarship, which afforded me the inspiration and exemplars to showcase the diversity and calibre of research interest.

CONTENTS

CHAPTER SUPPLEMENTS AVAILABLE ON thePoint

1 Introduction to Nursing Research in an Evidence-Based Practice Environment

Learning Objectives

On completing this chapter, you will be able to:

- Understand why research is important in nursing
- Discuss the need for evidence-based practice
- Describe broad historical trends and future directions in nursing research
- Identify alternative sources of evidence for nursing practice
- Describe major characteristics of the positivist and constructivist paradigm
- Compare the traditional scientific method (quantitative research) with constructivist methods (qualitative research)
- Identify several purposes of quantitative and qualitative research
- Define new terms in the chapter

Key Terms

- Assumption
- Cause-probing
- Clinical nursing research
- Clinical significance
- Constructivist paradigm
- Empirical evidence
- Evidence-based practice
- Generalizability
- Journal club
- Nursing research
- Paradigm
- Positivist paradigm
- Qualitative research
- Quantitative research
- Research
- Research methods
- Scientific method
- Systematic review

NURSING RESEARCH IN PERSPECTIVE

We know that many of you readers are not reading this book because you plan to become nurse researchers. Yet, we are also confident that many of you *will* participate in research-related activities during your careers, and virtually all of you will be expected to use research at a basic level. Although you may not yet grasp the relevance of research in your career as a nurse, we hope that you will come to see the value of nursing research and will be inspired by the efforts of the thousands of nurse researchers now working worldwide to improve patient care. You are embarking on a lifelong journey in which research will play a role. We hope to prepare you to enjoy the voyage.

What Is Nursing Research?

Whether you know it or not, you have already done a lot of research. When you use the Internet to find the "best deal" on a laptop or an airfare, you start with a question (e.g., Who has the best deal for what I want?), collect the information by searching different websites, and then come to a conclusion. This "everyday research" has much in common with formal research—but, of course, there are important differences, too.

As a formal enterprise, **research** is *systematic* inquiry that uses structured methods to answer questions and solve problems. The ultimate goal of formal research is to gain knowledge that would be useful for many people. **Nursing research** is systematic inquiry designed to develop trustworthy evidence about issues of importance to nurses and their clients. In this book, we emphasize **clinical nursing research**, which is research designed to guide nursing practice. Clinical nursing research typically begins with questions that are raised in day-to-day clinical practice—problems you may have already encountered.

Examples of nursing research questions •
- What is it like for older people to manage their health problems in the community in Canada? (Ploeg et al., 2017)
- Does Internet-based education improve chronic pain management? (Perry et al., 2017)

 TIP You may have the impression that research is abstract and irrelevant to practising nurses. But nursing research is about *real* people with *real* problems, and studying those problems offers opportunities to understand, then solve or address them through improvements to nursing care.

The Importance of Research to Evidence-Based Nursing

Nursing has experienced many changes in the past few decades. Nurses are increasingly expected to understand and undertake research and to base their practice on evidence from research—that is, to adopt an **evidence-based practice (EBP)**. EBP, broadly defined, is the use of the best evidence in making patient care decisions. Such evidence typically comes from research conducted by nurses and other health care professionals. Nurse leaders recognize the need to use evidence to make specific nursing decisions that are clinically appropriate and cost effective and result in positive client outcomes.

In Canada, research plays an important role in accreditation process and status. For example, the Registered Nurses' Association of Ontario (RNAO) has developed the Best Practice Spotlight Organizations (BPSOs) programme to recognize health care organizations that make a commitment to EBP. Changes to nursing practice are happening every day because of EBP efforts.

Example of evidence-based practice •
Many clinical practice changes arise from research. For example, "kangaroo care," the holding of preterm infants skin-to-skin, chest-to-chest by parents, is now widely practised in neonatal intensive care units (NICUs), but in the early 1990s, only a minority of

NICUs offered kangaroo care options. The adoption of this practice reflects good evidence that early skin-to-skin contact has clinical benefits and no negative side effects (Cong, Ludington-Hoe, & Walsh, 2011; Moore et al., 2012). Some of this evidence comes from rigorous studies by Canadian nurse researchers (Benoit et al., 2016; Campbell-Yeo et al., 2013; Johnston et al., 2009, 2013).

Roles of Nurses in Research

In the current EBP environment, every nurse is likely to engage in one or more activities along a continuum of research participation. At one end of the continuum are users or *consumers of nursing research*—nurses who read research reports to keep up-to-date on findings that may affect their practice. EBP depends on well-informed nursing research consumers.

At the other end of the continuum are the *producers of nursing research:* nurses who actively design and undertake studies. At one time, most nurse researchers were academics or professors who taught in schools of nursing, but research is increasingly being conducted by nurses at the bedside who want to find what works best for their clients.

Between these two end points on the continuum lie a variety of research-related activities in which nurses can participate. Even if you never conduct a study, you may do one of the following:

1. Identify an idea for a clinical inquiry
2. Assist in collecting research information
3. Offer advice to clients about participating in a study
4. Search for research evidence
5. Discuss the implications of a study in a **journal club** in your practice setting, which involves meetings to discuss research articles

In all research-related activities, nurses who have some research skills are more able than those without them to contribute to nursing and to EBP. Thus, with the research skills you gain from this book, *you* will be prepared to contribute to the advancement of nursing.

NURSING RESEARCH: PAST AND PRESENT

Most people agree that research in nursing began with Florence Nightingale in the mid-19th century. Based on her skilful analysis of factors affecting soldier mortality and morbidity during the Crimean War, she was successful in bringing about changes in nursing care and in public health. For many years after Nightingale's work, however, research was absent from the nursing literature. Studies began to appear in the early 1900s, but most concerned nurses' education.

From the 1950s to the mid-1960s, a lack of federal research funding was a major barrier to the growth of nursing research in Canada. During the 1960s, practice-oriented research began to emerge, and research-oriented journals started publication in several countries. In 1971, the launching of the first national conference on nursing research marked an important milestone in the Canadian nursing history. The focus of the conference was on nursing education and administration. Soon after that, Health and Welfare Canada provided substantial funding to establish the first Center for Nursing Research at McGill University in 1979. In the 1980s, nursing research was strengthened largely due to an increased investment by federal funding agencies such as the Medical Research Council of Canada (MRC) and the National Health Research and Development Program

(NHRDP) of Health Canada. The 1990s witnessed the birth of several more journals for nurse researchers, and specialty journals increasingly came to publish research articles. International cooperation in integrating EBP into nursing also developed in the 1990s. For example, Sigma Theta Tau International sponsored the first international research utilization conference, in cooperation with the faculty of the University of Toronto, in 1998. In 1999, the federal government established the Canadian Health Services Research Foundation (CHSRF), which created the Nursing Research Fund, a $25 million initiative to promote nursing research over a period of 10 years. In 2004, the Office of Nursing Policy, Health Canada, organized a meeting with five national nursing organizations, including the Canadian Nurses Association (CNA), Canadian Association of Schools of Nursing (CASN), Canadian Nurses Foundation (CNF), Academy of Canadian Executive Nurses (ACEN), and the Canadian Association of Nurse Researchers (CANR), with the purpose to discuss different strategies to promote research in nursing. The success of the meeting was marked by the establishment of the Canadian Consortium for Nursing Research and Innovation (CCNRI). The purpose of the CCNRI was to create a strong, unified voice to promote nursing research and to develop a framework for building nursing research capacity in Canada.

 TIP For those interested in learning more about the history of nursing research in the United States, we offer an expanded summary in the Supplement to this chapter on thePoint website.

Future Directions for Nursing Research

Nursing research continues to develop at a rapid pace and will undoubtedly flourish in the 21st century. Among the trends we foresee for the near future are the following:

- *Continued focus on EBP.* Encouragement for nurses to use research findings in practice is sure to continue. There is a need to improve the quality of nursing studies and nurses' skills in locating, understanding, critiquing, and using relevant study results. Relatedly, emerging interest is placed on *translational research*—research on how findings from studies can best be translated into practice (http://cihr-irsc.gc.ca).
- *Stronger evidence through confirmatory strategies.* Practising nurses rarely adopt an innovation on the basis of poorly designed or isolated studies. Strong research designs are essential, and confirmation is usually needed through *replication* (i.e., repeating) of studies in different clinical settings to validate the findings.
- *Continued emphasis on systematic reviews.* **Systematic reviews** are a cornerstone of EBP and have assumed increasing importance in all health disciplines. Systematic reviews rigorously integrate a wide scope of research information on a topic to determine if the evidence is weak or strong.
- *Expanded local research in health care settings.* Small studies designed to solve relevant problems will likely increase.
- *Expanded dissemination of research findings.* The Internet and other technological advances have had a big impact on the dissemination of research information, which in turn helps to promote EBP.
- *Increased focus on diversity issues and health disparities.* The issue of health disparities has emerged as a central concern, and this in turn has raised questions whether health interventions are sensitive to the diversity of Canada's population. Research must be sensitive to gender, religious affiliations, sexual orientation, abilities, economic status, and values of culturally and linguistically diverse populations.

- *Clinical significance and patient-oriented research.* Research findings increasingly must meet the test of being clinically significant, and patients have taken centre stage in efforts to define **clinical significance**. A major challenge in the years ahead will involve incorporating both research evidence and patient preferences into clinical decisions.
- *Interprofessional collaboration and health research.* Nurses function within an interprofessional environment. To answer complex questions in practice, there is a need for nurses to work closely with other professional groups.

What are nurse researchers likely to be studying in the future? Although there is tremendous diversity in research interests, research priorities have been articulated by CNF, CIHR, Sigma Theta Tau International, and other nursing organizations. For example, in the document titled Pan-Canadian Vision and Strategy for Health Services and Policy Research, CIHR identified 10 research priorities including innovation, patient engagement, primary and community care integration, person-centred disease management, and older adult health services (http://www.cihr-irsc.gc.ca/e/47945.html).

 TIP All websites cited in this chapter, plus additional websites with useful content relating to the foundations of nursing research, are in the Internet Resources on thePoint website. This will allow you to simply use the "Control/Click" feature to go directly to the website, without having to type in the URL and risk a typographical error. Websites corresponding to the content of all chapters of the book are also on thePoint.

SOURCES OF EVIDENCE FOR NURSING PRACTICE

Nurses make clinical decisions based on a large repertoire of knowledge. As a nursing student, you are gaining skills on how to practise nursing from your instructors, textbooks, and clinical placements. Even after you have graduated, you will continue to learn from other nurses and health care professionals. Because evidence is constantly evolving, learning about best-practice nursing will persist throughout your career.

Some of what you have learned thus far is based on systematic research, but much of it is not. What *are* the sources of evidence for nursing practice? Where does knowledge for practice come from? Until fairly recently, knowledge primarily was handed down from one generation to the next based on clinical experience, trial and error, tradition, and expert opinion. These alternative sources of knowledge are different from research-based information.

Tradition and Authority

Some nursing interventions are based on untested traditions, customs, and "unit culture" rather than on sound evidence. Indeed, a recent analysis suggests that that some traditional routines are ineffective, yet they persist, even in a health care centre recognized as a leader in EBP (Hanrahan et al., 2015). Another common source of knowledge is an authority, a person with specialized expertise. Reliance on authorities (such as nursing faculty or textbook authors) is unavoidable. Authorities, however, can be wrong—particularly if their expertise is based primarily on personal experience; yet, their knowledge is often unchallenged.

Example of "myths" in nursing textbooks • • • • • • • • • • • • • • • • • • •
One study suggests that nursing textbooks may contain many "myths." In their analysis of 23 widely used undergraduate psychiatric nursing textbooks, Holman et al. (2010) found that all books contained at least one unsupported assumption (myth) about loss and grief—that is, assumptions not supported by current research evidence. And many evidence-based findings about grief and loss were not included in the textbooks.

 TIP The consequences of *not* using research-based evidence can be devastating. For example, from 1956 through the 1980s, Dr. Benjamin Spock published several editions of *Baby and Child Care,* a parental guide that sold over 19 million copies worldwide. As an authority figure, he wrote the following advice: "I think it is preferable to accustom a baby to sleeping on his stomach from the beginning if he is willing" (Spock, 1979, p. 164). Research has clearly demonstrated that this sleeping position is associated with heighted risk of sudden infant death syndrome (SIDS). In their systematic review of evidence, Gilbert et al. (2005) wrote: "Advice to put infants to sleep on the front for nearly half a century was contrary to evidence from 1970 that this was likely to be harmful" (p. 874). They estimated that if medical advice had been guided by research evidence, over 60,000 infant deaths might have been prevented.

Clinical Experience and Trial and Error

Clinical experience can be a reliable source of knowledge. Yet, personal experience has limitations as a source of evidence for practice because each nurse's experience is too narrow to be generally useful, and personal experiences are often coloured by biases. Trial and error involves trying different alternatives over time until a solution to a problem is found. Trial and error can be practical, but the method tends to be disorganized, and solutions may be idiosyncratic.

Assembled Information

In making clinical decisions, health care professionals also rely on information that has been assembled for various purposes. For example, local, national, and international *benchmarking data* provide information on such issues as the rates of using various procedures (e.g., rates of caesarean deliveries) or rates of clinical problems (e.g., nosocomial infections). *Quality improvement and risk data*, such as medication error reports, can be used to assess practices and determine the need for practice changes. Such sources offer useful information but provide no mechanism to actually guide improvements.

Disciplined Research

Disciplined research is considered the best method of acquiring reliable knowledge that humans have developed. Evidence-based health care requires nurses to base their clinical practice, to the extent possible, on rigorous research-based findings rather than on tradition, authority, or personal experience. However, nursing will always be a rich blend of art and science, especially when the evidence is not available or not directly applicable to your patients.

PARADIGMS AND METHODS FOR NURSING RESEARCH

The questions that nurse researchers ask and the methods they use to answer their questions spring from a researcher's view of how the world "works." A **paradigm** is a worldview,

TABLE 1.1 Major Assumptions of the Positivist and Constructivist Paradigms

Type of Assumption	Positivist Paradigm	Constructivist Paradigm
The nature of reality	Reality exists; there is a real world driven by real, natural causes.	Reality is multiple and subjective, mentally constructed by individuals.
Relationship between researcher and those being researched	The researcher is independent from those being researched.	The researcher interacts with those being researched; findings are the creation of the interactive process.
The role of values in the inquiry	Values and biases are to be held in check; objectivity is sought.	Subjectivity and values are inevitable and desirable.
Best methods for obtaining evidence	• Deductive processes → hypotheses testing • Emphasis on discrete, specific concepts • Focus on the objective and quantifiable • Corroboration of researchers' predictions • Fixed, pre-specified design • Controls over context • Measured, quantitative information • Statistical analysis • Seeks generalizations	• Inductive processes → hypothesis generation • Emphasis on the whole • Focus on the subjective and non-quantifiable • Emerging insight grounded in participants' experiences • Flexible, emergent design • Context-bound, contextualized • Narrative information • Qualitative analysis • Seeks in-depth understanding

a general perspective to explain the world's complexities. Disciplined inquiry in nursing has been conducted mainly within two broad but very different paradigms. This section describes the two paradigms and outlines the research methods associated with them.

The Positivist Paradigm

The paradigm that dominated science and nursing research for decades is called *positivism*. Positivism is rooted in the 19th-century thought, guided by such philosophers as Isaac Newton and John Locke. Positivistic thinking is logical, rational, and scientific.

As shown in Table 1.1, a fundamental assumption of positivists is that there is a reality *out there* that can be studied and known. An **assumption** is a principle that is believed to be true without solid proof. People who support positivism assume that nature is ordered and regular and that a reality exists independent of human observation. In other words, the real world is not affected by the human mind, the way we think, perceive, or experience. The assumption of *determinism* refers to the positivists' belief that phenomena do not happen by chance but they are controlled and produced by antecedent causes. If a person is in pain, a nurse in a positivist tradition assumes that there must be a direct, external stimuli for the pain, whether it is related to trauma, burn injury, or chemical irritation. Following this logic, the nurse can remove the source to relieve pain. Within the **positivist paradigm**, research activity is often aimed at understanding the underlying causes of natural phenomena.

 TIP What do we mean by *phenomena*? In a research context, *phenomena* are those things in which researchers are interested—such as a health event (e.g., a patient fall), a health outcome (e.g., pain), or a health experience (e.g., living with chronic wounds).

Because of their belief in objective reality, positivists attach great importance to objectivity. Their approach involves the use of orderly, disciplined procedures with tight controls over the research situation to test hunches about the nature of phenomena being studied and relationships among them.

Strict positivist thinking has been challenged, and only few researchers adhere to the principles of pure positivism. Post-positivists still believe in reality and seek to understand it, but they recognize the impossibility of total objectivity. Yet, they see objectivity as a goal and strive to be as unbiased as possible. Post-positivists also appreciate the barriers to knowing reality with certainty and therefore seek *probabilistic* evidence—that is, learning what the true state of a phenomenon *probably* is. This modified positivist position remains a dominant force in nursing research. For the sake of simplicity, we refer to it as positivism.

The Constructivist Paradigm

The **constructivist paradigm** (sometimes called the *naturalistic paradigm*) began as a countermovement to positivism with writers such as Max Weber and Immanuel Kant. The constructivist paradigm is a major alternative system for conducting research in nursing. Table 1.1 compares four major assumptions of the positivist and constructivist paradigms.

For the naturalistic inquirer, reality is not a fixed entity but rather a construction of the people participating in the research; reality exists within a context, and many constructions are possible. Naturalists take the position of relativism: If there are multiple interpretations of reality depending on how different people experience it, then there is nothing called the absolute truth.

The constructivist paradigm assumes that knowledge is maximized when the distance between the inquirer and participants in the study is minimized. The voices and interpretations of those under study are crucial to understanding the phenomenon of interest, and subjective interactions are the best way to access them. Findings from a constructivist inquiry are the product of the interaction between the inquirer and the participants. A nurse in a constructivist tradition understands that the pain experience is different even with similar stimuli. Following this logic, the nurse will need to explore the meaning and values of pain for optimal pain relief.

Paradigms and Methods: Quantitative and Qualitative Research

Research methods are the techniques researchers use to design a study and to gather and analyse relevant information. The two paradigms correspond to different methods of developing evidence. A key methodologic distinction is between **quantitative research**, which is most closely aligned with positivism, and **qualitative research**, which is associated with constructivist inquiry—although positivists sometimes undertake qualitative studies and constructivist researchers sometimes collect quantitative information. This section gives an overview of the methods linked to the two alternative paradigms.

The Scientific Method and Quantitative Research

The traditional, positivist **scientific method** involves using a set of orderly procedures to gather information. Quantitative researchers typically move in a systematic fashion from the definition of a problem to a solution. By *systematic*, we mean that investigators progress through a series of steps, according to a plan. Quantitative researchers use objective methods designed to control the research situation with the goal of minimizing *bias* and maximizing validity.

Quantitative researchers gather **empirical evidence**—evidence that is rooted in objective reality and gathered directly or indirectly through the senses rather than through personal beliefs or hunches. Evidence for a quantitative study is gathered systematically, using formal instruments or questionnaires to collect needed information.

Usually (but not always) the information is *quantitative*—that is, numeric information that results from some type of formal measurement and that is analysed statistically. Quantitative researchers strive to go beyond the specifics of a research situation; the goal is to generalize research findings to individuals other than those who took part in the study (referred to as **generalizability**).

Nurse researchers have used the traditional scientific method to study a wide range of questions. Yet, there are important limitations. For example, quantitative researchers must deal with problems of *measurement.* To study a phenomenon, scientists must measure it, that is, attach numeric values that express quantity. For example, if the phenomenon of interest was patient stress, researchers would want to assess whether stress is high or low, or higher under certain conditions for some people. Physiologic phenomena such as blood pressure and temperature can be measured with accuracy and precision, but the same cannot be said of most psychological phenomena, such as stress or resilience.

Another issue is that nursing research focuses on human beings, who are inherently complicated and diverse. The traditional scientific method typically focuses on a relatively small set of phenomena (e.g., weight gain, depression) in a study. Complex relationships are controlled and even ignored rather than studied directly, and this narrowness of focus can sometimes limit insights. Relatedly, quantitative research within the positivist paradigm has sometimes been accused of a narrowness of vision that does not capture the full breadth of human experience.

 TIP Students often find quantitative studies more intimidating and difficult than qualitative ones. Try not to worry too much about the jargon at first—remember that each study has a *story* to tell, and grasping the main point of the story is what is initially important.

Constructivist Methods and Qualitative Research

Researchers in constructivist traditions emphasize the inherent complexity of humans, their ability to shape and "construct" their own experiences, and the idea that truth is a collection of realities. Consequently, constructivist studies focus heavily on understanding the human experience as it is lived, through the careful collection and analysis of *qualitative* materials that are narrative and subjective.

Researchers are critical of the traditional scientific method because it is considered *reductionist*—that is, it reduces human experience to only the few concepts that are defined in advance by researchers rather than naturally emerging from the experiences of those under study. Constructivist researchers tend to emphasize and capture the dynamic, holistic, and individual aspects of human life within the context of those who are experiencing them.

Flexible, evolving procedures are used to obtain findings that emerge during the study, which typically is undertaken in naturalistic settings. The collection of information and its analysis usually progress concurrently. As researchers sift through information, they gain insights, form new questions, and seek further evidence to determine the validity of their insights. Through an inductive reasoning process (going from specifics to the general), researchers integrate information to develop a theory or description that explains the phenomena under observation.

Constructivist studies provide rich, in-depth information that can potentially clarify the varied dimensions (or *themes*) of a complicated phenomenon. Findings from qualitative research are typically grounded in the real-life experiences of people with first-hand knowledge of a phenomenon. Nevertheless, the approach has several limitations. Human beings are used directly as the instrument for gathering information, and humans, though highly intelligent, are fallible.

Another potential limitation is the subjectivity of constructivist inquiry, which sometimes raises concerns about the idiosyncratic nature of the conclusions. Would two constructivist researchers studying the same phenomenon in similar settings arrive at similar conclusions? The situation is challenged by the fact that most constructivist studies involve a small group of participants. Thus, the generalizability of findings from constructivist inquiries is an issue of potential concern.

 TIP Researchers often do not discuss or even mention the underlying paradigm of their studies in their reports. The paradigm provides context, without being explicitly referenced.

Multiple Paradigms and Nursing Research

Paradigms can be thought of as lenses that sharpen a researcher's focus on phenomena of interest, not blinders that limit curiosity. We think that the emergence of alternative paradigms for studying nursing problems is a desirable trend to generate new evidence for practice. Nursing knowledge would be thin if it were not for a rich array of methods—methods that are often complementary in their strengths and limitations.

We have emphasized differences between the two paradigms and associated methods so that distinctions would be easy to understand. It is equally important, however, to note that the two paradigms have many features in common, some of which are mentioned here:

- *Ultimate goals.* The ultimate aim of disciplined research, regardless of paradigm, is to answer questions and solve problems. Both quantitative and qualitative researchers seek to capture the truth of the phenomena in which they are interested.
- *External evidence.* The word *empiricism* is often associated with the scientific method, but researchers in both traditions collect and analyse evidence gathered empirically, that is, through their senses.
- *Reliance on human cooperation.* Human cooperation is essential in both quantitative and qualitative research. To understand people's characteristics and experiences, researchers must encourage people to participate in the study *and* to speak candidly.
- *Ethical constraints.* Research with human beings is guided by ethical principles that sometimes interfere with research goals. Ethical dilemmas often confront researchers, regardless of paradigms or methods.
- *Fallibility.* Virtually all studies have limitations. Every research question can be addressed in different ways, and inevitably, there are trade-offs. Financial constraints are often an issue, but limitations exist even in well-funded research. This means that *no single study can ever definitively answer a research question.* The fallibility of any single study makes it important to understand and critique researchers' methods when evaluating evidence quality.

Thus, despite philosophical and methodologic differences, researchers using the traditional scientific method or constructivist methods share basic goals and face many similar challenges. The selection of an appropriate method depends on researchers' philosophy and worldview but also on the research question. If a researcher asks, "What are the effects of cryotherapy on nausea and oral mucositis in patients undergoing chemotherapy?" the researcher needs to examine effects through the careful quantitative assessment of patients. On the other hand, if a researcher asks, "How do parents learn to cope with the death of a child?" the researchers would find it difficult to quantify such a process. Personal worldviews of researchers help to shape their questions.

In reading about the alternative paradigms, you likely were more attracted to one of the two paradigms—the one that corresponds most closely to your view of the world. It is important, however, to learn about and value both approaches to disciplined inquiry and to recognize their respective strengths and limitations.

HOW-TO-TELL TIP How can you tell if a study is quantitative or qualitative? As you progress through this book, you should be able to identify most studies as quantitative versus qualitative based simply on the study's title or on terms in the summary at the beginning of an article. At this point, though, it may be easiest to distinguish the two types of studies based on how many *numbers* appear in the article, especially in tables. Quantitative studies typically have several tables with numbers and statistical information. Qualitative studies may have no tables with quantitative information, or only one numeric table describing participants' characteristics (e.g., the percentage who were male or female). Qualitative studies often have "word tables" or diagrams and figures illustrating processes inferred from the narrative information gathered.

THE PURPOSES OF NURSING RESEARCH

Why do nurses do research? Several different systems have been devised to classify different research goals. We describe two such classification systems to illustrate the broad range of questions that are important for nurses and to show differences between quantitative and qualitative inquiries.

 TIP Sometimes a distinction is made between basic and applied research. *Basic research* is appropriate for discovering general principles of human behaviour and biophysiologic processes. *Applied research* is designed to examine how these principles can be used to solve problems in nursing practice.

Research to Achieve Varying Levels of Explanation

Research purposes are classified by the extent to which studies are designed to provide explanations. A fundamental distinction that is especially relevant in quantitative research is between studies whose primary goal is to *describe* phenomena and those that are **cause-probing**—that is, studies designed to illuminate the underlying causes of phenomena.

Using a descriptive/explanatory framework, the specific purposes of nursing research include identification, description, exploration, explanation, and prediction/control. When researchers state their study purpose, they often use these terms (e.g., The purpose of this study was to *explore*…). For each purpose, various types of question are addressed—some more amenable to quantitative than to qualitative inquiry, and vice versa.

Identification and Description

In quantitative research, researchers usually begin with a phenomenon that has been previously studied or defined. Qualitative researchers, by contrast, sometimes study phenomena that are not well understood. In some cases, so little is known that the phenomenon has yet to be clearly identified or named or has been inadequately defined. The in-depth, probing nature of qualitative research is well suited to answering such questions as "What is this phenomenon?" and "What is its name?" (Table 1.2).

Quantitative example of description
Palese et al. (2015) conducted a study to describe the average healing time of stage II pressure ulcers. They found that it took approximately 23 days to achieve complete re-epithelialization.

Qualitative example of identification •
Gagnon et al. (2016) studied the barriers and facilitators of using Electronic Personal Health Records (ePHR) in Canada. They interviewed representatives from six stakeholder groups in seven Canadian provinces. Adoption of ePHR was influenced by knowledge, system design, user capacities and attitudes, environmental factors, and legal and ethical issues.

Description of phenomena is an important purpose of research. In descriptive studies, researchers count, delineate, and classify. Nurse researchers have described a wide variety of phenomena, such as patients' stress, health beliefs, and so on. Quantitative description focuses on the prevalence, size, and measurable aspects of phenomena. Qualitative researchers describe the nature, dimensions, and salience of phenomena, as shown in Table 1.2.

Exploration

Exploratory research begins with a phenomenon of interest; but rather than simply describing it, exploratory researchers examine the nature of the phenomenon, the manner in which it is manifested, and other factors to which it is related—including factors that might be *causing* it. For example, a *descriptive* quantitative study of patients' preoperative stress might document how much stress patients experience. An *exploratory* study might ask: What factors increase or lower a patient's stress? Qualitative methods can be used to explore the nature of little understood phenomena and to shed light on how a phenomenon is expressed.

Qualitative example of exploration •
Roberts et al. (2016) used in-depth interviews to explore the use of a self-help workbook titled: *Mastering the Art of Coping in Good Times,* to help cancer patients cope with stress and engage in self-management.

TABLE 1.2 Purposes on the Descriptive–Explanatory Continuum and Types of Research Questions for Quantitative and Qualitative Research

Purpose	Types of Questions: Quantitative Research	Types of Questions: Qualitative Research
Identification		What is this phenomenon? What is its name?
Description	How prevalent is the phenomenon? How often does the phenomenon occur?	What are the dimensions or characteristics of the phenomenon? What is important about the phenomenon?
Exploration	What factors are related to the phenomenon? What are the antecedents of the phenomenon?	What is the full nature of the phenomenon? What is really going on here? What is the process by which the phenomenon evolves?
Prediction and control	If phenomenon X occurs, will phenomenon Y follow? Can the phenomenon be prevented or controlled?	
Explanation	What is the underlying cause of the phenomenon? Does the theory explain the phenomenon?	Why does the phenomenon exist? What does the phenomenon mean? How did the phenomenon occur?

Explanation

Explanatory research seeks to understand the underlying causes or full nature of a phenomenon. In quantitative research, *theories* or prior findings are used deductively (reasoning from general to specifics) to generate hypothesized explanations that are tested statistically. Qualitative researchers search for explanations about how or why a phenomenon exists or what a phenomenon means as a basis for *developing* a theory that is grounded in rich, in-depth, experiential evidence.

Quantitative example of explanation •
Lavoie et al. (2016) developed a questionnaire based on the Theory of Planned Behaviour to explore the psychosocial determinants that influenced nurses' intention to practise euthanasia in palliative care. A random sample of 445 nurses from the province of Quebec, Canada, participated in the study.

Prediction and Control

Many phenomena defy explanation, yet it is often possible to predict or control them based on research evidence. For example, research has shown that the incidence of Down syndrome in infants increases with maternal age. We can predict that a woman aged 40 years is at higher risk of bearing a child with Down syndrome than a woman aged 25 years. We can attempt to influence the outcome by educating women about the risks and offering amniocentesis to women older than 35 years of age. The ability to predict and control in this example does not rely on an explanation of what *causes* older women to be at a higher risk. In many quantitative studies, prediction and control are key goals. Although explanatory studies are powerful, studies whose purpose is prediction and control are also critical to EBP.

Quantitative example of prediction •
Metcalfe et al. (2017) conducted a study to examine demographic, clinical, and psychosocial predictors of delayed breast reconstruction in mastectomy patients with the long-term survivorship period. Women who experienced higher levels of distress, anxiety, and body concerns both before and after mastectomy were more likely to select delayed breast reconstruction.

Research Purposes Linked to Evidence-Based Practice

Another system for classifying studies has emerged to communicate EBP-related purposes (DiCenso, Guyatt, & Ciliska, 2005; Guyatt et al., 2008; Melnyk & Fineout-Overholt, 2015). Table 1.3 identifies some of the questions relevant for each EBP purpose and offers an actual nursing research example. In this classification scheme, the various purposes can best be addressed with quantitative research, with the exception of the last category (meaning/process), which requires qualitative research.

Therapy, Treatment, or Intervention

Studies focused on therapy are designed to identify effective treatments for improving or preventing health problems. Such studies range from evaluations of highly specific treatments (e.g., comparing two types of cooling blankets for febrile patients) to complex multicomponent interventions designed to affect behavioural changes (e.g., nurse-led smoking cessation interventions). Intervention research plays a critical role in EBP.

TABLE 1.3 Research Purposes Linked to Evidence-Based Practice (EBP) and Key Research Questions

EBP Purpose	Key Research Question	Nursing Research Example
Therapy/intervention	What therapy or intervention will result in better health outcomes or prevent an adverse health outcome?	Kwon, Shin, and Juon (2016) tested the effects of an acupressure wristband for postoperative nausea and vomiting among patients undergoing thyroidectomy.
Diagnosis/assessment	What test or assessment procedure will yield accurate diagnoses or assessments of critical patient conditions and outcomes?	Sitzer (2016) developed and evaluated an automated self-assessment questionnaire for assessing the risk of falling in hospitalized patients.
Prognosis	Does exposure to a disease or health problem increase the risk of subsequent adverse consequences?	Storey and Von Ah (2015) studied the prevalence and impact of hyperglycaemia on hospitalized leukaemia patients, in terms of such outcomes as neutropenia, infection, and length of hospital stay.
Aetiology/cause/harm	What factors cause or contribute to the risk of a health problem or disease?	Hagerty et al. (2015) undertook a study to identify risk factors for catheter-associated urinary tract infections in critically ill patients with subarachnoid haemorrhage. The risk factors examined included patients' blood sugar levels, patient age, and levels of anaemia requiring transfusion.
Meaning/process	What is the meaning of life experiences, and what is the process by which they unfold?	Pieters (2016) studied resilience as a multidimensional process among older women who had recently completed treatment for early-stage breast cancer.

Diagnosis and Assessment

Many nursing studies concern the rigorous development and testing of formal instruments to screen, diagnose, and assess patients and to measure clinical outcomes. High-quality instruments with documented accuracy are essential both for clinical practice and for research.

Prognosis

Studies of prognosis examine the consequences or outcomes of a disease or health problem, explore factors that can modify the prognosis, and examine when (and for which types of people) the consequences are most likely. Such studies facilitate the development of long-term care plans for patients. They also provide valuable information for guiding patients to make beneficial lifestyle choices or to be vigilant for key symptoms.

Aetiology (Causation) and Harm

It is difficult to prevent harm or treat health problems if we do not know what causes them. For example, there would be no smoking cessation programmes if research had not provided firm evidence that smoking cigarettes causes or contributes to many health problems. Thus, determining the factors and exposures that affect or cause illness, mortality, or morbidity is an important purpose of many studies.

Meaning and Processes

Many health care activities (e.g., motivating people to adhere with treatments, providing sensitive advice to patients, designing appealing interventions) can greatly benefit from understanding the clients' perspectives. Research that offers evidence about what health and illness mean to clients, what barriers they face to positive health practices, and what processes they experience in a transition through a health care crisis is important to evidence-based nursing practice.

 TIP Most EBP-related purposes (except *diagnosis* and *meaning*) involve *cause-probing* research. For example, research on interventions focuses on whether an intervention *causes* improvements in key outcomes. Prognosis research examines whether a disease or health condition *causes* subsequent adverse consequences. Aetiology research seeks explanations about the underlying *causes* of health problems.

ASSISTANCE FOR CONSUMERS OF NURSING RESEARCH

We hope that this book will help you develop skills that will allow you to read, appraise, and use nursing studies and to appreciate nursing research. In each chapter, we present information relating to methods used by nurse researchers and provide guidance in several ways. First, we offer tips on what you can expect to find in actual research articles, identified by the icon ☞. There are also special "how-to-tell" tips (identified with the icon ☞) that help with some potentially confusing issues in research articles. Second, we include guidelines for critiquing various aspects of a study. The guiding questions in Box 1.1 are designed to assist you in using the information in this chapter in a preliminary assessment of a research article. And third, we offer opportunities to apply your new skills. The critical thinking exercises at the end of each chapter guide you through appraisals of real research examples of both quantitative and qualitative studies. These activities also challenge you to think about how the findings from these studies could be used in nursing practice. Answers to many of these questions are on thePoint website. Some of these examples are featured in our interactive *Critical Thinking Activity* on thePoint website. Some of the journal articles are found in the appendices. The full-journal article for studies identified with ** in the references list of each chapter are available on thePoint website. ✦

Box 1.1 Questions for a Preliminary Overview of a Research Report

1. How relevant is the research problem to the actual practice of nursing?
2. Was the study quantitative or qualitative?
3. What was the underlying purpose (or purposes) of the study—identification, description, exploration, explanation, or prediction/control? Does the purpose correspond to an EBP focus such as therapy/treatment, diagnosis, prognosis, aetiology/harm, or meaning?
4. What might be some clinical implications of this research? To what type of people and settings is the research most relevant? If the findings were accurate, how mightI use the results of this study in my clinical work?

RESEARCH EXAMPLES WITH CRITICAL THINKING EXERCISES

This section presents examples of studies with different purposes. Read the research summaries for Examples 1 and 2 and then answer the critical thinking questions that follow, referring to the full research reports if necessary. The critical thinking questions for Exercises 3 and 4 are based on the studies that appear in their entirety in Appendices A and B of this book.

> **TIP**   Examples 1 and 2 are also featured in our interactive *Critical Thinking Activity* on thePoint website, where you can record, print, and e-mail your responses to your instructor. Our comments for the questions in Examples 3 and 4 are in the Student Resources section on thePoint.

EXAMPLE 1: QUANTITATIVE RESEARCH

Study: Psychological outcomes after a sexual assault video intervention: A randomized trial (Miller et al., 2015)

Study Purpose: The purpose of the study was to test whether a brief video-based intervention had positive effects on the mental health of victims of a sexual assault. The intervention provided psychoeducation and information about coping strategies to survivors at the time of a sexual assault nurse examination.

Study Methods: Female sexual assault victims who received forensic examinations within 72 hours of their victimization were assigned to one of two groups: (1) those receiving standard care plus the video intervention and (2) those receiving care as usual, without the video. A total of 164 women participated in the study. They completed mental health assessments 2 weeks and 2 months after the forensic examination.

Key Findings: The researchers found that women in both groups had lower anxiety at the follow-up assessments. However, women in the special intervention group had significantly lower levels of anxiety symptoms than those in the usual care group at both follow-ups.

Conclusions: Miller et al. (2015) concluded that forensic nurses have an opportunity to intervene immediately after a sexual assault with an effective and inexpensive intervention.

Critical Thinking Exercises

1. Answer the questions from Box 1.1 regarding this study.
2. Also, consider the following targeted questions, which may assist you in assessing aspects of the study's merit:
   a. Why do you think levels of anxiety improved over time in both the intervention and standard care groups?
   b. Could this study have been undertaken as a qualitative study? Why or why not?

EXAMPLE 2: QUALITATIVE RESEARCH

Study: The pain experience of patients hospitalized with inflammatory bowel disease (IBD): a phenomenological study (Bernhofer et al., 2017)

Study Purpose: The purpose of this study was to understand the unique experience of pain in hospitalized patients with an admitting diagnosis of IBD.

Study Methods: Sixteen men and women with diverse backgrounds (e.g., age, length of IBD diagnosis) were recruited from two colorectal units of a large academic medical centre. Patients participated in interviews that lasted about a half hour. The interviews, which were audiotaped and then transcribed, focused on what the patients' pain experiences were like in the hospital.

Key Findings: Five recurring themes emerged in the analysis of the interview data: (1) feeling discredited and misunderstood; (2) a desire to dispel the stigma; (3) frustration with constant pain; (4) a need for caregiver knowledge and understanding; and (5) nurses as the connector between the patient and physicians. Here is an excerpt from an interview that illustrates the second theme on stigma: "I've been judged on numerous amounts of occasions in regards to them thinking that I'm just simply seeking out some kind of pain medication when in reality, I'm seeking out to feel better, to make the pain go away" (p. 204).

Conclusions: The researchers concluded that nurses caring for hospitalized patients with IBD could provide better pain management if they understand the issues highlighted in these themes.

Critical Thinking Exercises

1. Answer the questions from Box 1.1 regarding this study.
2. Also, consider the following targeted questions, which may assist you in assessing aspects of the study's merit:
   a. Why do you think that the researchers audiotaped and transcribed their in-depth interviews with study participants?
   b. Do you think it would have been appropriate for the researchers to conduct this study using quantitative research methods? Why or why not?

EXAMPLE 3: QUANTITATIVE RESEARCH IN APPENDIX A

- Read the abstract and the introduction of Swenson and colleagues' (2016) study ("Parents' use of praise and criticism in a sample of young children seeking mental health services") in Appendix A of this book.

Critical Thinking Exercises

1. Answer the relevant questions in Box 1.1.
2. Also consider the following targeted questions:
   a. Could this study have been undertaken as a qualitative study? Why or why not?
   b. Who provided some financial support for this research? (This information appears on the first page of the report.)

EXAMPLE 4: QUALITATIVE RESEARCH IN APPENDIX B

- Read the abstract and the introduction of Beck and Watson's (2010) study ("Subsequent childbirth after a previous traumatic birth") in Appendix B of this book.

Critical Thinking Exercises

1. Answer the relevant questions in Box 1.1.
2. Also consider the following targeted questions:
   a. What gap in the existing research was the study designed to fill?
   b. Was Beck and Watson's study conducted within the positivist paradigm or the constructivist paradigm? Provide a rationale for your choice.

WANT TO KNOW MORE?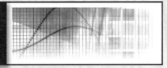
A wide variety of resources to enhance your learning and understanding of this chapter are available on thePoint.

- Interactive Critical Thinking Activity
- Chapter Supplement on the History of Nursing Research
- Answers to the Critical Thinking Exercises for Examples 3 and 4
- Internet Resources with useful websites for Chapter 1
- A Wolters Kluwer journal article on a topic related to this chapter

Summary Points

- **Nursing research** is systematic inquiry undertaken to develop evidence on problems of importance to nurses.
- Nurses in various settings are adopting an **EBP** that incorporates research findings into their decisions and interactions with clients.
- Knowledge of nursing research enhances the professional practice of all nurses—including both *consumers of research* (who read and evaluate studies) and *producers of research* (who design and undertake studies).
- Nursing research began with Florence Nightingale but developed slowly until its rapid acceleration in the 1950s. Since the 1980s, the focus has been on **clinical nursing research**—that is, on problems relating to clinical practice.
- The National Institute of Nursing Research (NINR), established at the U.S. National Institutes of Health in 1993, affirms the stature of nursing research in the United States.
- Future emphases of nursing research are likely to include EBP projects, *replications* of research, research integration through **systematic reviews**, expanded dissemination efforts, increased focus on health disparities, and a focus on the **clinical significance** of research results.
- Disciplined research stands in contrast to other knowledge sources for nursing practice,

such as tradition, authority, personal experience, and trial and error.
- Disciplined inquiry in nursing is conducted mainly within two broad **paradigms**—worldviews with underlying **assumptions** about reality: the positivist paradigm and the constructivist paradigm.
- In the **positivist paradigm**, it is assumed that there is an objective reality and that natural phenomena are regular and orderly. The related assumption of *determinism* refers to the belief that phenomena result from prior causes and are not haphazard.
- In the **constructivist paradigm**, it is assumed that reality is not a fixed entity but is rather a construction of human minds—and thus, "truth" is a composite of multiple constructions of reality.
- **Quantitative research** (associated with positivism) involves the collection and analysis of numeric information. Quantitative research is typically conducted within the traditional **scientific method**, which is systematic and controlled. Quantitative researchers base their findings on **empirical evidence** (evidence collected by way of the human senses) and strive for **generalizability** beyond a single setting or situation.
- Constructivist researchers emphasize understanding human experience as it is lived through the collection and analysis of subjective, narrative materials using flexible procedures; this paradigm is associated with **qualitative research**.

- A fundamental distinction that is especially relevant in quantitative research is between studies whose primary intent is to *describe* phenomena and those that are **cause-probing**—that is, designed to illuminate underlying causes of phenomena. Specific purposes on the description/explanation continuum include identification, description, exploration, explanation, and prediction/control.
- Many nursing studies can also be classified in terms of an EBP-related aim: therapy/treatment/intervention, diagnosis and assessment, prognosis, aetiology and harm, and meaning and process.

REFERENCES

Benoit, B., Campbell-Yeo, M., Johnston, C., Latimer, M., Caddell, K., & Orr, T. (2016). Staff nurse utilization of kangaroo care as an intervention for procedural pain in preterm infants. *Advances in Neonatal Care, 16*, 229–238.

Bernhofer, E., Masina, V., Sorrell, J., & Modic, M. (2017). The pain experience of patients hospitalized with inflammatory bowel disease: A phenomenological study. *Gastroenterology Nursing, 40*(3), 200–207.

*Campbell-Yeo, M., Johnston, C., Benoit, B., et al. (2013). Trial of repeated analgesia with kangaroo mother care (TRAKC trial). *BMC Pediatrics, 13*, 182.

Cong, X., Ludington-Hoe, S., & Walsh, S. (2011). Randomized crossover trial of kangaroo care to reduce biobehavioral pain responses in preterm infants: A pilot study. *Biological Research for Nursing, 13*, 204–216.

DiCenso, A., Guyatt, G., & Ciliska, D. (2005). Evidence-based nursing: A guide to clinical practice. St. Louis, MO: Elsevier Mosby.

Gagnon, M. P, Payne-Gagnon J., Breton E., et al. (2016). Adoption of electronic personal health records in Canada: Perceptions of stakeholders. *International Journal of Health Policy and Management, 5*, 425–433.

*Gilbert, R., Salanti, G., Harden, M., & See, S. (2005). Infant sleeping position and the sudden infant death syndrome: Systematic review of observational studies and historical review of recommendations from 1940 to 2002. *International Journal of Epidemiology, 34*, 874–887.

Guyatt, G., Rennie, D., Meade, M., & Cook, D. (2008). Users' guides to the medical literature: Essentials of evidence-based clinical practice (2nd ed.). New York: McGraw Hill.

Hagerty, T., Kertesz, L., Schmidt, J., et al. (2015). Risk factors for catheter-associated urinary tract infections in critically ill patients with subarachnoid hemorrhage. *Journal of Neuroscience Nursing, 47*, 51–54.

Hanrahan, K., Wagner, M., Matthews, G., et al. (2015). Sacred cow gone to pasture: A systematic evaluation and integration of evidence-based practice. *Worldviews on Evidence-Based Nursing, 12*, 3–11.

Holman, E., Perisho, J., Edwards, A., & Mlakar, N. (2010). The myths of coping with loss in undergraduate psychiatric nursing books. *Research in Nursing & Health, 33*, 486–499.

Johnston, C., Campbell-Yeo, M., Rich, B., et al. (2013). Therapeutic touch is not therapeutic for procedural pain in very preterm neonates: A randomized trial. *Clinical Journal of Pain, 29*, 824–829

Johnston, C. C., Filion, F., Campbell-Yeo, M., et al. (2009). Enhanced kangaroo mother care for heel lance in preterm neonates: A crossover trial. *Journal of Perinatology, 29*, 51–56.

Kwon, J. H., Shin, Y., & Juon, H. (2016). Effects of Nei-Guan (P6) acupressure wristband: On nausea, vomiting, and retching in women after thyroidectomy. *Cancer Nursing, 39*, 61–66.

Lavoie, M., Godin, G., Vézina-Im, L. A., Blondeau, D., Martineau, I., & Roy, L. (2016). Psychosocial determinants of nurses' intention to practise euthanasia in palliative care. *Nursing Ethics, 23*, 48–60.

Melnyk, B. M., & Fineout-Overholt, E. (2015). Evidence-based practice in nursing & healthcare: A guide to best practice (3rd ed.). Philadelphia, PA: Lippincott Williams & Wilkins.

Metcalfe, K. A., Semple, J., Quan, M. L., et al. (2017) Why some mastectomy patients opt to undergo delayed breast reconstruction: Results of a long-term prospective study. *Plastic Reconstruction Surgery, 139*(2), 267–275

**Miller, K., Cranston, C., Davis, J., et al. (2015). Psychological outcomes after a sexual assault video intervention: A randomized trial. *Journal of Forensic Nursing, 11*, 129–136.

*Moore, E., Anderson, G., Bergman, N., & Dowswell, T. (2012). Early skin-to-skin contact for mothers and their healthy newborn infants. *Cochrane Database of Systematic Reviews*, (5), CD003519.

Palese, A., Luisa, S., Ilenia, P., Laquintana, D., Stinco, G., & Di Giulio, P. (2015). What is the healing time of stage II pressure ulcers? Findings from a secondary analysis. *Advances in Skin & Wound Care, 28*, 69–75.

Perry, J., VanDenKerkhof, E. G., Wilson, R., & Tripp, D. A. (2017). Development of a guided internet-based psychoeducation intervention using cognitive behavioral therapy and self-management for individuals with chronic pain. *Pain Management in Nursing, 18*(2), 90–101.

Pieters, H. C. (2016). "I'm still here": Resilience among older survivors of breast cancer. *Cancer Nursing, 39*, E20–E28.

Ploeg, J., Matthew-Maich, N., Fraser, K., et al. (2017). Managing multiple chronic conditions in the community: A Canadian qualitative study of the experiences of older adults, family caregivers and healthcare providers. *BMC Geriatrics, 17*, 40

Roberts, N., Lee, V., Ananng, B., & Körner, A. (2016). Acceptability of bibliotherapy for patients with cancer: A qualitative, descriptive study. *Oncology Nursing Forum, 43*, 588–594.

Sitzer, V. (2016). Development of an automated self-assessment of fall risk questionnaire for hospitalized patients. *Journal of Nursing Care Quality, 31*, 46–53.

Spock, B. (1979). Baby and child care. New York: Dutton Publishing.

Storey, S., & Von Ah, D. (2015). Prevalence and impact of hyperglycemia on hospitalized leukemia patients. *European Journal of Oncology Nursing, 19*, 13–17.

*A link to this open-access article is provided in the Internet Resources section on thePoint website.

**This journal article is available on thePoint for this chapter.

Fundamentals of Evidence-Based Nursing Practice

2

Learning Objectives

On completing this chapter, you will be able to:

● Distinguish research utilization and evidence-based practice (EBP) and discuss their current status within nursing
● Identify several resources available to facilitate EBP in nursing practice
● List several models for implementing EBP
● Discuss the five major steps in undertaking an EBP effort for individual nurses
● Identify the components of a well-worded clinical question and be able to frame such a question
● Discuss broad strategies for undertaking an EBP project at the organizational level
● Distinguish EBP and quality improvement (QI) efforts
● Define new terms in the chapter

Key Terms

● Clinical practice guidelines
● Cochrane Collaboration
● Evidence hierarchies

● Evidence-based practice
● Implementation potential
● Meta-analysis
● Meta-synthesis

● Pilot test
● Quality improvement (QI)
● Systematic review

Learning about research methods provides a foundation for evidence based practice (EBP) in nursing.

This book will help you to develop methodologic skills for reading research articles and evaluating research evidence. Before we elaborate on methodologic techniques, we discuss key aspects of EBP to help you understand the key role that research plays in nursing.

BACKGROUND OF EVIDENCE-BASED NURSING PRACTICE

This section provides a context for understanding EBP and two closely related concepts: research utilization (RU) and knowledge translation (KT).

Definition of Evidence-Based Practice

Canadian pioneer David Sackett et al. (2000) defined **evidence-based practice** as "the integration of best research evidence with clinical expertise and patient values" (p. 1). The definition proposed by the Canadian Nurses Association (2010) is as follows: "the ongoing process that incorporates evidence from research, clinical expertise, client preferences and other available resources to make nursing decisions about clients. Decision-making in nursing practice is influenced by evidence and also by individual values, client choice, theories, clinical judgment, ethics, legislation, regulation, health-care resources and practice environments" (p. 3). A key ingredient in EBP is the effort to personalize "best evidence" to a specific patient's needs within a particular clinical context. A basic feature of EBP as a clinical problem-solving strategy is that it de-emphasizes decisions based on custom, authority, or ritual. The emphasis is on identifying the best available research evidence and *integrating* it with other factors in making clinical decisions. Advocates of EBP do not minimize the importance of clinical expertise. Rather, they advise that evidence-based decision making should integrate the best research evidence with clinical expertise, patient preferences, and local circumstances.

Because research evidence is constantly evolving based on new insights into human health and illness, EBP is a dynamic and ongoing process for identifying, understanding, and evaluating new information about patient care that can be integrated into practice.

Research Utilization

Research utilization (RU) is the use of findings from studies in a practical application that is unrelated to the original research. In RU, the emphasis is on translating new knowledge into real-world applications. EBP is a broader concept than RU because it integrates research findings with other contextual factors, as just noted. RU begins with the research itself (e.g., How can I put this new knowledge to good use in my clinical setting?), the starting point in EBP is a clinical question (e.g., What does the evidence say is the best approach to solving this clinical problem?).

During the 1980s, RU emerged as an important topic. In education, nursing schools began to include courses on research methods so that students would become skilful research consumers or knowledge users. In research, there was a shift in focus towards clinical nursing problems. Yet, concerns about the limited use of research evidence in the delivery of nursing care continued to grow.

The need to reduce the gap between research and practice led to formal RU projects, including the groundbreaking *Conduct and Utilization of Research in Nursing (CURN) Project*, a 5-year project undertaken by the Michigan Nurses Association in the 1970s. CURN's objectives were to increase the use of research findings in nurses' daily practice by disseminating current findings and facilitating organizational changes needed to implement innovations (Horsley, Crane, & Bingle, 1978). The CURN Project team concluded that RU by practising nurses was feasible but only if the research is relevant to practice and if the results are broadly disseminated.

During the 1980s and 1990s, RU projects were undertaken by numerous hospitals and organizations such as the Nursing Effectiveness, Utilization and Outcomes Research Unit that was funded by the Ontario Ministry of Health and located at both the University of Toronto and McMaster University. During the 1990s, however, the call for RU began to be superseded by the push for EBP.

The Evidence-Based Practice Movement

One keystone of the EBP movement is the Cochrane Collaboration, which was founded in the United Kingdom based on the work by British epidemiologist Archie Cochrane. Cochrane published a book in the 1970s that drew attention to the shortage of solid evidence about the effects of health care. He called for efforts to make research summaries about interventions available to health care providers. This led to the development of the

Cochrane Center in Oxford in 1993 and the international **Cochrane Collaboration**, with centres now established in locations throughout the world. Its aim is to help providers make good decisions by preparing and disseminating systematic reviews of the effects of health care interventions.

At about the same time that the Cochrane Collaboration was started, a group from McMaster Medical School in Canada developed a learning strategy they called *evidence-based medicine*. The evidence-based medicine movement, pioneered by Dr. David Sackett, has broadened to the use of the best evidence by *all* health care practitioners. In 1996, the Joanna Briggs Institute (JBI) was founded in Australia, the University of Adelaide. Since its inception, the institute has developed linkages across the world to promote and support EBP through systematic reviews, practice recommendations, and consumer information design. EBP has been considered a major paradigm shift in health care education and practice. With EBP, skilful clinicians can no longer rely on a repository of memorized information but rather must be adept in accessing, evaluating, and using new research evidence.

The EBP movement has advocates and critics. Supporters argue that EBP is a rational approach to providing the best possible care with the most cost-effective use of resources. Advocates also note that EBP provides a framework for self-directed lifelong learning that is essential in an era of rapid clinical advances and the information explosion. Critics worry that the advantages of EBP are exaggerated and that individual clinical judgements and patient inputs are being devalued. They are also concerned that insufficient attention is being paid to the role of qualitative research. Although there is a need for close scrutiny of how the EBP journey unfolds, an EBP path is the one that health care professions will almost surely follow in the years ahead.

TIP   A debate has emerged concerning whether the term *EBP* should be replaced with *evidence-informed practice* (EIP). Those who advocate for a different term have argued that the word "based" suggests a stance in which patient values and preferences are not sufficiently considered in EBP clinical decisions (Glasziou, 2005). Yet, as noted by Melnyk (2014), all current models of EBP incorporate clinicians' expertise and patients' preferences. She argued that "changing terms now will only create confusion at a critical time where progress is being made in accelerating EBP" (p. 348). We concur and we use EBP throughout this book.

Knowledge Translation

RU and EBP involve activities that can be undertaken at the level of individual nurses or at a higher organizational level (e.g., by nurse administrators), as we describe later in this chapter. A related movement emerged that mainly concerns system-level efforts to bridge the gap between knowledge generation and use. *Knowledge translation (KT)* is a term that is often associated with efforts to enhance systematic change in clinical practice. The Canadian Institutes of Health Research (CIHR) (2010) has defined KT as "a dynamic and iterative process that includes synthesis, dissemination, exchange and ethically-sound application of knowledge to improve the health of Canadians, provide more effective health services and products and strengthen the health care system."

TIP   *Translation science* (or implementation science) is a new discipline devoted to promoting KT. The knowledge to action (KTA) framework developed in Canada by Ian Graham and his colleagues has been used extensively to guide implementation projects. Several journals have emerged that are devoted to this field (e.g., the journal *Implementation Science*).

EVIDENCE-BASED PRACTICE IN NURSING

Before describing procedures relating to EBP in nursing, we briefly discuss some important issues, including the nature of "evidence," challenges to pursuing EBP, and resources available to address some of those challenges.

Types of Evidence and Evidence Hierarchies

There is no consensus about what constitutes usable evidence for EBP, but there is general agreement that findings from rigorous research are paramount. Yet, there is some debate about what constitutes "rigorous" research and what qualifies as "best" evidence.

Early in the EBP movement, there was a strong bias favouring evidence from a type of study called a *randomized controlled trial* (RCT). This bias reflected the Cochrane Collaboration's initial focus on evidence about the effectiveness of therapies rather than about broader health care questions. RCTs are especially well suited for drawing conclusions about the effects of health care interventions (see Chapter 9). The bias in ranking research approaches in terms of questions about effective therapies led to some resistance to EBP by nurses who felt that evidence from qualitative and non-RCT studies would be ignored.

Positions about the contribution of various types of evidence are less rigid than previously. Nevertheless, many published **evidence hierarchies** rank evidence sources according to the strength of the evidence they provide, and in most cases, RCTs are near the top of these hierarchies. We offer a modified evidence hierarchy that looks similar to others but is unique in illustrating that the ranking of evidence-producing strategies depends on the type of question being asked.

Figure 2.1 shows that **systematic reviews** are at the pinnacle of the hierarchy (Level I) because the strongest evidence comes from careful syntheses of multiple studies. The next highest level (Level II) depends on the nature of inquiry. For Therapy questions regarding the efficacy of a therapy or intervention (What works best for improving health outcomes?), individual RCTs constitute Level II evidence (systematic reviews of multiple RCTs are Level I). Going down the "rungs" of the evidence hierarchy for Therapy questions results in less reliable evidence. For example, Level III evidence comes from a type of study called quasi-experimental. In-depth qualitative studies are near the bottom, in terms of evidence regarding intervention effectiveness. (Terms in Figure 2.1 will be discussed in later chapters.)

For a Prognosis question, by contrast, Level II evidence comes from a single prospective cohort study, and Level III evidence is from a type of study called case control (Level I evidence is from a systematic review of cohort studies). Thus, contrary to what is often implied in discussions of evidence hierarchies, there really are multiple hierarchies. If one is interested in the best evidence for questions about meaning, an RCT would be a poor source of evidence, for example. Figure 2.1 illustrates these multiple hierarchies, with information on the right indicating the type of *individual study* that would offer the best evidence (Level II) for different questions. In all cases, appropriate systematic reviews are at the pinnacle.

Of course, *within* any level in an evidence hierarchy, evidence quality can vary considerably. For example, an individual RCT could be well designed, yielding strong Level II evidence for Therapy questions, or it could be so flawed that the evidence would be weak.

Thus, in nursing, *best evidence* refers to research findings that are methodologically appropriate, rigorous, and clinically relevant for answering pressing questions. These questions not only cover the efficacy, safety, ethics, and cost effectiveness of nursing interventions, but also the reliability of nursing assessment tests, the causes and consequences of health

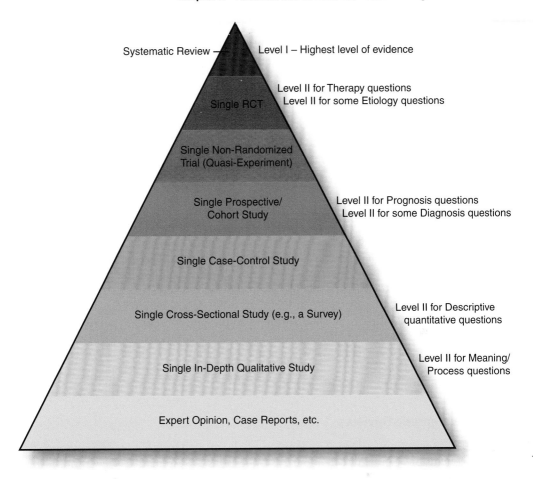

Figure 2.1 Evidence hierarchy: levels of evidence for different EBP questions.

problems, and the meaning and nature of patients' experiences. Confidence in the evidence is enhanced when the research methods are compelling, when there have been multiple confirmatory studies, and when the evidence has been carefully evaluated and synthesized.

Evidence-Based Practice Challenges

Studies that have explored barriers to evidence-based nursing have yielded similar results in many countries. Most barriers fall into one of three categories: (1) quality and nature of the research, (2) characteristics of nurses, and (3) organizational factors.

With regard to the research itself, one problem is the limited availability of strong research evidence for some practice areas. The need for research that directly addresses relevant clinical problems and for replicating studies in a range of practice settings remains a challenge. Also, nurse researchers need to improve their ability to communicate evidence to practising nurses. In non–English-speaking countries, another impediment is that most studies are reported in English.

Nurses' attitudes and education are also potential barriers to EBP. Studies have found that some nurses do not value or understand research, and others simply resist change. And, among the nurses who *do* appreciate research, many do not have the skills for accessing high-quality research evidence or for evaluating it for possible use in clinical decision making.

Finally, many challenges to using research in practice are organizational. "Unit culture" can undermine research use, and administrative or organizational barriers also play a major role. Although many organizations support the idea of EBP in theory, they do not always provide the necessary supports in terms of staff release time and provision of resources. Strong leadership in health care organizations is essential to making EBP happen.

RESOURCES FOR EVIDENCE-BASED PRACTICE

In this section, we describe some of the resources that are available to support EBP and to address some of the challenges.

Pre-Appraised Evidence

Research evidence comes in various forms, the most basic of which is from individual studies. While *primary studies* published in journals may have gone through a peer review process, they are not preprocessed (pre-appraised) for quality and use in practice. The term "preprocessed" refers to evidence that has been summarized and synthesized by other reviewers.

DiCenso, Guyatt, and Ciliska (2005) have described a hierarchy of preprocessed evidence. On the first rung above primary studies are synopses of single studies, followed by systematic reviews, and then synopses of systematic reviews. Clinical practice guidelines are at the top of the hierarchy. At each successive step in the hierarchy, there is a greater ease in applying the evidence to clinical practice. We describe several types of pre-appraised evidence sources in this section.

Systematic Reviews

EBP relies on meticulous integration of all key evidence on a topic so that well-grounded conclusions can be drawn about EBP questions. A systematic review is not just a literature review. A systematic review is in itself a methodical, scholarly inquiry that follows many of the same steps as those for other studies.

Systematic reviews can take various forms. One form is a narrative (qualitative) integration that merges and synthesizes findings, much like a rigorous literature review. For integrating evidence from quantitative studies, narrative reviews increasingly are being replaced by a type of systematic review known as a meta-analysis.

Meta-analysis is a technique for integrating quantitative research findings statistically. In essence, meta-analysis treats the findings from a study as one piece of information. The findings from multiple studies on the same topic are combined and then all of the information is analysed statistically in a manner similar to that in a usual study. Thus, instead of study participants being the *unit of analysis* (the most basic entity for the analysis), individual studies are the unit of analysis in a meta-analysis. Meta-analysis provides an objective method of integrating a body of findings and of observing patterns that might not have been detected.

> **Example of a meta-analysis** •
> Johnston and colleagues (2017) conducted a meta-analysis of the evidence to explore the effect of skin-to-skin care (SSC) on pain in neonates. Twenty-five studies including a total of 2,001 infants were included. SSC was considered effective in reducing pain as measured by both physiologic and behavioural indicators.

For qualitative studies, integration may take the form of a **meta-synthesis**. A meta-synthesis, however, is distinct from a quantitative meta-analysis: a meta-synthesis is less about reducing information and more about interpreting it.

> **Example of a meta-synthesis** •
> Leung and colleagues (2016) undertook a meta-synthesis of studies exploring the experience of transitioning from acute care to end-of-life care for patients with chronic critical illness in intensive care units.
>
> Their meta-synthesis of five qualitative studies conducted in Canada and the United States identifies the need for patients and families to understand that chronic critical illness is part of active dying.

Systematic reviews are increasingly available. Such reviews are published in professional journals that can be accessed using standard literature search procedures (see Chapter 7) and are also available in databases that are dedicated to such reviews. In particular, the Cochrane Database of Systematic Reviews (CDSR) and JBI database of systemic reviews and implementation reports contain thousands of systematic reviews relating to health care interventions.

 TIP Websites with useful content relating to EBP, including ones for locating systematic reviews, are in the Internet Resources for Chapter 2 on thePoint for you to access simply by using the "Control/Click" feature.

Clinical Practice Guidelines and Care Bundles

Evidence-based **clinical practice guidelines** distil a body of evidence into a usable form. Unlike systematic reviews, clinical practice guidelines (which often are *based* on systematic reviews) give specific concrete recommendations for evidence-based decision making. Guideline development typically involves the consensus of a group of researchers, experts, and clinicians. The use or adaptation of a clinical practice guideline is often an ideal focus for an EBP project.

Also, organizations are developing and adopting *care bundles*—a concept developed by the Institute for Healthcare Improvement and adopted by the Canadian Patient Safety Institute—that encompass a set of interventions to promote patient safety (http://www.patientsafetyinstitute.ca). There is growing evidence that a combination or bundle of strategies produces better outcomes than a single intervention.

> **Example of a care bundle project** •
> Tayyib, Coyer, and Lewis (2015) studied the effectiveness of a pressure ulcer prevention care bundle in reducing the incidence of pressure ulcers in critically ill patients. Patients who received the bundled interventions had a significantly lower incidence of pressure ulcers than patients who did not.

Finding care bundles and clinical practice guidelines can be challenging because there is no single guideline repository. A standard search in a bibliographic database such as MEDLINE (see Chapter 7) will yield many references; however, the results are likely to include not only the actual guidelines but also commentaries, implementation studies, and so on.

A recommended approach is to search in guideline databases or through specialty organizations that have sponsored guideline development. A few of the many possible sources deserve mention. In Canada, the Registered Nurses' Association of Ontario (RNAO) (www.rnao.org/bestpractices) maintains information about clinical practice guidelines. In the United States, nursing and health care guidelines are maintained by the National Guideline Clearinghouse (www.guideline.gov). Two sources in the United Kingdom are the Translating Research into Practice (TRIP) database and the National Institute for Clinical Excellence (NICE).

Although multiple guidelines often exist for the same topic, there are still many areas for which practice guidelines have not yet been developed. Worse yet, because of differences in the rigor of guideline development, update frequency, and interpretation of evidence, different guidelines sometimes offer different or even conflicting recommendations (Lewis, 2001). Thus, those who wish to adopt clinical practice guidelines should carefully appraise them to identify ones that are based on the strongest evidence, have been meticulously developed, are user friendly, and are appropriate for local use or adaptation.

Several appraisal instruments are available to evaluate clinical practice guidelines. One with broad support is the Appraisal of Guidelines Research and Evaluation (AGREE) Instrument, now in its second version (AGREE Collaboration, 2001; Brouwers et al., 2010; www. agreecollaboration.org). The AGREE II instrument has ratings for 23 dimensions within 6 domains (e.g., scope and purpose, rigor of development, presentation). As examples, a dimension in the scope and purpose domain is "The population (patients, public, etc.) to whom the guideline is meant to apply is specifically described," and one in the rigor of development domain is "The guideline has been externally reviewed by experts prior to its publication." The AGREE tool should be applied to a guideline by a team of two to four appraisers. More information about the AGREE II instrument is provided in the supplement to this chapter on thePoint website. ⚡

Example of using AGREE II •
Fisher (2014) evaluated clinical practice guidelines for urinary care of stroke patients in acute and rehabilitation settings. An expert panel of 25 local and regional experts in stroke and continence care assessed the selected guidelines using the AGREE II instrument.

    TIP   For those interested in learning more about the AGREE II instrument, we offer more information in the chapter supplement on thePoint website. ⚡

Models of the Evidence-Based Practice Process

EBP models offer frameworks for designing and implementing EBP projects in practice settings. Some models focus on the use of research by individual clinicians (e.g., the Stetler Model, one of the oldest models that originated as an RU model), but most focus on institutional EBP efforts (e.g., the Iowa Model). The many worthy EBP models are too numerous to list comprehensively but include the following:

- Advancing Research and Clinical Practice Through Close Collaboration (ARCC) Model (Melnyk & Fineout-Overholt, 2015)
- Diffusion of Innovations Model (Rogers, 1995)
- Iowa Model of Evidence-Based Practice to Promote Quality Care (Titler, 2010)
- Johns Hopkins Nursing Evidence-Based Practice Model (Dearholt & Dang, 2012)
- Promoting Action on Research Implementation in Health Services (PARiHS) Model (Rycroft-Malone, 2010; Rycroft-Malone et al., 2013)
- Stetler Model of Research Utilization (Stetler, 2010)

For those wishing to follow a formal EBP model, the cited references should be consulted. Several are also nicely synthesized by Melnyk and Fineout-Overholt (2015). Each model offers different perspectives on how to translate research findings into practice, but several steps and procedures are similar across the models. We provide an overview of key activities and processes in EBP efforts, based on a distillation of common elements from the various models, in a subsequent section of this chapter. We rely heavily on the Iowa Model, shown in Figure 2.2.

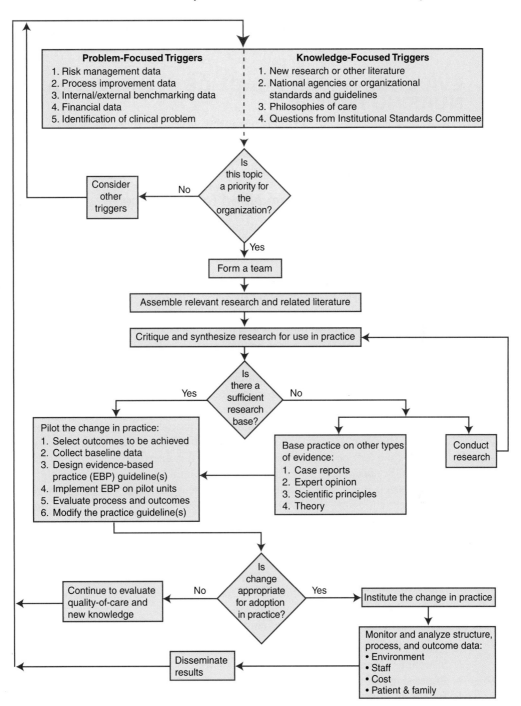

Figure 2.2 Iowa model of evidence-based practice to promote quality care. (Adapted with permission from Titler, M. G., Kleiber, C., Steelman, V., et al. (2001). The Iowa model of evidence-based practice to promote quality care. *Critical Care Nursing Clinics of North America, 13,* 497–509.)

TIP   Gawlinski and Rutledge (2008) offer suggestions for selecting an EBP model.

EVIDENCE-BASED PRACTICE IN INDIVIDUAL NURSING PRACTICE

This and the following section provide an overview of how research can be put to use in clinical settings. We first discuss strategies and steps for individual clinicians and then describe activities used by organizations or teams of nurses.

Clinical Scenarios and the Need for Evidence

Individual nurses make many decisions and are called upon to provide health care advice, and so they have ample opportunity to put research into practice. Here are four clinical scenarios that provide examples of such opportunities:

- Clinical Scenario 1. You work on an ICU and notice that *Clostridium difficile* infection has become more prevalent among surgical patients in your hospital. You want to know whether there is a reliable screening tool for assessing the risk of infection so that preventive measures can be initiated in a more timely and effective manner.
- Clinical Scenario 2. You work in an allergy clinic and notice how difficult it is for many children to undergo allergy scratch tests. You wonder whether an interactive distraction intervention would help reduce children's pain when they are being tested for allergens.
- Clinical Scenario 3. You work in a rehabilitation hospital, and one of your elderly patients, who had total hip replacement, tells you she is planning a long airplane trip. You know that a long plane ride will increase her risk of deep vein thrombosis and wonder whether compression stockings are an effective in-flight treatment. You decide to look for the best possible evidence to answer this question.
- Clinical Scenario 4. You are caring for a hospitalized cardiac patient who tells you that he has sleep apnea. He confides in you that he is reluctant to undergo continuous positive airway pressure (CPAP) treatment because he worries it will hinder intimacy with his wife. You wonder if there is any evidence about what it is like to undergo CPAP treatment so that you can better understand how to address your patient's concerns.

In these and thousands of other clinical situations, research evidence can be put to good use to improve nursing care. Some situations might lead to unit-wide or institution-wide scrutiny of current practices, but in other situations, individual nurses can personally examine evidence to help address specific problems.

For individual EBP efforts, the major steps in EBP include the following:

1. Asking clinical questions that can be answered with research evidence
2. Searching for and retrieving relevant evidence
3. Appraising and synthesizing the evidence
4. Integrating the evidence with your own clinical expertise, patient preferences, and local context
5. Assessing the effectiveness of the decision, intervention, or advice

Asking Well-Worded Clinical Questions: PIO and PICO

A crucial first step in EBP involves asking relevant clinical questions about uncertainties in clinical practice. Some EBP writers distinguish between background and foreground questions. *Background questions* are foundational questions about a clinical issue, such as:

What is cancer cachexia (progressive body wasting), and what is its pathophysiology? Answers to such questions are typically found in textbooks. *Foreground questions*, by contrast, are those that can be answered based on the current best research evidence on diagnosing, assessing, or treating patients, or on understanding the meaning or prognosis of their health problems. For example, we may wonder, is a fish oil–enhanced nutritional supplement effective in stabilizing weight in patients with advanced cancer? The answer to such a question may provide guidance on how best to address the needs of patients with cachexia.

Most guidelines for EBP use the acronyms PIO or PICO to help practitioners develop well-worded questions that facilitate a search for evidence. In the most basic PIO form, the clinical question is worded to identify three components:

1. P: The *population* or *patients* (What are the characteristics of the patients or people?)
2. I: The *intervention, influence*, indicator or *exposure* (What are the interventions or therapies of interest? or What are the potentially harmful influences/exposures of concern?)
3. O: The *outcomes* (What are the outcomes or consequences in which we are interested?)

Applying this scheme to our question about cachexia, our *population* (P) is cancer patients with cachexia, the *intervention* (I) is fish oil–enhanced nutritional supplements, and the *outcome* (O) is weight stabilization. As another example, in the second clinical scenario about scratch tests cited earlier, the population is children being tested for allergies, the intervention is interactive distraction, and the outcome is pain.

For questions that can best be answered with qualitative information (e.g., about the meaning of an experience or health problem), two components are most relevant:

1. The *population* (What are the characteristics of the patients or clients?)
2. The *situation* (What conditions, experiences, or circumstances are we interested in understanding?)

For example, suppose our question was: What is it like to suffer from cachexia? In this case, the question calls for rich qualitative information; the *population* is patients with advanced cancer and the *situation* is the experience of cachexia.

In addition to the basic PIO components, other components are sometimes important in an evidence search. In particular, a comparison (C) component may be needed, when the intervention or influence of interest is contrasted with a specific alternative. For example, we might be interested in learning whether fish oil–enhanced supplements (I) are better than melatonin (C) in stabilizing weight (O) in cancer patients (P). When a *specific* comparison is of interest, a PICO question is required; but if we were interested in uncovering evidence about *all* alternatives to an intervention of primary interest, then PIO components are sufficient. (By contrast, when asking questions to undertake an actual *study*, the "C" must always be specified.)

 TIP Other components may be relevant, such as a time frame in which an intervention might be appropriate (adding a "T" for PICOT questions) or a setting (adding an "S" for PICOS questions).

Table 2.1 offers templates for asking well-worded clinical questions for different types of foreground questions. The far right column includes questions with an explicit comparison (PICO), whereas the middle column does not have a comparison (PIO). The questions are categorized in a manner similar to that discussed in Chapter 1 (EBP Purpose), as featured in Table 1.3. One exception is that we have added description as a category. Note that although there are some differences in components across question types, there is always a P component.

TABLE 2.1 Question Templates for Selected Clinical Foreground Questions: PIO and PICO

Type of Question	PIO Question Template (Questions Without an Explicit Comparison)	PICO Question Template (Questions With an Explicit Comparison)
Therapy/treatment/ intervention	In ___ (**P**opulation), what is the effect of ___ (**I**ntervention) on ___ (**O**utcome)?	In ___ (**P**opulation), what is the effect of ___ (**I**ntervention), in comparison to ___ (**C**omparative/ alternative intervention), on ___ (**O**utcome)?
Diagnosis/assessment	For ___ (**P**opulation), does ___ (**I**dentifying tool/procedure) yield accurate and appropriate diagnostic/assessment information about ___ (**O**utcome)?	For ___ (**P**opulation), does ___ (**I**dentifying tool/procedure) yield more accurate or more appropriate diagnostic/assessment information than ___ (**C**omparative tool/ procedure) about ___ (**O**utcome)?
Prognosis	For ___ (**P**opulation), does ___ (**E**xposure to disease or condition) increase the risk of ___ (**O**utcome)?	For ___ (**P**opulation), does ___ (**E**xposure to disease or condition), relative to ___ (**C**omparative disease or condition) increase the risk of ___ (**O**utcome)?
Etiology/harm	In (**P**opulation), does ___ (**I**nfluence, exposure, or characteristic) increase the risk of ___ (**O**utcome)?	Does (**I**nfluence, exposure, or characteristic) increase the risk of ___ (**O**utcome) compared to ___ (**C**omparative influence, exposure or condition) in ___ (**P**opulation)?
Description (prevalence/incidence)	In ___ (**P**opulation), how prevalent is ___ (**O**utcome)?	*Explicit comparisons are not typical, except to compare different populations.*
Meaning or process	What is it like for ___ (**P**opulation) to experience ___ (condition, illness, circumstance)? **OR** What is the process by which ___ (**P**opulation) cope with, adapt to, or live with ___ (condition, illness, circumstance)?	*Explicit comparisons are not typical in these types of questions.*

 TIP It is crucial to practise asking clinical questions—it is the starting point for evidence-based nursing. Take some time to fill in the blanks in Table 2.1 for each question category. Do not be too self-critical at this point. Your comfort in developing questions will increase over time.

Finding Research Evidence

By wording clinical queries as PIO or PICO questions, you should be able to search the research literature for the information you need. Using the templates in Table 2.1, the information you insert into the blanks are *keywords* that can be used in an electronic search.

For an individual EBP endeavour, the best place to begin is by searching for evidence in a systematic review, clinical practice guideline, or other preprocessed source. This approach can lead to a quicker answer and potentially a superior answer if your methodologic skills are limited. Researchers who prepare reviews and clinical guidelines typically are well trained in research methods and use rigorous standards in evaluating the evidence. Moreover, preprocessed evidence is often prepared by a team, which means that the conclusions are cross-checked and fairly objective. Thus, when preprocessed evidence is available to answer a clinical question, you may not need to look any farther unless the review is outdated. When preprocessed evidence cannot be located or is old, you will need to look for best evidence in primary studies, using strategies we describe in Chapter 7.

 TIP Searching for evidence for an EBP project has been greatly simplified in recent years. Guidance on doing a search for evidence on clinical questions is available in the supplement for Chapter 7 (the chapter on literature reviews) on the book's website thePoint. ⁘

Appraising the Evidence for Evidence-Based Practice

Evidence should be appraised before clinical action is taken. The critical appraisal of evidence for the purposes of EBP may involve several types of assessments (Box 2.1) but often focuses primarily on evidence quality.

Evidence Quality

The overriding appraisal issue is whether the findings are *valid*. That is, were the study methods sufficiently rigorous that the evidence can be trusted? Ideally, you would find pre-appraised evidence, but a goal of this book is to help you evaluate research evidence yourself. If there are several primary studies and no existing systematic review, you would need to draw conclusions about the entire body of evidence. Clearly, you would want to put most weight on the most rigorous studies.

Magnitude of Effects

You would also need to assess whether study findings are clinically important and meaningful. The study results should be "real" and demonstrate a powerful effect. For example, consider clinical scenario 3 cited earlier, which suggests this question: Does the use of compression stockings lower the risk of flight-related deep vein thrombosis for high-risk patients? In our search, we found a relevant systematic review in the nursing literature—a meta-analysis of nine RCTs (Hsieh & Lee, 2005)—and others in the Cochrane database (Clarke et al., 2006; O'Meara et al., 2012). The conclusion of these reviews, based on reliable evidence, was that compression stockings are effective and the magnitude of the risk-reducing effect is fairly substantial. Thus, advice about using compression stockings may be appropriate, pending an appraisal of other factors. The magnitude of effects can be quantified, and several methods are described later in this book. The magnitude of effects also has a bearing on *clinical significance*, which we also discuss in a later chapter.

Box 2.1 Questions for Appraising the Evidence

1. What is the quality of the evidence—i.e., how rigorous and reliable is it?
2. What *is* the evidence—what is the magnitude of effects?
3. How precise is the estimate of effects?
4. What evidence is there of any side effects/side benefits?
5. What is the financial cost of applying (and not applying) the evidence?
6. Is the evidence relevant to my particular clinical situation?

Precision of Estimates

When the evidence is quantitative, another consideration is how precise the estimate of effect is. This type of appraisal requires some statistical knowledge, and so we postpone our discussion of *confidence intervals* to Chapter 14. Suffice it to say that research results provide only an *estimate* of effects, and it is useful to understand not only the exact estimate but also the range that includes the actual effect.

Peripheral Effects

Even if the evidence is judged to be valid and the magnitude of effects is sizeable, peripheral benefits and costs may be important in guiding decisions. In framing your clinical question, you would have identified the outcomes (O) in which you were interested—for example, weight stabilization for an intervention to address cancer cachexia. Research on this topic, however, would likely have considered other outcomes that need to be taken into account— for example, effects on quality of life.

Financial Costs

Another issue concerns the costs of applying the evidence. Costs may be small or non-existent. For example, in clinical scenario 4 concerning the experience of CPAP treatment, nursing action would be cost-neutral because the evidence would be used to reassure and inform patients. When interventions and assessments are costly, however, the resources needed to put the best evidence into practice should be factored into any decision. Of course, although the cost of a clinical decision needs to be considered, the cost of *not* taking action is equally important.

Clinical Relevance

Finally, it is important to appraise the evidence in terms of its relevance for the clinical situation at hand—that is, for *your* patient in a specific clinical setting. Best practice evidence can most readily be applied to an individual patient in your care if he or she is sufficiently similar to people in the study or studies under review. Would your patient have qualified for participation in the study—or would some factor (e.g., age, illness severity, comorbidities) have disqualified him or her? DiCenso et al. (2005) have provided some useful tips to help clinicians decide whether there is a compelling reason to conclude that results may *not* be applicable in their clinical situation.

Actions Based on Evidence Appraisals

Appraisals of the evidence may lead you to different courses of action. You may reach this point and conclude that the evidence base is not sufficiently sound, or that the likely effect is too small, or that the cost of applying the evidence is too high. The evidence appraisal may suggest that "usual care" is the best strategy. If, however, the initial appraisal of evidence suggests a promising clinical action, then you can proceed to the next step.

Integrating Evidence in Evidence-Based Practice

Research evidence needs to be integrated with other types of information, including your own clinical expertise and knowledge of your clinical setting. You may be aware of factors that would make implementation of the evidence, no matter how sound and how promising, inadvisable. Patient preferences and values are also important. A discussion with the patient may reveal negative attitudes towards a potentially beneficial course of action, contraindications (e.g., comorbidities), or possible impediments (e.g., lack of financial resources).

One final issue is the desirability of integrating evidence from qualitative research. Qualitative research can provide rich insights about how patients experience a problem, or about barriers to treatment adherence. A potentially beneficial intervention may fail to achieve desired outcomes if it is not implemented with sensitivity to the patients' perspectives. As Morse (2005) so aptly noted, evidence from an RCT may tell us whether a pill is effective, but qualitative research can help us understand why patients may not swallow the pill.

Implementing the Evidence and Evaluating Outcomes

After the first four steps of the EBP process have been completed, you can use the resulting information to make an evidence-based decision or to provide evidence-based advice. Although the steps in the process, as just described, may seem complicated, in reality, the process can be quite straightforward—*if* there is adequate evidence, and especially if it has been skilfully preprocessed. EBP is most challenging when findings from research are contradictory, inconclusive, or "thin"—that is, when better quality evidence is needed.

The last step in an individual EBP effort is evaluation. Part of the evaluation process involves following up to determine whether your actions achieved the desired outcome. Another part, however, concerns an evaluation of how well you are performing EBP. Sackett et al. (2000) offer self-evaluation questions that relate to the previous EBP steps, such as asking answerable questions (Am I asking any clinical questions at all? Am I asking well-worded questions?) and finding external evidence (Do I know the best sources of current evidence? Am I efficient in my searching?). A self-appraisal may lead to the conclusion that at least some of the clinical questions of interest to you are best addressed as a group effort.

EVIDENCE-BASED PRACTICE IN AN ORGANIZATIONAL CONTEXT

For some clinical scenarios, individual nurses may be able to implement EBP strategies on their own (e.g., giving advice about compression stockings). Many situations, however, require decision making by an organization, or by a team of nurses working to solve a recurrent problem. This section describes some issues that are relevant to institutional efforts at EBP—efforts that will lead to the development of a formal policy or protocol affecting the practice of many nurses.

Many steps in organizational EBP projects are similar to the ones described in the previous section. For example, gathering and appraising evidence are key activities in both, as shown in the Iowa Model in Figure 2.2 (assemble relevant research; critique and synthesize research). Additional issues are relevant at the organizational level, however, including the selection of a problem; an assessment of whether the topic is an organizational priority; deciding whether to test an EBP innovation on a trial basis; and deciding, based on a trial, whether the innovation should be adopted. We briefly discuss some of these topics.

Selecting a Problem for an Institutional Evidence-Based Practice Project

Some EBP projects originate in discussions among clinicians who have encountered a recurrent problem and seek a resolution. Others, however, are "top-down" efforts in which administrators take steps to stimulate the use of research evidence among clinicians.

Several models of EBP, such as the Iowa model, distinguish two types of stimulus ("triggers") for an EBP endeavour: (1) *problem-focused triggers*—the identification of a clinical practice problem in need of solution, or (2) *knowledge-focused triggers*—new findings in the research literature. The problem identification approach is likely to be clinically relevant and to have staff support if the problem is one that numerous nurses have encountered.

A second catalyst for an EBP project is a knowledge-focused trigger, which is akin to RU. The catalyst might be a new clinical guideline or a research article discussed in a journal club. With knowledge-focused triggers, the clinical relevance of the research might need to be assessed. In order to get the buy-in from the knowledge users, the central issue is whether a problem of significance to nurses in a particular setting will be solved by introducing an innovation.

Appraising Implementation Potential

With either type of trigger, the feasibility of undertaking an organizational EBP project needs to be assessed. In the Iowa model (Fig. 2.2), the first major decision point involves determining whether the organization considers practice change is a priority. Titler et al. (2001) advised considering the following issues before finalizing a topic for EBP: the topic's fit with the organization's strategic plan, the magnitude of the problem, the number of people invested in the problem, support of nurse leaders and of those in other disciplines, costs and availability of resources, and possible barriers to change.

Some EBP models involve a formal assessment of organizational "fit," often called **implementation potential** (or *environmental readiness*). In assessing the implementation potential of an innovation, several issues should be considered, particularly the transferability of the innovation (i.e., the extent to which the innovation might be appropriate in new settings), the feasibility of implementing it, and its cost–benefit ratio. If the implementation assessment suggests that there might be problems in testing the innovation in a particular practice setting, then the team can either identify a new problem and begin the process anew or develop a plan to improve the implementation potential (e.g., seeking external resources if costs are too high).

Evidence Appraisals and Subsequent Actions

In the Iowa model, the second major factor to consider is the synthesis and appraisal of research evidence. The key question focuses on whether the research base is sufficient to justify an evidence-based change—for example, whether a new clinical practice guideline is of sufficient quality that it can be used or adapted, or whether the research evidence is rigorous enough to recommend a practice innovation.

Assessments about the adequacy of the evidence can lead to different action paths. If the research evidence is weak, the team could assemble non-research evidence (e.g., through consultation with experts or client surveys) to determine the benefit of a practice change. Another option is to conduct an original study to address the practice question, thereby gathering new evidence. This course of action may be impractical and would result in years of delay.

If, on the other hand, there is a solid research base or a high-quality clinical practice guideline, then the team would develop plans to implement a practice innovation. A key activity usually involves developing or adapting a local evidence-based clinical practice protocol or guideline. Strategies for developing clinical practice guidelines are suggested in DiCenso et al. (2005) and Melnyk and Fineout-Overholt (2015).

Implementing and Evaluating the Innovation

Once the EBP product has been developed, the next step is to **pilot test** it (give it a trial run) and evaluate the outcome. Building on the Iowa model, this phase of the project likely would involve the following activities:

1. Developing an evaluation plan (e.g., identifying outcomes to be achieved, determining how many clients to include, deciding when and how often to measure outcomes)

2. Measuring client outcomes prior to implementing the innovation, so that there is a base-line for comparison against the outcomes of the innovation

3. Training relevant staff in the use of the new guideline and, if necessary, "marketing" the innovation to users

4. Trying the guideline out on one or more units or with a group of clients

5. Evaluating the pilot project, in terms of both process (e.g., How was the innovation received? What problems were encountered? What are the barriers?) and outcomes (e.g., How were client outcomes affected? What were the costs?)

A fairly informal evaluation may be adequate, but formal efforts are often appropriate and provide opportunities for dissemination to others at conferences or in professional journals.

 TIP Every nurse can play a role in using research evidence. Here are some strategies:

- Read widely and critically.
- Attend professional conferences.
- Become involved in a journal club.
- Pursue and participate in EBP projects.

QUALITY IMPROVEMENT

We conclude this chapter with a brief discussion of **quality improvement (QI)** (or quality assurance) projects, which are efforts ongoing in many health care settings and which some-times involve nurses. In recent years, there has been a lot of discussion in health journals about the differences and similarities between QI projects and research. And in nursing, efforts have been made to distinguish QI, research, and EBP projects (Shirey et al., 2011). All three have much in common, notably the use of systematic methods of solving health problems with an overall aim of fostering improvements in health care. Often, the research methods used overlap: Patient data are used in all three, and statistical analyses—sometimes combined with analysis of qualitative data—are also used in all three.

The definitions of QI, research, and EBP activities are distinct, and yet it is not always easy to distinguish them in real-world projects, resulting in confusion. QI has been defined by Health Council of Canada (HCC) as "systematic approach to making changes that improve clinical practice and health system performance, enhance professional and/or organizational development, and improve patient and population health outcomes" (HCC, 2003). According to the *Tri-Council Policy Statement: Ethical Conduct for Research Involving Humans*, research is defined as "an undertaking which involves a systematic investigation to establish facts, principles, or generalizable knowledge" (Government of Canada, http://www.pre.ethics.gc.ca/eng/archives/policy-politique/reports-rapports/trdr-vdrr/). And EBP projects, as we have seen, are efforts to translate "best evidence" into protocols to guide the actions of health care staff to maximize good outcomes for clients. Shirey et al. (2011) summarize the differences between the three as follows: "All three have an important, but different, relationship with knowledge: research generates it, EBP translates it, and QI incorporates it" (p. 60).

QI projects are discussed briefly in Chapter 13. Here, we note a few characteristics of QI:

- In QI efforts, the intervention or protocol can change as it is being evaluated to incor-porate new ideas or insights.
- The purpose of a QI project is often to effect immediate improvement in health care delivery.
- QI is designed with the intent of sustaining an improvement.

- QI is a necessary, integral activity for a health care institution; research is not.
- A literature review may not be undertaken in a QI project.
- QI projects are not externally funded.

Example of a nurse-led quality improvement project • • • • • • • • • • • • • • •

Fabbruzzo-Cota and colleagues (2016) undertook a QI project in an acute care hospital to reduce hospital-acquired pressure ulcers based on recommendations from the Registered Nurses' Association of Ontario Best Practice Guideline Risk Assessment & Prevention of Pressure Ulcers. The project involved initiatives such as documentation standardization, development of staff education and patient and family educational resources, initiation of a hospital-wide inventory for support surfaces, and procurement of equipment.

RESEARCH EXAMPLES WITH CRITICAL THINKING EXERCISES

Hundreds of projects to translate research evidence into nursing practice are underway worldwide. Those that have been described in the nursing literature offer good information about planning and implementing such an endeavour. In this section, we summarize one such project.

Read the research summary for Example 1 and then answer the critical thinking questions that follow, referring to the full research report if necessary (this example is featured on the interactive *Critical Thinking Activity* on thePoint website). The critical thinking questions for Exercises 2 and 3 are based on the studies that appear in their entirety in Appendices A and B of this book. Our comments for these exercises are in the Student Resources section on thePoint.

EXAMPLE 1: EVIDENCE-BASED PRACTICE PROJECT

Study: Implementation of the ABCDE bundle to improve patient outcomes in the intensive care unit in a rural community hospital (Kram et al., 2015)

Purpose: A team of nurses undertook an EBP to implement an existing care bundle designed to manage delirium—the ABCDE bundle—in a rural community ICU. The bundle incorporates **a**wakening, **b**reathing, **c**oordination (or **c**hoice of sedative), **d**elirium monitoring and management, and **e**arly mobility on a daily basis. The question for this EBP project was: Does the implementation of the ABCDE bundle care, versus the usual care (absence of the ABCDE bundle components), reduce the incidence of delirium, decrease patient length of stay (LOS) in the ICU, decrease patient total hospital LOS, and decrease length of mechanical ventilation of patients, thus decreasing costs in the ICU?

Framework: The project used the Johns Hopkins Nursing Evidence-Based Practice Model as its guiding framework.

Approach: The team began by reviewing the current body of evidence on the ABCDE bundle. They also undertook an organizational assessment and identified which practice changes were required. Key stakeholder support was sought. Approval was obtained from the nurse executive committee, the chief medical officer, and from physicians with ICU admitting privileges. Educational sessions, using various instructional methods, were conducted with staff from nursing, respiratory therapy, and rehabilitation services. The ABCDE bundle was implemented for all adult patients admitted to the ICU starting in October 2014.

Evaluation: To assess the effects of the ABCDE bundle, the team collected and organized relevant information for two periods: from October 2013 to January 2014 (pre-bundle) and from October 2014 to January 2015 (post-bundle). The outcomes of interest included rate of compliance to bundle elements by direct care providers, changes in hospital and ICU LOS between the two periods, changes in the number of ventilator days from pre-bundle to post-bundle, and prevalence of post-bundle delirium. Information was obtained for 47 patients in the pre-bundle group and 36 patients in the post-bundle group.

Findings and Conclusions: The team found that compliance with the bundle protocols was high. The average hospital stay was 1.8 days lower after the implementation of the bundle. Mechanical ventilation was lower by an average of 1 day in the post-bundle group. A baseline delirium prevalence rate of 19% was established as a baseline after the bundle was implemented. The EBP team concluded that the ABCDE bundle "can be implemented in rural, community-based hospitals and provides a safe, cost-effective method for enhancing ICU patient outcomes" (p. 250).

Critical Thinking Exercises

1. Of the EBP-focused research purposes (Table 1.3), which purpose was the central focus of this project?
2. What is the clinical question that the EBP team asked in this project? Identify the components of the question using the PICO framework.
3. Discuss how this project could have been based on either a knowledge-focused or problem-focused trigger.

EXAMPLE 2: QUANTITATIVE RESEARCH IN APPENDIX A

- Read the abstract and the introduction of Swenson and colleagues' (2016) study ("Parents' use of praise and criticism in a sample of young children seeking mental health services") in Appendix A of this book.

Critical Thinking Exercises

1. Identify one or more clinical foreground questions that, if posed, would be addressed by this study. Which PIO or PICO components does your question capture?
2. How, if at all, might evidence from this study be used in an EBP project (individual or organizational)?

EXAMPLE 3: QUALITATIVE RESEARCH IN APPENDIX B

- Read the abstract and the introduction of Beck and Watson's (2010) study ("Subsequent childbirth after a previous traumatic birth") in Appendix B of this book.

Critical Thinking Exercises

1. Identify one or more clinical foreground questions that, if posed, would be addressed by this study. Which PIO or PICO components does your question capture?
2. How, if at all, might evidence from this study be used in an EBP project (individual or organizational)?

Summary Points

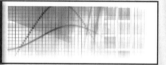

- **EBP** is the conscientious use of current best evidence in making clinical decisions about patient care; it is a clinical problem-solving strategy that de-emphasizes decision making based on custom and emphasizes the integration of research evidence with clinical expertise and patient preferences.
- **RU** and EBP are overlapping concepts that concern efforts to use research as a basis for clinical decisions, but RU *starts* with a research-based innovation that gets evaluated for possible use in practice. **KT** is a term used primarily about system-wide efforts to effect systematic change in clinical practice or policies.
- Two underpinnings of the EBP movement are the **Cochrane Collaboration** (which is based on the work of British epidemiologist Archie Cochrane) and the clinical learning strategy developed at the McMaster Medical School called *evidence-based medicine.*
- EBP involves evaluating evidence to determine *best evidence.* Often an **evidence hierarchy** is used to rank study findings according to the strength of evidence provided, but different hierarchies are appropriate for different types of questions. In all evidence hierarchies, however, *systematic reviews* are at the pinnacle.

- **Systematic reviews** are rigorous integrations of research evidence from multiple studies on a topic. Systematic reviews can involve either narrative approaches to integration (including **meta-synthesis** of qualitative studies) or quantitative methods (**meta-analysis**) that integrate findings statistically.
- Evidence-based **clinical practice guidelines** combine an appraisal of research evidence with specific recommendations for clinical decisions.
- Many models of EBP have been developed, including models that provide a framework for individual clinicians (e.g., the *Stetler Model*) and others for organizations or teams of clinicians (e.g., the *Iowa Model*).
- Individual nurses have opportunities to put research into practice. The five basic steps for individual EBP are (1) asking an answerable clinical question, (2) searching for relevant research-based evidence, (3) appraising and synthesizing the evidence, (4) integrating evidence with other factors, and (5) assessing effectiveness of actions.
- One scheme for asking well-worded clinical questions involves four primary components, an acronym for which is PICO: population (P), intervention or influence (I), comparison (C), and outcome (O). When there is no explicit comparison, the acronym is PIO.
- An appraisal of the evidence involves such considerations as the validity of study findings, their clinical importance, the magnitude

and precision of effects, associated costs and risks, and utility in a particular clinical situation.

- EBP in an organizational context involves many of the same steps as individual EBP efforts but is more formalized and must take organizational factors into account.

- *Triggers* for an organizational project include both pressing clinical problems (*problem-focused*) and existing knowledge (*knowledge- focused*).

- Before an EBP-based guideline or protocol can be tested, there should be an assessment of its **implementation potential**, which includes the issues of transferability, feasibility, and the cost–benefit ratio of implementing a new practice in a clinical setting.

- Once an evidence-based protocol or guideline has been developed and deemed worthy of implementation, the EBP team can move forward with a **pilot test** of the innovation and an assessment of the outcomes prior to widespread adoption.

- The purpose of **QI** is to improve practices and processes within a specific organization—not to generate new knowledge that can be generalized. QI does not typically involve translating "best evidence" into a protocol.

REFERENCES

*Brouwers, M., Kho, M., Browman, G., et al.; for the AGREE Next Steps Consortium. (2010). AGREE II: Advancing guideline development, reporting and evaluation in health care. *Canadian Medical Association Journal, 182,* E839–E842.

Canadian Nurses Association. (2010). *Evidence-informed decision-making and nursing practice [Position statement]*. Ottawa: Author.

Clarke, M., Hopewell, S., Juszczak, E., Eisinga, A., & Kjeldstrøm, M. (2006). Compression stockings for preventing deep vein thrombosis in airline passengers. *Cochrane Database of Systematic Reviews, (2)*, CD004002.

Dearholt, D., & Dang, D. (Eds.). (2012). *Johns Hopkins nursing evidence-based practice: Model and guidelines* (2nd ed.). Indianapolis, IN: Sigma Theta Tau International.

DiCenso, A., Guyatt, G., & Ciliska, D. (2005). *Evidence-based nursing: A guide to clinical practice*. St. Louis, MO: Elsevier Mosby.

Fisher, A. R. (2014). Development of clinical practice guidelines for urinary continence care of adult stroke survivors in acute and rehabilitation settings. *Canadian Journal of Neuroscience Nursing, 36*(3), 16–31.

Fabbruzzo-Cota C., Frecea M., Kozell K., et al. (2016). A Clinical Nurse Specialist-Led Interprofessional Quality Improvement Project to Reduce Hospital-Acquired Pressure Ulcers. *Clinical Nurse Specialist, 30*(2), 110–116.v

Gawlinski, A., & Rutledge, D. (2008). Selecting a model for evidence-based practice changes. *AACN Advanced Critical Care, 19*, 291–300.

Glasziou, P. (2005). Evidence-based medicine: Does it make a difference? Make it evidence informed with a little wisdom. *British Medical Journal, 330*(7482), 92.

Health Council of Canada. (2003). Which way to quality? Key perspectives on quality improvement in Canadian health care systems. Retrieved from http://accreditation.ca/sites/default/files/qireport_eng_fa.pdf

Horsley, J. A., Crane, J., & Bingle, J. D. (1978). Research utilization as an organizational process. *Journal of Nursing Administration, 8*, 4–6.

Hsieh, H. F., & Lee, F. P. (2005). Graduated compression stockings as prophylaxis for flight-related venous thrombosis: Systematic literature review. *Journal of Advanced Nursing, 51*, 83–98.

Johnston, C., Campbell-Yeo, M., Disher, T., et al. (2017). Skin-to-skin care for procedural pain in neonates. *Cochrane Database of Systematic Reviews, 2*, CD008435. doi: 10.1002/14651858.CD008435.pub3. Review.

**Kram, S., DiBartolo, M., Hinderer, K., & Jones, R. (2015). Implementation of the ABCDE bundle to improve patient outcomes in the intensive care unit in a rural community hospital. *Dimensions of Critical Care Nursing, 34*, 250–258.

Leung, A. K., To, M. J., Luong, L., et al. (2017). The Effect of Advance Directive Completion on Hospital Care Among Chronically Homeless Persons: a Prospective Cohort Study. *Journal of Urban Health, 94*(1), 43–53. doi: 10.1007/s11524-016-0105-2.

Lewis, S. (2001). Further disquiet on the guidelines front. *Canadian Medical Association Journal, 165*, 180–181.

Melnyk, B. M. (2014). Evidence-based practice versus evidence-informed practice: A debate that could stall forward momentum in improving healthcare quality, safety, patient outcomes, and costs. *Worldviews on Evidence-Based Nursing, 11*, 347–349.

Melnyk, B. M., & Fineout-Overholt, E. (2015). *Evidence-based practice in nursing and healthcare* (3rd ed.). Philadelphia, PA: Lippincott Williams & Wilkins.

Morse, J. (2005). Beyond the clinical trial: Expanding criteria for evidence. *Qualitative Health Research, 15*, 3–4.

O'Meara, S., Cullum, N., Nelson, E., & Dumville, J. (2012). Compression for venous ulcers. *Cochrane Database of Systematic Reviews, (1)*, CD000265.

Rogers, E. M. (1995). *Diffusion of innovations* (4th ed.). New York: Free Press.

Rycroft-Malone, J. (2010). Promoting Action on Research Implementation in Health Services (PARiHS). In J. Rycroft-Malone & T. Bucknall (Eds.), *Models and frameworks for implementing evidence-based practice: Linking evidence to action* (pp. 109–133). Malden, MA: Wiley-Blackwell.

*Rycroft-Malone, J., Seers, K., Chandler, J., et al. (2013). The role of evidence, context, and facilitation in an implementation trial: Implications for the development of the PARIHS framework. *Implementation Science, 8*, 28.

Sackett, D. L., Straus, S. E., Richardson, W. S., Rosenberg, W., & Haynes, R. B. (2000). *Evidence-based medicine: How to practice and teach EBM* (2nd ed.). Edinburgh: Churchill Livingstone.

Shirey, M., Hauck, S., Embree, J., et al. (2011). Showcasing differences between quality improvement, evidence-based practice, and research. *Journal of Continuing Education in Nursing, 42*, 57–68.

Stetler, C. B. (2010). Stetler model. In J. Rycroft-Malone & T. Bucknall (Eds.), *Models and frameworks for implementing evidence-based practice: Linking evidence to action* (pp. 51–77). Malden, MA: Wiley-Blackwell.

Tayyib, N., Coyer, F., & Lewis, P. (2015). A two-arm cluster randomized control trial to determine the effectiveness of a pressure ulcer prevention bundle for critically ill patients. *Journal of Nursing Scholarship, 47*, 237–247.

Titler, M. (2010). Iowa model of evidence-based practice. In J. Rycroft-Malone & T. Bucknall (Eds.), *Models and frameworks for implementing evidence-based practice: Linking evidence to action* (pp. 137–144). Malden, MA: Wiley-Blackwell.

Titler, M. G., Kleiber, C., Steelman, V., et al. (2001). The Iowa model of evidence-based practice to promote quality care. *Critical Care Nursing Clinics of North America, 13*, 497–509.

*A link to this open-access article is provided in the Internet Resources section on thePoint website.

**This journal article is available on thePoint for this chapter.

3

Key Concepts and Steps in Quantitative and Qualitative Research

Learning Objectives

On completing this chapter, you will be able to:

- Define new terms associated with quantitative and qualitative research
- Distinguish between experimental and non-experimental research
- Identify the three main disciplinary traditions for qualitative nursing research
- Describe the flow and sequence of activities in quantitative and qualitative research and discuss how they differ

Key Terms

- Cause-and-effect (causal) relationship
- Clinical trial
- Concept
- Conceptual definition
- Construct
- Data
- Dependent variable
- Emergent design
- Ethnography
- Experimental research
- Gaining entrée
- Grounded theory
- Hypothesis
- Independent variable
- Informant
- Intervention protocol
- Literature review
- Non-experimental research
- Observational study
- Operational definition
- Outcome variable
- Phenomenology
- Population
- Qualitative data
- Quantitative data
- Relationship
- Research design
- Sample
- Saturation
- Statistical analysis
- Study participant
- Subject
- Theme
- Theory
- Variable

THE BUILDING BLOCKS OF RESEARCH

Research, like any discipline, has its own language—its own *jargon*—and that jargon can sometimes be intimidating. We readily admit that the jargon can be confusing. Some research jargon used in nursing research has its roots in the social sciences, but sometimes different terms are used in medical research. Also, some terms are used by both quantitative and qualitative researchers, but others are used mainly by one or the other group. Please bear with us as we cover key terms that you will likely encounter in the research literature.

The Faces and Places of Research

When researchers answer a question through disciplined research, they are doing a *study* (or an *investigation*). Studies with humans involve two sets of people: those who do the research

TABLE 3.1 Key Terms in Quantitative and Qualitative Research

Concept	Quantitative Term	Qualitative Term
Person contributing information	Subject Study participant —	— Study participant Informant, key informant
Person undertaking the study	Researcher Investigator	Researcher Investigator
That which is being investigated	— Concepts Constructs Variables	Phenomena Concepts — —
Information gathered	Data (numerical values)	Data (narrative descriptions)
Connections between concepts	Relationships (cause-and-effect, associative)	Patterns of association
Logical reasoning processes	Deductive reasoning	Inductive reasoning

and those who provide the information. In a quantitative study, the people being studied are called **subjects** or **study participants**, as shown in Table 3.1. In a qualitative study, the people cooperating in the study are called study participants or **informants**. The person who conducts the research is the *researcher* or *investigator*. Studies are often undertaken by a research team rather than by a single researcher.

HOW-TO-TELL TIP How can you tell if an article appearing in a nursing journal is a *study*? In journals that specialize in research (e.g., *Canadian Journal of Nursing Research*), most articles are original research reports, but in specialty journals, there is usually a mix of research and non-research articles. Sometimes you can tell by the title, but sometimes you cannot. You can tell, however, by looking at the major headings of an article. If there is no heading called "Method" or "Research Design" (the section that describes what a researcher *did*) and no heading called "Findings" or "Results" (the section that describes what a researcher *learned*), then it is probably not a study.

Research can be undertaken in a variety of *settings* (the types of place where information is gathered), like in hospitals, homes, or other community settings. A *site* is the specific location for the research—it could be an entire community (e.g., a Haitian neighbourhood in Montreal) or an institution (e.g., a clinic in Vancouver). Researchers sometimes do *multisite studies* because the use of multiple sites offers a larger and often more diverse group of participants.

Concepts, Constructs, and Theories

Research involves real-world problems, but studies tend to concentrate on ideas in abstract terms. For example, *pain, fatigue,* and *obesity* are abstractions of human characteristics. These abstractions are called *phenomena* (especially in qualitative studies) or **concepts**.

Researchers sometimes use the term **construct**, which also refers to an abstraction, but often one that is deliberately invented (or constructed). For example, *self-care* in Orem's model of health maintenance is a construct. The terms *construct* and *concept* are sometimes used interchangeably, but a construct often refers to a more complex abstraction than a concept.

A **theory** is an explanation of some aspect of reality. In a theory, concepts are linked together by intricate relationships to describe or explain some aspect of the world. Theories play a role in both quantitative and qualitative research. In a quantitative study, researchers often start with a hypothesis and, using deductive reasoning, make predictions about how phenomena would behave in the real world *if the hypothesis were true.* The specific predictions are then tested. In qualitative studies, theory often is the *product* of the research: The investigators use information from study participants inductively to develop a theory rooted in the participants' experiences.

 TIP The reasoning process of *deduction* is associated with quantitative research, and *induction* is associated with qualitative research. The supplement for Chapter 3 on thePoint website explains and illustrates the distinction.

Variables

In quantitative studies, concepts are usually called **variables**. A variable, as the name implies, is something that varies. Weight, anxiety, and fatigue are all variables—they vary from one person to another, and from time to time. Most human characteristics are variables. If everyone weighed 150 pounds, weight would not be a variable; it would be a *constant*. But it is precisely because people and conditions *do* vary that most research is conducted. Quantitative researchers seek to understand how or why things vary and to learn how changes in one variable relate to changes in another. For example, in lung cancer research, lung cancer is a variable because not everybody has this disease. Researchers have studied factors that might be linked to lung cancer, such as cigarette smoking. Smoking is also a variable because not everyone smokes. A variable, then, is any quality of a person, group, or situation that varies or takes on different values. Variables are the central building blocks of quantitative studies.

 TIP Every study focuses on one or more phenomena, concepts, or variables, but these terms per se are not necessarily used in research reports. For example, a report might say, "The purpose of this study is to examine the effect of nurses' workload on hand hygiene adherence." Although the researcher did not explicitly label anything a variable, the variables under study are *workload* and *hand hygiene adherence*. Key concepts or variables are often indicated in the study title.

Characteristics of Variables

Variables are often inherent human characteristics, such as age or weight, but sometimes researchers *create* a variable. For example, if a researcher tests the effectiveness of patient-controlled analgesia compared to intramuscular analgesia in relieving pain after surgery, some patients would be given one type of analgesia, and some would receive the other. In the context of this study, method of pain management is a variable because different patients receive analgesic by different methods.

Some variables take on a wide range of values that can be represented on a continuum (e.g., a person's age or weight). Other variables take on only a few values; sometimes such variables convey quantitative information (e.g., number of children), but others simply involve placing people into categories (e.g., male, female; or blood type A, B, AB, or O).

Dependent and Independent Variables

As noted in Chapter 1, many studies seek to understand causes of phenomena. Does a nursing intervention *cause* improvements in patient outcomes? Does smoking *cause* lung cancer? The presumed cause is the **independent variable**, and the presumed effect is the **dependent** or **outcome variable**. In other words, the independent variable affects how the dependent variable will behave. The dependent variable is the outcome that researchers want to understand, explain, or predict. In terms of the PICOT (scheme discussed in Chapter 2), patient population or setting corresponds to the "P," the dependent variable corresponds to the "O" (outcome). The independent variable corresponds to the "I" (the intervention, influence, indication, or exposure), plus the "C" (the comparison) and the T (time frame).

 TIP   In searching for evidence, a nurse might want to learn about the effects of an intervention or influence (I), compared to *any* alternative, on a designated outcome. In a cause-probing study, however, researchers always specify what the comparative intervention or influence (the "C") is at the beginning of a study.

The terms *independent variable* and *dependent variable* also can be used to indicate *direction of influence* rather than cause and effect. For example, suppose we compared levels of depression among men and women diagnosed with pancreatic cancer and found men to be more depressed. We could not conclude that depression was *caused* by gender. Yet there is a relationship between gender and depression: It makes no sense to suggest that patient's depression influenced their gender. In this situation, it is appropriate to consider depression as the outcome variable and gender as the independent variable.

 TIP   Few research reports explicitly label variables as dependent and independent. Moreover, variables (especially independent variables) are sometimes not fully spelled out. Take the following research question: What is the effect of exercise on heart rate? In this example, heart rate is the dependent variable. Exercise, however, is not in itself a variable. Rather, exercise versus something else (e.g., no exercise) is a variable; "something else" is implied rather than stated in the research question.

Many outcomes have multiple causes or influences. If we were studying factors that influence people's body mass index, the independent variables might be height, physical activity, and diet. And, two or more outcome variables may be of interest. For example, a researcher may compare two alternative dietary interventions in terms of participants' weight, lipid profile, and self-esteem. It is common to design studies with multiple independent and dependent variables.

Variables are not *inherently* dependent or independent. A dependent variable in one study could be an independent variable in another. For example, a study might examine the effect of an exercise intervention (the independent variable) on osteoporosis (the dependent variable) to answer a therapy question. Another study might investigate the effect of osteoporosis (the independent variable) on bone fracture incidence (the dependent variable) to address a prognosis question. In short, whether a variable is independent or dependent is determined by how the research question is structured.

Example of independent and dependent variables • • • • • • • • • • • • • • • •
Research question (Aetiology/Harm question): Among older people with dementia, is delirium associated with accelerated cognitive decline? (Davis et al., 2017).
Independent variable: delirium
Dependent variables: cognitive functioning

Conceptual and Operational Definitions

The concepts of interest to researchers are abstractions, and they are defined by researchers' worldviews. A **conceptual definition** is the theoretical meaning of a concept. Researchers need to conceptually define even seemingly straightforward terms. A classic example is the concept of *caring.* Morse et al. (1990) examined how researchers and theorists defined *caring* and identified five categories of conceptual definitions: as a human trait, a moral imperative, an affect, an interpersonal relationship, and a therapeutic intervention. Researchers undertaking studies of caring need to clarify what aspects of caring are examined.

In qualitative studies, conceptual definitions of key phenomena may be a major end product that comes from those being studied. In quantitative studies, however, researchers must define concepts at the outset because they must decide how the variables will be measured. An **operational definition** indicates what the researchers specifically must do to measure the concept and collect needed information.

Readers of research articles may not agree with how researchers conceptualized and operationalized variables. However, clarity and precision of the definition are important in communicating what concepts mean within the context of the study.

Example of conceptual and operational definitions · · · · · · · · · · · · · · · ·

Oliffe et al. (2015) studied the relation between social stigma, depression, and suicidal ideation among men in British Columbia. The researchers defined stigma conceptually as "negative stereotypes that individuals and communities in a society hold about and/ or invoke on persons experiencing mental illness" (p. 303). They defined stigma operationally by a set of nine statements on the Depression Stigma Scale. Participants were asked to indicate how people view depression (e.g., most people believe that people with depression could snap out of it if they wanted). Participants were asked to respond on a scale from 0 (strongly disagree) to 4 (strongly agree).

Data

Research **data** (singular, datum) are the pieces of information gathered in a study. In quantitative studies, researchers identify and define their variables and then collect relevant data from study participants. The actual *values* of the study variables constitute the data. Quantitative researchers collect primarily **quantitative data**—information in numeric form. For example, if we conducted a quantitative study in which a key variable was *depression*, we would need to measure the severity of depression experienced by participants. We might ask, "Thinking about the past week, how depressed would you say you have been on a scale from 0 to 10, where 0 means 'not at all' and 10 means 'the most possible'?" Box 3.1 presents quantitative data for three fictitious people. The subjects provided a number along the 0 to 10 continuum corresponding to their degree of depression—9 for subject 1 (a high level of depression), 0 for subject 2 (no depression), and 4 for subject 3 (little depression).

In qualitative studies, researchers collect primarily **qualitative data**, that is, narrative descriptions. Narrative data can be obtained by talking to participants, by making notes about their behaviour in naturalistic settings, or by obtaining narrative records, such as diaries. Suppose we were studying depression qualitatively. Box 3.2 presents qualitative data for three participants responding conversationally to the question "Tell me about how you've

---

Box 3.1 Example of Quantitative Data

Question:	Thinking about the past week, how depressed would you say you have been on a scale from 0 to 10, where 0 means "not at all" and 10 means "the most possible"?
Data:	9 (Subject 1)
	0 (Subject 2)
	4 (Subject 3)

Box 3.2 Example of Qualitative Data

Question: Tell me about how you've been feeling lately—have you felt sad or depressed at all, or have you generally been in good spirits?

Data: "Well, actually, I've been pretty depressed lately, to tell you the truth. I wake up each morning and I can't seem to think of anything to look forward to. I mope around the house all day, kind of in despair. I just can't seem to shake the blues and I've begun to think I need to go see a shrink." (Participant 1)

"I can't remember ever feeling better in my life. I just got promoted to a new job that makes me feel like I can really get ahead in my company. And I've just gotten engaged to a really great guy who is very special." (Participant 2)

"I've had a few ups and downs the past week but basically things are on a pretty even keel. I don't have too many complaints." (Participant 3)

---

been feeling lately—have you felt sad or depressed at all, or have you generally been in good spirits?" Here, the data consist of rich narrative descriptions of participants' emotional state. In reports on qualitative studies, researchers include excerpts from their narrative data to support or illustrate their interpretations.

Relationships

Researchers usually study phenomena in relation to other phenomena—they examine relationships. A **relationship** is a connection between phenomena or variables; for example, researchers repeatedly have found that there is a *relationship* between frequency of turning bedridden patients and the incidence of pressure ulcers. Quantitative and qualitative studies examine relationships in different ways.

In quantitative studies, researchers are interested in the relationship between independent variables and outcomes. Relationships are often expressed in quantitative terms, such as *more than* or *less than*. For example, consider a person's weight as our outcome variable. What variables are related to (associated with) a person's weight? Some possibilities include height, caloric intake, and exercise. For each independent variable, we can make a prediction about its relationship to the outcome:

Height: Tall people will weigh more than short people.
Caloric intake: People with high caloric intake will be heavier than those with low caloric intake.
Exercise: The lower the amount of exercise, the greater will be the person's weight.

Each statement expresses a predicted relationship between weight (the outcome) and a measurable independent variable (predictor). Most quantitative research is conducted to assess whether relationships exist among variables and to measure how strong the relationship is.

 TIP Relationships are expressed in two basic forms. First, relationships can be expressed as "if more of Variable X, then more of (or less of) Variable Y." For example, there is a relationship between height and weight: With greater height, there tends to be greater weight, that is, tall people tend to weigh more than short people. The second form involves relationships expressed as group differences. For example, there is a relationship between gender and height: Men tend to be taller than women.

Variables can be related to one another in different ways, including **cause-and-effect (or causal) relationships**. Within the positivist paradigm, natural phenomena are assumed to have antecedent causes that are discoverable. For example, we might speculate that there is a causal relationship between caloric intake and weight: All else being equal, eating more calories causes greater weight. As noted in Chapter 1, many quantitative studies are *cause-probing*—they seek to understand the causes of phenomena.

Example of a study of causal relationships

Woo (2015) studied whether anticipation of pain and anxiety would intensify pain at dressing change among patients with chronic wounds. The results from this study indicate high anxiety and anticipatory pain can increase pain at dressing change.

Not all relationships can be explained by cause and effect. There is a relationship, for example, between a person's pulmonary artery and tympanic temperatures: People with high readings on one tend to have high readings on the other. We cannot say, however, that pulmonary artery temperature *caused* tympanic temperature, or vice versa. This type of relationship is sometimes referred to as an *associative* (or *functional*) *relationship* rather than a causal one.

Example of a study of associative relationships

Karunanayake (2016) studied risk factors of ear infections in First Nations and rural school-aged children between 6 and 17 years old in the province of Saskatchewan.

Ear infection was associated with younger age; firstborn in the family; and history of tonsillitis, asthma, and any respiratory related allergy.

Qualitative researchers are not concerned with quantifying relationships or in testing and confirming causal relationships. Rather, qualitative researchers may seek patterns of association as a way of illuminating the underlying meaning and dimensionality of phenomena of interest. Patterns of interconnected concepts are identified as a means of understanding the whole.

Example of a qualitative study of patterns

Dhaliwal and colleagues (2017) studied the impact of financial barriers on patients' ability to follow recommendations for the prevention of coronary artery disease. Financial barriers prevent people from accessing: medications, cardiac rehabilitation and exercise, psychological support, transportation, and parking.

MAJOR CLASSES OF QUANTITATIVE AND QUALITATIVE RESEARCH

Researchers usually work within a paradigm that is consistent with their world view and that gives rise to the types of question that excite their curiosity. In this section, we briefly describe broad categories of quantitative and qualitative research.

Quantitative Research: Experimental and Non-experimental Studies

A basic distinction in quantitative studies is between experimental and non-experimental research. In **experimental research**, researchers actively introduce an intervention or treatment—most often, to address therapy questions. In **non-experimental research**, on the other hand, researchers are bystanders or observers—they collect data without actively introducing treatments (most often, to address aetiology, prognosis, or diagnosis questions). For example, if a researcher gave bran flakes to one group of subjects and prune juice to another to evaluate which method facilitated elimination more effectively, the study would be experimental because the researcher intervened. If, on the other hand, a researcher compared elimination patterns of two groups whose regular eating patterns differed, the study would be non-experimental because there is no intervention. In medical and epidemiologic research, experimental studies usually are called **clinical trials**, and non-experimental inquiries are called **observational studies**.

Experimental studies are explicitly designed to test causal relationships—to test whether an intervention *caused* changes in the outcome. Sometimes non-experimental studies also explore causal relationships, but causal inferences in non-experimental research are tricky and less conclusive, for reasons we explain in a later chapter.

Example of experimental research ●
Schindel Martin et al. (2017) described their experimental study testing the impact of an education programme on staff self-efficacy to provide dementia care in an acute care hospital. There was a significant improvement in self-efficacy among nurses in the intervention group who received the education; no significant change was observed among nurses who did not receive the education.

In this example, the researchers intervened by delivering the intervention to eon group of nurses and no special intervention to other group. In other words, the researcher *controlled* the independent variable, which in this case was the education intervention.

Example of non-experimental research ●
Mann et al. (2017) compared high and low clinic and emergency room (ER) use among patients with chronic pain. High ER users reported lower pain, self-efficacy, and more comorbidities.

In this non-experimental study to address a prognosis question, the researchers did not intervene in any way. They were interested in a similar population as in the previous example (patients with chronic pain), but their intent was to explore relationships among existing conditions rather than to test a potential solution to a problem.

Qualitative Research: Disciplinary Traditions

Many qualitative nursing studies are rooted in research traditions that originated in anthropology, sociology, and psychology. Three such traditions are briefly described here. Chapter 10 provides a fuller discussion of these and other traditions and the methods associated with them.

The **grounded theory** tradition seeks to describe and understand key social psychological processes. Grounded theory was developed in the 1960s by two sociologists, Glaser and Strauss (1967). The focus of most grounded theory studies is on the social and psychological experiences that characterize a particular event or episode. A major component of grounded theory is the discovery of a *core variable* (the main concern) to explain what is going on in that social scene. Grounded theory researchers strive to generate explanations of phenomena that are grounded in reality.

Example of a grounded theory study •
Sinclair et al. (2016) used grounded theory methods to understand the meaning of sympathy, empathy, and compassion among hospitalized patients with advanced cancer in Calgary. Empathy as a core variable was described as an affective response to individual's suffering whereas sympathy was perceived as an unwanted, pity-based response to a distress.

Phenomenology is concerned with people's lived experiences. Phenomenology is an approach to thinking about what life experiences of people are like and what they mean. The phenomenologic researcher asks the questions: What is the *essence* of this phenomenon as experienced by these people? or What is the meaning of the phenomenon to those who experience it?

Example of a phenomenologic study •
McWilliams et al. (2016) used an interpretive phenomenologic approach in their study of the experiences of women seeking care at the emergency department while having a miscarriage. Five themes emerged from the lived experiences of eight women: "Pregnant/Life: Miscarriage/Death"; "Deciding to go to the emergency department: Something's wrong"; "Not an illness: A different kind of trauma"; "Need for acknowledgement"; and "Leaving the emergency department: What now?"

Ethnography, the primary research tradition in anthropology, provides a framework for studying the patterns and lifeways of a defined cultural group in a holistic fashion. Ethnographers typically engage in extensive *fieldwork*, often participating in the life of the culture under study. Ethnographers strive to learn from members of a cultural group, to understand their world view, and to describe their customs and norms.

Example of an ethnographic study •
Sandvoll et al. (2015) used ethnographic methods to explore how nursing home staff members managed unpleasant resident behaviours in two public nursing homes in Norway.

MAJOR STEPS IN A QUANTITATIVE STUDY

In quantitative studies, researchers move from the beginning point of a study (asking a question) to the end point (obtaining an answer) in a reasonably linear sequence of steps that is broadly similar across studies (Fig. 3.1). This section describes that flow, and the next section describes how qualitative studies differ.

Phase 1: The Conceptual Phase

The early steps in a quantitative study typically involve activities with a strong conceptual element. During this phase, researchers call on such skills as creativity, deductive reasoning, and a grounding in research evidence on the topic of interest.

Step 1: Formulating and Delimiting the Problem

Quantitative researchers begin by identifying an interesting research problem and formulating *research questions*. The research questions identify what the study variables are. In developing questions, nurse researchers must attend to substantive issues (Is this problem important?), theoretical issues (Is there a conceptual framework for this problem?), clinical

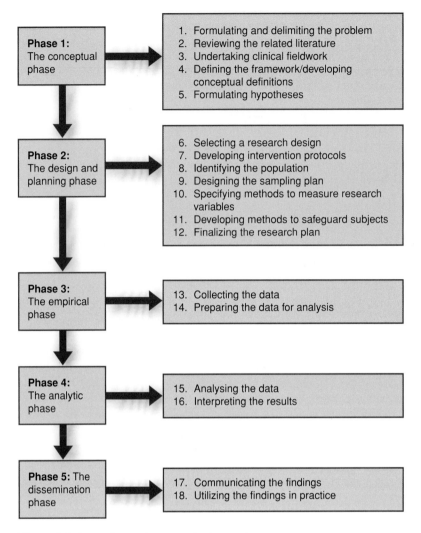

Figure 3.1 Flow of steps in a quantitative study.

issues (Will findings be useful in clinical practice?), methodologic issues (How can this question be answered to yield high-quality evidence?), and ethical issues (Can this question be addressed in an ethical manner?).

Step 2: Reviewing the Related Literature

Quantitative research is guided by previous knowledge. Quantitative researchers typically strive to understand what is already known about a topic by undertaking a thorough **literature review** before any data are collected.

Step 3: Undertaking Clinical Fieldwork

Researchers embarking on a clinical study often benefit from spending time in relevant clinical settings (in the *field*), discussing the topic with clinicians (knowledge users) and observing current practices. Such clinical fieldwork allows the researcher to understand the issue from clinicians' and clients' viewpoints.

Step 4: Defining the Framework and Developing Conceptual Definitions

When quantitative research is performed within the context of a theoretical framework, the findings may have broader significance and utility. Even when the research question is not embedded in a theory, researchers should have a conceptual rationale and a clear vision of the concepts under study.

Step 5: Formulating Hypotheses

Hypotheses state researchers' expectations about specific relationships between study variables. Hypotheses are predictions of the relationships researchers expect to observe in the study data. The research question identifies the concepts of interest and asks how the concepts might be related; a hypothesis is the predicted answer. Most quantitative studies are designed to test hypotheses through statistical analysis.

Phase 2: The Design and Planning Phase

In the second major phase of a quantitative study, researchers decide on the methods they will use to address the research question. Researchers make many methodologic decisions that have crucial implications for the quality of the study evidence.

Step 6: Selecting a Research Design

The **research design** is the overall plan for obtaining answers to the research questions. Quantitative designs tend to be well structured and controlled, with the goal of minimizing bias. Research designs also indicate how often data will be collected and what types of comparisons will be made. The research design is like a recipe that outline the steps involved in the study.

Step 7: Developing Protocols for the Intervention

In experimental research, researchers create the independent variable, which means that participants are exposed to different treatments. An **intervention protocol** for the study must be developed, specifying exactly what the intervention will entail (e.g., who will administer it, over how long a period the treatment will last, and so on) *and* what the alternative condition will be. This step is not necessary in non-experimental research.

Step 8: Identifying the Population

Quantitative researchers need to specify the characteristics of study participants—that is, they must identify the population to be studied. A **population** is *all* the individuals or objects with common, defining characteristics (the "P" component in PICO questions).

Step 9: Designing the Sampling Plan

Researchers typically collect data from a **sample**, which is a subset of the population. The researcher's *sampling plan* specifies how the sample will be selected and how many subjects will be included. The risk is that the sample might not adequately reflect the population's traits.

Step 10: Specifying Methods to Measure Variables

Quantitative researchers must find methods to measure the research variables accurately. A variety of quantitative data collection approaches exist; the primary methods are *self-reports* (e.g., interviews and questionnaires), *observations* (e.g., watching and recording people's behaviour), and *biophysiologic measurements*. The task of measuring research variables and developing a *data collection plan* is complex and challenging.

Step 11: Developing Methods to Safeguard Human/Animal Rights

Most nursing research involves human subjects, although some involve animals. In either case, procedures need to be developed to ensure that the study adheres to ethical principles.

Step 12: Reviewing and Finalizing the Research Plan

Before collecting data, researchers often undertake assessments to ensure that procedures will work smoothly. For example, they may evaluate the *readability* of written materials to see if participants with low reading skills can comprehend them. Researchers usually have their research plan critiqued by reviewers to obtain clinical or methodologic feedback. Researchers seeking financial support submit a *proposal* to a funding source, and reviewers usually suggest improvements.

Phase 3: The Empirical Phase

The third phase of quantitative studies involves collecting the research data. This phase is often the most time-consuming part of the study. Data collection may require months of work.

Step 13: Collecting the Data

The actual collection of data in a quantitative study often proceeds according to a pre-established plan. The plan typically spells out procedures for training data collection staff, for actually collecting data (e.g., where and when the data will be gathered), and for recording information.

Step 14: Preparing the Data for Analysis

Data collected in a quantitative study must be prepared for analysis. For example, one preliminary step is *coding*, which involves translating verbal data into numeric form (e.g., coding gender information as "1" for females and "2" for males).

Phase 4: The Analytic Phase

Quantitative data must be subjected to analysis and interpretation, which occur in the fourth major phase of a project.

Step 15: Analyzing the Data

To answer research questions and test hypotheses, researchers analyze their data in a systematic fashion. Quantitative data are analyzed through **statistical analyses**, which include some simple procedures (e.g., computing an average) as well as more complex, sophisticated methods.

Step 16: Interpreting the Results

Interpretation involves making sense of study results and examining their implications. Researchers attempt to explain the findings in light of prior evidence, theory, and clinical experience and in light of the limitations and potential error of the methods they used in the study. Interpretation also involves coming to conclusions about the *clinical significance* of the new evidence.

Phase 5: The Dissemination Phase

In the analytic phase, researchers come full circle: The questions posed at the outset are answered. The researchers' job is not completed, however, until study results are disseminated.

Step 17: Communicating the Findings

A study cannot contribute evidence to nursing practice if the results are not communicated. Another—and often final—task of a research project is the preparation of a *research report* that can be shared with others. We discuss research reports in the next chapter.

Step 18: Putting the Evidence into Practice

Ideally, the concluding step of a high-quality study is to plan for its use in practice settings. Although nurse researchers may not implement a plan for using research findings, they can contribute to the process by developing recommendations on how the evidence could be used in practice, by ensuring that adequate information has been provided for a meta-analysis, and by pursuing opportunities to disseminate the findings to practicing nurses (e.g., conference presentations, publications).

ACTIVITIES IN A QUALITATIVE STUDY

Quantitative research involves a fairly linear progression of tasks—researchers plan what steps to take and then follow those steps. In qualitative studies, by contrast, the progression is closer to a circle than to a straight line. Qualitative researchers continually examine and interpret data and make decisions about how to proceed based on what has been discovered (Fig. 3.2).

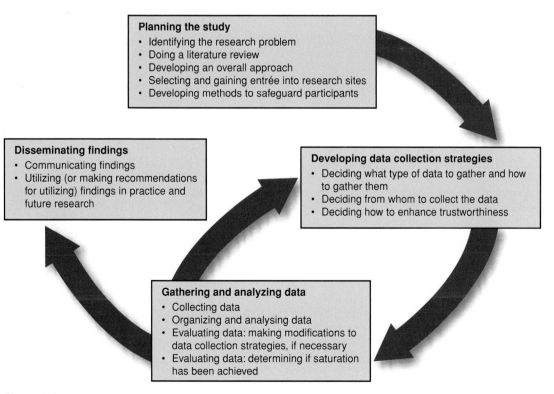

Figure 3.2 Flow of activities in a qualitative study.

Because qualitative researchers have a flexible approach, we cannot show the flow of activities precisely—the flow varies from one study to another, and researchers themselves may not know in advance how the study will unfold. We provide a general sense of qualitative studies by describing major activities and indicating when they might be performed.

Conceptualizing and Planning a Qualitative Study

Identifying the Research Problem

Qualitative researchers usually begin with a broad topic, often focusing on an aspect about which little is known. Qualitative researchers often proceed with a fairly broad initial question that allows the focus to be sharpened and delineated more clearly once the study is underway.

Doing a Literature Review

Some qualitative researchers avoid consulting the literature before collecting data. They worry that prior studies might influence the conceptualization of the phenomenon under study, which they believe should be based on participants' viewpoints rather than on prior findings. Others believe that researchers should conduct at least a brief literature review at the outset. In any case, qualitative researchers typically find a relatively small body of relevant work because of the type of questions they ask.

Selecting and Gaining Entrée into Research Sites

Before going into the field, qualitative researchers must identify an appropriate site. For example, if the topic is the health beliefs of the urban poor, an inner-city neighbourhood with a concentration of low-income residents must be identified. In some cases, researchers may have access to the selected site, but in others, they need to **gain entrée** into it. Gaining entrée typically involves negotiations with *gatekeepers* (e.g., administrators, programme directors, president of an organization) who have the authority to permit entry into their world.

 TIP The process of gaining entrée is usually associated with doing fieldwork in qualitative studies, but quantitative researchers often need to gain entrée into sites for collecting data as well.

Developing an Overall Approach

Quantitative researchers do not collect data before finalizing their research design. Qualitative researchers, by contrast, use an **emergent design** that develops and evolves during data collection. Certain design features are guided by the study's qualitative tradition, but qualitative studies rarely have rigid designs that prohibit changes while in the field.

Addressing Ethical Issues

Qualitative researchers must also develop plans for addressing ethical issues—and, indeed, there are special concerns in qualitative studies because of the more intimate nature of the relationship that typically develops between researchers and participants.

Conducting a Qualitative Study

In qualitative studies, the tasks of sampling, data collection, data analysis, and interpretation typically take place on a cyclic and repetitive basis. Qualitative researchers begin by talking with people who have the first-hand experience of the phenomenon under study. The discussions and observations are loosely structured, allowing participants to express a full range of beliefs, feelings, and behaviours. Analysis and interpretation are ongoing activities that guide choices about "next steps."

The process of data analysis involves putting together related narrative information into a coherent picture. Through inductive reasoning, researchers identify **themes** and categories, which are used to build a rich description or theory of the phenomenon. Data gathering becomes increasingly purposeful: As conceptualizations develop, researchers seek participants to confirm and enrich theoretical understandings or challenge them.

Quantitative researchers decide in advance how many subjects to include in the study, but qualitative researchers' sampling decisions are guided by the data. Many qualitative researchers use the principle of **saturation**, which occurs when the same themes and categories are recurring, such that no new information can be gleaned by further data collection.

Quantitative researchers seek to collect high-quality data by measuring their variables with standardized instruments that have been demonstrated to be accurate and valid. Qualitative researchers, by contrast, *are* the main data collection instrument and must take steps to demonstrate the *trustworthiness* of the data. The central feature of these efforts is to ensure that the findings accurately reflect the participants' viewpoints rather than researchers' perceptions. One confirmatory activity, for example, involves going back to participants, sharing preliminary interpretations with them, and asking them to evaluate whether the researcher's thematic analysis is consistent with their experiences.

Qualitative nursing researchers also strive to share their findings at conferences and in journal articles. Qualitative studies help to shape nurses' perceptions of a problem, their conceptualizations of potential solutions, and their understanding of patients' concerns and experiences.

 TIP An emerging trend is for researchers to design *mixed-methods (MM) studies* that involve the collection, analysis, and integration of quantitative and qualitative data. *MM research* is discussed in Chapter 13.

GENERAL QUESTIONS IN REVIEWING A STUDY

Box 3.3 presents some further suggestions for performing a preliminary overview of a research report, drawing on concepts explained in this chapter. These guidelines supplement those presented in Box 1.1 (Chapter 1).

Box 3.3 Additional Questions for a Preliminary Review of a Study

1. What was the study all about? What were the main phenomena, concepts, or constructs under investigation?
2. If the study was quantitative, what were the independent and dependent variables?
3. Did the researcher examine relationships or patterns of association among variables or concepts? Did the report imply the possibility of a causal relationship?
4. Were key concepts defined, both conceptually and operationally?
5. What type of study does it appear to be, in terms of types described in this chapter—experimental or non-experimental/observational? Grounded theory, phenomenologic, or ethnographic?
6. Did the report provide information to suggest how long the study took to complete?

RESEARCH EXAMPLES WITH CRITICAL THINKING EXERCISES

In this section, we illustrate the progression of activities and discuss the time schedule of a study conducted by an author of this book. Read the research summary and then answer the critical thinking questions that follow, referring to the full research report if necessary. This example is featured in our interactive *Critical Thinking Activity* on thePoint website. The critical thinking questions for Examples 2 and 3 are based on the studies that appear in their entirety in Appendices A and B of this book. Our comments for these exercises are in the Student Resources section on thePoint.

EXAMPLE 1: PROJECT SCHEDULE FOR A QUANTITATIVE STUDY

Study: Postpartum depressive symptomatology: Results from a two-stage US national survey (Beck et al., 2011).

Study Purpose: Beck et al. (2011) undertook a study to estimate the prevalence of mothers with elevated postpartum depressive (PPD) symptom levels in the United States and factors associated with differences in symptom levels.

Study Methods: This study took a little less than 3 years to complete. Key activities and methodologic decisions included the following:

Phase 1. Conceptual Phase: 1 Month. Beck had been a member of the Listening to Mothers II National Advisory Council. The data for their national survey (the Childbirth Connection: Listening to Mothers II U.S. National Survey) had already been collected when Beck was approached to analyse the variables in the survey relating to PPD symptoms. The first phase took only 1 month because data collection was already completed, and Beck, a world expert on PPD, just needed to update a review of the literature.

Phase 2. Design and Planning Phase: 3 Months. The design phase entailed identifying which of the hundreds of variables on the national survey the researchers would focus on in their analysis. Also, their research questions were formalized during this phase. Approval from a human subjects committee also was obtained during this phase.

Phase 3. Empirical Phase: 0 Months. In this study, the data from nearly 1,000 postpartum women had already been collected.

Phase 4. Analytic Phase: 12 Months. Statistical analyses were performed to (1) estimate the percentage of new mothers experiencing elevated PPD symptom levels and (2) identify which demographic, antepartum, intrapartum, and postpartum variables were significantly related to elevated symptom levels.

Phase 5. Dissemination Phase: 18 Months. The researchers prepared and submitted their report to the *Journal of Midwifery & Women's Health* for possible publication. It was accepted within 5 months and was "in press" (awaiting publication) another 4 months before being published. The article received the *Journal of Midwifery & Women's Health* 2012 Best Research Article Award.

Critical Thinking Exercises

1. Answer the relevant questions from Box 3.3 regarding this study.
2. Also consider the following targeted questions:
   a. Would you describe the method of data collection as *self-report* or *observation*?
   b. How would you evaluate Beck and colleagues' dissemination plan?
   c. Do you think an appropriate amount of time was allocated to the various phases and steps in this study?
   d. Would it have been appropriate for the researchers to address the research question using qualitative research methods? Why or why not?
3. If the results of this study are valid and generalizable, what might be some of the uses to which the findings could be put in clinical practice?

EXAMPLE 2: QUANTITATIVE RESEARCH IN APPENDIX A

- Read the abstract and introduction of Swenson and colleagues' (2016) study ("Parents' use of praise and criticism in a sample of young children seeking mental health services") in Appendix A of this book.

Critical Thinking Exercises

1. Answer the relevant questions in Box 3.3.
2. Also consider the following targeted questions:
   a. Comment on the composition of research team for this study.
   b. Did this report present any actual *data* from the study participants?
   c. Would it have been possible for the researchers to use an experimental design for this study?

EXAMPLE 3: QUALITATIVE RESEARCH IN APPENDIX B

- Read the abstract and the introduction of Beck and Watson's (2010) study ("Subsequent childbirth after a previous traumatic birth") in Appendix B of this book.

Critical Thinking Exercises

1. Answer the relevant questions in Box 3.3.
2. Also consider the following targeted questions:
   a. Find an example of actual *data* in this study. (You will need to look at the "Results" section of this study.)
   b. How long did it take Beck and Watson to collect the data for this study? (You will find this information in the "Procedure" section.)
   c. How much time elapsed between when the paper was accepted for publication and when it was actually published? (You will find relevant information at the end of the paper.)

WANT TO KNOW MORE?

A wide variety of resources to enhance your learning and understanding of this chapter are available on thePoint.

- Interactive Critical Thinking Activity
- Chapter Supplement on Deductive and Inductive Reasoning
- Answers to the Critical Thinking Exercises for Examples 2 and 3
- Internet Resources with useful websites for Chapter 3
- A Wolters Kluwer journal article on a topic related to this chapter

Summary Points

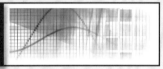

- The people who provide information to the researchers in a **study** are called **subjects** or **study participants** in quantitative research or study participants or **informants** in qualitative research; collectively, they comprise the **sample**.
- The *site* is the location for the research; researchers sometimes engage in multisite studies.
- Researchers investigate **concepts** and *phenomena* (or **constructs**), which are abstractions inferred from people's behaviour or characteristics.
- Concepts are the building blocks of **theories**, which are systematic explanations of some aspect of the real world.
- In quantitative studies, concepts are called variables. A **variable** is a characteristic or quality that takes on different values (i.e., varies from one person or object to another).
- The **dependent** (or **outcome**) **variable** is the behaviour, characteristic, or outcome the researcher is interested in explaining, predicting, or affecting (the "O" in the PICO scheme). The **independent variable** is the presumed cause of or influence on the dependent variable. The independent variable corresponds to the "I" and the "C" components in the PICO scheme.
- A **conceptual definition** describes the abstract meaning of a concept being studied. An **operational definition** specifies how the variable will be measured.
- **Data**—the information collected during the course of a study—may take the form of numeric values (**quantitative data**) or narrative information (**qualitative data**).
- A **relationship** is a connection (or pattern of association) between variables. Quantitative researchers study the relationship between independent variables and outcome variables.
- When the independent variable causes or affects the outcome, the relationship is a **cause-and-effect** (or **causal**) **relationship**. In an *associative* (or *functional*) *relationship*, variables are related in a non-causal way.
- A key distinction in quantitative studies is between **experimental research**, in which researchers actively intervene to test an intervention or therapy, and **non-experimental** (or **observational**) **research**, in which researchers collect data about existing phenomena without intervening.
- Qualitative research often is rooted in research traditions that originate in other disciplines. Three such traditions are grounded theory, phenomenology, and ethnography.
- **Grounded theory** seeks to describe and understand key social psychological processes that occur in a social setting.
- **Phenomenology** focuses on the lived experiences of humans and is an approach to gaining insight into what the life experiences of people are like and what they mean.

- **Ethnography** provides a framework for studying the meanings, patterns, and life-ways of a culture in a holistic fashion.
- In a quantitative study, researchers usually progress in a linear fashion from asking research questions to answering them. The main phases in a quantitative study are the conceptual, planning, empirical, analytic, and dissemination phases.
- The *conceptual phase* involves (1) defining the problem to be studied, (2) doing a **literature review**, (3) engaging in *clinical fieldwork* for clinical studies, (4) developing a framework and conceptual definitions, and (5) formulating **hypotheses** to be tested.
- The *planning phase* entails (6) selecting a **research design**, (7) developing **intervention protocols** if the study is experimental, (8) specifying the **population**, (9) developing a plan to select a **sample**, (10) specifying a *data collection plan* and methods to measure variables, (11) developing strategies to safeguard subjects' rights, and (12) finalizing the research plan.
- The *empirical phase* involves (13) collecting data and (14) preparing data for analysis (e.g., *coding* data).
- The *analytic phase* involves (15) performing **statistical analyses** and (16) interpreting the results.

- The *dissemination phase* entails (17) communicating the findings and (18) promoting the use of the study evidence in nursing practice.
- The flow of activities in a qualitative study is more flexible and less linear. Qualitative studies typically involve an **emergent design** that evolves during data collection.
- Qualitative researchers begin with a broad question regarding a phenomenon of interest, often focusing on a little-studied aspect. In the early phase of a qualitative study, researchers select a site and seek to **gain entrée** into it, which typically involves enlisting the cooperation of *gatekeepers* within the site.
- Once in the field, researchers select informants, collect data, and then analyze and interpret them in an iterative fashion; experiences during data collection help in an ongoing fashion to shape the design of the study.
- Early analysis in qualitative research leads to refinements in sampling and data collection, until **saturation** (redundancy of information) is achieved. Analysis typically involves a search for critical **themes** or categories.
- Both quantitative and qualitative researchers disseminate their findings, most often by publishing their research reports in professional journals.

REFERENCES

Beck, C. T., Gable, R. K., Sakala, C., & Declercq, E. R. (2011). Postpartum depressive symptomatology: Results from a two-stage U.S. national survey. *Journal of Midwifery & Women's Health, 56*, 427–435.

Davis, D. H., Muniz-Terrera, G., Keage, H. A., et al; Epidemiological Clinicopathological Studies in Europe (EClipSE) Collaborative Members. (2017). Association of delirium with cognitive decline in late life: A neuropathologic study of 3 population-based cohort studies. *JAMA Psychiatry, 74*, 244–251.

Demirel, G., & Guler, H. (2015). The effect of uterine and nipple stimulation on induction with oxytocin and the labor process. *Worldviews on Evidence-Based Nursing, 12*, 273–280.

Dhaliwal, K. K., King-Shier, K., Manns, B. J., et al. (2017). Exploring the impact of financial barriers on secondary prevention of heart disease. *BMC Cardiovascular Disorders, 17*(1), 61.

Glaser, B. G., & Strauss, A. L. (1967). The discovery of grounded theory: Strategies for qualitative research. Piscataway, NJ: Aldine.

Karunanayake, C. P., Albritton, W., Rennie, D. C., et al.; Project Research Team TF, Study Team TS. (2016). Ear infection and its associated risk factors in First Nations and rural school-aged Canadian children. *International Journal of Pediatrics*, 2016:1523897.

Keogh, B., Callaghan, P., & Higgins, A. (2015). Managing preconceived expectations: Mental health service users' experiences of going home from hospital: A grounded theory study. *Journal of Psychiatric and Mental Health Nursing, 22*, 715–723.

Lai, Y., Hung, C., Stocker, J., Chan, T., & Liu, Y. (2015). Postpartum fatigue, baby-care activities, and maternal-infant attachment of vaginal and cesarean births following rooming-in. *Applied Nursing Research*, 28, 116–120.

MacWilliams, K., Hughes, J., Aston, M., Field, S., & Moffatt, F. W. (2016). Understanding the experience of miscarriage in the emergency department. *Journal of Emergency Nursing*, 42, 504–512.

Mann, E. G., Johnson, A., Gilron, I., & VanDenKerkhof, E. G. (2017). Pain management strategies and health care use in community-dwelling individuals living with chronic pain. *Pain Medicine*. doi: 10.1093/pm/pnw341. [Epub ahead of print]

Morse, J. M., Solberg, S. M., Neander, W. L., Bottorff, J. L., & Johnson, J. L. (1990). Concepts of caring and caring as a concept. *Advances in Nursing Science*, 13, 1–14.

Oliffe, J. L, Ogrodniczuk, J. S, Gordon, S. J, et al. (2016). Stigma in male depression and suicide: A Canadian sex comparison study. *Community Mental Health Journal*, 52, 302–310.

*Sandvoll, A., Grov, E., Kristoffersen, K., & Hauge, S. (2015). When care situations evoke difficult emotions in nursing staff members: An ethnographic study in two Norwegian nursing homes. *BMC Nursing*, 14, 40.

Schindel Martin L, Gillies L, Coker E, et al. (2016). An education intervention to enhance staff self-efficacy to provide dementia care in an acute care hospital in Canada: A nonrandomized controlled study. *American Journal of Alzheimers Disease and Other Dementia*, 31, 664–677.

Shih, F. F., Chen, C., Chiao, C., Li, C., Kuo, P., & Lai, T. (2015). Comparison of pregnancy stress between in vitro fertilization/embryo transfer and spontaneous pregnancy in women during early pregnancy. *The Journal of Nursing Research*, 23, 280–289.

Sinclair, S., Beamer, K., Hack, T. F., et al. (2016). Sympathy, empathy, and compassion: A grounded theory study of palliative care patients' understandings, experiences, and preferences. *Palliative Medicine*,. doi: 026921631666349

Stoddard, S., Varela, J., & Zimmerman, M. (2015). Future expectations, attitude toward violence, and bullying perpetration during early adolescence: A mediation evaluation. *Nursing Research*, 64, 422–433.

*Tornøe, K., Danbolt, L., Kvigne, K., & Sørlie, V. (2015). The challenge of consolation: Nurses' experiences with spiritual and existential care for the dying—a phenomenological hermeneutical study. *BMC Nursing*, 14, 62.

Woo, K. Y. (2015). Unravelling nocebo effect: the mediating effect of anxiety between anticipation and pain at wound dressing change. *Journal of Clinical Nursing*, 24(13–14), 1975–1984.

*A link to this open-access article is provided in the Internet Resources section on thePoint website.

**This journal article is available on thePoint for this chapter.

4 Reading and Critiquing Research Articles

Learning Objectives

On completing this chapter, you will be able to:

- Identify and describe the major sections in a research journal article
- Characterize the style used in quantitative and qualitative research reports
- Read a research article and broadly grasp its "story"
- Describe aspects of a research critique
- Understand the many challenges researchers face and identify some tools for addressing methodologic challenges
- Define new terms in the chapter

Key Terms

- Abstract
- Bias
- Blinding
- Confounding variable
- Credibility
- Critique
- Findings
- IMRAD format

- Inference
- Journal article
- Level of significance
- *p*
- Placebo
- Randomness
- Reflexivity
- Reliability

- Research control
- Scientific merit
- Statistical significance
- Statistical test
- Transferability
- Triangulation
- Trustworthiness
- Validity

Evidence from nursing studies is communicated through research reports that describe what was studied, how it was studied, and what was found. Research reports are often daunting to readers without research training. This chapter aims to make research reports more understandable and to provide some guidance regarding critiques of research reports.

TYPES OF RESEARCH REPORTS

Nurses are most likely to encounter research evidence in journals or at professional conferences. Research **journal articles** are descriptions of studies published in professional journals. Competition for journal space is keen, so research articles are brief—generally only 10 to 20 double-spaced pages. This means that researchers must condense a lot of information about the study into a short report.

Usually, manuscripts are reviewed by two or more *peer reviewers* (other researchers) who make recommendations about acceptance or revisions to the manuscript. Reviews are usually *blind*—reviewers are not told researchers' names, and authors are not told reviewers' names. Consumers thus have some assurance that journal articles have been vetted by other impartial nurse researchers. Nevertheless, publication does not mean that the findings can be uncritically accepted. Research method courses help nurses to evaluate the quality of evidence reported in journal articles.

At conferences, research findings are presented as oral presentations or poster sessions. In an *oral presentation*, researchers are typically allotted 10 to 20 minutes to describe key features of their study to an audience. In *poster sessions*, many researchers simultaneously present visual displays summarizing their studies, and conference attendees walk around the room looking at the displays. Conferences offer an opportunity to network and dialogue: Attendees can ask questions to help them better understand what the findings mean; moreover, they can offer the researcher's suggestions relating to clinical implications of the study. Thus, professional conferences are a valuable forum for clinical audiences.

THE CONTENT OF RESEARCH JOURNAL ARTICLES

Many research articles follow an organization called the **IMRAD format**. This format organizes content into four main sections—Introduction, Method, Results, and Discussion. The paper is preceded by a title and an abstract and concludes with references.

The Title and Abstract

Research reports have a title that succinctly conveys key information. In qualitative studies, the title normally includes the central phenomenon and specific individuals under investigation. In quantitative studies, the title communicates key variables and the population (in other words, PICO components).

The **abstract** is a brief description (usually fewer than 250 words) of the study placed at the beginning of the article. The abstract answers questions like the following: What were the research questions? What methods were used to address those questions? What were the key findings? and What are the implications for nursing practice? Readers can review an abstract to judge whether to read the full report.

The Introduction

The introduction to a research article presents readers with the research problem and its context. This section usually describes the following:

- The central phenomena, issues/problems, concepts, or variables under study
- The study purpose and research questions or hypotheses
- A review of the related literature
- The theoretical or conceptual framework
- The significance of and need for the study

Thus, the introduction lets readers know the problem and appreciate the rationale behind the study.

Example of an introductory material ·
In Canada, more than 42,000 total knee arthroplasty (TKA) surgeries were performed from 2012 to 2013 (Canadian Institute for Health Information, 2014)....The purpose of joint replacement for these patients is to reduce pain and knee joint stiffness, and thereby increase mobility and function.... An individualized preoperative education approach has been used successfully to reduce symptoms in patients with cancer.

Further, systematic reviews have recommended individualization of preoperative edu-cational content. However, no studies were found that used an individualized approach to preoperative patient education for patients with TKA.... This study aimed to inves-tigate the impact of an individually delivered preoperative education intervention on pain-related interference, pain, and nausea for patients undergoing unilateral TKA (Wilson et al., 2016).

In this paragraph, the researchers described the central concept of interest (patients who had undergone TKA surgeries), the need for the study (the fact that little is known about the effectiveness of individualized approach to preoperative patient education), and the study purpose.

 TIP   The introduction section of many reports is not specifically labelled "Introduc-tion." The report's introduction immediately follows the abstract.

The Method Section

The method section describes the methods used to answer the research questions. In a quan-titative study, the method section usually describes the following, which may be presented in labelled subsections:

- The research design
- The sampling plan (setting of the study, criteria for participant recruitment)
- Methods of measuring variables and collecting data
- Study procedures, including procedures to protect human rights
- Data analysis methods

Qualitative researchers discuss many of the same issues but with different emphases. For example, a qualitative study often provides more information about the research setting and the background of the study. Reports of qualitative studies also describe the researchers' efforts to enhance the integrity of the study.

The Results Section

The results section presents the **findings** that were obtained by analysing the study data. The text presents a narrative summary of key findings, often accompanied by tables or charts to summarize detailed information. Virtually all results sections contain descriptive information, including a description of the participants (e.g., average age, percent male and female).

In quantitative studies, the results section also reports the following information relating to statistical tests performed:

- *The names of statistical tests used.* Researchers test their hypotheses and estimate the prob-ability that the results are right using **statistical tests**. For example, if the researcher finds that the average birth weight of drug-exposed infants in the sample is lower than the birth weight of infants not exposed to drugs, how probable is it that the same would be true for other infants not in the sample? A statistical test helps answer the question: Is the relationship between prenatal drug exposure and infant birth weight *real or happen by chance*, and would it likely be observed with a new sample from the same population? Statistical tests are based on common principles; you do not have to know the names of all statistical tests to comprehend the findings.
- *The value of the calculated statistic.* Computers are used to calculate a numeric value for the particular statistical test used. The value allows researchers to reach conclusions about

their hypotheses. The *actual* value of the statistic, however, is not inherently meaningful and needs not concern you.

● *Statistical significance.* A critical piece of information is whether the statistical tests were significant (not to be confused with clinically important). If a researcher reports that the results are **statistically significant**, it means the findings are probably true (not happen by chance) and replicable with a new sample. Research reports also indicate the **level of significance**, which is an index of how *probable* it is that the findings are reliable. For example, if a report indicates that a finding was significant at the .05 probability level (symbolized as *p*), this means that only 5 times out of 100 (5 ÷ 100 = .05) would the obtained result be totally different. In other words, 95 times out of 100, similar results would be obtained with a new sample. Readers can thus have a high degree of confidence—but not total assurance—that the results are accurate.

> ### Example from the results section of a quantitative study · · · · · · · · · · · · ·
> Park, Chun, and Gang (2015) tested the effects of a 16-session Patient-Centered Environment Programme (PCEP) on a variety of outcomes for home-dwelling patients with dementia. Here is a sentence adapted from the reported results: "Findings showed that agitation ($t = 2.91$, $p < .02$) and pain ($t = 4.51$, $p < .002$) improved after receiving the PCEP" (p. 40).

In this example, the researchers indicated that both agitation and pain were *significantly* improved after the PCEP intervention was introduced. The changes in agitation and pain were not likely to have been haphazard and probably would be replicated with a new sample. These findings are very reliable. For example, with regard to pain reduction, the finding would occur just as a "fluke" less than 2 times in 1,000 ($p < .002$). Note that to comprehend this finding, you do not need to understand what a *t*-statistic is, or do you need to concern yourself with the actual value of the *t* statistic, 4.51.

 TIP   Results are *more* reliable if the *p*-value is *smaller*. For example, there is a higher probability that the results are accurate when $p = .01$ (1 in 100 chance of a different result) than when $p = .05$ (5 in 100 chances of a different result). Researchers sometimes report an exact probability (e.g., $p = .03$) or a probability below conventional thresholds (e.g., $p < .05$—less than 5 in 100).

In qualitative reports, researchers often organize findings according to the major themes, processes, or categories that were identified in the data. The results section of qualitative reports sometimes has several subsections with headings correspond to labels for the themes. Excerpts from the *raw data* (the actual words of participants) are presented to support and provide a rich description of the thematic analysis. The results section of qualitative studies may also present the researcher's emerging theory about the phenomenon under study.

> ### Example from the results section of a qualitative study · · · · · · · · · · · · ·
> Shahram et al. (2017) studied the social determinants of substance use among young pregnant aboriginal women in Canada. The women expressed a need for approval and acceptance due to a lack of cultural connection and belonging when growing up. Here is an excerpt illustrating that feeling: *I struggled with like who I was, my identity because I was bounced around so much... my identity was a big one for me. I just couldn't Figure out where I belong so I just drank because I didn't really care about too much. And that had to do with like residential [school] so... the more I learnt about it and the more I go to like, with all the workshops they have going on, and hearing everybody's stories and just knowing... has helped* (p. 5).

The Discussion Section

In the discussion, the researcher presents conclusions about the meaning and implications of the findings, that is, what the results mean, why things turned out the way they did, how the findings fit with other evidence, and how the results can be used in practice. The discussion in both quantitative and qualitative reports may include the following elements:

- An interpretation of the results
- Clinical and research implications
- Study limitations and credibility of the results

Researchers must be alert to deficiencies in their own studies and present them openly. A discussion section that presents the researcher's grasp of study limitations demonstrates to readers that the authors were aware of the limitations and probably took them into account in interpreting the findings.

References

Research articles conclude with a list of the books and articles that were referenced. If you are interested in additional reading on a topic, the reference list of a recent study is a good place to begin.

THE STYLE OF RESEARCH JOURNAL ARTICLES

Research reports tell a story. However, the style in which many research journal articles are written—especially for quantitative studies—makes it difficult for some readers to understand or become interested in the story.

Why Are Research Articles So Hard to Read?

To some readers, research reports may seem confusing. Four factors should be considered:

1. *Compactness.* Journal space is limited, so authors compress a lot of information into a small space. Interesting, personalized aspects of the investigation cannot be reported, and, in qualitative studies, only a handful of supporting quotes can be included.
2. *Jargon.* The authors of research articles use research terms that may be technical.
3. *Objectivity.* Quantitative researchers tend to avoid any impression of subjectivity, so they tell their research stories in a way that makes them sound impersonal. Most quantitative research articles are written in the passive voice, which tends to make the articles less inviting and lively. Qualitative reports, by contrast, are often written in a more conversational style.
4. *Statistical information.* In quantitative reports, numbers and statistical symbols may intimidate readers who do not have statistical training.

A goal of this textbook is to assist you in understanding the content of research reports and in overcoming anxieties about jargon and statistical information.

 HOW-TO-TELL TIP How can you tell if the voice is active or passive? In the active voice, the article would say what the researchers *did* (e.g., "We used a mercury sphygmomanometer to measure blood pressure"). In the passive voice, the article indicates what *was done,* without indicating who did it, although it is implied that the researchers were the agents ("e.g., A mercury sphygmomanometer *was used* to measure blood pressure").

Tips on Reading Research Articles

As you progress through this book, you will acquire skills for evaluating research articles, but the skills involved in critical appraisal take time to develop. Here are some hints on how to get better at understanding research reports.

- Grow accustomed to the style of research articles by reading them frequently, even though you may not yet understand the technical points.
- Read journal articles slowly. It may be useful to skim the article first to get the major points and then read the article more carefully a second time.
- On the second reading, train yourself to become an *active* reader. Reading actively means that you constantly monitor yourself to verify that you understand what you are reading. If you have difficulty, you can ask someone for help. In most cases, that "someone" will be your instructor, but also consider contacting the researchers themselves.
- Keep this textbook with you as a reference when you read articles so that you can look up unfamiliar terms in the glossary or index.
- Try not to get bogged down in (or scared away by) statistical information. Try to grasp the gist of the story without letting symbols and numbers frustrate you.

CRITIQUING RESEARCH REPORTS

A critical reading of a research article involves a careful appraisal of the researcher's major conceptual and methodologic decisions. It will be difficult to criticize these decisions at this point, but your skills will improve as you progress through this book.

What Is a Research Critique?

A research **critique** is an objective assessment of a study's strengths and limitations. Critiques usually conclude with the reviewer's summary of the study's contribution, recommendations regarding the value of the evidence, and suggestions about improving the study or the report.

Research critiques of individual studies are prepared for various reasons, and they vary in scope. Peer reviewers who are asked to prepare a written critique for a journal considering publication of a manuscript may evaluate the strengths and weaknesses in terms of substantive issues (Was the research problem significant to nursing?), theoretical issues (Were the conceptual underpinnings sound?), methodologic decisions (Were the methods rigorous, yielding believable evidence?), interpretive (Did the researcher reach defensible conclusions?), ethics (Were participants' rights protected?), and style (Is the report clear, grammatical, and well organized?). In short, peer reviewers do a comprehensive review to provide feedback to the researchers and to journal editors about the merit of both the study and the report and typically offer suggestions for revisions.

Critiques designed to inform evidence-based nursing practice are seldom comprehensive. For example, it is of little consequence to evidence-based practice (EBP) that an article is ungrammatical. A critique of the clinical utility of a study focuses on whether the research method is rigorous and whether the evidence is accurate, believable, and clinically relevant.

Students taking a research methods course also may be asked to critique a study. Such critiques are often intended to cultivate critical thinking and to induce students to apply newly acquired skills in research methods.

Critiquing Support in This Textbook

We provide several types of support for research critiques. First, detailed critiquing suggestions relating to chapter content are included at the end of most chapters. Second, it is always helpful to have a good model, so we prepared critiques of two studies, one quantitative, the other qualitative. The two studies in their entirety and the critiques are in Appendices C and D.

Third, we offer a set of key critiquing guidelines for quantitative and qualitative reports in this chapter, in Tables 4.1 and 4.2, respectively. The questions in the guidelines concern

TABLE 4.1 Guide to a Focused Critique of Evidence Quality in a Quantitative Research Report

Aspect of the Report	Critiquing Questions	Detailed Critiquing Guidelines
Method Research design	• Was the most rigorous possible design used, given the purpose of the research? • Were appropriate comparisons made to enhance interpretability of the findings? • Was the number of data collection points appropriate? • Did the design minimize biases and threats to the validity of the study (e.g., was blinding used, was attrition minimized)?	Box 9.1, page 160
Population and sample	• Was the population identified and described? Was the sample described in sufficient detail? • Was the best possible sampling design used to enhance the sample's representativeness? Were sample biases minimized? • Was the sample size adequate? Was a power analysis used to estimate sample size needs?	Box 10.1, page 172
Data collection and measurement	• Were key variables operationalized using the best possible method (e.g., interviews, observations, and so on)? • Are the specific instruments adequately described, and were they good choices, given the study purpose and study population? • Did the report provide evidence that the data collection methods yielded data that were high on reliability and validity?	Box 10.2, page 183
Procedures	• If there was an intervention, was it adequately described, and was it properly implemented? Did most participants allocated to the intervention group actually receive it? • Were data collected in a manner that minimized bias? Were the staff who collected data appropriately trained?	Box 9.1, page 160
Results Data analysis	• Were appropriate statistical methods used? • Was the most powerful analytic method used? (e.g., did the analysis control for confounding variables)? • Were Type I and Type II errors avoided or minimized?	Box 14.1, page 261
Findings and interpretation	• Was information about statistical significance presented? • Was information about effect size and precision of estimates (confidence intervals) presented? • Was the clinical significance of the findings discussed?	Box 15.1, page 280
Summary assessment	• Despite limitations, do the study findings appear to be valid—do you have confidence in the *truth* value of the results? • Does the study contribute any meaningful evidence that can be used in nursing practice or that is useful to the nursing discipline?	

TABLE 4.2 **Guide to a Focused Critique of Evidence Quality in a Qualitative Research Report**

Aspect of the Report	Critiquing Questions	Detailed Critiquing Guidelines
Method Research design and research tradition	• Is the identified research tradition (if any) congruent with the methods used to collect and analyze data? • Was an adequate amount of time spent in the field or with study participants? • Was there evidence of reflexivity in the design?	Box 11.1, page 200
Sample and setting	• Was the group or population of interest adequately described? Were the setting and sample described in sufficient detail? • Was the best possible method of sampling used to enhance information richness? • Was the sample size adequate? Was saturation achieved?	Box 12.1, page 209
Data collection	• Were the methods of gathering data appropriate? Were data gathered through two or more methods to achieve triangulation? • Did the researcher ask the right questions or make the right observations? • Was there a sufficient amount of data? Were they of sufficient depth and richness?	Box 12.2, page 214
Procedures	• Do data collection and recording procedures appear appropriate? • Were data collected in a manner that minimized bias? Were the people who collected data appropriately trained?	Box 12.2, page 214
Enhancement of trustworthiness	• Did the researchers use strategies to enhance the trustworthiness/integrity of the study, and were those strategies adequate? • Do the researchers' clinical and methodologic qualifications and experience enhance confidence in the findings and their interpretation?	Box 17.1, page 315
Results Data analysis	• Was the data analysis strategy compatible with the research tradition and with the nature and type of data gathered? • Did the analysis yield an appropriate "product" (e.g., a theory, taxonomy, thematic pattern)? • Did the analytic procedures suggest the possibility of biases?	Box 16.2, page 298
Findings	• Were the findings effectively summarized, with good use of excerpts from the data and supporting arguments? • Did the themes adequately capture the meaning of the data? Does it appear that the researcher satisfactorily conceptualized the themes or patterns in the data? • Did the analysis yield an insightful, provocative, authentic, and meaningful picture of the phenomenon under investigation?	Box 16.2, page 298
Summary assessment	• Do the study findings appear to be trustworthy—do you have confidence in the *truth* value of the results? • Does the study contribute any meaningful evidence that can be used in nursing practice or that is useful to the nursing discipline?	

the rigor with which the researchers dealt with critical research challenges, some of which we outline in the next section.

 TIP For those undertaking a comprehensive critique, we offer more inclusive critiquing guidelines in the Supplement to this chapter on the Point website.

The second columns of Tables 4.1 and 4.2 list some key critiquing questions, and the third column cross-references the more detailed guidelines in the various chapters of the book. The question wording in these guidelines calls for a yes or no answer (although it may well be that the answer sometimes will be "Yes, *but…*"). In all cases, the desirable answer is *yes*; that is, a *no* suggests a possible limitation and a *yes* suggests a strength. Therefore, the more *yeses* a study gets, the stronger it is likely to be. Cumulatively, then, these guidelines can suggest a global assessment: A report with 10 *yeses* is likely to be superior to one with only two. However, these guidelines are not intended to yield a formal quality "score."

We acknowledge that our critiquing guidelines have shortcomings. In particular, they are generic even though critiquing cannot use a one-size-fits-all list of questions. Important critiquing questions that are relevant to certain studies (e.g., those that have a Therapy purpose) do not fit into a set of general questions for all quantitative studies. Thus, you need to use some judgment about whether the guidelines are sufficiently comprehensive for the type of study you are critiquing. We also note that there are questions in these guidelines for which there are no totally objective answers. Even experts sometimes disagree about methodological strategies.

 TIP Just as a careful clinician seeks research evidence that certain practices are or are not effective, you as a reader should demand the researchers use sound methodology to generate evidence.

Critiquing With Key Research Challenges in Mind

In critiquing a study, it is useful to be aware of the challenges that confront researchers. For example, they face ethical challenges (e.g., Can the study achieve its goals without infringing on human rights?), practical challenges (Will I be able to recruit enough participants?), and methodologic challenges (Will the methods I use yield results that can be trusted?). Most of this book provides guidance relating to the last question, and this section highlights key methodologic challenges. This provides an opportunity to introduce important terms and concepts that are relevant in a critique. The worth of a study's evidence for nursing practice often relies on how well researchers deal with these challenges.

Inference

Inference is an integral part of doing and critiquing research. An **inference** is a conclusion drawn from the study evidence using logical reasoning and taking into account the methods used to generate that evidence.

Inference is necessary because researchers use representatives or proxies that "stand in" for things that are fundamentally of interest. Theoretically, a sample of participants is a representative of an entire population. People who are assigned to a control group and the general population should display the same outcome if they did not receive an intervention.

Researchers face the challenge of using methods that yield good and persuasive evidence in support of inferences that they wish to make. Readers must draw their own inferences based on a critique of methodologic decisions.

Reliability, Validity, and Trustworthiness

Researchers want their inferences to correspond to the *truth*. Research cannot contribute evidence to guide clinical practice if the findings are inaccurate, biased, or fail to represent the experiences of the target group.

Quantitative researchers use several criteria to assess the quality of a study, sometimes referred to as its **scientific merit**. Two especially important criteria are reliability and validity. **Reliability** refers to the accuracy and consistency of information obtained in a study. The term is most often associated with the methods used to measure variables. For example, if a thermometer measured a patient's temperature as 371°C 1 minute and as 39.5°C the next minute, the thermometer would be unreliable.

Validity is a more complex concept that broadly concerns the *soundness* of the study's evidence. Like reliability, validity is an important criterion for evaluating methods to measure variables. In this context, the validity question is whether the methods are really measuring the concepts that they claim to measure. Is a paper-and-pencil measure of depression *really* measuring depression? Or is it measuring something else, such as loneliness or stress? Researchers strive for solid conceptual definitions of research variables and valid methods to operationalize them.

Another aspect of validity concerns the quality of evidence about the relationship between the independent variable and the dependent variable. Did a nursing intervention *really* bring about improvements in patients' outcomes—or were other factors responsible for patients' progress? Researchers make numerous methodologic decisions that can influence this type of study validity.

Qualitative researchers use different criteria and terminology in evaluating a study's integrity. In general, qualitative researchers discuss methods of enhancing the **trustworthiness** of the study's data and findings (Lincoln & Guba, 1985). Trustworthiness encompasses several different dimensions—credibility, transferability, confirmability, dependability, and authenticity—which are described in Chapter 17.

Credibility is an especially important aspect of trustworthiness. Credibility is the extent to which readers can be confident about the reported results being truthful and accurate. Credibility in a qualitative study can be enhanced in several ways, but one strategy merits early discussion because it has implications for the design of all studies, including quantitative ones. **Triangulation** is the use of multiple sources or referents to draw conclusions about what constitutes the truth. In a quantitative study, this might mean having two ways to measure an outcome, to assess whether results are similar. In a qualitative study, triangulation might involve efforts to understand the complexity of a phenomenon by using multiple data collection methods to grasp the truth (e.g., having in-depth discussions with participants, as well as watching their behaviour in natural settings). Nurse researchers are also beginning to triangulate across paradigms—that is, to integrate both quantitative and qualitative data in a single study to enhance the validity of the conclusions. We discuss such *mixed-methods* research in Chapter 13.

Example of triangulation ·
Puts et al. (2017) from University of Toronto explored how comorbidities, frailty, and functional impairment may influence the way that older people with cancer, their families, and health care providers make decisions about chemotherapy. The

researchers triangulated data from interviews and surveys with people aged ≥70 years with advanced prostate, breast, colorectal, or lung cancer, their family members, oncologists, and family physicians.

Nurse researchers need to design their studies in such a way that threats to the reliability, validity, and trustworthiness of their studies are minimized, and users of research must evaluate if they were successful.

TIP In reading and critiquing research articles, it is appropriate to have a "show me" attitude—that is, to expect researchers to build and present a solid case for the merit of their inferences. They do this by demonstrating the findings are reliable and valid or trustworthy.

Bias

Bias can threaten a study's validity and trustworthiness. A **bias** is a distortion or influence that can lead to an error in inference. Bias can be caused by various factors, including study participants' lack of honesty, researchers' preconceptions, or faulty methods of collecting data.

Some bias is random and affects only small segments of the data. As an example, a few study participants might provide inaccurate information because they were tired at the time of data collection. *Systematic bias* results when the bias is consistent or uniform. For example, if a scale consistently measured people's weight as being 2 pounds heavier than their true weight, there would be systematic bias in the data on weight. Rigorous research methods aim to eliminate or minimize bias (whether random or systematic).

Researchers adopt a variety of strategies to address bias. Triangulation is one such approach that uses multiple sources of information or points of view to identify biases. In quantitative research, research control is a common method to minimize bias.

Research Control

A central feature of most quantitative studies is that they involve efforts to control aspects of the research. **Research control** usually involves keeping the outcome variable constant so that the true relationship between the independent and outcome variables can be understood. In other words, research control attempts to eliminate contaminating factors that might cloud the relationship between the variables that are of central interest.

Contaminating factors, often called **confounding (or *extraneous*) variables**, can best be illustrated with an example. Suppose we were studying whether urinary incontinence (UI) leads to depression. Prior evidence suggests that this is the case, but previous studies have not clarified whether it is UI per se or other factors that contribute to risk of depression. The question is whether UI itself (the independent variable) contributes to higher levels of depression or whether there are other factors that can account for the relationship between UI and depression. We need to design a study to control other determinants of the outcome—determinants that are also related to the independent variable, UI.

One confounding variable here is age. Depressive symptoms tend to be more common in older people, and people with UI tend to be older than those without this problem. In other words, perhaps age is the *real* cause of depression in people with UI. The true causal relationship between UI and depression can only be clarified when age is properly controlled.

There are three possible explanations for the relationship outlined schematically as follows:

1. UI → depression
2. Age → UI → depression
3.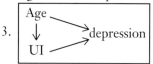

The arrows symbolize a causal mechanism or influence. In model 1, UI directly affects depression, independently of other factors. In model 2, UI is a *mediating variable*—the effect of age on depression is *mediated* by UI. According to this representation, age affects depression *through* the effect that age has on UI. In model 3, both age and UI have separate effects on depression, and age also increases the risk of UI. Some research is specifically designed to test paths of mediation and multiple causations, but in the present example, age is extraneous to the research question. We want to design a study that tests the first explanation. Age must be controlled if our goal is to explore model 1 suggesting that having UI makes a person more vulnerable to depression no matter what a person's age.

How can we impose such control? There are a number of ways, as we discuss in Chapter 9, but the general principle underlying each alternative is that the confounding variable must be *held constant*. The confounding variable must somehow be handled, so it is not related to the independent variable or the outcome. As an example, let us say we wanted to compare the average scores on a depression scale for those with and without UI. We would want to design a study in such a way that the ages of those in the UI and non-UI groups are comparable, even though, in general, the groups are not usually comparable in terms of age.

By exercising control over age, we would be taking a step towards understanding the relationship between UI and depression. The world is complex, and many variables are interrelated in complicated ways. The value of evidence in quantitative studies is often related to how well researchers control confounding influences.

Research rooted in the constructivist paradigm does not impose controls. With their emphasis on holism and individual human experience, qualitative researchers typically believe that imposing controls removes some of the meaning of reality.

Bias Reduction: Randomness and Blinding

For quantitative researchers, a powerful tool for eliminating bias involves **randomness**—having certain features of the study established by chance rather than by researcher preference. When people are selected *at random* to participate in a study, for example, each person in the initial pool has an equal chance of being selected. This, in turn, means that there are no systematic biases in the make-up of the sample. For example, men and women, the young and the old, the rich and the poor have an equal chance of being selected. Similarly, if participants are allocated *at random* to two comparison groups (e.g., a special intervention and "usual care" group), then there is no systematic biases in the groups' composition. Randomness is a compelling method of controlling confounding variables and reducing bias.

Another bias-reducing strategy is called **blinding** (or *masking*), which is used in some quantitative studies to prevent biases as a result of people's awareness. Blinding involves hiding information from participants, data collectors, or care providers to increase objectivity. For example, if study participants are aware of whether they are getting an experimental drug or a sham drug (a **placebo**), then their outcomes could be influenced by their expectations of the new drug's efficacy. Blinding involves disguising or withholding information about participants' status in the study (e.g., whether they are in a certain group) or about the study hypotheses.

Example of randomness and blinding •
Da Silva et al. (2015) studied the effect of foot reflexology on tissue integrity and impairment of the feet among people with type 2 diabetes mellitus. Their sample of 45 people with diabetes was randomly assigned to one of two groups—one group received guidelines on foot care plus 12 sessions of foot reflexology, and the other group received the guidelines only. The person who assessed foot impairment was blinded to which group the participants were in.

Qualitative researchers do not consider randomness or blinding to be necessary to understand phenomena. A researcher's judgement is viewed as an indispensable tool for uncovering the complexities of the phenomena of interest.

Reflexivity

Qualitative researchers are also interested in discovering the truth about human experience. Qualitative researchers often rely on reflexivity to limit personal bias. **Reflexivity** is the process that involves critically and careful consideration about how personal values could affect data collection and interpretation. Qualitative researchers are trained to explore these issues, to be reflective about decisions made during the study, and to record their thoughts in personal diaries and memos.

Example of reflexivity •
Sanon, Spigner, and McCullagh (2016) examined the role of transnationalism (maintenance of relationships and activities that transcend borders across countries) among Haitian immigrants in terms of hypertension self-management. By means of reflexivity, the primary researcher "considered her historical, social, and political context and position as they influenced her reflections, and the meanings she ascribed to the participants' accounts" (p. 150). The researcher also reflected on the inequality in power relationship between the participants and herself.

 TIP Reflexivity can be a useful exercise in quantitative as well as qualitative research—self-awareness and introspection can enhance the quality of any study.

Generalizability and Transferability

Nurses increasingly rely on evidence from disciplined research as a guide in their clinical practice. EBP is based on the assumption that study findings are not unique to the people, places, or circumstances of the original research.

As noted in Chapter 1, *generalizability* is the criterion used in quantitative studies to assess the extent to which the findings can be applied to other groups and settings. How do researchers improve the generalizability of a study? First and foremost, they must design studies strong in reliability and validity. There is little point in wondering whether results are generalizable if they are not accurate or valid. In selecting participants, researchers must also give thought to the types of people to whom results might be generalized—and then select subjects accordingly. If a study is intended to have implications for male and female patients, then men and women should be included as participants.

Qualitative researchers do not specifically aim for generalizability, but they do want to generate knowledge that might be useful in similar situations. Lincoln and Guba (1985), in their influential book on naturalistic inquiry, discuss the concept of **transferability**, the extent to which qualitative findings can be transferred to other settings, as another aspect of trustworthiness. An important mechanism for promoting transferability is the amount of rich descriptive information qualitative researchers provide about study background.

RESEARCH EXAMPLES WITH CRITICAL THINKING EXERCISES

Abstracts for a quantitative and a qualitative nursing study are presented in the following sections. Read the abstracts for Examples 1 and 2 and then answer the critical thinking questions that follow. Exercises 1 and 2 are featured on the interactive *Critical Thinking Activity* on website. The critical thinking questions for Exercises 3 and 4 are based on the studies that appear in their entirety in Appendices A and B of this book. Our comments for these exercises are in the Student Resources section on thePoint. ⋆

EXAMPLE 1: QUANTITATIVE RESEARCH

Study: Relationships among daytime napping and fatigue, sleep quality, and quality of life (QOL) in cancer patients (Sun & Lin, 2015). ⋆

Background: The relationships among napping and sleep quality, fatigue, and QOL in cancer patients are not clearly understood.

Objective: The aim of the study was to determine whether daytime napping is associated with night-time sleep, fatigue, and QOL in cancer patients.

Methods: In total, 187 cancer patients were recruited. Daytime napping, night-time self-reported sleep, fatigue, and QOL were assessed using a questionnaire. Objective sleep parameters were collected using a wrist actigraph.

Results: According to waking-after-sleep-onset measurements, patients who napped during the day experienced poorer night-time sleep than did patients who did not ($t = -2.44$, $p = .02$). Daytime napping duration was significantly negatively correlated with QOL. Patients who napped after 4 pm had poorer sleep quality ($t = -1.93$, $p = .05$) and a poorer Short-Form Health Survey mental component score ($t = 2.06$, $p = .04$) than did patients who did not. Fatigue, daytime napping duration, and sleep quality were significant predictors of the mental component score and physical component score, accounting for 45.7% and 39.3% of the variance, respectively.

Conclusions: Daytime napping duration was negatively associated with QOL. Napping should be avoided after 4 pm.

Implications for Practice: Daytime napping affects the QOL of cancer patients. Future research can determine the role of napping in the sleep hygiene of cancer patients.

Critical Thinking Exercises

1. Consider the following targeted questions:
   a. What were the independent and dependent variables in this study? What are the PICO components?
   b. Is this study experimental or non-experimental?
   c. How, if at all, was *randomness* used in this study?
   d. How, if at all, was *blinding* used in this study?
   e. Did the researchers use any statistical tests? If yes, were any of the results statistically significant?
2. If the results of this study are valid and generalizable, what might be some of the uses to which the findings could be put in clinical practice?

EXAMPLE 2: QUALITATIVE RESEARCH

Study: Adolescents' lived experiences while hospitalized after surgery for ulcerative colitis (Olsen et al., 2015)

Abstract: Adolescents are in a transitional phase of life characterized by major physical, emotional, and psychological challenges. Living with ulcerative colitis is experienced as a reduction of their life quality. Initial treatment of ulcerative colitis is medical, but surgery may be necessary when medical treatment ceases to have an effect. No research-based studies of adolescents' experience of the hospital period after surgery for ulcerative colitis exist. The objective of the study was to identify and describe adolescents' live experiences while hospitalized after surgery for ulcerative colitis. This qualitative study was based on interviews with eight adolescents. Analysis and interpretation were based on a hermeneutic interpretation of meaning. Three themes were identified: Body: Out of order, Seen and understood, and Where are all the others? The adolescents experience a postoperative period characterized by physical and mental impairment. Being mentally unprepared for such challenges, they shun communication and interaction. The findings demonstrate the importance of individualized nursing care on the basis of the adolescent's age, maturity, and individual needs. Further study of adolescent patients' hospital stay, focusing on the implications of being young and ill at the same time, is needed.

Critical Thinking Exercises

1. Consider the following targeted questions:
   a. On which qualitative research tradition, if any, was this study based?
   b. Is this study experimental or non-experimental?
   c. How, if at all, was *randomness* used in this study?
   d. Is there any indication in the abstract that *triangulation* was used? *Reflexivity*?

2. If the results of this study are trustworthy and transferable, what might be some of the uses to which the findings could be put in clinical practice?

3. Compare the two abstracts in Examples 1 and 2. The first is structured, with specific headings, whereas the second is a more "traditional" format consisting of a single paragraph. Which do you prefer? Why?

EXAMPLE 3: QUANTITATIVE RESEARCH IN APPENDIX A

- Read the introduction and methods section of Swenson and colleagues' (2016) study ("Parents' use of praise and criticism in a sample of young children seeking mental health services") in Appendix A of this book.

Critical Thinking Exercises

1. Answer the following targeted questions:
   a. Did this article follow a traditional IMRAD format? Where does the introduction to this article begin and end?
   b. How, if at all, was *randomness* used in this study?
   c. How, if at all, was *blinding* used?
   d. Comment on the possible generalizability of the study findings.

EXAMPLE 4: QUALITATIVE RESEARCH IN APPENDIX B

- Read the abstract of Beck and Watson's (2010) study ("Subsequent childbirth after a previous traumatic birth") in Appendix B of this book.

Critical Thinking Exercises

1. Answer the following targeted questions, which may assist you in assessing aspects of the study's merit:
   a. Where does the introduction to this article begin and end?
   b. How, if at all, was *randomness* used in this study?
   c. Is there any indication in the abstract that *triangulation* was used? *Reflexivity*?
   d. Comment on the possible transferability of the study findings.

WANT TO KNOW MORE? ✳️

A wide variety of resources to enhance your learning and understanding of this chapter are available on thePoint.

- Interactive Critical Thinking Activity
- Chapter Supplement on Guides to Overall Critiques of Research Reports
- Answers to the Critical Thinking Exercises for Examples 3 and 4
- Internet Resources with useful websites for Chapter 4
- A Wolters Kluwer journal article on a topic related to this chapter

---

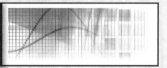

Summary Points

- Both quantitative and qualitative researchers disseminate their findings, most often by publishing reports of their research as **journal articles,** which concisely describe what researcher did and what they found.

- Journal articles often consist of an **abstract** (a synopsis of the study) and four major sections that often follow the **IMRAD format:** an **I**ntroduction (the research problem and its context); **M**ethod section (the strategies used to answer research questions); **R**esults (study findings); and **D**iscussion (interpretation and implications of the findings).

- Research reports are often difficult to read because they are dense, concise, and contain jargon. Quantitative research reports may be intimidating at first, because, compared to qualitative reports, they are more impersonal and report on statistical tests.

- **Statistical tests** are used to test hypotheses and to evaluate the reliability of the findings. Findings that are **statistically significant** have a high probability of being "real."

- A goal of this book is to help students to prepare a research **critique,** which is a critical appraisal of the strengths and limitations of a study, often to assess the worth of the evidence for nursing practice.

- Researchers face numerous challenges, the solutions to which must be considered in critiquing a study because they affect the inferences that can be made.

- An **inference** is a conclusion drawn from the study evidence, taking into account the methods used to generate that evidence. Researchers strive to have their inferences correspond to the *truth.*

- **Reliability** (a key challenge in quantitative research) refers to the accuracy of information obtained in a study. **Validity** broadly concerns the *soundness* of the study's evidence—that is, whether the findings are convincing and well grounded.

- **Trustworthiness** in qualitative research encompasses several different dimensions, including credibility, dependability, confirmability, transferability, and authenticity.
- **Credibility** is achieved to the extent that the methods engender confidence in the truth of the data and in the researchers' interpretations. **Triangulation,** the use of multiple sources to draw conclusions about the truth, is one approach to enhancing credibility.
- A **bias** is an influence that produces a distortion in the study results. In quantitative studies, research control is an approach to addressing bias. **Research control** is used to *hold constant* outside influences on the dependent variable so that the relationship between the independent and dependent variables can be better understood.
- Researchers seek to control **confounding** (or *extraneous*) **variables**—variables that are extraneous to the purpose of a specific study.

- For quantitative researchers, **randomness**—having certain features of the study established by chance—is a powerful tool to eliminate bias.
- **Blinding** (or *masking*) is sometimes used to avoid biases stemming from participants' or research agents' awareness of study hypotheses or research status.
- **Reflexivity,** the process of reflecting critically on the self and of scrutinizing personal values that could affect data collection and interpretation, is an important tool in qualitative research.
- **Generalizability** in a quantitative study concerns the extent to which the findings can be applied to other groups and settings.
- A similar concept in qualitative studies is **transferability,** the extent to which qualitative findings can be transferred to other settings. One mechanism for promoting transferability is a rich and thorough description of the research context so that others can make inferences about contextual similarities.

REFERENCES

Canadian Institute for Health Information. 2014 Annual Report [Internet]. Ottawa: CIHI; June, 2014. [cited September 14, 2015]. Hip and knee replacements in Canada: Canadian Joint Replacement Registry. Available from: https://secure. cihi.ca/free_products/CJRR%202014%20Annual% 20Report_EN-web.pdf. Retrieved on October 14, 2017.

*da Silva, N., Chaves, É., de Carvalho, E., Carvalho, L., & Iunes, D. (2015). Foot reflexology in feet impairment of people with type 2 diabetes mellitus: Randomized trial. *Revista Latino-Americana de Enfermagem, 23,* 603–610.

Larimer, K., Durmus, J., & Florez, E. (2015). Experiences of young adults with pacemakers and/or implantable cardioverter defibrillators. *Journal of Cardiovascular Nursing.* Advance online publication.

Lincoln, Y. S., & Guba, E. G. (1985). *Naturalistic inquiry.* Newbury Park, CA: Sage.

Montreuil, M., Butler, K., Stachura, M., & Pugnaire-Gros, C. (2015). Exploring helpful nursing care in pediatric mental health settings: The perceptions of children with suicide risk factors and their parents. *Issues in Mental Health Nursing, 36,* 849–859.

Olsen, I., Jensen, S., Larsen, L., & Sørensen, E. (2015). Adolescents' lived experiences while hospitalized after surgery for ulcerative colitis. *Gastroenterology Nursing.* Advance online publication.

Park, H., Chun, Y., & Gang, M. (2015). Effects of the Patient-Centered Environment Program on behavioral and emotional problems in home-dwelling patients with dementia. *Journal of Gerontological Nursing, 41,* 40–48.

Puts, M. T., Sattar, S., McWatters, K, et al. (2017). Chemotherapy treatment decision-making experiences of older adults with cancer, their family members, oncologists and family physicians: A mixed methods study. *Supportive Care in Cancer, 25,* 879–886.

Sanon, M. A., Spigner, C., & McCullagh, M. C. (2016). Transnationalism and hypertension self-management among Haitian immigrants. *Journal of Transcultural Nursing, 27,* 147–156.

Shahram, S. Z., Bottorff, J. L, Oelke N. D, Kurtz, D. L, Thomas, V., & Spittal, P. M; For The Cedar Project Partnership. (2017). Mapping the social determinants of substance use for pregnant-involved young aboriginal women. *International Journal of Qualitatively Studies and Health Well-being, 12,* 1275155.

**Sun, J. L., & Lin, C. C. (2015). Relationships among daytime napping and fatigue, sleep quality, and quality of life in cancer patients. *Cancer Nursing.* Advance online publication.

Wilson, R. A., Watt-Watson, J., Hodnett E., et al. (2016). A Randomized Controlled Trial of an Individualized Preoperative Education Intervention for Symptom Management After Total Knee Arthroplasty. *Orthopaedic Nursing, 35*(1), 20–29.

*A link to this open-access article is provided in the Internet Resources section on thePoint website.

**This journal article is available on thePoint for this chapter.

5   Ethics in Research

Learning Objectives

On completing this chapter, you will be able to:

- Discuss the historical background that led to the creation of various codes of ethics
- Understand the potential for ethical dilemmas stemming from conflicts between ethics and research demands
- Identify the three primary ethical principles articulated in the *Belmont Report* and the important dimensions encompassed by each
- Identify procedures for adhering to ethical principles and protecting study participants
- Given sufficient information, evaluate the ethical dimensions of a research report
- Define new terms in the chapter

Key Terms

- Anonymity
- Assent
- *Belmont Report*
- Beneficence
- Code of ethics
- Confidentiality
- Consent form

- Debriefing
- Ethical dilemma
- Full disclosure
- Informed consent
- Research Ethics Board (REB)
- Minimal risk

- Risk/benefit assessment
- Stipend
- Vulnerable group

ETHICS AND RESEARCH

In any research with human beings or animals, researchers must address ethical issues. Ethical concerns are especially prominent in nursing research because the line between what constitutes the expected practice of nursing and the collection of research data sometimes gets blurred. This chapter discusses ethical principles that should be kept in mind when reading a study.

Historical Background

We might like to think that violations of moral principles among researchers occurred centuries ago, but this is not the case. The Nazi medical experiments of the 1930s and 1940s are the most recognized example of recent disregard for ethical conduct. The Nazi programme of research involved using prisoners of war and "racial enemies" in medical experiments. The studies were unethical not only because they exposed people to harm but also because subjects could not refuse participation.

There are more recent examples. For instance, between 1932 and 1972, the Tuskegee Syphilis Study, sponsored by the U.S. Public Health Service, investigated the effects of syphilis among 400 poor African-American men. Medical treatment was deliberately withheld to study the course of the untreated disease. It was revealed in 1993 that US federal agencies had sponsored radiation experiments since the 1940s on hundreds of people, many of them prisoners or elderly hospital patients. And, in 2010, it was revealed that a US doctor who worked on the Tuskegee study inoculated prisoners in Guatemala with syphilis in the 1940s. In 1998, Andrew Wakefield published a case series in *The Lancet*, which suggested a link between the measles, mumps, and rubella (MMR) vaccine and autism and behavioural regression in children. In 2004, investigation by *Sunday Times* reporter documented that Wakefield had failed to disclose financial conflicts of interest. The British General Medical Council (GMC) conducted an inquiry into allegations of misconduct against Wakefield. In 2010, Wakefield was charged with misconduct for subjecting his study participants unnecessary invasive medical procedures such as colonoscopies and lumbar punctures and deliberating falsifying results in the publication. In Canada, unethical nutrition experiments were performed by the Department of Indian Affairs of Canada on aboriginal children at six residential schools between 1942 and 1952. In one of the experiments, children were given a flour mix containing added thiamine, riboflavin, niacin, and bone meal. Despite the increase in the number of children who developed anaemia leading to deaths and developmental delay, the experiment continued. Dental care was withheld for the researchers to explore the relationship between malnutrition and dental caries and gingivitis.

The Truth and Reconciliation Commission of Canada was established and spent 6 years travelling to all parts of Canada to hear from the indigenous people about the residential school experiences, impacts, and consequences. The truth telling and reconciliation process is an acknowledgement of the injustices and harms experienced by the indigenous people and the need for continued healing. The Commission had a clear mandate to create a national research centre at the University of Manitoba where relevant documents are archived and accessible to survivors, their families, and communities, as well as to the general public.

Other examples of studies with ethical transgressions have emerged to give ethical concerns the high visibility they have today.

Codes of Ethics

In response to human rights violations, various **codes of ethics** have been developed. The ethical standards known as the Nuremberg Code was developed in 1949 in response to the Nazi atrocities. Several other international standards have been developed, including the Declaration of Helsinki, which was adopted in 1964 by the World Medical Association and was most recently revised in 2013.

Most disciplines, such as medicine and nursing, have established their own code of ethics. In Canada, the Canadian Nurses Association (CAN) published its *Ethical Guidelines for Nurses in Research Involving Human Participants* in 2002. The CAN published *Code of Ethics for Registered Nurses*, a document that covers ethical issues for practising nurses primarily but also includes principles that apply to nurse researchers. The CNA is working with registered nurses, nurse practitioners, and licensed practical nurses (registered practical nurses in Ontario) to revise the code of ethics that will be launched in 2017.

In the United States, the American Nurses Association (ANA) issued *Ethical Guidelines in the Conduct, Dissemination, and Implementation of Nursing Research* in 1995 (Silva, 1995). And, the International Council of Nurses (ICN) developed the *ICN Code of Ethics for Nurses*, which was updated in 2012.

TIP   Many useful websites are devoted to ethics and research, links to some of which are listed in the Internet Resources for this chapter on thePoint website.

Government Regulations for Protecting Study Participants

Governments throughout the world fund research and establish rules for adhering to ethical principles. In the United States, an important code of ethics was adopted by the National Commission for the Protection of Human Subjects of Biomedical and Behavioral Research. The commission issued a report in 1978, known as the **Belmont Report**, which provided a model for many guidelines adopted by the Medical Research Council of Canada (MRC) and the Social Sciences and Humanities Research Council (SSHRC) in Canada. In 2001, Canada's three federal research agencies (tri-council), the Canadian Institutes of Health Research (CIHR), the Natural Sciences and Engineering Research Council of Canada (NSERC), and the Social Sciences and Humanities Research Council of Canada (SSHRC), jointly created the Interagency Advisory Panel on Research Ethics (PRE or the Panel).

Tri-Council Policy Statement (TCPS): Ethical conduct for research involving humans is a joint policy first published in 1998 and updated recently in 2014 to provide guidance on the ethical conduct of research involving human. The purpose of the TCPS is to balance between the potential benefits of research and protection of participants from research-related harm. Research involving humans should be conducted in a manner that is sensitive and respect human dignity through three core principles—Respect for Persons, Concern for Welfare, and Justice.

- Respecting for persons: Researchers understand that a person is autonomous and he or she should be free to choose without interference.
- Concern for Welfare: Researchers should aim to protect the welfare of participants from any potential risks associated with the research.
- Justice: Researchers have the obligation to treat people fairly and equitably. No groups in the population is overly burdened by the harms of research or denied the benefits of the knowledge generated from it.

These statements clearly spell out the need to maintain free, informed, and ongoing consent throughout the research process to build and maintain the trust of participants and the public in the research process.

Ethical Dilemmas in Conducting Research

Research that violates ethical principles typically occurs because a researcher believes that knowledge is potentially beneficial in the long run. For research problems, participants' rights and study quality are put in direct conflict, posing **ethical dilemmas** for researchers. Here are examples of research problems in which the desire for rigor conflicts with ethical considerations:

1. *Research question:* Does a new medication prolong life in patients with AIDS?
   Ethical dilemma: The best way to test the effectiveness of an intervention is to administer the medication to some participants but withhold it from others to see if the groups have different outcomes. However, the group receiving the intervention may be exposed to potentially hazardous side effects. On the other hand, the group *not* receiving the drug may be denied a beneficial treatment.
2. *Research question:* Are nurses equally empathic in their treatment of male and female patients in the intensive care unit (ICU)?
   Ethical dilemma: Ethics require that participants be aware of their role in a study. Yet if the researcher informs nurse participants that their empathy in treating male and female

ICU patients will be scrutinized, will their behaviour be "normal"? If the nurses' usual behaviour is altered because of the known presence of research observers, then the findings will be inaccurate.

3. *Research question:* How do parents cope when their children have a terminal illness?
   Ethical dilemma: To answer this question, the researcher may need to probe into parents' psychological state at a vulnerable time, yet knowledge of the parents' coping mechanisms might help to design effective ways of addressing parents' grief and stress.

4. *Research question:* What is the process by which adult children adapt to the day-to-day stress of caring for a parent with Alzheimer's disease?
   Ethical dilemma: Sometimes, especially in qualitative studies, a researcher may get so close to participants that they become willing to share "secrets" and privileged information. Interviews can become confessions—sometimes of unseemly or illegal behaviour. In this example, suppose a woman admitted to physically abusing her mother—how does the researcher respond to that information without undermining a pledge of confidentiality? And, if the researcher divulges the information to authorities, how can a pledge of confidentiality be given in good faith to other participants?

As these examples suggest, researchers are sometimes in a bind. Their goal is to develop high-quality evidence for practice, but they must also adhere to rules for protecting human rights. Another type of dilemma may arise if nurse researchers face conflict-of-interest situations, in which their expected behaviour as nurses conflicts with standard research behaviour (e.g., deviating from a research protocol to assist a patient). It is precisely because of such dilemmas that codes of ethics are needed to guide researchers' efforts.

ETHICAL PRINCIPLES FOR PROTECTING STUDY PARTICIPANTS

The *Belmont Report* articulated three primary ethical principles on which standards of ethical research conduct are based: beneficence, respect for human dignity, and justice. We briefly discuss these principles and then describe methods researchers use to comply with them.

Beneficence

Beneficence imposes a duty on researchers to minimize harm and maximize benefits. Human research should be intended to produce benefits for participants or, more typically, for others. This principle covers multiple aspects.

The Right to Freedom From Harm and Discomfort

Researchers have an obligation to prevent or minimize harm in studies with humans. Participants must not be subjected to unnecessary risks of harm or discomfort, and their participation in research must be necessary for achieving societally important aims. In research with humans, *harm* and *discomfort* can be physical (e.g., injury), emotional (e.g., stress), social (e.g., loss of social support), or financial (e.g., loss of wages). Ethical researchers must use strategies to minimize all types of harms and discomforts, even ones that are temporary.

Protecting human beings from physical harm is often straightforward, but it may be more difficult to address psychological issues. For example, participants may be asked questions about their personal lives. Such queries might lead people to reveal deeply personal information. The need for sensitivity may be greater in qualitative studies, which often involve in-depth exploration into highly personal areas. Researchers need to be aware of the nature of the intrusion on people's psyches.

The Right to Protection From Exploitation

Involvement in a study should not place participants at a disadvantage. Participants need to be assured that their participation, or information they provide, will not be used against them. For example, people describing their economic situation should not risk loss of public health benefits; people reporting drug abuse should not fear being reported for a crime.

Study participants enter into a special relationship with researchers, and this relationship should not be exploited. Because nurse researchers may have a nurse–patient (in addition to a researcher–participant) relationship, special care may be needed to avoid exploiting that bond. Patients' consent to participate in a study may result from their understanding of the researcher's role as *nurse*, not as *researcher*.

In qualitative research, psychological distance between researchers and participants often declines as the study progresses. The emergence of a pseudo-therapeutic relationship is not uncommon, which could create additional risks that exploitation could inadvertently occur. On the other hand, qualitative researchers often are in a better position than quantitative researchers to *do good*, rather than just to avoid doing harm, because of the close relationships they develop with participants.

Example of therapeutic research experiences • • • • • • • • • • • • • • • • • •
Goulet et al. (2017) conducted a case study involving the development, implementation, and evaluation of a post-seclusion and/or restraint review with the healthcare team and patients in an acute psychiatric care unit. The review was perceived as a learning opportunity. Nurses reported that they took the time to explore patient's feelings. Which helped to build therapeutic relationship. One participant said, "This was the first time I really took the time to get the patient's feedback and talk about it."

Respect for Human Dignity

Respect for human dignity is the second ethical principle in the *Belmont Report*. This principle includes the right to self-determination and the right to full disclosure.

The Right to Self-Determination

The principle of *self-determination* means that prospective participants have the right to decide voluntarily whether to participate in a study, without risking harmful treatment. It also means that people have the right to ask questions, refuse answering questions, and drop out of the study.

A person's right to self-determination includes freedom from coercion. *Coercion* involves explicit or implicit threats of penalty from failing to participate in a study or excessive rewards from agreeing to participate. The issue of coercion requires careful thought when researchers are in a position of authority or influence over potential participants, as might be the case in a nurse–patient relationship. Coercion can be subtle. For example, a generous monetary incentive (or **stipend**) to encourage the participation of a low-income group (e.g., the homeless) might be considered mildly coercive because such incentives may be seen as a form of pressure.

The Right to Full Disclosure

Respect for human dignity encompasses people's right to make informed decisions about study participation, which requires full disclosure. **Full disclosure** means that the researcher has fully described the study, the person's right to refuse participation, and potential risks and benefits. The right to self-determination and the right to full disclosure are the two elements that establish informed consent (discussed later in this chapter).

Full disclosure is not always straightforward because it can create biases and sample recruitment problems. Suppose we were testing the hypothesis that high school students with a high absentee rate are more likely to be substance abusers than students with good attendance. If we approached potential participants and fully explained the study's purpose, some students might refuse to participate, and non-participation would be selective; students who are substance abusers—the group of primary interest—might be least likely to participate. Moreover, by knowing the study purpose, those who participate might not give candid responses. In such a situation, full disclosure could undermine the study.

As a solution, researchers sometimes use *covert data collection* (*concealment*), which is collecting data without participants' knowledge and thus without their consent. This might happen if a researcher wanted to observe people's behaviour and was worried that doing so openly would change the behaviour of interest. Researchers might choose to obtain needed information through hidden methods, such as observing while pretending to be engaged in other activities.

A more controversial technique is the use of *deception*, which can involve deliberately withholding information about the study or providing participants with false information. For example, in studying high school students' use of drugs, we might describe the research as a study of students' health practices, which is a mild form of misinformation.

Deception and concealment are problematic ethically because they interfere with people's right to make truly informed decisions about personal costs and benefits of participation. Some people think that deception is never justified, but others believe that if the study involves minimal risk yet offers benefits to society, then deception may be justified.

Full disclosure has emerged as a concern in connection with data collected over the Internet (e.g., analysing the content of messages posted to blogs or social media sites). The issue is whether such messages can be used as data without the authors' consent. Some researchers believe that anything posted electronically is in the public domain, but others feel that the same ethical standards must apply in cyberspace research and that researchers must carefully protect the rights of individuals who are participants in "virtual" communities.

Justice

The third principle articulated in the *Belmont Report* concerns justice, which includes participants' right to fair treatment and their right to privacy.

The Right to Fair Treatment

One aspect of justice concerns the equitable distribution of benefits and burdens of research. The selection of participants should be based on research requirements and not on people's vulnerabilities. For example, groups with lower social standing (e.g., prisoners) have sometimes been selected as study participants, raising ethical concerns.

Potential discrimination is another aspect of distributive justice. During the 1990s, it was found that women and minorities were being excluded from many clinical studies. In Canada, this led to policies (e.g., sex and gender-based analysis policy) requiring that researchers who seek funding from the CIHR include women to demonstrate that biological, economic, and social differences between gender and sex have created differences in health risk, health system interaction, and health outcomes. On the other hand, the CIHR published guidelines to carry out ethical and culturally competent research involving aboriginal people as study participants.

The right to fair treatment encompasses other obligations. For example, researchers must treat people who decline to participate in a study in a non-prejudicial manner, they must honour all agreements made with participants, they must show respect for the beliefs of people from different backgrounds, and they must treat participants courteously and thoughtfully at all times.

The Right to Privacy

Research with humans involves intrusions into people's lives. Researchers should ensure that their research is not more intrusive than it needs to be and that privacy is protected. Participants have the right to expect that any data they provide will be kept in strict confidence.

Privacy issues have become even more salient in the Canadian health care community since the Privacy Act, which governs the personal information-handling practices by federal government departments and agents, and the Personal Information Protection and Electronic Documents Act (PIPEDA), which outlines how private sector organizations must handle personal information. As for the public sector, each province and territory has established its own legislation and commissioner or ombudsman. In addition, privacy legislation pertaining to health information are articulated in the Personal Health Information Protection Act (PHIPA) in Ontario, the Personal Health Information Privacy and Access Act in New Brunswick, and the Personal Health Information Act in Newfoundland and Labrador.

PROCEDURES FOR PROTECTING STUDY PARTICIPANTS

Now that you are familiar with ethical principles for conducting research, you need to understand the procedures researchers use to adhere to them. It is these procedures that should be evaluated in critiquing the ethical aspects of a study.

 TIP   Information about ethical considerations is usually presented in the method section of a research report, often in a subsection labelled "Procedures."

Risk/Benefit Assessments

One strategy that researchers use to protect participants is to conduct a **risk/benefit assessment**. Such an assessment is designed to evaluate whether the benefits of participating in a study are in line with the costs—that is, whether the *risk/benefit ratio* is acceptable. Box 5.1 summarizes major costs and benefits of research participation to study participants. Benefits to society and to nursing should also be taken into account. The selection of a significant topic that has the potential to improve patient care is the first step in ensuring that research is ethical.

 TIP   In evaluating the risk/benefit ratio of a study, you might want to consider how comfortable *you* would have felt about being a study participant.

In some cases, risks may be negligible. **Minimal risk** is a risk expected to be no greater than those ordinarily encountered in daily life or during routine procedures. When the risks are not minimal, researchers must proceed with caution, taking every step possible to reduce risks and maximize benefits.

Informed Consent

An important procedure for safeguarding participants involves obtaining their informed consent. **Informed consent** means that participants have adequate information about the

> **Box 5.1 Potential Benefits and Risks of Research to Participants**
>
> **Major Potential Benefits to Participants**
> - Access to a potentially beneficial intervention that might otherwise be unavailable
> - Comfort in being able to discuss their situation or problem with a friendly, objective person
> - Increased knowledge about themselves or their conditions
> - Escape from normal routine
> - Satisfaction that information they provide may help others with similar problems
> - Direct gains through stipends or other incentives
>
> **Major Potential Risks to Participants**
> - Physical harm, including unanticipated side effects
> - Physical discomfort, fatigue, or boredom
> - Emotional distress from self-disclosure, discomfort with strangers, embarrassment relating to questions being asked
> - Social risks, such as the risk of stigma, negative effects on personal relationships
> - Loss of privacy
> - Loss of time
> - Monetary costs (e.g., for transportation, child care, time lost from work)

study, comprehend the information, and have the power of free choice, enabling them to consent to or decline participation voluntarily.

Researchers usually document informed consent by having participants sign a **consent form**. This form includes information about the study purpose, specific expectations regarding participation (e.g., how much time will be required), the voluntary nature of participation, and potential costs and benefits.

 TIP The Chapter Supplement on website provides additional information about the content of informed consent forms as well as an actual example from a study by one of the book's authors (Beck).

Example of informed consent •
Dube and her team (2016) explored the scope and accessibility of youth-oriented HIV/ HCV prevention initiatives in Atlantic Canada. The study included semi-structured interviews with 47 key informants from all sectors to explore their perceptions of HIV, gender, sex, diversity, and equity. Written informed consent was obtained from study participants.

Researchers may not obtain written informed consent when data collection is through self-administered questionnaires. Researchers often assume *implied consent* (i.e., the return of a completed questionnaire implies the person's consent to participate).

In qualitative studies that involve repeated data collection, it may be difficult to obtain meaningful consent at the outset. Because the design emerges during the study, researchers may not know what the risks and benefits will be. In such situations, consent may be an ongoing process, called *process consent*, which involves ongoing renegotiation.

Confidentiality Procedures

Study participants have the right to expect that the data they provide will be kept in strict confidence. Participants' right to privacy is protected through confidentiality procedures.

Anonymity

Anonymity, the most secure means of protecting confidentiality, occurs when the researcher cannot link participants to their data. For example, if questionnaires were distributed to a group of nursing home residents and were returned without any identifying information, responses would be anonymous.

Example of anonymity •
Lavoie and colleagues (2016) conducted a study to identify psychosocial factors that influenced nurses' intention to practice euthanasia in palliative care. A random sample of 154 nurses form the province of Quebec completed an anonymous questionnaire. The perceived social pressure to practice euthanasia and the appropriateness of practicing euthanasia according to one's personal and moral values were significant determinants of intention to practice euthanasia in palliative care among nurses.

Confidentiality in the Absence of Anonymity

When anonymity is not possible, other confidentiality procedures are required. A promise of **confidentiality** is a pledge that any information participants provide will not be publicly reported in a manner that identifies them and will not be made accessible to others.

Researchers can take a number of steps to ensure that a *breach of confidentiality* does not occur. These include maintaining identifying information in locked files, substituting *identification (ID) numbers* for participants' names on records, and reporting only aggregate data for groups of participants.

Confidentiality is especially important in qualitative studies because of their in-depth nature, yet anonymity is rarely possible. Qualitative researchers also face the challenge of adequately disguising participants in their reports. Because the number of respondents is small and because rich descriptive information is presented, qualitative researchers must be especially careful in safeguarding participants' identity.

 TIP   As a means of enhancing individual and institutional privacy, research articles frequently avoid giving information about the locale of the study. For example, a report might say that data were collected in a 200-bed, private nursing home, without mentioning its name or location.

Confidentiality sometimes creates tension between researchers and legal authorities, especially if participants engage in criminal activity like substance abuse.

Example of confidentiality procedures •
Hayes (2015) studied the life patterns of incarcerated women. The 18 women who participated selected pseudonyms for themselves. The interviews were conducted in private rooms in the prison. The researcher made certain that the rooms did not have cameras or microphones in them and that no correctional staff were nearby.

Debriefings and Referrals

Researchers should show respect for participants during the interactions they have with them. For example, researchers should be polite and respectful of cultural, linguistic, and lifestyle diversity.

Formal strategies for communicating respect for participants' well-being are also available. For example, it is sometimes advisable to offer **debriefing** sessions following data collection so that participants can ask questions or share concerns. Researchers can also demonstrate their interest in participants by offering to share study findings with them after the data have been analysed. Finally, researchers may need to assist participants by making referrals to appropriate health, social, or psychological services.

Example of referrals •
Stremler and colleagues (2017) studied the factors associated with anxiety, depressive symptoms, and decisional conflict in parents of children hospitalized in the paediatric intensive care units. A total of 74 mothers and 44 fathers participated in the study.

The primary investigator notified and recommended participants with high score of anxiety and depression on the standardized questionnaires to visit a family physician or health professional specializing in mental health. A referral to a PICU social worker was arranged if the parent agreed.

Treatment of Vulnerable Groups

Adherence to ethical standards is often straightforward. The rights of special **vulnerable groups**, however, may need extra protections. Vulnerable populations may be incapable of giving fully informed consent (e.g., cognitively impaired people) or may be at high risk of unintended side effects (e.g., pregnant women). You should pay particular attention to the ethical dimensions of a study when vulnerable people are involved. Among the groups that should be considered as being vulnerable are the following:

- *Children.* Legally and ethically, children do not have the competence to give informed consent, and so the consent of children's parents or guardians should be obtained. However, it is appropriate—especially if the child is at least 7 years of age—to obtain the child's assent as well. **Assent** refers to the child's affirmative agreement to participate.
- *Mentally or emotionally disabled people.* Individuals whose disability makes it impossible for them to make informed decisions (e.g., people in a coma) also cannot legally provide informed consent. In such cases, researchers should obtain the consent of a legal guardian.
- *Severely ill or physically disabled people.* For patients who are very ill or undergoing certain treatments (e.g., mechanical ventilation), it might be necessary to assess their ability to make reasoned decisions about study participation.
- *The terminally ill.* Terminally ill people can seldom expect to benefit personally from research, and thus the risk/benefit ratio needs to be carefully assessed.
- *Institutionalized people.* Nurses often conduct studies with hospitalized or institutionalized people (e.g., prisoners) who might feel that their care would be jeopardized by failure to cooperate. Researchers studying institutionalized groups need to emphasize the voluntary nature of participation.
- *Pregnant women.* The Canadian government has issued additional requirements governing research with pregnant women and foetuses. These requirements reflect a desire to safeguard both the pregnant woman, who may be at heightened physical or psychological risk, and the foetus, who cannot give informed consent.

Example of research with a vulnerable group • • • • • • • • • • • • • • • • • • •
McGilton and other researchers (2017) studied the effects of a communication intervention on residents' quality of life, as well as care providers' perceived knowledge, mood, and burden. To protect the resident, a facility staff member reviewed clinical records to confirm the diagnosis of dementia and communication difficulties. Prospective participants were asked if the research assistant could speak to them about the study. The research assistant approached the participants and/or their proxy to obtain written, informed consent.

External Reviews and the Protection of Human Rights

Researchers may not be objective in developing procedures to protect participants' rights. Biases may arise from their commitment to an area of knowledge and their desire to conduct a rigorous study. Because of the risk of a biased evaluation, the ethical dimensions of a study are usually subjected to external review.

Most hospitals, universities, and other institutions where research is conducted have established formal committees for reviewing research plans. In Canada, the committee is often called an **Research Ethics Board (REB)**. Before undertaking a study, researchers must submit research plans to the REB and must also undergo formal training based on the Tri-Council Policy Statements (TCPS2) (e.g., Course on Research ethics or CORE). An REB can approve the proposed plans, require modifications, or disapprove them.

Example of REB approval •
Varcoe and co-researchers (2017) tested a health promotion intervention for indigenous women who have experienced intimate partner violence. The interventions were facilitated by nurses and an Elder who used ceremony and traditional practices to help the participants identify and address their health and safety priorities. The study received approval from the Ethics Review Boards of the investigators' universities.

A total of 21 women participated in the study. Based on individual and focus group interviews, participants found the intervention acceptable and some aspects were especially helpful including prayer and traditional teachings, smudging, the talking feather, traditional activities, food, and access to nurses.

Ethical Issues in Using Animals in Research

Some nurse researchers who focus on biophysiologic phenomena use animals as their subjects. Ethical considerations are clearly different for animals and humans; for example, *informed consent* is not relevant for animals. The Canadian Council on Animal Care was established in 1982 to oversee the use experimental animals. The Guide to the Care and Use of Experimental Animals articulate principles for the proper care and treatment of animals used in research, covering such issues as the transport of research animals, pain and distress in animal subjects, the use of appropriate anaesthesia, and euthanizing animals under certain conditions during or after the study.

Example of research with animals •
Kaur and co-researchers (2016) studied the effect of bromelain or pineapple extract on blood coagulability in mice. The Queen's University Animal Care Committee approved all procedures, and the study adhered to Animals for Research Act and the guidelines of the Canadian Council on Animal Care.

CRITIQUING THE ETHICAL ASPECTS OF A STUDY

Guidelines for critiquing the ethical aspects of a study are presented in Box 5.2. Members of an REB are provided with sufficient information to answer all these questions, but research articles do not always include detailed information about ethics because of space constraints in journals. Thus, it may be difficult to critique researchers' adherence to ethical guidelines. Nevertheless, we offer a few suggestions for considering ethical issues.

Many research reports do acknowledge that the study procedures were reviewed by an REB. When a report mentions a formal review, it is usually safe to assume that a panel of concerned people thoroughly reviewed ethical issues raised by the study.

You can also come to some conclusions based on a description of the study methods. There may be sufficient information to judge, for example, whether study participants were subjected to harm or discomfort. Reports do not always state whether informed consent was secured, but you should decide whether the same data could have been gathered as described if participation were purely voluntary (e.g., if data were gathered unobtrusively).

In thinking about the ethical aspects of a study, you should also consider who the study participants were. For example, if the study involves vulnerable groups, there should be more information about protective procedures. You might also need to attend to the study participants who were *not included*. For example, there has been considerable concern about the omission of certain groups (e.g., minorities) from clinical research.

RESEARCH EXAMPLES WITH CRITICAL THINKING EXERCISES

Brief summaries of a quantitative and a qualitative nursing study are presented in the following sections. Read the research summaries and then answer the critical thinking questions about the ethical aspects of the studies that follow, referring to the full research report if necessary. Examples 1 and 2 are featured on the interactive *Critical Thinking Activity* on website. The critical thinking questions for Examples 3 and 4 are based on the studies that appear in their entirety in Appendices A and B of this book. Our comments for these exercises are in the Student Resources section on thePoint.

EXAMPLE 1: QUANTITATIVE RESEARCH

Study: Family typology and appraisal of preschoolers' behaviour by female caregivers (Coke & Moore, 2015) ⚙–

Study Purpose: The purpose of the study was to explore family factors associated with appraisal of a child's behaviour by a primary female caregiver, the extent to which the caregiver's appraisal is distorted, and the child's risk of having a behaviour problem.

Research Methods: Data were collected by means of a questionnaire completed by female family caregivers of 117 preschoolers who attended a rural Head Start preschool programme for low-income families. The questionnaires, which took about 30 minutes to complete, included questions about caregiver stress, appraisal and ratings of children's behaviours, and social support. No participant needed assistance in completing the questionnaire due to reading or language problems. The researchers decided to focus on female caregivers "because recruitment of male caregivers of young children is problematic" (p. 446). The sample of caretakers included African American (83%), White (15%), Hispanic (2%), and Native American (1%) women.

Ethics-Related Procedures: The caretakers were recruited during a parent–child field day and a parent–teacher orientation at the Head Start programme. The lead researcher met with all volunteering caretakers. Each participant was assigned a unique ID number to protect her identity, and the listing that linked the participant to the ID number was kept separate from the questionnaires under lock and key. After completed the questionnaire, each participant was given a gift bag with a $5 gift card to a local store and health-related education materials for the children. The study was approved by the County Board of Education and the IRB of the researchers' university prior to recruitment.

Key Findings: Distortion of the caregiver's rating of her child's behaviour was associated with a higher risk of having a child with behavioural problems. Vulnerable families were significantly more likely to have a child with high risk of behaviour problems than families classified as secure.

Critical Thinking Exercises

1. Answer the relevant questions from Box 5.2 regarding this study.
2. Also consider the following targeted questions:
   a. Could the data for this study have been collected anonymously?
   b. Comment on the appropriateness of the participant stipend in this study.
3. If the results of this study are valid and generalizable, what might be some of the uses to which the findings could be put in clinical practice?

EXAMPLE 2: QUALITATIVE RESEARCH

Study: Grief interrupted: The experience of loss among incarcerated women (Harner et al., 2011)

Study Purpose: The purpose of the study was to explore the experiences of grief among incarcerated women following the loss of a loved one.

Study Methods: The researchers used phenomenologic methods in this study. They recruited 15 incarcerated women who had experienced the loss of a loved one during their confinement. In-depth interviews about the women's experience of loss lasted 1 to 2 hours.

Ethics-Related Procedures: The researchers recruited women by posting flyers in the prison's dayroom. The flyers were written at the 4.5 grade level. Because the first author was a nurse practitioner at the prison, the researchers used several strategies to "diffuse any perceived coercion" (p. 457), such as not posting flyers near the health services unit and not offering any monetary or work-release incentives to participate. Written informed consent was obtained, but because of high rates of illiteracy, the informed consent document was read aloud to all potential participants. During the consent process, and during the interviews, the women were given opportunities to ask questions. They were informed that participation would have no effect on sentence length, sentence structure, parole, or access to health services. They were also told they could end the interview at any time without fear of reprisals. Furthermore, they were told that the researcher was a mandated reporter and would report any indication of suicidal or homicidal ideation. Participants were not required to give their names to the research team. During the interview, efforts were made to create a welcoming and nonthreatening environment. The research team received approval for their study from a university IRB and from the Department of Corrections Research Division.

Key Findings: The researchers revealed four themes, which they referred to as existential life worlds: Temporality: frozen in time; Spatiality: no place, no space to grieve; Corporeality: buried emotions; and Relationality: never alone yet feeling so lonely.

Critical Thinking Exercises

1. Answer the relevant questions from Box 5.2 regarding this study.
2. Also consider the following targeted questions:
   a. The researchers did not offer any stipend—was this ethically appropriate?
   b. Might the researchers have benefited from obtaining a Certificate of Confidentiality for this research?
3. If the results of this study are trustworthy and transferable, what might be some of the uses to which the findings could be put in clinical practice?

EXAMPLE 3: QUANTITATIVE RESEARCH IN APPENDIX A

- Read the method section of Swenson and colleagues' (2016) study ("Parents' use of praise and criticism in a sample of young children seeking mental health services") in Appendix A of this book.

Critical Thinking Exercises

1. Answer the relevant questions in Box 5.2.
2. Also consider the following targeted questions:
   a. Where was information about ethical issues located in this report?
   b. What additional information regarding the ethical aspects of their study could the researchers have included in this article?

EXAMPLE 4: QUALITATIVE RESEARCH IN APPENDIX B

- Read the method section of Beck and Watson's (2010) study ("Subsequent childbirth after a previous traumatic birth") in Appendix B of this book.

Critical Thinking Exercises

1. Answer relevant questions in Box 5.2.
2. Also consider the following targeted questions:
   a. Where was information about the ethical aspects of this study located in the report?
   b. What additional information regarding the ethical aspects of Beck and Watson's study could the researchers have included in this article?

WANT TO KNOW MORE?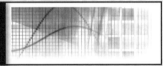

A wide variety of resources to enhance your learning and understanding of this chapter are available on thePoint.

- Interactive Critical Thinking Activity
- Chapter Supplement on Informed Consent
- Answers to the Critical Thinking Exercises for Examples 3 and 4
- Internet Resources with useful websites for Chapter 5
- A Wolters Kluwer journal article on a topic related to this chapter

---

Summary Points

- Because research has not always been conducted ethically and because of genuine **ethical dilemmas** that researchers face in designing studies that are both ethical and rigorous, **codes of ethics** have been developed to guide researchers.
- Three major ethical principles from the *Belmont Report* are incorporated into many guidelines: beneficence, respect for human dignity, and justice.
- **Beneficence** involves the performance of some good and the protection of participants from physical and psychological harm and exploitation.
- Respect for human dignity involves the participants' right to self-determination, which includes participants' right to participate in a study voluntarily.

- **Full disclosure** means that researchers have fully described to prospective participants their rights and the costs and benefits of the study. When full disclosure poses the risk of biased results, researchers sometimes use *concealment* (the collection of information without participants' knowledge) or *deception* (withholding information or providing false information).
- Justice includes the right to fair treatment and the right to privacy. In the United States, privacy has become a major issue because of the Privacy Rule regulations that resulted from the Health Insurance Portability and Accountability Act (HIPAA).
- Procedures have been developed to safeguard study participants' rights, including the performance of a risk/benefit assessment, the implementation of informed consent procedures, and taking steps to safeguard participants' confidentiality.
- In a **risk/benefit assessment,** the potential benefits of the study to individual participants

and to society are weighed against the costs to individuals.

- **Informed consent** procedures, which provide prospective participants with information needed to make a reasoned decision about participation, normally involve signing a **consent form** to document voluntary and informed participation.
- Privacy can be maintained through **anonymity** (wherein not even researchers know participants' identities) or through formal **confidentiality procedures** that safeguard the participants' data.
- Researchers sometimes offer **debriefing** sessions after data collection to provide participants with more information or an opportunity to air complaints.

- **Vulnerable groups** require additional protection. These people may be vulnerable because they are not able to make an informed decision about study participation (e.g., children), because of diminished autonomy (e.g., prisoners), or because their circumstances heighten the risk of harm (e.g., pregnant women, the terminally ill).
- External review of the ethical aspects of a study by a human subjects committee or **Institutional Review Board (IRB)** is highly desirable and is often required by universities and organizations from which participants are recruited.

REFERENCES

A pilot study of "post-seclusion and/or restraint review" intervention with patients and staff in a mental health setting. (2017). *Perspectives in Psychiatric Care.* doi: 10.1111/ppc.12225. [Epub ahead of print]

Canadian Nurses Association. (2002). *Ethical guidelines for nurses in research involving human participants.* Ottawa: Author.

**Coke, S. P., & Moore, L. (2015). Family typology and appraisal of preschoolers' behavior by female caregivers. *Nursing Research, 64,* 444–451.

Dube, A., Harris, G., Gahagan, J., et al. (2016). Bridging the silos in HIV and Hepatitis C prevention: a cross-provincial qualitative study. *International Journal of Public Health.*

*Harner, H., Hentz, P., & Evangelista, M. (2011). Grief interrupted: The experience of loss among incarcerated women. *Qualitative Health Research, 21,* 454–464.

Hayes, M. O. (2015). The life pattern of incarcerated women: The complex and interwoven lives of trauma, mental illness, and substance abuse. *Journal of Forensic Nursing, 11,* 214–222.

Kaur, H., Corscadden, K., Lott, C., et al. (2016). Bromelain has paradoxical effects on blood coagulability: a study using thromboelastography. *Blood Coagulation & Fibrinolysis, 27*(7), 745–752.

Lavoie, M., Godin, G., Vézina-Im, L. A., et al. (2015). Psychosocial determinants of physicians' intention to practice euthanasia in palliative care. *BMC Medical Ethics, 16,* 6.

McGilton, K. S., Rochon, E., Sidani, S., et al. (2017). Can We Help Care Providers Communicate More Effectively With Persons Having Dementia Living in Long-Term Care Homes? *American Journal of Alzheimer's Disease & Other Dementias, 32*(1), 41–50.

Silva, M. C. (1995). *Ethical guidelines in the conduct, dissemination, and implementation of nursing research.* Washington, DC: American Nurses Association.

Stremler, R., Haddad, S., Pullenayegum, E., et al. (2017). Psychological Outcomes in Parents of Critically Ill Hospitalized Children. *Journal of Pediatric Nursing, 34,* 36–43.

Varcoe, C., Browne, A. J., Ford-Gilboe, M., et al. (2017). Reclaiming Our Spirits: Development and Pilot Testing of a Health Promotion Intervention for Indigenous Women Who Have Experienced Intimate Partner Violence. *Research in Nursing & Health, 40*(3), 237–254.

*A link to this open-access article is provided in the Internet Resources section on thePoint website.

**This journal article is available on thePoint for this chapter.

6 Research Problems, Research Questions, and Hypotheses

Learning Objectives

On completing this chapter, you will be able to:

- Describe the process of developing and refining a research problem
- Distinguish the functions and forms of statements of purpose and research questions for quantitative and qualitative studies
- Describe the function and characteristics of research hypotheses
- Critique statements of purpose, research questions, and hypotheses in research reports with respect to their placement, clarity, wording, and importance
- Define new terms in the chapter

Key Terms

- Directional hypothesis
- Hypothesis
- Nondirectional hypothesis
- Null hypothesis
- Problem statement
- Research hypothesis
- Research problem
- Research question
- Statement of purpose

OVERVIEW OF RESEARCH PROBLEMS

Research studies begin in much the same fashion as an evidence-based practice (EBP) effort—as problems that need to be solved or questions that need to be answered. This chapter discusses research problems and research questions. We begin by clarifying some terms.

Basic Terminology

Researchers begin with a *topic* of interest. Examples of research topics are claustrophobia during magnetic resonance imaging (MRI) tests and pain management for sickle cell disease. Within broad topic areas are many possible research problems. In this section, we illustrate various terms using the topic *side effects of chemotherapy*.

A **research problem** arises from a condition, issue, or subject area that is poorly understood. The purpose of research is to "solve" the problem—or to contribute to its solution—by

TABLE 6.1 Terms Relating to Research Problems With Examples

Term	Example
Topic	Side effects of chemotherapy
Research problem (problem statement)	Nausea and vomiting are common side effects among patients on chemotherapy, and interventions to date have been only moderately successful in reducing these effects. New interventions that can reduce or prevent these side effects need to be identified.
Statement of purpose	The purpose of the study is to compare the effectiveness of patient-controlled versus nurse-administered antiemetic therapy for controlling nausea and vomiting in patients on chemotherapy.
Research question	What is the relative effectiveness of patient-controlled antiemetic therapy versus nurse-controlled antiemetic therapy with regard to (1) medication consumption and (2) control of nausea and vomiting in patients on chemotherapy?
Hypotheses	Subjects receiving antiemetic therapy by a patient-controlled pump will (1) be less nauseous, (2) vomit less, and (3) consume less medication than subjects receiving nurse-administered therapy.

gathering relevant data. A **problem statement** articulates the problem and an *argument in a sentence* that explains the need for a study. Table 6.1 presents a simplified problem statement related to the topic of side effects of chemotherapy.

Many reports provide a **statement of purpose** (or *purpose statement*), which is a summary of an overall goal. Sometimes the words *aim* or *objective* are used in lieu of purpose. **Research questions** are the specific queries researchers want to answer. Researchers indicate specific predictions about answers to research in **hypotheses** that are tested in the study.

These terms are not always consistently defined in research textbooks. Table 6.1 illustrates the interrelationships among terms as we define them.

Research Problems and Paradigms

Some research problems are better suited to qualitative than quantitative inquiry. Quantitative studies usually involve concepts that are well developed and methods of measurement that have been (or can be) developed. For example, a quantitative study might be undertaken to assess whether people with chronic illness are more depressed than people without a chronic illness. There are relatively good measures of depression that would yield quantitative data about the level of depression in those with and without a chronic illness.

Qualitative studies are undertaken because a researcher wants to develop a rich, context-bound understanding of a phenomenon. Qualitative methods would not be well suited to comparing levels of depression among those with and without chronic illness, but they would be ideal for exploring the *meaning* of depression among chronically ill people. In evaluating a research report, one consideration is whether the research problem is suitable for the chosen paradigm.

Sources of Research Problems

Where do ideas for research problems come from? At the most basic level, research topics originate with researchers' interests.

Researchers may be inspired by nurses' clinical experience, readings in the nursing literature, and theories from nursing and other disciplines. Also, topics are sometimes suggested by global, social, or political issues of relevance to the health care community (e.g., health disparities). Additionally, researchers who have developed a *program of research* may get inspiration for "next steps" from their own findings or from a discussion of those findings with others. Because research is a time-consuming enterprise, curiosity about and interest in a topic are essential to a project's success.

Example of a problem source for a quantitative study • • • • • • • • • • • • •
Sawhney is a nurse practitioner and she has developed a strong research interest in pain management for patients who had undergone total knee arthroplasty (TKA). Nerve blocks are commonly used in clinical practice to provide pain relief. Adductor canal (AC) peripheral nerve blocks may be effective to manage pain after TKA, but peri-articular infiltration (PI) of the knee joint has been shown to preserve better motor function. Sawhney (2016) led a research project to compare the two techniques and their effects on pain and postoperative mobilization. The researchers found that participants who received AC block reported significantly higher pain scores at rest and during knee bend than PI.

Development and Refinement of Research Problems

Developing a research problem is a creative process. Researchers often begin with interests in a broad topic area and then develop a more specific researchable problem or question. For example, suppose a hospital nurse begins to wonder why some patients complain about having to wait for pain medication when certain nurses are assigned to them. The general topic is differences in patients' complaints about pain medications. The nurse might ask, Why is there a discrepancy? This broad question may lead to other questions, such as How do the nurses differ? or What are the common characteristics of patients who complained about pain? The nurse may then observe that the ethnic background of the patients and nurses could be relevant. This may direct the nurse to look at the literature on nursing behaviors and ethnicity, or it may lead to a discussion with peers. These efforts may result in several research questions, such as the following:

- What are the major complaints among patients of different ethnic backgrounds?
- Is there a relationship between the nurses' ethnic background and the frequency they dispense pain medication?
- Does the number of patient complaints increase when patients and nurses are of different ethnic backgrounds?

These questions stem from the same problem, yet each would be studied differently; for example, some suggest a qualitative approach, and others suggest a quantitative one. Both ethnicity and nurses' dispensing behaviors are variables that can be measured reliably. A qualitative researcher would be more interested in understanding the *essence* of patients' complaints, patients' *experience* of frustration, or the *process* by which the problem got resolved. These aspects of the problem would be difficult to measure. Researchers choose a problem to study based on its perceived significance and on its fit with a paradigm of preference.

COMMUNICATING RESEARCH PROBLEMS AND QUESTIONS

Every study needs a problem statement that articulates what is problematic and what must be solved. Most research reports also present either a statement of purpose, research questions, or hypotheses, and often combinations of these three elements are included.

Many students do not really understand problem statements and may have trouble identifying them in a research article. A problem statement is presented early and often begins with the first sentence after the abstract. Research questions, purpose statements, or hypotheses appear later in the introduction.

Problem Statements

A good problem statement includes a clear description of what the problem is, what "needs fixing," or what is poorly understood. Problem statements, especially for quantitative studies, often have most of the following six components:

1. *Problem identification:* What is wrong with the current situation?
2. *Background:* What is the nature of the problem, or the context of the situation, that readers need to understand?
3. *Scope of the problem:* How big a problem is it, and how many people are affected?
4. *Consequences of the problem:* What is the cost of *not* fixing the problem?
5. *Knowledge gaps:* What information about the problem is lacking?
6. *Proposed solution:* How will findings of the new study help solve the problem?

Let us suppose that our topic was humor as a complementary therapy for reducing stress in hospitalized patients with cancer. One research question (discussed later in this section) might be "What is the effect of nurses' use of humor on stress and natural killer cell activity in hospitalized cancer patients?" Box 6.1 presents a rough draft of a problem statement for such a study. This problem statement is a reasonable draft, but it could be improved.

Box 6.2 illustrates how the problem statement could be made stronger by adding information about scope (component 3), long-term consequences (component 4), and possible solutions (component 6). This second draft builds a more compelling *argument* for new research: Millions of people are affected by cancer, and the disease has adverse consequences not only for patients and their families but also for society. The revised problem statement also suggests a basis for the new study by describing a possible solution.

 HOW-TO-TELL TIP   How can you tell a problem statement? Problem statements are rarely explicitly labeled. The first sentence of a research report is often the starting point of a problem statement. The problem statement is usually interwoven with findings from the research literature. Prior findings provide a rationale to support the problem statement and highlight gaps in knowledge. In many articles, it is difficult to disentangle the problem statement from the literature review, unless there is a subsection specifically labeled "Literature Review" or something similar.

Box 6.1 Draft Problem Statement on Humor and Stress

A diagnosis of cancer is associated with high levels of stress. Sizeable numbers of patients who receive a cancer diagnosis describe feelings of uncertainty, fear, anger, and loss of control. Interpersonal relationships, psychological functioning, and role performance have all been found to suffer following cancer diagnosis and treatment.

A variety of alternative/complementary therapies have been developed in an effort to decrease the harmful effects of cancer-related stress on psychological and physiologic functioning, and resources devoted to these therapies have increased in recent years. However, many of these therapies have not been carefully evaluated to assess their efficacy, safety, or cost effectiveness. For example, the use of humor has been recommended as a therapeutic device to improve quality of life, decrease stress, and perhaps improve immune functioning, but the evidence to justify its advocacy is scant.

> ### Box 6.2 Some Possible Improvements to Problem Statement on Humor and Stress
>
> Each year, thousands of Canadians are diagnosed with cancer, which remains one of the top causes of death among both men and women (Xie, Semenciw, & Mery, 2015).* Numerous studies have documented that a diagnosis of cancer is associated with high levels of stress. Sizeable numbers of patients who receive a cancer diagnosis describe feelings of uncertainty, fear, anger, and loss of control (Richardson, et al., 2017). Interpersonal relationships, psychological functioning, and role performance have all been found to suffer following cancer diagnosis and treatment (citations). These stressful outcomes can, in turn, adversely affect health, long-term prognosis, and medical costs among cancer survivors (citations).
>
> A variety of alternative/complementary therapies have been developed in an effort to decrease the harmful effects of cancer-related stress on psychological and physiologic functioning, and resources devoted to these therapies (money and staff) have increased in recent years (Onishi, 2016). However, many of these therapies have not been carefully evaluated to determine their efficacy, safety, or cost-effectiveness. For example, the use of humor has been recommended as a therapeutic device to improve quality of life, decrease stress, and perhaps improve immune functioning (Beach & Prickett, 2017), but the evidence to justify its advocacy is scant. Preliminary findings from a recent small-scale endocrinology study with a healthy sample exposed to a humorous intervention (citation), however, hold promise for further inquiry with immunocompromised populations.

*Reference citations would be inserted to support the statements.

Problem statements for a qualitative study similarly express the nature of the problem, its context, its scope, and information needed to address it. The statements often incorporate terms and concepts that suggest the research tradition. For example, a problem statement for a phenomenologic study might note the need to know more about people's experiences or meanings they attribute to those experiences.

Statements of Purpose

Many researchers discuss their research goals as a statement of purpose. The purpose statement establishes the general direction of the inquiry and captures the study's substance. It is usually easy to identify a purpose statement because the word *purpose* is explicitly stated: "The purpose of this study was ..."—although sometimes the words *aim*, *goal*, or *objective* are used instead, as in "The aim of this study was ...."

In a quantitative study, a statement of purpose identifies the key study variables and their possible interrelationships as well as the population of interest (i.e., all the PICO elements).

Example of a statement of purpose from a quantitative study • • • • • • • •
The purpose of this study was to examine the effects of an education–support intervention delivered in home settings to people with chronic heart failure, in terms of their functional status, self-efficacy, quality of life, and self-care ability (Clark et al., 2015).

This purpose statement identifies the population (P) of interest as patients with heart failure living at home. The key study variables were the patients' exposure or nonexposure to the special intervention (the independent variable encompassing the I and C components) and the patient's functional status, self-efficacy, quality of life, and self-care ability (the dependent variables or Os).

In qualitative studies, the statement of purpose indicates the nature of the inquiry; the key concept or phenomenon; and the group, community, or setting under study.

Example of a statement of purpose from a qualitative study • • • • • • • • •
The aim of this study was to examine the experiences of access to primary health care by African immigrant and refugee families in Manitoba.

(Woodgate et al., 2017)

This statement indicates that the group under study is African immigrant and refugee families and the central phenomenon is the immigrants' experiences in their quest to access primary health care in Canada.

Researchers often communicate information about their approach through their choice of words. A study whose purpose is to *explore* or *describe* some phenomenon is likely to be an investigation of a little-researched topic, often involving a qualitative approach such as phenomenology or ethnography. A statement of purpose for a qualitative study—especially a grounded theory study—may also use words such as *understand*, *discover*, or *generate*. Statements of purpose in qualitative studies also may "encode" the tradition of inquiry through certain terms or "buzz words" associated with those traditions, as follows:

- *Grounded theory:* processes; social structures; social interactions
- *Phenomenologic studies:* experience; lived experience; meaning; essence
- *Ethnographic studies:* culture; roles; lifeways; cultural behavior

Quantitative researchers also use certain words to communicate the nature of the inquiry. A statement indicating that the study purpose is to *test* or *evaluate* something (e.g., an intervention) suggests an experimental design, for example. A study whose purpose is to *examine* or *explore* the relationship between two variables is more likely to involve a non-experimental design. Sometimes the word is ambiguous: If a purpose statement states that the researcher's intent is to *compare* two things, the comparison could involve alternative treatments (using an experimental design) or two pre-existing groups such as smokers and nonsmokers (using a nonexperimental design). In any event, words such as *test*, *evaluate*, and *compare* suggest quantifiable variables and designs with scientific controls.

A purpose statement should use language that communicates neutrality and objectivity. A study goal that is written to *prove*, *demonstrate*, or *show* something suggests a bias.

Research Questions

Research questions are, in some cases, direct rewordings of statements of purpose, phrased as a question rather than a statement, as in the following example:

- *Purpose:* The purpose of this study is to assess the relationship between the functional dependence level of renal transplant recipients and their rate of recovery.
- *Question:* What is the relationship between the functional dependence level (I) of renal transplant recipients (P) and their rate of recovery (O)?

Some research articles omit a statement of purpose and state only research questions, but in many cases, the opposite is true. Some researchers use research questions to add greater clarity to a global purpose statement.

Research Questions in Quantitative Studies

In Chapter 2, we discussed clinical foreground questions to guide an EBP inquiry. The EBP question templates in Table 2.1 could guide a research project as well, but *researchers* design their questions in terms of their *variables*. Take, for example, the first question in Table 2.1:

"In (population), what is the effect of (intervention) on (outcome)?"A researcher would be more likely to think of the question in these terms: "In (population), what is the effect of (independent variable) on (dependent variable)?" Thinking in terms of variables helps to guide researchers' decisions about how to operationalize or define them. Thus, in quantitative studies, research questions identify the population (P) under study, the key study variables (I, C, and O components), and relationships among the variables.

Most research questions concern relationships among variables, and thus, many quantitative research questions could be written using a general question template: "In (population), what is the relationship between (independent variable or IV) and (dependent variable or DV)?" Examples of variations include the following:

- *Treatment, intervention:* In (population), what is the effect of (IV: intervention vs. an alternative) on (DV)?
- *Prognosis:* In (population), does (IV: disease or illness vs. its absence) affect or increase the risk of (DV)?
- *Etiology/harm:* In (population), does (IV: exposure vs. nonexposure) cause or increase risk of (DV)?

Not all research questions are about relationships—some are descriptive. As examples, here are two descriptive questions that could be answered in a quantitative study on nurses' use of humor:

- How often do nurses use humor as a complementary therapy with hospitalized cancer patients?
- What are the characteristics of nurses who use humor as a complementary therapy with hospitalized cancer patients?

Answers to such questions might be useful in developing effective strategies for reducing stress in patients with cancer.

Example of a research question from a quantitative study • • • • • • • • • • •
Scott and colleagues (2017) undertook a study that addressed the following question: Is there a relationship between sexual orientation and depression in the Canadian population?

In this example, the question asks about the relationship between an independent variable (sexual orientation) and a dependent variable (depression) in Canadians living in the 10 provinces.

Research Questions in Qualitative Studies

Research questions in qualitative studies stipulate the phenomenon and the population of interest. Grounded theory researchers are likely to ask *process* questions, phenomenologists tend to ask *meaning* questions, and ethnographers generally ask *descriptive* questions about cultures. The terms associated with the various traditions, discussed previously in connection with purpose statements, are likely to be incorporated into the research questions.

Example of a research question from a phenomenologic study • • • • • • • • •
What is the lived experience of intensive care for critically ill patients who experienced delirium?

(Whitehorne et al., 2015)

Not all qualitative studies are linked to a specific research tradition. Many researchers use constructivist methods to describe or explore phenomena without focusing on cultures, meaning, or social processes.

Example of a research question from a descriptive qualitative study • • • • •
In their descriptive qualitative study, Girard et al. (2016) explored actual activities carried out by primary care nurses for **patients with chronic disease and mental disorders** in the Province of Quebec. **Participants described five types of activities: assessment, care planning, interprofessional collaboration, therapeutic relationship, and health promotion.**

In qualitative studies, research questions may change during the study. Researchers begin with a *focus* that defines the broad boundaries of the inquiry, but the boundaries are not cast in stone. The question can be modified as new information makes it relevant to do so.

 TIP Researchers most often state their purpose or research questions at the end of the introduction or immediately after the review of the literature. Sometimes, a separate section of a research article is devoted to formal statements about the research problem formally and might be labeled "Purpose," "Statement of Purpose," "Research Questions," or, in quantitative studies, "Hypotheses."

RESEARCH HYPOTHESES

A hypothesis is a prediction, usually involving a predicted relationship between two or more variables. Qualitative researchers do not have formal hypotheses because qualitative researchers want the inquiry to be guided by participants' viewpoints rather than by their own hunches. The following discussion focuses on hypotheses in quantitative research.

Function of Hypotheses in Quantitative Research

Many research questions ask about relationships between variables, and hypotheses are predicted answers to these questions. For instance, the research question might ask, "Does sexual abuse in childhood affect the development of irritable bowel syndrome in women?" The researcher might predict the following: Women (P) who were sexually abused in childhood (I) have a higher incidence of irritable bowel syndrome (O) than women who were not abused (C).

Hypotheses are sometimes informed by a theory. Scientists reason from theories to *generate hypotheses that are tested in the real world* (Chapter 8). Even in the absence of a theory, hypotheses offer direction and suggest explanations. For example, suppose we hypothesized that the incidence of desaturation in low–birth-weight infants undergoing intubation and ventilation would be lower using the closed tracheal suction system (CTSS) than using partially ventilated endotracheal suction (PVETS). Our hypothesis might be based on prior studies or clinical observations.

Now let us suppose the hypothesis is not confirmed in a study—that is, we find that rates of desaturation are similar for both the PVETS and CTSS methods. *The failure of data to support a prediction forces researchers to analyze theory or previous research critically, to review study limitations, and to explore alternative explanations for the findings.* The use of hypotheses tends to promote critical thinking. Now suppose we conducted the study guided only by the question, Is there a relationship between suction method and rates of desaturation? Without a hypothesis, the researcher is seemingly prepared to accept any results. The problem is that it is almost always possible to explain something superficially after the fact, no matter what the findings are. Hypotheses reduce the possibility that any results will be misinterpreted as meaningful.

Characteristics of Testable Hypotheses

Research hypotheses usually state the expected relationship between the independent variable (the presumed cause or influence) and the dependent variable (the presumed outcome or effect) within a population.

Example of a research hypothesis •
Castonguay and colleagues (2017) studied breast cancer survivors' engagement in vigorous intensity physical activities. They hypothesized that body-related shame would predict low levels of activities over time; in contrast, feelings of guilt would be associated with physical activities. Only body-related shame was a significant predictor.

In this example, the population is breast cancer survivors. The IVs are body-related shame and guilt, and the outcome variable is participation in vigorous exercise. The hypothesis predicts that body-related shame and guilt are related to rates of exercise participation.

Hypotheses that do not make a relational statement are difficult to test. Take the following example: *Pregnant women who receive prenatal instruction about postpartum experiences are not likely to experience postpartum depression.* This statement expresses no anticipated relationship and cannot be tested using standard statistical procedures. In our example, how would we decide whether to accept or reject the hypothesis?

We could, however, modify the hypothesis as follows: Pregnant women who receive prenatal instruction are less likely than those who do not to experience postpartum depression. Here, the outcome variable (O) is postpartum depression, and the IV is receipt (I) versus nonreceipt (C) of prenatal instruction. The relational aspect of the prediction is embodied in the phrase *less than*. If a hypothesis lacks a phrase such as *more than, less than, different from, related to,* or something similar, it is not testable. To test the revised hypothesis, we could ask two groups of women with different prenatal instruction experiences to respond to questions on depression and then compare the groups' responses.

Wording of Hypotheses

Hypotheses can be stated in various ways, as in the following example:

1. Older patients are more likely to fall than younger patients.
2. There is a relationship between a patient's age and the likelihood of falling.
3. The risk of falling increases with the age of the patient.
4. Older patients differ from younger ones with respect to their risk of falling.

In each example, the hypothesis states the population (patients), the IV (age), the outcome variable (falling), and an anticipated relationship between them.

Hypotheses can be either directional or nondirectional. A **directional hypothesis** specifies the expected direction of the relationship between variables. In the four versions of the hypothesis, versions 1 and 3 are directional because they predict that older patients are more likely to fall than younger ones. A **nondirectional hypothesis** does not specify the direction of the relationship (versions 2 and 4). These versions predict that a patient's age and falling are related but do not indicate whether *older* or *younger* patients are predicted to be at greater risk.

 TIP Hypotheses can be either *simple hypotheses* (with a single independent variable and dependent variable) or *complex* (multiple independent or dependent variables). Information about this differentiation is available on the supplement to this chapter on thePoint website.

Another distinction is between research and null hypotheses. **Research hypotheses** are statements of expected relationships between variables. All the hypotheses presented thus far are research hypotheses that indicate actual expectations.

Statistical inference operates on a logic that may be counterintuitive. This logic requires that hypotheses be expressed to indicate the *absence* of a relationship. **Null hypotheses** state that there is no relationship between the independent and dependent variables. The null form of the hypothesis in our preceding example would be "Older patients are just as likely as younger patients to fall." The null hypothesis can be compared with the assumption of innocence in many systems of criminal justice. The variables are assumed to be "innocent" of a relationship until they can be shown "guilty" through statistical tests.

Research articles typically state research rather than null hypotheses. In statistical testing, underlying null hypotheses are assumed, without being stated.

 TIP If a researcher uses statistical tests (which is true in most quantitative studies), it means that there are underlying hypotheses—regardless of whether the researcher explicitly stated them—because statistical tests are designed to test hypotheses.

Hypothesis Testing and Proof

Hypotheses are formally tested through statistical analysis. Researchers use statistics to test whether their hypotheses have a high probability of being correct (i.e., has a probability less than 5% or less than 0.05, that the observed findings or the research hypothesis would have occurred by chance, supporting the decision to reject the null hypothesis). Statistical analysis does not offer proof; it only supports inferences that a hypothesis is *probably* correct (or not). Hypotheses are never *proved* or *disproved*; rather, they are *supported* or *rejected*. Hypotheses come to be increasingly supported with evidence from multiple studies.

To illustrate why this is so, suppose we hypothesized that height and weight are related. We predict that, on average, tall people weigh more than short people. Suppose we happened by chance to get a sample of short, heavy people and tall, thin people. Our results might indicate that there is no relationship between a person's height and weight, but we would not be reasonable in concluding that the study *proved* or *demonstrated* that height and weight are unrelated.

This example illustrates the difficulty of using observations from a sample to generalize to a population. Other issues, such as the accuracy of the measures and the effects of uncontrolled variables prevent researchers from concluding that hypotheses are proved.

CRITIQUING RESEARCH PROBLEMS, RESEARCH QUESTIONS, AND HYPOTHESES

In a comprehensive critique of a research article, you would evaluate whether researchers have adequately communicated their research problem. The problem statement, purpose,

> **Box 6.3 Guidelines for Critiquing Research Problems, Research Questions, and Hypotheses**
>
> 1. What was the research problem? Was the problem statement easy to locate and was it clearly stated? Did the problem statement build a cogent and persuasive argument for the new study?
> 2. Does the problem have significance for nursing?
> 3. Was there a good fit between the research problem and the paradigm (and tradition) within which the research was conducted?
> 4. Did the report formally present a statement of purpose, research question, and/or hypotheses? Was this information communicated clearly and concisely, and was it placed in a logical and useful location?
> 5. Were purpose statements or research questions worded appropriately (e.g., Were key concepts/variables identified and the population specified?)
> 6. If there were no formal hypotheses, was their absence justified? Were statistical tests used in analyzing the data despite the absence of stated hypotheses?
> 7. Were hypotheses (if any) properly worded—did they state a predicted relationship between two or more variables? Were they presented as research or as null hypotheses?

research questions, and hypotheses set the stage for describing what was done and what was learned. You should not have to dig too deeply to figure out the research problem or discover the questions.

A critique of the research problem involves multiple dimensions. Substantively, you need to consider whether the problem has significance for nursing. Studies that build on existing evidence in a meaningful way can make contributions to EBP. Also, research problems that address research priorities (Chapter 1) have a high likelihood of providing important evidence for nurses.

Another dimension in critiquing the research problem concerns methodologic issues—in particular, whether the research problem is compatible with the chosen research paradigm and its associated methods. You should also evaluate whether the statement of purpose or research questions provide clues to research inquiry.

If a research article describing a quantitative study does not state hypotheses, you should consider whether their absence is justified. If there are hypotheses, you should evaluate whether the hypotheses are sensible and consistent with existing evidence or relevant theory. Also, hypotheses are valid guideposts in scientific inquiry only if they are testable. To be testable, hypotheses must predict a relationship between two or more measurable variables.

Specific guidelines for critiquing research problems, research questions, and hypotheses are presented in Box 6.3.

RESEARCH EXAMPLES WITH CRITICAL THINKING EXERCISES

This section describes how the research problem and research questions were communicated in two nursing studies, one quantitative and one qualitative. Read the summaries and then answer the critical thinking questions that follow, referring to the full research report if necessary. Exercises 1 and 2 are featured on the interactive *Critical Thinking Activity* on website. The critical thinking questions for Exercises 3 and 4 are based on the studies that appear in their entirety in Appendices A and B of this book. Our comments for these exercises are in the Student Resources section on thePoint.

EXAMPLE 1: QUANTITATIVE RESEARCH

Study: Association of maternal and infant salivary testosterone and cortisol and infant gender with mother–infant interaction in very low–birth-weight infants (Cho et al., 2015).

Problem Statement (excerpt): "Prematurity-related health and developmental problems are more common in male VLBW (very low–birth weight, less than 1,500 g) infants than in females.... Furthermore, male VLBW infants experience less positive mother–infant interactions than females do. These associations raise important questions about whether the vulnerability of male VLBW infants to suboptimal mother–infant interactions is due to factors beyond gender socialization.... Based on the association of elevated testosterone in infants.... with negative cognitive and behavioral outcomes and of high or low cortisol with infant health and development, both hormones may affect mother–infant interactions" (pp. 357–359).

Statement of Purpose: "The purpose of this...study was to examine possible associations between these steroid hormonal levels and mother–VLBW-infant interactions and their potential importance for gender differences" (p. 359).

Research Questions: One of the research questions for this study was "Are elevated levels of salivary testosterone and cortisol negatively associated with the quality of mother–VLBW infant interactions at 3 and 6 months?" (p. 359).

Hypothesis: "We hypothesized that the levels of testosterone and cortisol in VLBW infants would be negatively associated with mother–infant interactions, especially among male infants" (p. 359).

Study Methods: The study participants were 62 mother–VLBW infant pairs recruited from a level IV neonatal intensive care unit. Data were collected through infant record review, interviews with the mothers, biochemical measurements of both mothers and infants, and observation of mother–infant interactions at 40 weeks' postmenstrual age and at 3 and 6 months corrected age.

Key Findings: Higher maternal testosterone and infant cortisol were associated with more positive and more frequent maternal interactive behaviors. Mothers interacted with their infants more frequently when the infants had lower levels of testosterone.

Critical Thinking Exercises

1. Answer the relevant questions from Box 6.3 regarding this study.
2. Also consider the following targeted questions:
   a. Where in the research report do you think the researchers presented the hypotheses? Where in the report would the results of the hypothesis tests be placed?
   b. Was the stated hypothesis directional or nondirectional?
   c. Was the researchers' hypothesis supported in the statistical analysis?
3. If the results of this study are valid and generalizable, what are some of the uses to which the findings might be put in clinical practice?

EXAMPLE 2: QUALITATIVE RESEARCH

Study: Adolescent and young adult survivors of childhood brain tumours: Life after treatment in their own words (Hobbie et al., 2016).

Problem Statement (excerpt): "Although 5-year survival rates for children diagnosed with brain tumours have improved to 75%, survivors report late effects that can be acute or long term, episodic, or progressive.... Gaps exist in evidence regarding the perspectives of AYA (adolescents and young adults) regarding their HRQOL (health-related quality of life)...To date, there are few studies that examine the perspectives of AYA survivors of childhood brain tumours in terms of their sense of self and their role in their families" (p. 135).

Statement of Purpose: "The aim of this study was to describe how adolescent and young adult survivors of childhood brain tumours describe their health-related quality of life—that is, their physical, emotional, and social functioning" (p. 134).

Research Question: "We specifically asked: How do AYA survivors of childhood brain tumours describe their HRQOL (physical, emotional, and social functioning)?" (p. 135).

Method: The researchers recruited a sample of 41 adolescents and young adult survivors of a childhood brain tumour, who were living with their families. In-depth interviews were conducted in a private setting at the homes of study participants. Participants were asked several conversational questions, such as "Tell me about yourself" and "What parts of your life are most challenging?"

Key Findings: The researchers found that the survivors struggled for normalcy in the face of changed functioning due to their cancer and the late effects of their treatment.

Critical Thinking Exercises

1. Answer the relevant questions from Box 6.3 regarding this study.
2. Also consider the following targeted questions:
   a. Where in the research report do you think the researchers presented the statement of purpose and research questions?
   b. Does it appear that this study was conducted within one of the three main qualitative traditions? If so, which one?
3. If the results of this study are trustworthy, what are some of the uses to which the findings might be put in clinical practice?

EXAMPLE 3: QUANTITATIVE RESEARCH IN APPENDIX A

- Read the abstract and introduction of Swenson and colleagues' (2016) study ("Parents' use of praise and criticism in a sample of young children seeking mental health services") in Appendix A of this book.

Critical Thinking Exercises

1. Answer the relevant questions from Box 6.3 regarding this study.
2. Also answer the following question: What might a hypothesis for this study be? State it as a research hypothesis and as a null hypothesis.

EXAMPLE 4: QUALITATIVE RESEARCH IN APPENDIX B

● Read the abstract and introduction of Beck and Watson's (2010) study ("Subsequent childbirth after a previous traumatic birth") in Appendix B of this book.

Critical Thinking Exercises

1. Answer the relevant questions from Box 6.3 regarding this study.

2. Also consider the following targeted questions:

   a. Do you think that Beck and Watson provided a sufficient rationale for the significance of their research problem?

   b. In their argument for their study, did Beck and Watson say anything about the fourth element of an argument identified in the book—that is, the consequences of the problem?

WANT TO KNOW MORE? ☀

A wide variety of resources to enhance your learning and understanding of this chapter are available on thePoint.

- Interactive Critical Thinking Activity
- Chapter Supplement on Simple and Complex Hypotheses
- Answers to the Critical Thinking Exercises for Examples 3 and 4
- Internet Resources with useful websites for Chapter 6
- A Wolters Kluwer journal article on a topic related to this chapter

---

Summary Points

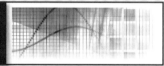

- A **research problem** is a perplexing or troubling situation that a researcher wants to address through disciplined inquiry.
- Researchers usually identify a broad *topic*, narrow the scope of the problem, and then identify research questions consistent with a paradigm of choice.
- Researchers communicate their aims in research articles as problem statements, statements of purpose, research questions, or hypotheses.
- The **problem statement** articulates the nature, context, and significance of a problem to be studied. Problem statements typically include several components: problem identification; background, scope, and consequences of the problem; knowledge gaps; and possible solutions to the problem.
- A **statement of purpose,** which summarizes the overall study goal, identifies the key concepts (variables) and the study group or population. Purpose statements often communicate, through the choice of verbs and other key terms, aspects of the study design or the research tradition.
- **Research questions** are the specific queries researchers want to answer in addressing the research problem.
- A **hypothesis** states predicted relationships between two or more variables—that is, the anticipated association between independent and dependent variables.

- **Directional hypotheses** predict the direction of a relationship; **nondirectional hypotheses** predict the existence of relationships, not their direction.
- **Research hypotheses** predict the existence of relationships; **null hypotheses**, which express the absence of a relationship, are the hypotheses subjected to statistical testing.
- Hypotheses are never proved or disproved—they are accepted or rejected, supported or not supported by the data.

REFERENCES

Beck, C. T., & Watson, S. (2010). Subsequent childbirth after a previous traumatic birth. *Nursing Research*, 59(4), 241–249.

Beach, W. A., & Prickett, E. (2016). Laughter, humor, and cancer: Delicate moments and poignant interactional circumstances. *Health Communication*, 32(7), 791–802.

Castonguay, A. L., Wrosch, C., Pila, E., & Sabiston, C. M. (2017). Body-Related Shame and Guilt Predict Physical Activity in Breast Cancer Survivors Over Time. *Oncology Nursing Forum*, 44(4), 465–475.

Cho, J., Su, X., Phillips, V., & Holditch-Davis, D. (2015). Association of maternal and infant salivary testosterone and cortisol and infant gender with mother-infant interaction in very-low-birthweight infants. *Research in Nursing & Health*, 38, 357–368.

*Clark, A., McDougall, G., Riegel, B., et al. (2015). Health status and self-care outcomes after an education-support intervention for people with chronic heart failure. *Journal of Cardiovascular Nursing*, 30, S3–S13.

Girard, A., Hudon, C., Poitras, M. E., Roberge, P., & Chouinard, M. C. (2016). Primary care nursing activities with patients affected by physical chronic disease and common mental disorders: A qualitative descriptive study. *Journal of Clinical Nursing*, 26(9–10), 1385–1394.

**Hobbie, W., Ogle, S., Reilly, M., et al. (2016). Adolescent and young adult survivors of childhood brain tumors: Life after treatment in their own words. *Cancer Nursing*, 39, 134–143.

Judge, M., Beck, C. T., Durham, H., McKelvey, M., & Lammi-Keefe, C. (2014). Pilot trial evaluating maternal docosahexaenoic acid consumption during pregnancy: Decreased postpartum depressive symptomatology. *International Journal of Nursing Sciences*, 1, 339–345.

Onishi K. (2016). Complementary therapy for cancer survivors: Integrative nursing care. *Asia Pacific Journal of Oncology Nursing*, 3(1), 41–44.

Richardson, E. M., Scott, J. L., Schüz, N., Sanderson, K., & Schüz, B. (2017). Qualitatively comparing the support needs of people with cancer based on their history of anxiety/depression. *Oncology and Therapy*, 5(1), 41–51.

Sawhney, M., Mehdian, H., Kashin, B., et al. (2016). Pain After Unilateral Total Knee Arthroplasty: A Prospective Randomized Controlled Trial Examining the Analgesic Effectiveness of a Combined Adductor Canal Peripheral Nerve Block with Periarticular Infiltration Versus Adductor Canal Nerve Block Alone Versus Periarticular Infiltration Alone. *Anesthesia & Analgesia*, 122(6), 2040–2046.

Scott, R. L., Lasiuk, G., Norris, C. M. (2017). Sexual orientation and depression in Canada. *Canadian Journal of Public Health*, 107(6), e545–e549.

*Swall, A., Ebbeskog, B., Lundh Hagelin, C., & Fagerberg, I. (2015). Can therapy dogs evoke awareness of one's past and present life in persons with Alzheimer's disease? *International Journal of Older People Nursing*, 10, 84–93.

Swenson, S., Ho, G. W., Budhathoki, C., et al. (2016). Parents' Use of Praise and Criticism in a Sample of Young Children Seeking Mental Health Services. *Journal of Pediatric Health Care*, 30(1), 49–56.

*Thomas, T., Blumling, A., & Delaney, A. (2015). The influence of religiosity and spirituality on rural parents' health decision-making and human papillomavirus vaccine choices. *Advances in Nursing Science*, 38, E1–E12.

Whitehorne, K., Gaudine, A., Meadus, R., & Solberg, S. (2015). Lived experience of the intensive care unit for patients who experienced delirium. *Am J Crit Care*, 24(6), 474–479.

Woodgate, R. L., Busolo, D. S., Crockett, M., Dean, R. A., Amaladas, M. R., & Plourde, P. J. (2017). A qualitative study on African immigrant and refugee families' experiences of accessing primary health care services in Manitoba, Canada: It's not easy! *International Journal for Equity in Health*, 16(1), 5.

Xie, L., Semenciw, R., & Mery, L. (2015). Cancer incidence in Canada: Trends and projections (1983-2032). *Health Promotion and Chronic Disease Prevention in Canada*, 35(Suppl 1), 2–186

Yeager, K., Sterk, C., Quest, T., Dilorio, C., Vena, C., & Bauer-Wu, S. (2016). Managing one's symptoms: A qualitative study of low-income African Americans with advanced cancer. *Cancer Nursing*, 39(4), 303–312.

*A link to this open-access article is provided in the Internet Resources section on thePoint website.

**This journal article is available on thePoint for this chapter.

7 | Finding and Reviewing Research Evidence in the Literature

Learning Objectives

On completing this chapter, you will be able to:

- Understand the steps involved in doing a literature review
- Identify bibliographic aids for retrieving nursing research reports and locate references for a research topic
- Understand the process of screening, abstracting, critiquing, and organizing research evidence
- Evaluate the style, content, and organization of a literature review
- Define new terms in the chapter

Key Terms

- Bibliographic database
- CINAHL database
- Google Scholar
- Keyword
- Literature review
- MEDLINE database
- MeSH
- Primary source
- PubMed
- Secondary source

A **literature review** is a written summary of evidence on a research problem. It is useful for consumers of nursing research to acquire skills for reading, critiquing, and preparing written evidence summaries.

BASIC ISSUES RELATING TO LITERATURE REVIEWS

Before discussing the activities involved in undertaking a research-based literature review, we briefly discuss some general issues. The first concerns the purposes of doing a literature review.

Purposes of Research Literature Reviews

The primary purpose of literature reviews is to summarize evidence on a topic—to sum up what is known and what is not known. Literature reviews are sometimes stand-alone reports intended to communicate the state of evidence to others, but reviews are also used to lay the foundation for new studies and to help researchers interpret their findings.

In qualitative research, there are different opinions regarding literature reviews. Grounded theory researchers typically begin to collect data before examining the literature. As a theory takes shape, researchers turn to the literature to see how prior findings relate to the theory. Phenomenologists and ethnographers often undertake a literature search at the outset of a study.

Regardless of when they perform the review, researchers usually include a brief summary of relevant literature in their introductions. The literature review summarizes current evidence on a topic and explains the significance of the new study. Literature reviews will often contain the problem statement as part of the argument for the study.

Types of Information to Seek for a Research Review

Findings from previous studies are used for a research review. If you are preparing a literature review, you should rely mostly on **primary sources**, which are original descriptions of studies written by the researchers who conducted them. **Secondary source** research documents are descriptions of studies prepared by someone else. Literature reviews are secondary sources. Recent reviews are a good place to start because they offer an overview and a valuable bibliography. If you are doing your own literature review, however, secondary sources should not substitute for primary sources because secondary sources do not provide sufficient detail and may not be completely objective.

 TIP For an evidence-based practice (EBP) project, a recent, high-quality systematic review may be sufficient to provide the needed information about the evidence base, although it is usually a good idea to search for studies published after the review. We provide more explicit guidance on searching for evidence for an EBP query in the Chapter Supplement on thePoint website.

A literature search may yield non-research references, including opinion articles, case reports, and clinical anecdotes. Such materials may broaden the understanding of a problem or demonstrate a need for research. These writings, however, may have limited utility in research reviews because they do not address the central question: What is the current state of *evidence* on this research problem?

Major Steps and Strategies in Doing a Literature Review

Conducting a literature review is a little bit like doing a study: A reviewer starts with a question and then must gather, analyse, and interpret the information. Figure 7.1 depicts the literature review process and shows that there are potential feedback loops, with opportunities to go back to earlier steps in search of more information.

Reviews should be unbiased, thorough, and up-to-date. Also, high-quality reviews are systematic. Decision rules for including a study should be explicit because a good review

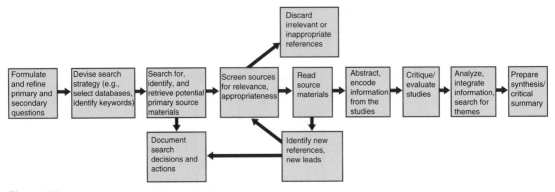

Figure 7.1 Flow of tasks in a literature review.

should be reproducible. This means that another diligent reviewer would be able to apply the same decision rules and come to similar conclusions about the state of evidence on the topic.

> **TIP** Locating all relevant information on a research question is like being a detective. The literature retrieval tools we discuss in this chapter are helpful, but there is still a need to do some digging for, and sifting of, the clues to evidence on a topic.

Doing a literature review is in some ways similar to undertaking a qualitative study. It is useful to have a flexible approach to "data collection" and to think creatively about opportunities for new sources of information.

LOCATING RELEVANT LITERATURE FOR A RESEARCH REVIEW

An early step in a literature review is developing a strategy to locate relevant studies. The ability to locate evidence on a topic is an important skill that requires adaptability—rapid technologic changes mean that new methods of searching the literature are introduced continuously. We urge you to consult with librarians or faculty at your institution for updated suggestions.

Developing a Search Strategy

Having good search skills is important. A particular productive approach is to search for evidence in bibliographic databases, which we discuss next. Reviewers also use the *ancestry approach* ("footnote chasing"), using citations from relevant studies to track down earlier research (the "ancestors"). A third strategy, the *descendancy approach*, involves finding a pivotal early study and searching forward to find more recent studies ("descendants") that cited the key study.

> **TIP** You may be tempted to begin a literature search through an Internet search engine, such as Yahoo, Google, or Bing. Such a search is likely to yield a lot of "hits" on your topic but is unlikely to give you full bibliographic information on *research* literature on your topic.

Decisions must also be made about limiting the search. For example, reviewers may constrain their search to reports written in one language. You may also want to limit your search to studies conducted within a certain time frame (e.g., within the past 10 years).

Searching Bibliographic Databases

Bibliographic databases are accessed by computer. Most databases can be accessed through user-friendly software with menu-driven systems and on-screen support so that minimal instruction is needed to generate a list of appropriate citations. Your school or hospital library probably has subscriptions to these services.

Getting Started With an Electronic Search

Before searching a bibliographic database electronically, you should become familiar with the features of the software you are using to access it. The software has options for restricting or expanding your search, combining two searches, saving your search, and so on. Most programmes have tutorials, and most also have Help buttons.

An early task in an electronic search is identifying keywords to launch the search (although an *author search* for prominent researchers in a field is also possible). A **keyword** is a word or phrase that captures key concepts in your question. For quantitative studies, the keywords are usually the independent or dependent variables (i.e., at a minimum, the "I" and "O" of the PICO components) and perhaps the population. For qualitative studies, the keywords are the central phenomenon and the population. If you use the question templates for asking clinical questions in Table 2.1, the words you enter in the blanks are likely to be good keywords.

 TIP   If you want to identify all research reports on a topic, you need to be flexible and to think broadly about keywords. For example, if you are interested in anorexia, you might look up *anorexia, eating disorders,* and *weight loss,* and perhaps *appetite, eating behaviour, food habits, bulimia,* and *body weight changes.*

There are various search approaches for a bibliographic search. All citations in a database have to be coded so they can be retrieved. Each database and programme uses their own indexing systems that use specific *subject headings* (subject codes) to categorize entries.

You can undertake a *subject search* by entering a subject heading into the search field. You do not have to worry about knowing the subject codes because most software has mapping capabilities. *Mapping* is a feature that allows you to search for topics using your own keywords rather than the exact subject heading used in the database. The software translates ("maps") your keywords into the most plausible subject heading and then retrieves citation records that have been coded with that subject heading.

When you enter a keyword into the search field, the programme likely will launch both a subject search and a textword search. A *textword search* looks for your keyword in the text fields of the records, that is, in the title and the abstract. Thus, if you searched for *lung cancer* in the MEDLINE database (which we describe in a subsequent section), the search would retrieve citations coded for the subject code of *lung neoplasms* (the MEDLINE subject heading used to code entries) and also any entries in which the words *lung cancer* appeared, even if it had not been coded for the *lung neoplasm* subject heading.

Some features of an electronic search are similar across databases. One feature is that you usually can use *Boolean operators* to expand or delimit a search. Three widely used Boolean operators are AND, OR, and NOT (in all caps). The operator *AND* restricts a search. If we searched for *pain AND children,* the software would retrieve only records that have both terms. The operator *OR* expands the search: *pain OR children* could be used in a search to retrieve records with either term. Finally, *NOT* narrows a search: *pain NOT children* would retrieve all records with pain that did not include the term *children.*

Wildcard and truncation symbols are other useful tools. A *truncation symbol* (often an asterisk, *) expands a search term to include all forms of a root. For example, a search for *child** would instruct the computer to search for any word that begins with "child" such as children, childhood, or childrearing. In some databases, *wildcard symbols* (often ? or *) inserted in the middle of a search term permits a search for alternative spellings. For example, a search for *behavio?r* would retrieve records with either *behavior* or *behaviour.* For each database, it is important to learn what these special symbols are and how they work. Note that the use of special symbols, while useful, may turn off a software's mapping feature.

One way to force a textword search is to use quotation marks around a phrase, which yields citations in which the exact phrase appears in text fields. In other words, *lung cancer* and "lung cancer" might yield different results. A thorough search strategy might entail doing a search with and without wildcard characters and with and without quotation marks.

Two especially useful electronic databases for nurses are CINAHL (**C**umulative **I**ndex to **N**ursing and **A**llied **H**ealth **L**iterature) and MEDLINE (**Med**ical Literature On-**Line**), which we discuss in the next sections. We also briefly discuss Google Scholar. Other useful bibliographic databases for nurses include the Cochrane Database of Systematic Reviews, Web of Knowledge, Scopus, and EMBASE (the Excerpta Medica database). The Web of Knowledge database is useful for a descendancy search strategy because of its strong citation indexes.

 TIP If your goal is to conduct a *systematic* review, you will need to establish an explicit formal plan about your search strategy and keywords, as discussed in Chapter 18.

The CINAHL Database

CINAHL is an important electronic database for nurses. It covers references to hundreds of nursing and allied health journals as well as to books and dissertations. CINAHL contains about three million records.

CINAHL provides information for locating references (i.e., the author, title, journal, year of publication, volume, and page numbers) and abstracts for most citations. Links to actual articles are often provided. We illustrate features of CINAHL but note that some features may be different at your institution and changes are introduced periodically.

A "basic search" in CINAHL involves entering keywords in the search field (more options for expanding and limiting the search are available in the "Advanced Search" mode). You can restrict your search to records with certain features (e.g., only ones with abstracts), to specific publication dates (e.g., only those after 2010), to those published in English, or to those coded as being in a certain subset (e.g., nursing). The basic search screen also allows you to expand the search by clicking the option "Apply related words."

To illustrate with a concrete example, suppose we were interested in research on the effect of music on agitation in people with dementia. We entered the following terms in the search field and placed only one limit on the search—only records with abstracts:

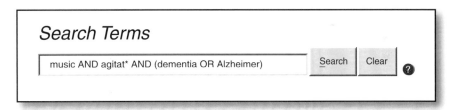

```
Search Terms

  music AND agitat* AND (dementia OR Alzheimer)     Search   Clear   ?
```

By clicking the Search button, we got dozens of "hits" (citations). Note that we used two Boolean operators. The use of "AND" ensured that retrieved records had to include all three keywords, and the use of "OR" allowed either dementia or Alzheimer to be the third keyword. Also, we used a truncation symbol * in the second keyword. This instructed the computer to search for any word that begins with "agitat" such as agitated or agitation.

By clicking the Search button, all of the identified references would be displayed on the monitor, and we could view and print full information for ones that seemed promising. An example of a shortened CINAHL record entry for this search report is presented in Figure 7.2. The title of the article and author information is displayed, followed by source information. The source indicates the following:

- Name of the journal (*Geriatric Nursing*)
- Year and month of publication (Jan/Feb 2016)
- Volume (37)
- Issue (1)
- Page numbers (25–29)

Title:	A personalized multimedia device to treat **agitated** behavior and improve mood in people with **dementia**: A pilot study
Authors:	Davison, Tanya E.; Nayer, Kanvar; Coxon, Selby; de Bono, Arthur; Eppingstall, Barbara; Jeon, Yun-Hee; van der Ploeg, Eva S.; O'Connor, Daniel W.
Affiliation:	Department of Psychiatry, Monash University, Australia; Department of Design, Monash University, Australia; Nursing School, University of Sydney, Australia
Source:	Geriatric Nursing (GERIATR NURS), Jan/Feb2016; 37(1): 25-29. (5p)
Major Subjects:	Multimedia -- Utilization -- In Old Age; Dementia -- Therapy -- In Old Age; Agitation -- Therapy -- In Old Age; Therapy, Computer Assisted -- In Old Age
Minor Subjects:	Anxiety -- Therapy; Depression -- Therapy; Aged; Inpatients; Middle Age; Neuropsychological Tests; Scales; Paired T-Tests; Data Analysis Software; Patient Satisfaction; Pilot Studies; Treatment Outcomes; Funding Source
Journal Subset:	Core Nursing; Nursing; Peer Reviewed; **USA**
Abstract:	**Agitated** behaviors and dysphoric moods in nursing home residents with **dementia** may be a response to a lack of personalized, meaningful activity and stimulation. To address this deficiency, a personal computer was adapted to play favorite **music** and display photographs, movies and messages that were selected or made by family members. The system (called Memory Box) is accompanied by a simplified interface to help people with **dementia** access material independently. The system's ability to reduce **agitation**, and improve symptoms of depression and anxiety, was tested by means of an eight-week randomized, single-blinded, cross-over trial comparing Memory Box with a control condition that offered equivalent contact with research staff. Eleven nursing home residents with mild to severe **dementia** and persistent, daily **agitated** behaviors completed the study. Outcome measures included ratings of anxiety, depression and **agitated** behavior made by knowledgeable staff members in collaboration with researchers. Memory Box was well utilized and highly rated by residents, families and staff members. There were significant reductions in depressive and anxiety symptoms during the course of the intervention. The system shows promise as a tool to assist families and nursing home staff to improve the wellbeing of cognitively impaired older people with **agitated** behaviors.
Instrumentation:	Mini-Mental Status Examination (MMSE) (Folstein et al) 38-point Cornell Scale for Depression in **Dementia** (CSDD) 60-point Rating for Anxiety in Dementia (RAID)
MEDLINE Info:	*PMID:* 26412509 *NLM UID:* 8309633
Accession Number:	113169588

Figure 7.2 Example of a printout from a Cumulative Index to Nursing and Allied Health Literature search (CINAHL).

Figure 7.2 also shows the CINAHL major and minor subject headings that were coded for this particular study. Any of these headings could have been used in a subject heading search to retrieve this reference. Note that the subject headings include substantive headings such as *Agitation–Therapy—In Old Age* as well as methodologic (e.g., *Paired T-Tests*) and sample characteristic headings (e.g., *Aged; Inpatients*). The subject terms have hyperlinks so that we could expand the search by clicking on them (we could also click on the author's name or on the journal). The abstract for the study is then presented, with the search terms (music, agitated, agitation, and dementia) bolded. Next, the names of any formal instruments used in the study are printed under "Instrumentation." Based on the abstract, we would then decide whether this reference was pertinent to our inquiry. Note that there is also a sidebar link in each record called *Times Cited in this Database*, which would retrieve records for articles that had cited this paper (for a descendancy search).

The MEDLINE Database

The **MEDLINE database**, developed by the U.S. National Library of Medicine, is the premier source for bibliographic coverage of the biomedical literature. MEDLINE covers about 5,600 medical, nursing, and health journals and has more than 24 million records. MEDLINE can be accessed for free on the Internet at the **PubMed** website. PubMed is a life-long resource regardless of your institution's access to bibliographic databases.

MEDLINE uses a controlled vocabulary called **MeSH** (Medical Subject Headings) to index articles. MeSH terminology provides a consistent way to retrieve information that may use different terminology for the same concepts. Once you have begun a search, a field on the right side of the screen labelled "Search Details" lets you see how the keywords you entered mapped onto MeSH terms, which might lead you to pursue other leads.

When we did a PubMed search of MEDLINE analogous to the one we described earlier for CINAHL, using the same keywords and restrictions, 90 records were retrieved. The list of records in the two PubMed and CINAHL searches overlapped considerably, but new references were found in each search. Both searches, however, retrieved the study by Davison—the CINAHL record for which was shown in Figure 7.2. The PubMed record for the same reference is presented in Figure 7.3. As you can see, the MeSH terms in Figure 7.3 are different than the CINAHL subject headings in Figure 7.2.

 TIP After you have found a study that is good exemplar of what you are looking for, you can search for other similar studies in the database. In PubMed, after identifying a key study, you could click on "Similar articles" on the right of the screen to locate similar studies. In CINAHL, you would click on "Find Similar Results."

Geriatr Nurs. 2016 Jan-Feb;37(1):25-9. doi: 10.1016/j.gerinurse.2015.08.013. Epub 2015 Sep 26.

A personalized multimedia device to treat agitated behavior and improve mood in people with dementia: A pilot study.

Davison TE[1], Nayer K[2], Coxon S[2], de Bono A[2], Eppingstall B[1], Jeon YH[3], van der Ploeg ES[1], O'Connor DW[4].

Abstract

Agitated behaviors and dysphoric moods in nursing home residents with dementia may be a response to a lack of personalized, meaningful activity and stimulation. To address this deficiency, a personal computer was adapted to play favorite music and display photographs, movies, and messages that were selected or made by family members. The system (called Memory Box) is accompanied by a simplified interface to help people with dementia access material independently. The system's ability to reduce agitation, and improve symptoms of depression and anxiety, was tested by means of an eight-week randomized, single-blinded, cross-over trial comparing Memory Box with a control condition that offered equivalent contact with research staff. Eleven nursing home residents with mild to severe dementia and persistent, daily agitated behaviors completed the study. Outcome measures included ratings of anxiety, depression and agitated behavior made by knowledgeable staff members in collaboration with researchers. Memory Box was well utilized and highly rated by residents, families and staff members. There were significant reductions in depressive and anxiety symptoms during the course of the intervention. The system shows promise as a tool to assist families and nursing home staff to improve the wellbeing of cognitively impaired older people with agitated behaviors.

KEYWORDS: Agitation; Controlled trial; Dementia; Mood; Treatment
PMID: 26412509

Preliminary MeSH terms

- Aged
- Anxiety/prevention & control
- Behavioral Symptoms/therapy
- Cross-Over Studies
- Dementia*
- Depression/prevention & control
- Humans
- Music Therapy/methods*
- Nursing Homes
- Nursing Evaluation Research
- Photography
- Pilot Projects
- Psychiatric Status Rating Scales
- Psychomotor Agitation*
- Psychomotor Agitation/therapy

Figure 7.3 Example of printout from PubMed search.

Google Scholar

Google Scholar (GS) is a popular bibliographic search engine that was launched in 2004. GS includes articles in journals from scholarly publishers in all disciplines and also includes books, technical reports, and other documents. One advantage of GS is that it is accessible free of charge over the Internet. Like other bibliographic search engines, GS allows users to search by topic, by a title, and by author, and uses Boolean operators and other search conventions. Also, like PubMed and CINAHL, GS has a *Cited By* feature for a descendancy search and a *Related Articles* feature to locate other sources with relevant content to an identified article. Because of its expanded coverage of material, GS can provide greater access to free full-text publications.

In the field of medicine, GS has generated controversy, with some arguing that it has the same utility and quality as popular medical databases and others urging caution in depending only on GS. The capabilities and features of GS may improve in the years ahead, but at the moment, it may be risky to depend on GS exclusively. For a full literature review, we think it is best to combine searches using GS with searches of other databases.

Example of a bibliographic search •
Zuckerman (2016) did a literature review on the use of oral chlorhexidine to prevent ventilator-associated pneumonia. She searched for relevant studies in four bibliographic databases: CINAHL, PubMed, Scopus, and EMBASE. A total of 47 articles were initially identified; only 16 were duplicates. (This journal article is available on thePoint.)

Screening, Documentation, and Abstracting

After searching for and retrieving references, there are several important steps before a synthesis can begin.

Screening and Gathering References

References that have been identified in the search need to be screened for relevance. You can usually know the relevance by reading the abstract. When you find a relevant article, try to obtain a full copy rather than relying on information in the abstract only.

    TIP   The *open-access journal* movement is gaining momentum in health care publishing. Open-access journals provide articles free of charge online. When an article is not available online, you may be able to access it by communicating with the lead author, either directly through an e-mail or through a resource called *Research Gate* (www.researchgate.net).

Documentation in Literature Retrieval

Search strategies are often complex, so it is wise to document your search actions and results. You should make note of databases searched, keywords used, limits instituted, and any other information that would help you keep track of what you did. Part of your strategy can be documented by printing your search history from the electronic databases. Documentation will promote efficiency by preventing unintended duplication and will also help you to assess what else needs to be tried.

Abstracting and Recording Information

Once you have retrieved useful articles, you need a strategy to organize the information in the articles. For simple reviews, it may be sufficient to make notes about key features of the

Example of a Mini-Protocol for a Literature Review (Therapy Question)

Citation and Abstract   (copy and paste information from bibliographic database)

Variables: Intervention (Independent Variable): _____
                     Outcome Variable: _____
Framework/Theory: _____
Design Type: ☐ Experimental   ☐ Quasi-experimental
                    Specific Design: _____
                    Control for confounding variables: _____
                    Blinding? ☐ No ☐ Yes Who blinded? _____
                    Intervention description: _____
                    _____
                    Control group condition: _____
Sample: Size: ____ Sampling method: _____
                    Sample characteristics: _____
                    _____
Data Sources: ☐ Self-report ☐ Observational ☐ Biophysiologic ☐ Other
                    Description of measures: _____
                    _____
                    Data Quality: _____
Key Findings: _____
                    _____
                    _____
                    _____

Figure 7.4 Example of a mini-protocol for a literature review (therapy question).

retrieved studies and to base your review on these notes. When a literature review involves a large number of studies, a formal system of recording information from each study may be needed. One mechanism that we recommend for complex reviews is to *code* the characteristics of each study and then record codes in a set of tables, a system that we describe in detail elsewhere (Polit & Beck, 2016).

Another approach is to "copy and paste" each abstract and citation information from the bibliographic database into a word processing document. Then, the bottom of each page could have a "mini-protocol" for recording important information that you want to record consistently across studies. There is no fixed format for such a protocol—you must decide what elements are important to record systematically to help you organize and analyse information. We present an example for a half-page protocol in Figure 7.4, with entries that would be most suitable for Therapy/Intervention questions. Although many of the terms on this protocol are probably not familiar to you at this point, you will learn their meaning in subsequent chapters.

EVALUATING AND ANALYSING THE EVIDENCE

In drawing conclusions about a body of evidence, reviewers must make judgements about the quality of the studies. Thus, an important part of a doing a literature review is evaluating the body of completed studies and integrating the evidence across studies.

Evaluating Studies for a Review

In reviewing the literature, you would not undertake a comprehensive critique of each study, but you would need to assess the quality of each study so that you could draw conclusions about the overall body of evidence and about gaps in the evidence. Critiques for a literature review tend to focus on study methods, so the critiquing guidelines in Tables 4.1 and 4.2 might be useful.

In literature reviews, methodologic features of the studies under review is evaluated by a broad question: To what extent do the findings reflect the *truth* (the true state of affairs) or, conversely, to what extent do flaws undermine the believability of the evidence? The "truth" is most likely to be discovered when researchers use powerful designs, good sampling plans, high-quality data collection procedures, and appropriate analyses.

Analysing and Synthesizing Information

Once relevant studies have been retrieved and critiqued, the information has to be analysed and synthesized. We find the analogy between doing a literature review and doing a qualitative study useful: In both, the focus is on the identification of important *themes*.

A thematic analysis essentially involves detecting patterns and regularities as well as inconsistencies. A number of different types of themes can be identified in a literature review analysis, three of which are as follows:

- *Substantive themes:* What is the pattern of evidence—what are the key findings? How much evidence is there? How consistent is the body of evidence? What gaps are there in the evidence?
- *Methodologic themes:* What methods have been used to address the question? What are major methodologic deficiencies and strengths?
- *Generalizability/transferability themes:* To what population does the evidence apply? Do the findings vary for different types of people (e.g., men vs. women) or setting (e.g., urban vs. rural)?

In preparing a review, you would need to determine which themes are most relevant for the purpose at hand. Most often substantive themes are of greatest interest.

PREPARING A WRITTEN LITERATURE REVIEW

Writing literature reviews can be challenging, especially when large volume of information and thematic analyses must be condensed into a few pages. We offer some suggestions, but we recognize that skills in writing literature reviews develop over time.

Organizing the Review

Organization is crucial in preparing a written review. When literature on a topic is extensive, it is useful to summarize information in a table. The table could include columns with headings such as Author, Sample Characteristics, Design, and Key Findings. Such a table provides a quick overview that allows you to make sense of a mass of information.

Most writers find an outline helpful. Unless the review is very simple, it is important to have an organizational plan so that the review has a meaningful and understandable flow. Although the specifics of the organization differ from topic to topic, the goal is to structure the review that will lead to a logical conclusion about the state of evidence on the topic. After finalizing an organizing structure, you should review your notes or protocols to decide where a particular reference fits. If some references do not seem to fit anywhere, they may need to be deleted. Remember that the number of references is not as important as their relevance.

Writing a Literature Review

It is beyond the scope of this textbook to offer detailed guidance on writing research reviews, but we offer a few comments on their content and style. Additional assistance is provided in books such as those by Fink (2014) and Garrard (2014).

Content of the Written Literature Review

A written research review should provide readers with an objective synthesis of current evidence on a topic. Although key studies may be described, it is not necessary to provide details for every reference. Studies with comparable findings often can be summarized together, as illustrated in the third paragraph of Example 1 at the end of this chapter.

Findings should be summarized in your own words. The review should demonstrate that you have considered the cumulative worth of the body of research. Stringing together quotes from articles does not indicate that previous research has been assimilated and understood.

The review should be as unbiased as possible. The review should not overlook a study because its findings contradict those of other studies or conflict with your ideas. Inconsistent results should be analysed and the supporting evidence evaluated objectively.

A literature review typically concludes with a summary of current evidence on the topic. The summary should recap key findings, assess their credibility, and point out gaps in the evidence. When the literature review is conducted for a new study, the summary should demonstrate the need for the research and provide an explanation for any hypotheses.

As you read this book, you will become increasingly proficient in critically evaluating the research literature. We hope you will understand how to conduct a research review once you have completed this chapter, but we do not expect that you will be in a position to write a state-of-the-art review until you have acquired more skills in research methods.

Style of a Research Review

Students preparing research reviews often have trouble writing in an acceptable style. Remember that hypotheses cannot be proved or disproved by statistical testing, and no question can be definitely answered in a single study. Strictly speaking, hypotheses are not proved or verified; they are *supported* by research findings.

 TIP Phrases indicating the conditional nature of research results, such as the following, are appropriate:

- Several studies have *found . . .*
- Findings thus far *suggest . . .*
- The results *are consistent* with the conclusion that . . .
- There *appears* to be fairly strong evidence that . . .

Also, a literature review should include few opinions and should explicitly reference the source. Reviewers' own opinions do not belong in a review, with the exception of assessments of study quality.

CRITIQUING RESEARCH LITERATURE REVIEWS

Some nurses never prepare a written research review, and perhaps you will never be required to do one. Most nurses, however, do *read* research reviews (including the literature review sections of research reports), and they should be prepared to evaluate such reviews critically.

It is often difficult to critique a research review if you are not familiar with the topic. You may not be able to judge whether the author has included all relevant literature and has adequately summarized knowledge on that topic. Certain areas of a research review, however, can be evaluated by general readers who are not experts on the topic. A few suggestions for critiquing research reviews are presented in Box 7.1. Extra critiquing questions are relevant for systematic reviews, as we discuss in Chapter 18.

Box 7.1 Guidelines for Critiquing Literature Reviews

1. Does the review seem thorough and up-to-date? Did it include major studies on the topic? Did it include recent research?
2. Did the review rely mainly on research reports, using primary sources?
3. Did the review critically appraise and compare key studies? Did it identify important gaps in the literature?
4. Was the review well organized? Is the development of ideas clear?
5. Did the review use appropriate language, suggesting the tentativeness of prior findings? Is the review objective?
6. If the review was in the introduction for a new study, did the review support the need for the study?
7. If the review was designed to summarize evidence for clinical practice, did it draw appropriate conclusions about practice implications?

In assessing a literature review, the overarching question is whether it summarizes the current state of research evidence. If the review is written as part of an original research report, an equally important question is whether the review lays a solid foundation for the new study.

 TIP Literature reviews in the introductions of research articles are almost always very brief and are unlikely to present a thorough critique of existing studies. Knowledge gaps should be identified.

RESEARCH EXAMPLES WITH CRITICAL THINKING EXERCISES

The best way to learn about the style, content, and organization of a research literature review is to read reviews that appear in the nursing literature. We present an excerpt from a review for a mixed-method study—one involving the collection and analysis of both quantitative and qualitative data. The excerpt is followed by some questions to guide critical thinking—you can refer to the entire report if needed. Example 1 is featured on the interactive *Critical Thinking Activity* on thePoint website. The critical thinking questions for Examples 2 and 3 are based on the studies that appear in their entirety in Appendices A and B of this book. Our comments for these exercises are in the Student Resources section on thePoint.

EXAMPLE 1: LITERATURE REVIEW FROM A MIXED-METHOD STUDY

Study: Symptoms in women with peripartum cardiomyopathy (PPCM): A mixed-method study (Patel et al., 2016)

Statement of Purpose: The purpose of this study was to explore and describe women's experiences of symptoms in PPCM.

Literature Review (excerpt): "Peripartum cardiomyopathy (PPCM) is idiopathic disease, rare in high income countries and a diagnosis of exclusion. It is associated with, at times, severe heart failure (HF) occurring toward the end of pregnancy or in the months following birth. The left ventricle may not be dilated but the left ventricle ejection fraction is nearly always reduced below 45%. The Heart Failure Association of the European Society of Cardiology Working Group on PPCM defined it as: *An idiopathic cardio-myopathy presenting with HF secondary to left ventricle systolic dysfunction towards the end of pregnancy or in the months following delivery, where no other cause of HF is found. It is a diagnosis of exclusion. The left ventricle may not be dilated, but the ejection fraction is nearly always reduced below 45%* (Sliwa et al., 2017).

The incidence and prognosis of PPCM varies globally (Elkayam, 2011). The true incidence is unknown, as the clinical presentation varies. Current estimates range between 1:299 (Haiti), 1:1,000 (South Africa), and 1:2,500–4,000 births (United States) (Elkayam, 2011; Garg, Palaniswamy, & Lanier, 2015; Sliwa et al., 2017). No data exist on the prevalence of the disease in Europe (Hilfiker-Kleiner et al., 2015). Assuming an incidence of 1:3,500 to 1:1,400 births would yield an expected incidence of up to 300 patients per year in Germany, with severe, critical cardiac failure in around 30 (Hilfiker-Kleiner et al., 2015). The incidence in Sweden has been estimated to be 1:9,191 births (Barasa et al., 2017).

The anatomical and physiologic changes in the mother associated with normal pregnancy are profound, and this may result in symptoms and signs that overlap with those usually associated with disease out-side of pregnancy. The main/cardinal symptoms of PPCM are those of HF and include fatigue, shortness of breath, and fluid retention, and thus diagnosis is often missed or delayed as initial symptoms are similar to those of hemodynamic changes in normal pregnancy or early postpartum period (Ersbøll et al., 2016; Garg, Palaniswamy, & Lanier, 2015; Sliwa et al., 2010). An analysis of Internet narratives of women with PPCM showed that symptoms overlap with normal discomforts of pregnancy, and thus create space for clinicians to overlook the seriousness of their situation (Dekker et al., 2016). A survey of women with PPCM participating in an online support group showed their frustration with the nursing staff (Hess & Weinland, 2012) for being ignored, dismissed, and neglected. Only 4% of the posts on the forum described interactions with health care professionals as positive.

The causes, risk factors, aetiology, treatment, and prognosis of PPCM have been described elsewhere (Ersbøll et al., 2016; Garg, Palaniswamy, & Lanier, 2015; Hilfiker-Kleiner, 2015; Sliwa et al., 2017). There are, however, a lot more questions that remain unanswered, and women's experiences of symptoms of PPCM are rarely explored. As understanding specific conditions from the 'sufferers' perspective is a foundational starting point for caring (Watson & Brewer, 2015), it is important to understand the subjective experience and meaning of PPCM from the affected person's perspective. "The lack of research in this area points to the need for knowledge acquirement from those who are affected, to assist with differential and early diagnosis of PPCM" (pp. 14–15).

Critical Thinking Exercises

1. Answer the relevant questions from Box 7.1 regarding this literature review.
2. Also consider the following targeted questions, which may further sharpen your critical thinking skills and assist you in understanding this study:
   a. In performing the literature review, what keywords might the researchers have used to search for prior studies?
   b. Using the keywords, perform a computerized search to see if you can find a recent relevant study to aug-ment the review.

EXAMPLE 2: QUANTITATIVE RESEARCH IN APPENDIX A

- Read the introduction to Swenson and colleagues' (2016) study ("Parents' use of praise and criticism in a sample of young children seeking mental health services") in Appendix A of this book.

Critical Thinking Exercises

1. Answer the relevant questions from Box 7.1 regarding this study.
2. Also consider the following targeted questions:
   a. In performing the literature review, what keywords might have been used to search for prior studies?
   b. Using the keywords, perform a computerized search to see if you can find a recent relevant study to augment the review.

EXAMPLE 3: QUALITATIVE RESEARCH IN APPENDIX B

- Read the abstract and introduction of Beck and Watson's (2010) study ("Subsequent childbirth after a previous traumatic birth") in Appendix B of this book.

Critical Thinking Exercises

1. Answer the relevant questions from Box 7.1 regarding this study.
2. Also consider the following targeted questions:
   a. What was the central phenomenon in this study? Was that phenomenon adequately covered in the literature review?
   b. In performing their literature review, what keywords might Beck and Watson have used to search for prior studies?

WANT TO KNOW MORE? ☀

A wide variety of resources to enhance your learning and understanding of this chapter are available on thePoint.

- Interactive Critical Thinking Activity
- Chapter Supplement on Finding Evidence for an EBP Inquiry in PubMed
- Answers to the Critical Thinking Exercises for Examples 2 and 3
- Internet Resources with useful websites for Chapter 7
- A Wolters Kluwer journal article on a topic related to this chapter

---

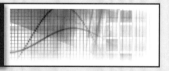

Summary Points

- A research **literature review** is a written summary of the state of evidence on a research problem.
- The major steps in preparing a written research review include formulating a question, devising a search strategy, searching and retrieving relevant sources, abstracting and encoding information, critiquing studies, analysing and integrating the information, and preparing a written synthesis.
- Research reviews rely primarily on findings in research reports. Information in non-research references (e.g., opinion articles, case reports) may broaden understanding of a problem but has limited utility in summarizing evidence.
- A **primary source** is the original description of a study prepared by the researcher

who conducted it; a **secondary source** is a description of a study by another person. Literature reviews should rely mostly on primary source material.

- Strategies for finding studies on a topic include the use of bibliographic tools but also include the *ancestry approach* (tracking down earlier studies cited in a reference list of a report) and the *descendancy approach* (using a pivotal study to search forward to subsequent studies that cited it).

- Key resources for a research literature search are the **bibliographic databases** that can be searched electronically. For nurses, the **CINAHL** and **MEDLINE** databases are especially useful.

- In searching a bibliographic database, users can do a **keyword** search that looks for terms in *text fields* of a database record (or that *maps* keywords onto the database's subject

codes) or can search according to the *subject heading* codes themselves.

- Retrieved references must be screened for relevance, and then pertinent information can be abstracted and encoded for subsequent analysis. Studies must also be critiqued to assess the strength of evidence in existing research.

- The analysis of information from a literature search essentially involves the identification of important *themes*—regularities and patterns in the information.

- In preparing a written review, it is important to organize materials coherently. Preparation of an outline is recommended. The reviewers' role is to point out what has been studied, how adequate and dependable the studies are, and what gaps exist in the body of research.

REFERENCES

Barasa, A., Rosengren, A., Sandström, T. Z., et al. (2017). Heart Failure in Late Pregnancy and Postpartum: Incidence and Long-Term Mortality in Sweden From 1997 to 2010. *Journal of Cardiac Failure, 23*(5), 370–378.

Dekker, R. L., Morton, C. H., Singleton, P., & Lyndon, A. (2016). Women's Experiences Being Diagnosed With Peripartum Cardiomyopathy: A Qualitative Study. *Journal of Midwifery & Women's Health, 61*(4), 467–473.

Ersbøll, A. S., Damm, P., Gustafsson, F., et al. (2016). Peripartum cardiomyopathy: a systematic literature review. *Acta Obstetricia et Gynecologica Scandinavica, 95*(11), 1205–1219.

Fink, A. (2014). *Conducting research literature reviews: From the Internet to paper* (4th ed.). Thousand Oaks, CA: Sage.

Garg, J., Palaniswamy, C., & Lanier, G. M. (2015). Peripartum cardiomyopathy: definition, incidence, etiopathogenesis, diagnosis, and management. *Cardiology in Review, 23*(2), 69–78.

Garrard, J. (2014). *Health sciences literature review made easy: The matrix method* (4th ed.). Burlington, MA: Jones & Bartlett Learning.

Hess, R. F., & Weinland, J. A. (2012). The life-changing impact of peripartum cardiomyopathy: an analysis of online postings. *MCN: The American Journal of Maternal/Child Nursing, 37*(4), 241–246.

Hilfiker-Kleiner, D., Haghikia, A., Nonhoff, J., & Bauersachs, J. (2015). Peripartum cardiomyopathy: current management and future perspectives. *European Heart Journal, 36*(18), 1090–1097.

Li, W., Li, H., Long, Y. (2016). Clinical Characteristics and Long-term Predictors of Persistent Left Ventricular Systolic Dysfunction in Peripartum Cardiomyopathy. *Canadian Journal of Cardiology, 32*(3), 362–368.

*Patel, H., Berg, M., Barasa, A., Begley, C., & Schaufelberger, M. (2016). Symptoms in women with peripartum cardiomyopathy: A mixed method study. *Midwifery, 32*, 14–20.

Polit, D., & Beck, C. (2016). *Nursing research: Generating and assessing evidence for nursing practice* (10th ed.). Philadelphia, PA: Wolters Kluwer.

Sliwa, K., Mebazaa, A., Hilfiker-Kleiner, D., et al. (2017). Clinical characteristics of patients from the worldwide registry on peripartum cardiomyopathy (PPCM): EURObservational Research Programme in conjunction with the Heart Failure Association of the European Society of Cardiology Study Group on PPCM. *European Journal of Heart Failure, 19*(9), 1131–1141.

Watson, J., & Brewer, B. B. (2015). Caring science research: criteria, evidence, and measurement. *Journal of Nursing Administration, 45*(5), 235–236.

**Zuckerman, L. M. (2016). Oral chlorhexidine use to prevent ventilator-associated pneumonia in adults: Review of the current literature. *Dimensions of Critical Care Nursing, 35*, 25–36.

*A link to this open-access article is provided in the Internet Resources section on the**Point** website.

This journal article is available on the Point** for this chapter.

Theoretical and Conceptual Frameworks

Learning Objectives

On completing this chapter, you will be able to:

- Identify major characteristics of theories, conceptual models, and frameworks
- Identify several conceptual models or theories frequently used by nurse researchers
- Describe how theory and research are linked in quantitative and qualitative studies
- Critique the appropriateness of a theoretical framework—or its absence—in a study
- Define new terms in the chapter

Key Terms

- Conceptual framework
- Conceptual map
- Conceptual model
- Descriptive theory
- Framework
- Middle-range theory
- Model
- Schematic model
- Theoretical framework
- Theory

High-quality studies typically achieve a high level of *conceptual integration*. This happens when the research questions fit the chosen methods, when the questions are consistent with existing evidence, and when there is a plausible conceptual rationale for expected outcomes—including a rationale for any hypotheses or interventions. For example, suppose a research team hypothesized that a nurse-led smoking cessation intervention would reduce smoking among patients with cardiovascular disease. Why would they make this prediction—what is the "theory" about how the intervention might change people's behaviour? Do the researchers predict that the intervention will change patients' knowledge? attitudes? motivation? The researchers' view of how the intervention would "work" should drive the design of the intervention and the study.

Studies are not developed in a vacuum—there must be an underlying conceptualization of people's behaviours and characteristics. In some studies, the underlying conceptualization is fuzzy or unstated, but in good research, a defensible conceptualization is made explicit. This chapter discusses theoretical and conceptual contexts for nursing research problems.

THEORIES, MODELS, AND FRAMEWORKS

Many terms are used in connection with conceptual contexts for research, such as theories, models, frameworks, schemes, and maps. These terms are interrelated but are used differently by different writers. We offer guidance in distinguishing these terms as we define them.

Theories

In nursing education, the term *theory* is used to refer to content covered in classrooms, as opposed to actual nursing practice. In both lay and scientific language, *theory is an abstraction of the reality.*

Theory is often defined as an abstract generalization that describes and explains how phenomena are interrelated. As classically defined, theories consist of two or more concepts and a set of logical connections, providing a tool for deducing hypotheses. To illustrate, according to *reinforcement theory*, behaviour that is reinforced (i.e., rewarded) tends to be repeated and learned. The proposition allows hypothesis generation. For example, we could deduce from the theory that hyperactive children who are rewarded when they engage in quiet play will exhibit less acting-out behaviours than unrewarded children. This prediction, as well as others based on reinforcement theory, could be tested in a study.

The term *theory* is also used less restrictively to refer to a broad characterization of a phenomenon. A **descriptive theory** explains and thoroughly describes a phenomenon. Descriptive theories are inductive, observation-based abstractions that describe or classify characteristics of individuals, groups, or situations by summarizing their commonalities. Such theories are important in qualitative studies.

Theories can help interpret research findings. Theories may guide researchers' understanding not only of the "what" of natural phenomena but also of the "why" of their occurrence. Theories can also help to stimulate research by providing direction and impetus.

Theories vary in their level of generality. *Grand theories* (or *macrotheories*) claim to explain large segments of human experience. In nursing, there are grand theories that offer explanations of the whole of nursing and that characterize the nature and mission of nursing practice, as distinct from other disciplines. An example of a nursing theory that has been described as a grand theory is Parse's Humanbecoming Paradigm (Parse, 2014). Theories of relevance to researchers are often less abstract than grand theories. **Middle-range theories** attempt to explain such phenomena as stress, comfort, and health promotion. Middle-range theories, compared to grand theories, are more specific and easier for empirical testing.

Models

A **conceptual model** deals with abstractions (concepts) that are relevant to a common theme. Conceptual models provide a conceptual perspective on interrelated phenomena, but they are more loosely structured than theories and do not link concepts in a logical deductive system. A conceptual model broadly presents an understanding of a phenomenon and reflects the assumptions of the model's designer. Conceptual models can serve as springboards for generating hypotheses.

Some writers use the term **model** to define a phenomenon with a minimal use of words, which can convey different meanings to different people. Two types of models used in research contexts are schematic models and statistical models. *Statistical models*, not discussed here, are equations that mathematically express relationships among a set of variables and that are tested statistically.

Schematic models (or **conceptual maps**) visually represent relationships among phenomena and are used in both quantitative and qualitative research. Concepts and linkages between them are depicted graphically through boxes, arrows, or other symbols. As an example of a schematic model, Figure 8.1 shows *Pender's Health Promotion Model* (HPM), which is a model for explaining and predicting the health-promotion component of lifestyle (Pender et al., 2015). Schematic models are appealing as visual summaries of complex ideas.

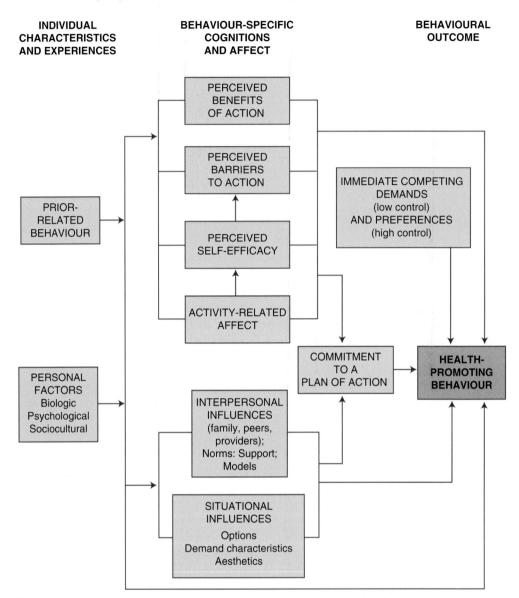

Figure 8.1 The Health Promotion Model. (Adapted from Pender, N. J. (2011). The Health Promotion Model. Retrieved from http://www.nursing.umich.edu/faculty/pender/chart.gif.)

Frameworks

A **framework** is the conceptual foundation of a study. Not every study is based on a theory or model, but every study has a framework. In a study based on a theory, the framework is called the **theoretical framework**; in a study based on a conceptual model, the framework may be called the **conceptual framework**. However, the terms *conceptual framework, conceptual model,* and *theoretical framework* are often used interchangeably.

A study's framework is often implicit (i.e., not formally acknowledged or described). Worldviews shape how concepts are defined, but researchers often fail to clarify the conceptual foundations of their concepts. By clarifying conceptual definitions of key variables, researchers provide important information about the study's framework.

Quantitative researchers are less likely to identify their frameworks than qualitative researchers. The framework is usually part of a research tradition that defines qualitative research. For example, ethnographers generally begin within a theory of culture. Grounded theory researchers incorporate sociologic principles into their framework and approach. The questions raised by qualitative researchers reflect certain theoretical formulations.

In recent years, *concept analysis* has become an important enterprise among students and nurse scholars. Several methods have been proposed for undertaking a concept analysis and clarifying conceptual definitions (Walker & Avant, 2011). Efforts to analyse concepts of relevance to nursing should facilitate greater conceptual clarity among nurse researchers.

Example of developing a conceptual definition • • • • • • • • • • • • • • • • •
Krishnan (2017) used Walker and Avant's (2011) eight-step concept analysis methods to conceptually define *good death in long-term care residents.* She searched and analysed national and international databases and found 151 relevant articles and 7 books. They proposed the following definition: "The attributes of spiritual care are healing presence, therapeutic use of self, intuitive sense, exploration of the spiritual perspective, patient centredness, meaning-centred therapeutic intervention and creation of a spiritually nurturing environment" (p. 211).

The Nature of Theories and Conceptual Models

Theories, conceptual frameworks, and models are not *discovered;* they are created. Theory building depends not only on observable evidence but also on a theorist's creativity in pulling evidence together and making sense of it. A theory cannot be proved—a theory represents a theorist's best efforts to describe and explain phenomena. Through research, theories evolve and are sometimes rejected. This may happen if new evidence challenges a previously accepted theory. Or, a new theory might integrate new observations with an existing theory to yield a more precise explanation of a phenomenon.

Theory and research have a reciprocal relationship. Theories are built inductively from observations including research. Hypotheses deductive from the theory, in turn, must be tested by systematic inquiry. Thus, research plays a dual and continuing role in theory building and testing.

CONCEPTUAL MODELS AND THEORIES USED IN NURSING RESEARCH

Nurse researchers have used both nursing and non-nursing frameworks as conceptual contexts for their studies. This section briefly discusses several frameworks that have been found useful by nurse researchers.

Conceptual Models of Nursing

Several nurses have formulated conceptual models representing explanations of what the nursing discipline is and what the nursing process entails. As Fawcett and DeSanto-Madeya (2013) have noted, four concepts are central to models of nursing: *human beings, environment, health,* and *nursing.* The various conceptual models define these concepts differently, link them in diverse ways, and emphasize different relationships among them. Moreover, the models emphasize different processes as being central to nursing.

The conceptual models were not developed primarily as a base for nursing research. Indeed, most models have had more impact on nursing education and clinical practice than on research. Nevertheless, nurse researchers have turned to these conceptual frameworks for inspiration in formulating research questions and hypotheses.

 TIP The Supplement to Chapter 8 on thePoint website includes a table of several prominent conceptual models in nursing. The table describes the model's key features and identifies a study that claimed the model as its framework.

Let us consider one conceptual model of nursing that has received research attention, Roy's Adaptation Model. In this model, humans are viewed as biopsychosocial adaptive systems who cope with environmental change through the process of adaptation (Roy & Andrews, 2009). Within the human system, there are four subsystems: physiologic/physical, self-concept/group identity, role function, and interdependence. These subsystems are adaptive modes that provide mechanisms for coping with environmental stimuli and change. Health is viewed as both a state and a process of being and becoming integrated and whole that reflects the interaction between persons and environment. The goal of nursing, according to this model, is to promote client adaptation. Nursing interventions usually take the form of increasing, decreasing, modifying, removing, or maintaining internal and external stimuli that affect adaptation. Roy's Adaptation Model has been the basis for several middle-range theories and dozens of studies.

Research example using Roy's Adaptation Model • • • • • • • • • • • • • • •
Alvarado García and Salazar Maya (2015) used Roy's Adaptation Model as a basis for their in-depth study of how elderly adults adapt to chronic benign pain.

Middle-Range Theories Developed by Nurses

In addition to conceptual models that describe and characterize the nursing process, nurses have developed middle-range theories and models that focus on more specific phenomena of interest to nurses. Examples of middle-range theories that have been used in research include Beck's (2012) Theory of Postpartum Depression; Kolcaba's (2003) Comfort Theory, Pender's (2011) HPM, and Mishel's (1990) Uncertainty in Illness Theory. The latter two are briefly described here.

Pender's (2011) (HPM) focuses on explaining health-promoting behaviours, using a wellness orientation. According to the model (see Fig. 8.1), *health promotion* entails activities directed towards developing resources that maintain or enhance a person's well-being. The model proposes a number of relationships that can be used in developing and testing interventions and understanding health behaviours. For example, one HPM proposition is that people engage in behaviours if they anticipate benefits, and another is that perceived competence (or *self-efficacy*) relating to a given behaviour increases the likelihood of performing the behaviour.

Example using the Health Promotion Model • • • • • • • • • • • • • • • • • •
Hanson and colleagues (2009) used the HPM as their framework for an integrative review of the quantitative and qualitative evidence concerning factors influencing the participation of Canadian women in mammography. They found that the most common barriers to screening were membership in an ethnic minority and concerns about pain, radiation, and embarrassment.

Mishel's Uncertainty in Illness Theory (Mishel, 1990) focuses on the concept of uncertainty—the inability of a person to determine the meaning of illness-related events. According to this theory, people develop subjective appraisals to assist them in interpreting the experience of illness and treatment. Uncertainty occurs when people are unable to recognize stimuli and develop a clear idea of the situation. A situation appraised as uncertain will mobilize individuals to use their resources to adapt to the situation. Mishel's conceptualization of uncertainty and her Uncertainty in Illness Scale have been used in many nursing studies.

Example using Uncertainty in Illness Theory • • • • • • • • • • • • • • • • • • •
Cypress (2016) used Mishel's Uncertainty in Illness Theory as a foundation for exploring uncertainty among chronically ill patients in the intensive care unit.

Other Models Used by Nurse Researchers

Many concepts in which nurse researchers are interested are not unique to nursing, and so their studies are sometimes linked to frameworks that are not models from nursing. Several alternative models have gained prominence in the development of nursing interventions to promote health-enhancing behaviours and life choices. Four non-nursing theories have frequently been used in nursing studies: Bandura's (2001) Social Cognitive Theory, Prochaska et al.'s (2002) Transtheoretical (Stages of Change) Model, the Health Belief Model (HBM) (Becker, 1974), and the Theory of Planned Behaviour (TPB) (Ajzen, 2005).

Social Cognitive Theory (Bandura, 2001), which is sometimes called *self-efficacy theory*, offers an explanation of human behaviour using the concepts of self-efficacy, outcome expectations, and incentives. Self-efficacy concerns people's belief in their own capacity to carry out particular behaviours (e.g., smoking cessation). Self-efficacy expectations determine the behaviours a person chooses to perform, their degree of perseverance, and the quality of the performance. For example, Lee et al. (2016) examined whether social cognitive theory–based factors, including self-efficacy, were determinants of physical activity maintenance in breast cancer survivors from the Breast Health Centre in Winnipeg after a physical activity intervention.

 TIP Self-efficacy is a key construct in several models discussed in this chapter. Self-efficacy can vary and it has repeatedly been found to affect people's behaviours. Self-efficacy enhancement is often a goal in interventions designed to change people's health-related behaviour.

In the Transtheoretical Model (Prochaska et al., 2002), the core construct is *stages of behavioural change*, which conceptualizes a continuum of motivational readiness to change. The five stages of change are precontemplation, contemplation, preparation, action, and maintenance. Studies have shown that successful self-changers use different processes at each particular stage, thus suggesting the desirability of interventions that are individualized to the person's stage of readiness for change. For example, Lee et al. (2014) tested a web-based self-management intervention for breast cancer survivors. The exercise and diet intervention programme incorporated transtheoretical model–based strategies.

Becker's (1974) Health Belief Model is a framework for explaining people's health-related behaviour, such as adherence with a medical regimen. According to the model, health-related behaviour is influenced by a person's perception of a threat posed by a health problem as well as by the value associated with actions aimed at reducing the threat (Becker, 1974). A revised HBM (RHBM) has incorporated the concept of self-efficacy (Rosenstock, Strecher, & Becker, 1988). Nurse researchers have used the HBM extensively. For example, Jeihooni et al. (2015) developed and tested an osteoporosis prevention program based on the HBM.

The Theory of Planned Behaviour (Ajzen, 2005), which is an extension of another theory called the Theory of Reasoned Action, offers a framework for understanding people's

behaviour and its psychological determinants. According to the theory, behaviour is chosen and determined by people's *intention* to perform that behaviour. Intentions, in turn, are
affected by attitudes towards the behaviour, subjective norms (i.e., perceived social pressure
to perform or not perform the behaviour), and perceived behavioural control (i.e., anticipated ease or difficulty of engaging in the behaviour). Forbes et al. (2015), for example, used
TPB as a framework in their study of **cancer survivors'** intentions towards strength exercise
in Nova Scotia.

Although the use of theories and models from other disciplines such as psychology
(*borrowed theories*) has stirred some controversy, nursing research is likely to continue on
its current path of conducting studies within an interdisciplinary perspective. A borrowed
theory that is tested and found to be useful in health-relevant situations of interest to nurses
becomes *shared theory*.

 TIP Links to websites devoted to several theories mentioned in this chapter are provided in the Internet Resources on thePoint website.

USING A THEORY OR FRAMEWORK IN RESEARCH

The ways in which theory is used by quantitative and qualitative researchers are elaborated
on in this section. The term *theory* is used in its broadest sense to include conceptual models,
formal theories, and frameworks.

Theories in Qualitative Research

Theory is almost always present in studies that are embedded in a qualitative research tradition such as ethnography or phenomenology. However, different traditions involve theory
in different ways.

Sandelowski (1993) distinguished between *substantive theory* (conceptualizations of
a specific phenomenon) and theory that conceptualizes human inquiry. Some qualitative
researchers insist on an atheoretical stance to minimize prior conceptualizations (substantive theories) that might bias their inquiry. For example, phenomenologists are committed
to theoretical naiveté and try to avoid preconceived views of the phenomenon. Nevertheless,
phenomenologists are guided by a framework that focuses their inquiry on certain aspects of
a person's life world—that is, lived experiences.

Ethnographers bring a cultural perspective to their studies, and this perspective shapes
their fieldwork. Cultural theories include *ideational theories*, which suggest that cultural
conditions are constructed by mental activity and ideas, and *materialistic theories*, which
view material conditions (e.g., resources, production) as the source of cultural develop-
ments (Fetterman, 2010).

The theoretical underpinning of grounded theory is a mixture of sociologic perspectives, the most prominent of which is *symbolic interaction* (or *interactionism*). Three underlying
principles include (1) humans act towards things based on the meanings that the things have
for them; (2) the meaning of things is derived from the human interactions; and (3) meanings are handled in, and modified through, an interpretive process (Blumer, 1986).

Example of a grounded theory study •
Hernandez and other researchers (2016) did a grounded theory study to explore the
experience of weight management in normal-weight individuals. The participants
described a combination of mindfulness related to what was being eaten as well as
automatic processes to maintain a self-defined specific weight target.

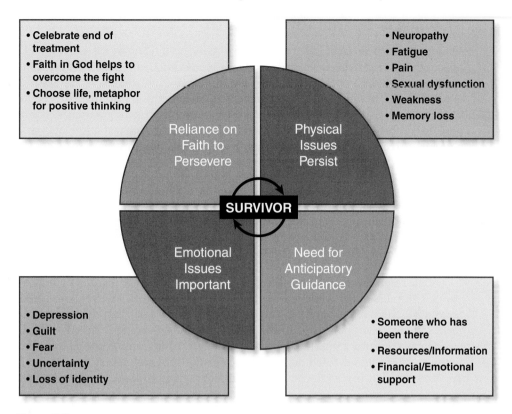

Figure 8.2 A grounded theory of the experience of transitioning into survivorship among African-American women with breast cancer. (Reprinted with permission from Mollica, M., & Nemeth, L. (2015). Transition from patient to survivor in African American breast cancer survivors. *Cancer Nursing, 38,* 16–22.)

Despite this theoretical perspective, grounded theory researchers, like phenomenologists, try to suspend prior substantive theory about the phenomenon until they develop their own theory. The goal of grounded theory is to understand a phenomenon that is *grounded* in actual observations. Once the theory starts to take shape, grounded theorists use previous literature for comparison with the emerging categories of the theory. Grounded theory researchers, who focus on social or psychological processes, often develop conceptual maps to explain a process. Figure 8.2 illustrates such a conceptual map for a study of the transition from patient to survivor in African-American breast cancer survivors (Mollica & Nemeth, 2015); this study is described at the end of this chapter.

In recent years, some qualitative nurse researchers have used *critical theory* as a framework in their research. Critical theory is a paradigm that involves a critique of society and societal processes and structures, as we discuss in Chapter 11.

Qualitative researchers sometimes use conceptual models of nursing or other formal theories as interpretive frameworks. For example, a number of qualitative nurse researchers acknowledge that their studies are rooted in nursing conceptual models such as those developed by Parse (2014), Roy (Roy & Andrews, 2009), Rogers (1994), or Newman (1997).

 TIP Systematic review of qualitative studies on a specific topic can lead to substantive theory development. In meta-syntheses, qualitative studies are combined to identify common elements. The findings from different sources are then used for theory building, as discussed in Chapter 18.

Theories in Quantitative Research

Quantitative researchers link research to theory or models in various ways. The classic approach is to test hypotheses deduced from an existing theory. For example, a nurse might read about Pender's (2011) HPM (see Fig. 8.1) and might reason as follows: If the HPM is valid, then I would expect that patients with osteoporosis who perceive the benefit of a calcium-enriched diet would be more likely to alter their eating patterns than those who perceive no benefits. This hypothesis could be tested through statistical analysis of data on patients' perceptions in relation to their eating habits. Repeated acceptance of hypotheses derived from a theory lends support to the theory.

 TIP When a quantitative study is based on a theory or model, the research article typically states this fact early—often in the abstract, or even in the title. Some reports also have a subsection of the introduction called "Theoretical Framework." The report usually includes a brief overview of the theory so that all readers can understand, in a broad way, the conceptual context of the study.

Some researchers test theory-based interventions. There are theories on how to influence people's attitudes or behaviour and hence their health outcomes. Interventions based on a solid conceptualization of human behaviour have a better chance of being effective than ones developed without a conceptual base. Interventions rarely affect outcomes directly—there are mediating factors that play a role in the pathway between the intervention and desired outcomes. For example, interventions based on Self-Determination Theory suggest that human behaviours are determined by perceived competence, autonomous motivation, and perceived relatedness.

Example of theory testing in an intervention study • • • • • • • • • • • • • • • •
Cossette and colleagues (2016) conducted a randomized controlled trial to test the effectiveness of theory-based (Self-Determination Theory) programme designed to enhance autonomy and motivation in self-care among patients with heart failure. In the treatment group, the project nurse fostered self-care by actively involving family caregivers. Caregiver involvement was found to be both a feasible and acceptable way to support self-care.

Many researchers who cite a theory or model as their framework are not directly *testing* the theory but may use the theory to provide an *organizing structure*. In such an approach, researchers *assume* that the model they adopt is valid and then use its constructs or schemas to provide an explanatory context.

Quantitative researchers also use findings from prior research to develop an original model. In some cases, the model combines elements or constructs from an existing theory.

Example of developing a new model •
Miranda and colleagues (2017) developed a web-based intervention to increase condom use among HIV-positive men who have sex with men. The intervention was based on their own conceptual model, which represented a synthesis of two theories: the TPB and Social Cognitive Theory.

CRITIQUING FRAMEWORKS IN RESEARCH REPORTS

It is often challenging to critique the theoretical context of a published research report—or its absence—but we offer a few suggestions.

In a qualitative study in which a grounded theory is developed, you may not have enough information to refute the proposed theory because the researchers present selected evidence to support the theory. You can, however, assess whether conceptualizations are insightful and whether the evidence is convincing. In a phenomenologic study, you should look for a discussion that links researchers' viewpoint and the philosophy of phenomenology.

For quantitative studies, the first task is to see whether the study has an explicit conceptual framework. If there is no mention of a theory, model, or framework (and often there is not), you should consider whether this absence diminishes the value of the study. Research often benefits from an explicit conceptual context, but some studies are so reasonable that the lack of a theory does not affect its utility. If, however, the study involves the test of a hypothesis or a complex intervention, the absence of a formal framework can lead to conceptual misunderstanding.

If the study does have an explicit framework, you can think about its appropriateness. You may not be able to challenge the researcher's use of a particular theory, but you can assess whether the link between the problem and the theory is genuine. Did the researcher present a convincing rationale for the framework used? In quantitative studies, did the hypotheses *flow* from the theory? Did the researcher interpret the findings within the context of the framework? If the answer to such questions is no, you may have grounds for criticizing the study's framework, even though you may not be able to suggest ways to improve the conceptual basis of the study. Some suggestions for evaluating the conceptual basis of a quantitative study are offered in Box 8.1.

TIP Some studies claim theoretical linkages that are not justified. This is most likely to occur when researchers first formulate the research problem and then later find a theoretical context to fit it. An after-the-fact linkage of theory to a research question is often artificial. If a research problem is truly linked to a conceptual framework, then the design of the study, the measurement of key constructs, and the analysis and interpretation of data will *flow* from that conceptualization.

Box 8.1 Guidelines for Critiquing Theoretical and Conceptual Frameworks

1. Did the report describe an explicit theoretical or conceptual framework for the study? If not, does the absence of a framework detract from the study's conceptual integration?
2. Did the report adequately describe the major features of the theory or model so that readers could understand the conceptual basis of the study?
3. Is the theory or model appropriate for the research problem? Does the purported link between the problem and the framework seem contrived?
4. Was the theory or model used for generating hypotheses, or is it used as an organizational or interpretive framework? Do the hypotheses (if any) naturally flow from the framework?
5. Were concepts defined in a way that is consistent with the theory? If there was an intervention, were intervention components consistent with the theory?
6. Did the framework guide the study methods? For example, was the appropriate research tradition used if the study was qualitative? If quantitative, do the operational definitions correspond to the conceptual definitions?
7. Did the researcher tie the study findings back to the framework at the end of the report? Were the findings interpreted within the context of the framework?

RESEARCH EXAMPLES WITH CRITICAL THINKING EXERCISES

This section presents two examples of studies that have strong theoretical links. Read the summaries and then answer the critical thinking questions, referring to the full research report if necessary. Examples 1 and 2 are featured on the interactive *Critical Thinking Activity* on thePoint website. The critical thinking questions for Examples 3 and 4 are based on the studies that appear in their entirety in Appendices A and B of this book. Our comments for these exercises are in the Student Resources section on thePoint. ⚙

EXAMPLE 1: THE HEALTH PROMOTION MODEL IN A QUANTITATIVE STUDY

Study: The effects of coping skills training (CST) among teens with asthma (Srof et al., 2012)

Statement of Purpose: The purpose of the study was to evaluate the effects of a school-based intervention, CST, for teenagers with asthma.

Theoretical Framework: The HPM, shown in Figure 8.1, was the guiding framework for the intervention. The authors noted that within the HPM, various behaviour-specific cognitions (e.g., perceived barriers to behaviour, perceived self-efficacy) influence health-promoting behaviour *and* are modifiable through an intervention. In this study, the overall behaviour of interest was asthma self-management. The CST intervention was a five-session small-group strategy designed to promote problem-solving, cognitive–behaviour modification, and conflict resolution using strategies to improve self-efficacy and reduce perceived barriers. The researchers hypothesized that participation in CST would result in improved outcomes in asthma self-efficacy, asthma-related quality of life, social support, and peak expiratory flow rate (PEFR).

Method: In this pilot study, 39 teenagers with asthma were randomly assigned to one of the two groups—one that participated in the intervention and the other that did not. The researchers collected data about the outcomes from all participants at two points in time: before the start of the intervention and 6 weeks later.

Key Findings: Teenagers in the treatment group scored significantly higher at the end of the study on self-efficacy, activity-related quality of life, and social support than those in the control group.

Conclusions: The researchers noted that the self-efficacy and social support effects of the intervention were consistent with the HPM model. They recommended that, although the findings were promising, replication of the study, and an extension to specifically examine asthma self-management behaviour would be useful.

Critical Thinking Exercises

1. Answer the relevant questions from Box 8.1 regarding this study.
2. Also consider the following targeted questions:
   a. In the model shown in Figure 8.1, which factors did the researchers predict that the intervention would affect, according to the abbreviated description in the textbook?
   b. Is there another model or theory that was described in this chapter that could have been used to study the effect of this intervention?
3. If the results of this study are valid and generalizable, what might be some of the uses to which the findings could be put in clinical practice?

EXAMPLE 2: A GROUNDED THEORY STUDY

Study: Transition from patient to survivor in African-American breast cancer survivors (Mollica & Nemeth, 2015).

Statement of Purpose: The purpose of the study was to examine the experience of African-American women as they transition between breast cancer patient and breast cancer survivor.

Theoretical Framework: A grounded theory approach was chosen because the researchers noted as a goal "the discovery of theory from data systematically obtained and analyzed" (p. 17). The researchers further noted the use of induction that is inherent in a grounded theory approach: "An open, exploratory approach was used to identify recurrent meaningful concepts through systematic, inductive analysis of content" (p. 17).

Method: Data were collected through interviews with 15 community-based African-American women who had completed treatment for primary breast cancer between 6 and 18 months prior to the interviews. Women were recruited from community settings in two American cities. The women were interviewed by telephone. Each interview, which lasted about 45 minutes, was audiotaped so that the interviews could be transcribed. The interviewer asked broad questions about the women's experiences following their treatment for breast cancer. Recruitment and interviewing continued until no new information was revealed—that is, until data saturation occurred.

Key Findings: Based on their analysis of the in-depth interviews, the researchers identified four main processes: perseverance through struggles supported by reliance on faith, dealing with persistent physical issues, needing anticipatory guidance after treatment, and finding emotional needs as important as physical ones. A schematic model for the substantive theory is presented in Figure 8.2.

Critical Thinking Exercises

1. Answer the relevant questions from Box 8.1 regarding this study.
2. Also consider the following targeted questions:
3. In what way was the use of theory different in the Mollica and Nemeth study than in the previous study by Srof and colleagues?
4. Comment on the utility of the schematic model shown in Figure 8.2.
5. If the results of this study are trustworthy, what might be some of the uses to which the findings could be put in clinical practice?

EXAMPLE 3: QUANTITATIVE RESEARCH IN APPENDIX A

- Read the Introduction of Swenson and colleagues' (2016) study ("Parents' use of praise and criticism in a sample of young children seeking mental health services") in Appendix A of this book.

Critical Thinking Exercises

1. Answer the relevant questions from Box 8.1 regarding this study.
2. Also consider the following question: Would any of the theories or models described in this chapter have provided an appropriate conceptual context for this study?

EXAMPLE 4: QUALITATIVE RESEARCH IN APPENDIX B

- Read the introduction of Beck and Watson's (2010) study ("Subsequent childbirth after a previous traumatic birth") in Appendix B of this book.

Critical Thinking Exercises

1. Answer the relevant questions from Box 8.1 regarding this study.
2. Also consider the following targeted questions:
   a. Do you think that a schematic model would have helped to present the findings in this report?
   b. Did Beck and Watson present convincing evidence to support their use of the philosophy of phenomenology?

WANT TO KNOW MORE?

A wide variety of resources to enhance your learning and understanding of this chapter are available on thePoint.

- Interactive Critical Thinking Activity
- Chapter Supplement on Prominent Conceptual Models of Nursing Used by Nurse Researchers
- Answers to the Critical Thinking Exercises for Examples 3 and 4
- Internet Resources with useful websites for Chapter 8
- A Wolters Kluwer journal article on a topic related to this chapter

Summary Points

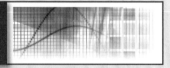

- High-quality research requires *conceptual integration,* one aspect of which is having a defensible theoretical rationale for the study.
- As classically defined, a **theory** is an abstract generalization that systematically explains relationships among phenomena. **Descriptive theory** thoroughly describes a phenomenon.
- *Grand theories* (or *macrotheories*) attempt to describe large segments of the human experience. **Middle-range theories** are specific to certain phenomena.

- Concepts are also the basic elements of **conceptual models,** but concepts are not linked in a logically ordered, deductive system.
- In research, the goals of theories and models are to make findings meaningful, to integrate knowledge into coherent systems, to stimulate new research, and to explain phenomena and relationships among them.
- **Schematic models** (or **conceptual maps**) are graphic representations of phenomena and their interrelationships using symbols or diagrams and a minimal use of words.
- A **framework** is the conceptual underpinning of a study, including an overall rationale and conceptual definitions of key concepts. In qualitative studies, the framework often springs from distinct research traditions.

● Several conceptual models of nursing have been used in nursing research. The concepts central to models of nursing are *human beings, environment, health,* and *nursing.* An example of a model of nursing used by nurse researchers is Roy's Adaptation Model.

● Non-nursing models used by nurse researchers (e.g., Bandura's Social Cognitive Theory) are referred to as *borrowed theories;* when the appropriateness of borrowed theories for nursing inquiry is confirmed, the theories become *shared theories.*

● In some qualitative research traditions (e.g., phenomenology), the researcher strives to suspend previously held *substantive* theories of the specific phenomena under study, but each tradition has rich theoretical underpinnings.

● Some qualitative researchers seek to develop *grounded theories,* data-driven explanations to account for phenomena under study through inductive processes.

● In the classical use of theory, researchers test hypotheses deduced from an existing theory. An emerging trend is the testing of theory-based interventions.

● In both quantitative and qualitative studies, researchers sometimes use a theory or model as an organizing framework, or as an interpretive tool.

REFERENCES

Ajzen, I. (2005). *Attitudes, personality, and behavior* (2nd ed.). Berkshire: Open University Press.

*Alvarado-García, A., & Salazar Maya, Á. (2015). Adaptation to chronic benign pain in elderly adults. *Investigación y Educación en Enfermería, 33,* 128–137.

Bandura, A. (2001). Social cognitive theory: An agentic perspective. *Annual Review of Psychology, 52,* 1–26.

Beck, C. T. (2012). Exemplar: Teetering on the edge: A second grounded theory modification. In P. L. Munhall (Ed.), *Nursing research: A qualitative perspective* (5th ed., pp. 257–284). Sudbury, MA: Jones & Bartlett Learning.

Becker, M. (1974). *The health belief model and personal health behavior.* Thorofare, NJ: Slack.

Blumer, H. (1986). *Symbolic interactionism: Perspective and method.* Berkeley: University of California Press.

Cossette, S., Belaid, H., Heppell, S., et al. (2016). Feasibility and acceptability of a nursing intervention with family caregiver on self-care among heart failure patients: a randomized pilot trial. *Pilot and Feasibility Studies, 2,* 34.

Cypress, B. S. (2016). Understanding uncertainty among critically ill patients in the intensive care unit using Mishel's Theory of Uncertainty of Illness. *Dimensions of Critical Care Nursing, 35,* 42–49.

Fawcett, J., & DeSanto-Madeya, S. (2013). *Contemporary nursing knowledge: Analysis and evaluation of nursing models and theories* (3rd ed.). Philadelphia, PA: F. A. Davis.

Fetterman, D. M. (2010). *Ethnography: Step-by-step* (3rd ed.). Thousand Oaks, CA: Sage.

Forbes, C. C., Blanchard, C. M., Mummery, W. K., & Courneya, K. (2015). Prevalence and correlates of strength exercise among breast, prostate, and colorectal cancer survivors. *Oncology Nursing Forum, 42*(2), 118–127

Hanson, K., Montgomery, P., Bakker, D., & Conlon, M. (2009). Factors influencing mammography participation in Canada: an integrative review of the literature. *Current Oncology, 16*(5), 65–75.

Hernandez, C. A., Hernandez, D. A., Wellington, C. M., & Kidd, A. (2016). The experience of weight management in normal weight adults. *Applied Nursing Research, 32,* 289–295.

*Jeihooni, A. K., Hidarnia, A., Kaveh, M., Hajizadeh, E., & Askari, A. (2015). Effects of an osteoporosis prevention program based on Health Belief Model among females. *Nursing and Midwifery Studies, 4,* e26731.

Kolcaba, K. (2003). *Comfort theory and practice: A vision for holistic health care and research.* New York, NY: Springer Publishing.

Krishnan, P. (2017). Concept analysis of good death in long term care residents. *International Journal of Palliative Nursing, 23*(1), 29–34.

Lee, C., Szuck, B., & Lau, Y. (2016). Determinants of physical activity maintenance in breast cancer survivors after a community-based intervention. *Oncology Nursing Forum, 43,* 93–102.

Lee, M. K., Yun, Y., Park, H., Lee, E., Jung, K., & Noh, D. (2014). A web-based self-management exercise and diet intervention for breast cancer survivors: Pilot randomized controlled trial. *International Journal of Nursing Studies, 51,* 1557–1567.

Miranda, J., & Côté, J. (2017). The Use of Intervention Mapping to Develop a Tailored Web-Based Intervention, Condom-HIM. *JMIR Public Health and Surveillance, 3*(2), e20.

Mishel, M. H. (1990). Reconceptualization of the uncertainty in illness theory. *Image, 22*(4), 256–262.

Mollica, M., & Nemeth, L. (2015). **Transition from patient to survivor in African American breast cancer survivors. *Cancer Nursing, 38,* 16–22.

Newman, M. (1997). Evolution of the theory of health as expanding consciousness. *Nursing Science Quarterly, 10,* 22–25.

Parse, R. R. (2014). *The Humanbecoming Paradigm: A transformational worldview.* Pittsburgh, PA: Discovery International.

Pender, N. J. (2011). The Health Promotion Model. Retrieved from http://www.nursing.umich.edu/faculty/pender/chart.gif

Pender, N. J., Murdaugh, C., & Parsons, M. A. (2015). *Health promotion in nursing practice* (7th ed.). Upper Saddle River, NJ: Prentice Hall.

Prochaska, J. O., Redding, C. A., & Evers, K. E. (2002). The transtheoretical model and stages of changes. In K. Glanz,

B. K. Rimer, & F. M. Lewis (Eds.), *Health behavior and health education: Theory, research, and practice* (pp. 99–120). San Francisco, CA: Jossey-Bass.

Rogers, M. E. (1994). The science of unitary human beings: Current perspectives. *Nursing Science Quarterly, 7,* 33–35.

Rosenstock, I., Strecher, V., & Becker, M. (1988). Social learning theory and the health belief model. *Health Education Quarterly, 15,* 175–183.

Roy, C., & Andrews, H. (2009). *The Roy adaptation model* (3rd ed.). Upper Saddle River, NJ: Prentice Hall.

Sandelowski, M. (1993). Theory unmasked: The uses and guises of theory in qualitative research. *Research in Nursing & Health, 16,* 213–218.

Srof, B., Velsor-Friedrich, B., & Penckofer, S. (2012). The effects of coping skills training among teens with asthma. *Western Journal of Nursing Research, 34,* 1043–1061.

Walker, L., & Avant, K. (2011). *Strategies for theory construction in nursing* (5th ed.). Upper Saddle River, NJ: Prentice Hall.

*A link to this open-access article is provided in the Internet Resources section on thePoint website.

**This journal article is available on thePoint for this chapter.

9 Quantitative Research Design

Learning Objectives

On completing this chapter, you will be able to:

- Discuss key research design decisions for a quantitative study
- Discuss the concepts of causality and identify criteria for causal relationships
- Describe and identify experimental, quasiexperimental, and nonexperimental designs
- Distinguish between cross-sectional and longitudinal designs
- Identify and evaluate alternative methods of controlling confounding variables
- Understand various threats to the validity of quantitative studies
- Evaluate a quantitative study in terms of its research design and methods of controlling confounding variables
- Define new terms in the chapter

Key Terms

- Attrition
- Baseline data
- Blinding
- Case-control design
- Cause
- Cohort design
- Construct validity
- Control (comparison) group
- Correlation
- Correlational study
- Crossover design
- Cross-sectional design
- Descriptive research
- Effect
- Experiment
- Experimental group
- External validity
- History threat
- Homogeneity
- Internal validity
- Intervention
- Longitudinal design
- Matching
- Maturation threat
- Mortality
- Nonequivalent control group
- Nonexperimental study
- Placebo
- Posttest data
- Pretest–posttest design
- Prospective design
- Quasiexperiment
- Randomization (random assignment)
- Randomized controlled trial (RCT)
- Research design
- Retrospective design
- Selection threat (self-selection)
- Statistical conclusion validity
- Statistical power
- Threats to validity
- Time-series design
- Validity

For quantitative studies, a study's methods have a huge impact on the validity of the results than the research design—particularly if the inquiry is *cause-probing*. This chapter has information about how you can draw conclusions about evidence quality in a quantitative study.

OVERVIEW OF RESEARCH DESIGN ISSUES

The **research design** of a study spells out the strategies that researchers adopt to answer their questions and test their hypotheses. This section describes some basic design issues.

Key Research Design Features

Table 9.1 describes seven key features that are typically addressed in the design of a quantitative study. Design decisions that researchers must make include the following:

- *Will there be an intervention?* A basic design issue is whether or not researchers will introduce an intervention and test its effects—the distinction between experimental and nonexperimental research.
- *What types of comparisons will be made?* Quantitative researchers often make some type of comparisons. Sometimes, the *same* people are compared at different points in time (e.g., preoperatively vs. postoperatively), but often, different people are compared (e.g., those getting vs. not getting an intervention).
- *How will confounding variables be controlled?* In quantitative research, efforts are often made to control factors extraneous to the research question. This chapter discusses techniques for controlling confounding variables.
- *Will **blinding** be used?* Researchers must decide if information about the study (e.g., who is getting an intervention) will be hidden from data collectors, study participants, or others to minimize the risk of *expectation bias*—that is, the risk that such knowledge could influence study outcomes.

TABLE 9.1 Key Design Features

Feature	Key Questions	Design Options
Intervention	Will there be an intervention?	Experimental (RCT), quasiexperimental, nonexperimental (observational) design
Comparisons	What type of comparisons will be made to illuminate relationships?	Same participants (at different times or conditions), different participants
Control over confounding variables	How will confounding variables be controlled? Which confounding variables will be controlled?	Randomization, crossover, homogeneity, matching, statistical control
Blinding	From whom will critical information be withheld to avert bias?	Blinding participants, interventionists, other staff, data collectors
Time frames	How often will data be collected? When, relative to other events, will data be collected?	Cross-sectional, longitudinal design
Relative timing	When will information on independent and dependent variables be collected—looking backward or forward?	Retrospective (case control), prospective (cohort)
Location	Where will the study take place?	Setting choice: single site versus multisite

- *How often will data be collected?* Data sometimes are collected from participants at a single point in time (*cross-sectionally*), but other studies involve multiple points of data collection over time (*longitudinally*).
- *When will "effects" be measured, relative to potential causes?* Some studies collect information about outcomes and then look back *retrospectively* for potential causes. Other studies begin with a potential cause and then observe the outcomes, in a *prospective* fashion.
- *Where will the study take place?* Data for quantitative studies are collected in various settings, such as in hospitals or people's homes. Another decision concerns how many different sites will be involved in the study—a decision that could affect the generalizability of the results.

Many design decisions are independent of the others. For example, both experimental and nonexperimental studies can compare different people or the same people at different times. This chapter describes the implications of design decisions on the study's rigor or quality.

 TIP Information about the research design usually appears early in the method section of a research article.

Causality

Many research questions are about *causes* and *effects*. For example, does turning patients cause reductions in pressure ulcers? Does exercise cause improvements in heart function? Causality is a hotly debated issue, but we all understand the general concept of a **cause**. For example, we understand that failure to sleep *causes* fatigue and that high caloric intake *causes* weight gain. Most phenomena are determined multiple factors. Weight gain, for example, can be a result of high caloric intake *or* other factors. Causes are seldom *deterministic;* they only increase the likelihood that an effect will occur. For example, smoking is a cause of lung cancer, but not everyone who smokes develops lung cancer, and not everyone with lung cancer smoked.

While it might be easy to grasp what researchers mean when they talk about a *cause,* what exactly is an **effect**? One way to understand an effect is by understanding a counterfactual (Shadish, Cook, & Campbell, 2002). A *counterfactual* is defined by what would happen to the same people if they were exposed and not exposed to a causative factor at the same time. An effect is the difference between what actually did happen with the exposure and what would have happened without it.

Three criteria for establishing causal relationships are attributed to John Stuart Mill.

1. *Temporal:* A cause must precede an effect in time. If we test the hypothesis that smoking causes lung cancer, we need to show that cancer occurred *after* smoking began.
2. *Relationship:* There must be an association between the presumed cause and the effect. In our example, we have to demonstrate an association between smoking and cancer—that more smokers than nonsmokers get lung cancer.
3. *Confounders:* The relationship cannot be explained as being *caused by a third variable.* Suppose that smokers tended to live predominantly in urban environments. There would then be a possibility that the relationship between smoking and lung cancer reflects an underlying causal connection between the environment and lung cancer.

Other criteria for causality have been proposed. One important criterion in health research is *biologic plausibility*—evidence from basic physiologic studies that a causal pathway is possible. Researchers investigating causal relationships must provide persuasive evidence regarding these criteria through their research design.

TABLE 9.2 Hierarchy of Designs for Different Cause-Probing Research Questions

Type of Question	Hierarchy of Designs
Therapy	RCT/Experimental > Quasiexperimental > Cohort > Case control > Descriptive correlational
Prognosis	Cohort > Case control > Descriptive correlational
Etiology/harm (prevention)	RCT/Experimental > Quasiexperimental > Cohort > Case control > Descriptive correlational

Research Questions and Research Design

Quantitative research is used to address different types of research questions, and different designs are appropriate for different questions. In this chapter, we focus primarily on designs for Therapy, Prognosis, Etiology/Harm, and Description questions (Meaning questions require a qualitative approach and are discussed in Chapter 11).

Except for Description, questions that call for a quantitative approach usually concern causal relationships:

- Does a telephone counselling intervention for patients with prostate cancer *cause* improvements in their psychological distress? (Therapy question)
- Do birth weights under 1,500 g *cause* developmental delays in children? (Prognosis question)
- Does salt *cause* high blood pressure? (Etiology/Harm question)

Some designs are better at revealing cause-and-effect relationships than others. In particular, experimental designs (**randomized controlled trials (RCTs)**) are the best possible designs for showing causal relationships—but it is not always possible to use such designs. Table 9.2 summarizes a "hierarchy" of designs for answering different types of causal questions and augments the evidence hierarchy presented in Figure 2.1.

EXPERIMENTAL, QUASIEXPERIMENTAL, AND NONEXPERIMENTAL DESIGNS

This section describes designs that differ with regard to whether or not there is an intervention.

Experimental Design: Randomized Controlled Trials

Early scientists learned that complexities occurring in nature can make it difficult to understand relationships through pure observation. This problem was addressed by isolating phenomena and controlling the conditions under which they occurred. These experimental procedures have been adopted by researchers interested in human physiology and behaviour.

Characteristics of True Experiments

A true **experiment** or RCT is characterized by the following properties:

- *Intervention*—The experimenter *does* something to some participants by manipulating the independent variable.
- *Control*—The experimenter introduces a control group that does not receive the intervention.
- *Randomization*—The experimenter assigns participants to a control or experimental condition on a random basis.

By introducing an **intervention**, experimenters consciously vary the independent variable and then observe its effect on the outcome. To illustrate, suppose we were investigating the effect of gentle massage (I), compared to no massage (C), on pain (O) in nursing home residents (P). One experimental design for this question is a **pretest–posttest design**, which involves observing the outcome (pain levels) before and after the intervention. Participants in the experimental group receive a gentle massage, whereas those in the control group do not. This design allows us to see if changes in pain were *caused* by the massage among people who received the treatment. In this example, we met the first criterion of a true experiment by varying massage receipt, the independent variable.

This example also meets the second requirement for experiments, use of a control group. Inferences about causality require a comparison, but not all comparisons yield equally persuasive evidence. For example, if we were to supplement the diet of premature babies (P) with special nutrients (I) for 2 weeks, their weight (O) at the end of 2 weeks would tell us nothing about the intervention's effectiveness. At a minimum, we would need to compare before and after treatment to see if weight had increased. But suppose we find an average weight gain of 450 g. Does this finding support an inference of a causal connection between the nutritional intervention (the independent variable) and weight gain (the outcome)? No, because infants normally gain weight as they grow. Without a control group—a group that does not receive the supplements (C)—it is impossible to separate the effects of maturation from those of the treatment. The term **control group** refers to a group of participants whose performance on an outcome is used to evaluate the performance of the **experimental group** (the group getting the intervention) on the same outcome.

Experimental designs also involve placing participants in groups at random. Through **randomization (random assignment)**, every participant has an equal chance of being included in any group. If people are randomly assigned, there is no systematic bias in the groups with regard to their characteristics that may affect the outcome. *Randomly assigned groups are expected to be comparable, on average, with respect to an infinite number of biologic, psychological, and social traits at the outset of the study.* Group differences on outcomes observed *after* randomization can therefore be inferred as being caused by the treatment.

Random assignment can be accomplished by flipping a coin or pulling names from a hat. Researchers typically use computers to perform the randomization.

TIP There is a lot of confusion about random assignment versus random sampling. Random assignment is a *signature* of an experimental design (RCT). If subjects are not randomly assigned to intervention groups, then the design is not a true experiment. Random *sampling,* by contrast, refers to a method of selecting people for a study, as we discuss in Chapter 10. Random sampling is *not* a signature of an experimental design. In fact, most RCTs do *not* involve random sampling.

Experimental Designs

The most basic experimental design involves randomizing people to different groups and then measuring outcomes. This design is sometimes called a *posttest-only design.* A more widely used design, discussed earlier, is the pretest–posttest design, which involves collecting *pretest data* (often called **baseline data**) on the outcome before the intervention and **posttest (outcome) data** after it.

Example of a pretest–posttest design

Stevens and the Canadian Institute of Health Research team in children's pain (2016) studied the sustained effectiveness of a multidimensional knowledge translation intervention on pain assessment and management in eight Canadian pediatric hospitals. After the implementation of the program, half of the participating hospital units were randomized to participate in teleconferences every 4 months. Pain practice outcomes were measured at baseline and at the end of the study.

 TIP Experimental designs can be described graphically using symbols to represent features of the design. Space does not permit us to present these diagrams here, but many are shown in the Supplement to this chapter on thePoint.

The people who are randomly assigned to different conditions usually are different people. For example, if we were testing the effect of music on agitation (O) in patients with dementia (P), we could give some residents music (I) and others no music (C). A **crossover design**, by contrast, involves exposing people to one treatment first, and then crossover to another treatment. Such studies are true experiments only if people are randomly assigned to different orderings of treatment. For example, if a crossover design were used to compare the effects of music on patients with dementia, some would be randomly assigned to receive music first followed by a period of no music, and others would receive no music first. In such a study, the three conditions for an experiment have been met: There is intervention, randomization, and control—with *participants serving as their own control group (no treatment)*.

A crossover design has the advantage of exposing the same people to different conditions. However, such designs are sometimes inappropriate because of possible *carryover effects*. When subjects are exposed to two different treatments, they may be influenced in the second condition by their experience in the first. However, when carryover effects are implausible, as when intervention effects are immediate and short-lived, a crossover design is powerful.

Example of a crossover design •
Kiddoo and colleagues (2015) used a crossover design to test whether single-use hydrophilic-coated catheters reduced urinary tract infections compared to multiple use polyvinylchloride catheters for children with neurogenic bladder due to spina bifida. Patients were randomly assigned to the two types of catheter for 24 weeks each. They concluded that single-use hydrophilic-coated catheters did not decrease the incidence of symptomatic urinary tract infection in community-dwelling chronic intermittent catheterization users when compared to clean multiple-use polyvinylchloride catheters.

Experimental and Control Conditions

Researchers need to design an intervention that is of sufficient intensity and duration to produce an expected outcome. The intervention is described carefully in formal *protocols* that stipulate exactly what the treatment is.

Researchers have choices about what to use as the control condition, and the decision affects the interpretation of the findings. Among the possibilities for the control condition are the following:

- "Usual care"—Standard or normal procedures are used to treat patients
- An alternative treatment (e.g., music vs. massage)
- A **placebo** or pseudointervention presumed to have no therapeutic value
- An *attention control condition* (the control group gets attention but not the intervention's active ingredients)
- *Delayed treatment* (i.e., control group members are *wait-listed* and exposed to the intervention at a later point)

Example of a delayed treatment •
Stern and Lindquist (2015) tested the clinical and cost-effectiveness of enhanced multidisciplinary teams (EMDTs) compared to "usual care" for the treatment of pressure ulcers in long-term care (LTC) facilities in Ontario, Canada. In a stepped wedge design, some facilities were exposed to the intervention toward the end of the study than in its early stages.

Ethically, the delayed treatment design is attractive but is not always feasible. Testing two alternative interventions is also appealing ethically, but it may be difficult to detect differential effects if both treatments were good.

Researchers must also consider possibilities for blinding. Many nursing interventions do not lend themselves easily to blinding. For example, if the intervention were a smoking cessation program, participants would know whether they were receiving the intervention, and the intervener would know who was in the program. It is usually possible and desirable, however, to blind the participants' group status from the people collecting outcome data.

Example of an experiment with blinding •
Chartrand, Tourigny, & MacCormick (2017) at the University of Ottawa studied the effect of an educational preoperative DVD on parents' anxiety, participation, and knowledge as well as its impact on children's distress, pain, and recovery after same-day surgery. The nurses caring for the participants, research assistants collecting data, and researchers were blinded to group assignments.

 TIP The term *double blind* is widely used when more than one group is blinded (e.g., participants and interventionists). However, this term is falling into disfavour because of its ambiguity, in favour of clear specifications about exactly who was blinded and who was not.

Advantages and Disadvantages of Experiments

RCTs are the "gold standard" for intervention studies (Therapy questions) because they yield the most persuasive evidence about the effects of an intervention. Through randomization to groups, researchers come as close as possible to attaining an "ideal" counterfactual.

The great strength of experiments lies in the potential to infer causal relationships with confidence. Through the controls imposed by intervening, comparing, and—especially—randomizing, alternative explanations can often be ruled out. For this reason, meta-analyses of RCTs, which integrate evidence from multiple experimental studies, are at the tip of evidence hierarchies for questions relating to causes (Fig. 2.1).

Despite the advantages of experiments, they have limitations. First, many interesting variables simply are not suitable for intervention. A large number of human traits, such as disease or health habits, do not occur at random. That is why RCTs are not at the top of the hierarchy for Prognosis questions (Table 9.2), which concern the consequences of health problems. For example, infants could not be randomly assigned to having cystic fibrosis to see if this disease causes poor psychosocial adjustment.

Second, many variables could technically—but not ethically—be manipulated experimentally. For example, there have been no RCTs to study the effect of cigarette smoking on lung cancer. Such a study would require people to be assigned randomly to a smoking group (people forced to smoke) or a nonsmoking group (people prohibited from smoking). Thus, although RCTs are technically at the top of the evidence hierarchy for Etiology/Harm questions (Table 9.2), many etiology questions cannot be answered using an experimental design.

Sometimes, RCTs are not feasible because of practical issues. It may, for instance, be impossible to secure the administrative approval to randomize people into groups. In summary, experimental designs have some limitations that restrict their use for some real-world problems; nevertheless, RCTs have a clear superiority to other designs for testing causal hypotheses.

 HOW-TO-TELL TIP   How can you tell if a study is experimental? Researchers usually indicate in the method section of their reports that they used an experimental or randomized design (RCT). If such terms are missing, you can conclude that a study is experimental if the article says that the study purpose was to *test the effects of* an intervention AND if participants were put into groups at random.

Quasiexperiments

Quasiexperiments (called *trials without randomization* in the medical literature) are also the implementation of an intervention without randomization, the signature of a true experiment. Some quasiexperiments even lack a control group.

Quasiexperimental Designs

A frequently used quasiexperimental design is the **nonequivalent control group** pretest–posttest design, which involves comparing two or more groups of people before and after implementing an intervention. For example, suppose we wished to study the effect of a chair yoga intervention (I) for older people (P) on quality of life (QOL) (O). The intervention is being offered to everyone at a community senior center, and randomization is not possible. For comparative purposes, we collect outcome data at a different senior centre that is not implementing the intervention (C). Data on QOL are collected from both groups at baseline and 10 weeks later.

This quasiexperimental design is identical to a pretest–posttest experimental design *except* people were not randomized to groups. The quasiexperimental design is weaker because, without randomization, *it cannot be assumed that the experimental and comparison groups are equivalent at the outset.* The design is, nevertheless, strong because the baseline data allow us to see whether elders in the two senior centers had similar QOL scores before the intervention. If the groups are comparable at baseline, we could be relatively confident inferring that posttest differences in QOL were the result of the yoga intervention. If QOL scores are different initially, however, postintervention differences are hard to interpret. Note that in quasiexperiments, the term **comparison group** is sometimes used in lieu of *control group* to refer to the group against which outcomes in the treatment group are evaluated.

Now suppose we had been unable to collect baseline data. Such a design (*nonequivalent control group posttest-only*) has a flaw that is hard to overcome. We no longer have information about initial equivalence. If QOL in the experimental group is higher than that in the control group at the posttest, can we conclude that the intervention *caused* improved QOL? There could be other explanations for the differences. In particular, QOL in the two centers might have differed initially. The hallmark of strong quasiexperiments is the effort to introduce some controls, such as baseline measurements.

Example of a nonequivalent control group design • • • • • • • • • • • • • • • •
Austen and colleagues (2017) used a nonequivalent control group pretest–posttest design to test whether a music video would promote and increase in comfort levels in viewing breastfeeding among young adults. Half of all participants were exposed to the music video whereas the remaining participants did not view the video. Breastfeeding comfort ratings were improved at posttest for participants who saw the video.

Some quasiexperiments have neither randomization nor a comparison group. Suppose a hospital implemented rapid response teams (RRTs) in its acute care units and wanted to learn the effects on patient outcomes (e.g., mortality). For the purposes of this example, assume no other hospital would be a good comparison, and so the only possible comparison is a before–after contrast. If RRTs were implemented in January, we could compare the mortality rate, for example, during the 3 months before RRTs with the mortality rate in the subsequent 3-month period.

This *one-group pretest–posttest design* seems logical, but it has weaknesses. What if one of the 3-month periods is atypical, apart from the RRTs? What about the effect of other changes introduced during the same period? What about the effects of external factors, such as seasonal morbidity? The design in question offers no way to control these factors.

However, the design could be modified so that some alternative explanations for changes in mortality could be ruled out. For example, the **time-series design** involves collecting data over an extended time period and introducing the treatment during that period. The present study could be designed with four observations before the RRTs are introduced (e.g., four quarters of mortality data for the prior year) and four observations after it (mortality for the next four quarters). Although a time-series design does not eliminate all interpretive problems, the extended time perspective strengthens the ability to attribute improvements to the intervention.

Example of a time-series design •
Lavoie-Tremblay et al. (2017) tested the effectiveness of a quality improvement program to enhance team's effectiveness, nosocomial infections, and patient experience in an academic health science centre in Montreal. The intervention was composed of independent learning modules, workshops, and hands-on learning. There was a significant reduction in the number of vancomycin-resistant *Enterococcus* (VRE) infection over a 19-month period. No significant change was observed in the patients' evaluation of nurse communication, responsiveness, cleanliness, and discharge information.

Advantages and Disadvantages of Quasiexperiments

One strength of quasiexperiments is their practicality. Nursing research often occurs in natural settings, where it is difficult to deliver an innovative treatment randomly to some people but not to others. Strong quasiexperimental designs introduce some research control when full experimental rigor is not possible.

Another issue is that people are not always willing to be randomized. Quasiexperimental designs, because they do not involve random assignment, are likely to be acceptable to more people. This, in turn, has implications for the generalizability of the results—but the results are less conclusive.

The major disadvantage of quasiexperiments is that causal inferences cannot be made as readily as with RCTs. A number of plausible alternative explanations can be used to interpret results of quasiexperiments. For example, suppose we administered a special diet to a group of frail nursing home residents to assess its impact on weight gain. If we use a nonequivalent control group and then observe a weight gain, we must ask: Is it *plausible* that some other factor caused the gain? Is it *plausible* that pretreatment differences between the intervention and comparison groups resulted in differential gain? Is it *plausible* that there was an average weight gain simply because the most frail died or were transferred to a hospital? If the answer to any of these *rival hypotheses* is yes, then inferences about the causal effect of the intervention are weakened. With quasiexperiments, there is almost always at least one plausible rival explanation.

HOW-TO-TELL TIP How can you tell if a study is quasiexperimental? Researchers do not always identify their designs as quasiexperimental. If a study involves an intervention and if the report does not explicitly mention random assignment, it is probably safe to conclude that the design is quasiexperimental.

Nonexperimental Studies

Many cause-probing research questions cannot be addressed with an RCT or quasiexperiment. For example, take this Prognosis question: Do birth weights under 1,500 g *cause* developmental delays in children? Clearly, we cannot manipulate birth weight, the independent variable. When researchers do not intervene by controlling the independent variable, the study is nonexperimental, or, in the medical literature, *observational*.

There are various reasons for doing a **nonexperimental study**, including situations in which the independent variable cannot be manipulated (Prognosis questions) or should not be manipulated for ethical reasons (some Etiology questions). Experimental designs are also not appropriate for Descriptive questions.

Types of Nonexperimental/Observational Studies

When researchers study the effect of a *cause* they cannot manipulate, they undertake a **correlational study** that examines relationships between variables. A **correlation** is an association between two variables, that is, a tendency for change in one variable to be related to change in another (e.g., people's height and weight). Correlations can be detected through statistical analyses.

It is risky to infer causal relationships in correlational research. In RCTs, investigators predict that purposeful variation of the independent variable will result in a change to the outcome variable. In correlational research, investigators do not control the independent variable, which has often already occurred. A famous research dictum is relevant: *Correlation does not prove causation.* The mere existence of a relationship between variables is not enough to conclude that one variable caused the other, even if the relationship is strong.

Correlational studies are weaker than RCTs for cause-probing questions, but different designs offer varying degrees of supportive evidence. The strongest design for Prognosis questions, and for Etiology questions when randomization is impossible, is a cohort design (Table 9.2). Observational studies with a **cohort design** (sometimes called a **prospective design**) start with a presumed cause and then go forward to evaluate the presumed effect. For example, in prospective lung cancer studies, researchers start with a cohort of adults (P) that includes smokers (I) and nonsmokers (C) and then compare subsequent lung cancer incidence (O) in the two groups.

Example of a cohort (prospective) design •
Dennis, Merry, & Gagnon (2017) studied the relationship between migration status and postpartum depression among recent refugee; asylum-seeking, nonrefugee immigrant; and Canadian-born women.

TIP Experimental studies are inherently prospective because the researcher institutes the intervention and subsequently examines its effect.

In correlational studies with a **retrospective design**, an effect (outcome) observed in the present is linked to a potential cause occurring in the past. For example, in retrospective lung cancer research, researchers begin with some people who have lung cancer and others who do not and then look for differences in previous behaviours or conditions, such as smoking habits. Such a study uses a **case-control design**—that is, *cases* with a certain condition such as lung cancer are compared to *controls* without it. In designing a case-control study, researchers try to identify controls who are as similar as possible to cases with regard to confounding variables (e.g., age, gender). The difficulty, however, is that the two groups are almost never comparable with respect to *all* factors influencing the outcome.

Example of a case-control design •
Marin & Woo (2017) conducted a study to identify clinical characteristics that differentiate arterial leg ulcers from venous leg ulcers. Individuals with arterial leg ulcers were associated with lower health-related QOL, greater mobility impairments, and more deficits in self-care and usual activities than those with venous leg ulcers.

Prospective studies are more costly, but stronger, than retrospective studies. For one thing, the temporal order of events is clear in prospective research (i.e., smoking is known to precede the lung cancer). In addition, samples are more likely to be representative of smokers and nonsmokers.

A second broad class of nonexperimental studies is **descriptive research**. The purpose of descriptive studies is to observe, describe, and document aspects of a situation. For example, an investigator may wish to discover the percentage of teenagers who smoke—that is, the *prevalence* of certain behaviours. Sometimes a study design is *descriptive correlational*, meaning that researchers seek to describe relationships among variables, without inferring causal connections. For example, researchers might be interested in describing the relationship between fatigue and psychological distress in HIV patients. In such situations, a descriptive nonexperimental design is appropriate.

Example of a descriptive correlational study •
Jin and colleagues (2017) conducted a descriptive correlational study of family caregivers for patients with stroke to examine relationships among perceptions of functional deficits, mood states, and empathic responses.

 TIP For Descriptive questions, the strongest design is a nonexperimental study that relies on random sampling of participants. Random sampling is discussed in Chapter 10.

Advantages and Disadvantages of Nonexperimental Research

The major disadvantage of nonexperimental studies is that they do not provide persuasive evidence for causal inferences. Correlational studies are designed to describe relationships, but they are often undertaken to discover causes. Yet correlational studies are susceptible to incorrect interpretation because groups being compared have formed through **self-selection**. A researcher doing a correlational study cannot assume that the comparison groups were similar before the occurrence of the independent variable.

As an example of such interpretive problems, suppose we studied differences in depression (O) of cancer patients (P) who do or do not have adequate social support (I and C). Suppose we found a correlation—that is, that patients without social support were more depressed than patients with social support. We could interpret this to mean that patients' emotional state is influenced by the adequacy of their social support, as diagrammed in Figure 9.1A. There are, however, alternative interpretations. Maybe a third variable influences *both* social support and depression, such as whether the patients are married. Having a spouse may affect patients' depression *and* the quality of their social support (Fig. 9.1B). A

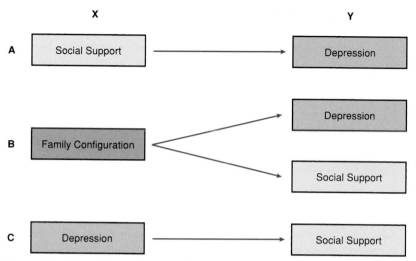

Figure 9.1 Alternative explanations for correlation between depression and social support in cancer patients.

third possibility is reversed causality (Fig. 9.1C). Depressed cancer patients may find it more difficult to elicit social support than patients who are cheerful. In this interpretation, the person's depression causes the amount of received social support, not the other way around. The point is that correlational results should be interpreted cautiously.

 TIP Be prepared to think critically when a researcher claims to be studying the "effects" of one variable on another in a nonexperimental study. For example, if a report title were "The Effects of Eating Disorders on Depression," the study would be nonexperimental (i.e., participants were not randomly assigned to an eating disorder). In such a situation, you might ask, Did the eating disorder have an effect on depression?—or did depression have an effect on eating patterns? or Did a third variable (e.g., childhood abuse) have an effect on both?

Nevertheless, nonexperimental studies play a big role in nursing because many interesting problems do not lend themselves to intervention. An example is whether smoking causes lung cancer. Despite the absence of any RCTs with humans, few people doubt that this causal connection exists. There is strong evidence of a relationship between smoking and lung cancer and, through prospective studies, that smoking precedes lung cancer. In numerous replications, researchers have been able to control for, and thus rule out, other possible "causes" of lung cancer.

Correlational research can offer an efficient way to collect large amounts of data about a problem. For example, it would be possible to collect information about people's health problems and eating habits. Researchers could then examine which problems correlate with which eating patterns. By doing this, many relationships could be discovered in a short time. By contrast, an experimenter looks at only a few variables at a time. For example, one RCT might manipulate cholesterol, whereas another might manipulate protein. Nonexperimental work is often necessary to support future interventional studies.

THE TIME DIMENSION IN RESEARCH DESIGN

Research designs incorporate decisions about when and how often data will be collected, and studies can be categorized in terms of how they deal with time. The major distinction is between cross-sectional and longitudinal designs.

Cross-Sectional Designs

In **cross-sectional designs**, data are collected at one point in time. For example, a researcher might study whether psychological symptoms in menopausal women are correlated with physiologic symptoms. Retrospective studies are usually cross-sectional: Data on the independent and outcome variables are collected at the same time (e.g., participants' lung cancer status and smoking habits), but the independent variable usually concerns events or behaviours occurring in the past.

Cross-sectional designs can be used to study time-related phenomena, but they are less persuasive than longitudinal designs. Suppose we were studying changes in children's health-promotion activities between ages 8 and 10 years. One way to investigate this would be to interview children at age 8 years and then 2 years later at age 10 years—a longitudinal design. Or, we could question two groups of children, ages 8 and 10 years, at one point in time and then compare responses—a cross-sectional design. If 10-year-olds engaged in more health-promoting activities than 8-year-olds, it might be inferred that children made healthier choices as they aged. To make this inference, we have to assume that the older children would have responded as the younger ones did had they been questioned 2 years earlier or, conversely, that 8-year-olds would report more health-promoting activities if they were questioned again 2 years later.

Cross-sectional designs are economical, but they pose problems for inferring changes over time. The amount of social and technologic change that characterizes our society makes it questionable to assume that differences in the behaviours or characteristics of different age groups are the result of the passage through time rather than cohort differences.

> **Example of a cross-sectional study** •
> Freeman and colleagues (2016) studied the relationship between expression of the desire to die and demographic factors—including age—in palliative home care services in Ontario, Canada. Four age groups were compared—those aged 18 to 64 years, 65 to 74 years, 75 to 84 years, and 85 years or older. Home care clients over the age of 85 years were three times more likely to express a desire to die than clients under the age of 65.

Longitudinal Designs

Longitudinal designs involve collecting data multiple times over an extended period. Such designs are useful for studying changes over time and for establishing the sequencing of phenomena, which is a criterion for inferring causality.

In nursing research, longitudinal studies are often *follow-up studies* of a clinical population, undertaken to assess the subsequent status of people with a specified condition or who received an intervention. For example, patients who received a smoking cessation intervention could be followed up to assess its long-term effectiveness. As a nonexperimental example, samples of premature infants could be followed up to assess subsequent motor development.

> **Example of a follow-up study** •
> Puts and coresearchers (2017) examined how comorbidity, frailty, and functional status influenced the decision-making process for chemotherapy treatments among older adults with cancer. Thirty-two participants completed the survey that assessed the degree of control an individual wanted when decisions are being made about medical treatment and satisfaction with decision. Similar evaluation was done 3 to 6 months after the treatment decision.

In longitudinal studies, researchers must decide the number of data collection points and the time intervals between them. When change is rapid, numerous data collection points at relatively short intervals may be required to understand transitions. By convention, however, the term *longitudinal* implies multiple data collection points over an extended period of time.

A challenge in longitudinal studies is the loss of participants (**attrition**) over time. Attrition is problematic because those who drop out of the study usually differ in important ways from those who continue to participate, resulting in potential biases and problems with generalizability.

 TIP   Not all longitudinal studies are prospective because sometimes the independent variable occurred even before the initial wave of data collection. And not all prospective studies are longitudinal in the classic sense. For example, an experimental study that collects data at 1, 2, and 4 hours after an intervention would be prospective but not longitudinal (i.e., data are not collected over a long time period).

TECHNIQUES OF RESEARCH CONTROL

A major goal of research design in quantitative studies is to maximize researchers' control over confounding variables. Two broad categories of confounders need to be controlled—those that are intrinsic to study participants and those that are situational factors.

Controlling the Study Context

External factors, such as the research context, can affect outcomes. In well-controlled quantitative research, steps are taken to achieve *constancy of conditions* so that outcomes reflect the effect of the independent variable and not the study context.

Researchers cannot totally control study contexts, but certain strategies worth consideration. For example, blinding is a way to control bias. By keeping data collectors and others unaware of group allocation, researchers minimize the risk that other people involved in the study will influence the results.

Most quantitative studies also standardize communications to participants. Formal scripts are often prepared to inform participants about the study purpose and methods. In intervention studies, researchers develop formal intervention protocols. Careful researchers pay attention to *intervention fidelity*—that is, they monitor whether an intervention is faithfully delivered in accordance with its plan and that the intended treatment was actually received.

> **Example of attention to intervention fidelity** ·
> Markle-Reid and colleagues (2016) described their efforts to support program fidelity in implementing an interprofessional, nurse-led program to promote self-management in older adults with type 2 diabetes and multiple chronic conditions. The investigators prepared a manual describing the program and provided training to all team members. To monitor implementation, the researchers met with the program team at monthly meetings.

Controlling Participant Factors

Outcomes of interest to nurse researchers are affected by dozens of attributes that are irrelevant to the research question. For example, suppose we were investigating the effects of a physical fitness program on the physical functioning of nursing home residents. In this study, variables such as the participants' age, gender, and smoking history would be confounding variables; each is likely to be related to the outcome variable (physical functioning), independent of the program. In other words, the effects that these variables have on the outcome are extraneous to the study. In this section, we review strategies researchers can use to control confounding variables.

Randomization

Randomization is the most effective way to control participants' characteristics. A critical advantage of randomization, compared with other control strategies, is that it controls *all* possible sources of extraneous variation, without any conscious decision about which variables should be controlled. In our example of a physical fitness intervention, random assignment of elders to an intervention or control group would yield groups presumably comparable in terms of age, gender, smoking history, and dozens of other characteristics that could affect the outcome. Randomization to different treatment orderings in a crossover design is especially powerful: Participants serve as their own controls, thereby controlling all confounding characteristics.

Homogeneity

When randomization is not feasible, other methods of controlling extraneous characteristics can be used. One alternative is **homogeneity**, in which only people who are similar with respect to confounding variables are included in the study. In the physical fitness example, if gender were a confounding variable, we could recruit only men (or women) as participants. If age was considered a confounder, participation could be limited to a specified age range. Using a homogeneous sample is easy, but one problem is limited generalizability.

> **Example of control through homogeneity** •
> Lambert et al. (2016) used a randomized controlled trial design to examine the effect of a self-directed coping skill and self-management interventions for couples managing prostate cancer. Several variables were controlled through homogeneity; inclusion criteria were patients diagnosed with early stage of prostate cancer in the past 4 months, receiving or planning to receive treatment, having no previous cancer diagnosis, and having a partner willing to participate in the study.

Matching

A third method of controlling confounding variables is **matching**, which involves consciously forming comparable groups. For example, suppose we began with a group of nursing home residents who agreed to participate in the physical fitness program. A comparison group of nonparticipating residents could be created by matching participants on the basis of important confounding variables (e.g., age and gender). This procedure results in groups known to be similar on specific confounding variables. Matching is often used to form comparable groups in case-control designs.

Matching has some drawbacks. To match effectively, researchers must know what the relevant confounders are. Also, after two or three variables, it becomes difficult to match. Suppose we wanted to control age, gender, and length of nursing home stay. In this situation, if a program participant were an 80-year-old woman whose length of stay was 5 years, we would have to seek another woman with these characteristics for comparison. With more than three variables, matching becomes difficult. Thus, matching is a control method used primarily when more powerful procedures are not feasible.

Example of control through matching •
Stavrinos et al. (2015) compared clinical characteristics, treatments, and outcomes of homeless to nonhomeless patients admitted to intensive care units. Sixty-three randomly selected homeless patients and 63 nonhomeless patients were matched for calendar year of admission sex, age, and admitting units. Homelessness was not an independent predictor of hospital mortality.

Statistical Control

Researchers can also control confounding variables statistically. Methods of statistical control are complex, and so a detailed description of powerful statistical control mechanisms, such as *analysis of covariance*, will not be attempted. However, you should recognize that nurse researchers are increasingly using powerful statistical techniques to control confounding variables. A brief description of methods of statistical control is presented in Chapter 14.

Evaluation of Control Methods

Random assignment is the most effective approach to controlling confounding variables because randomization tends to control individual variation on all possible confounders. Crossover designs are especially powerful, but they cannot be used in many situations because of the possibility of carryover effects. Two issues need to be addressed in other alternative designs. First, researchers must decide in advance which variables to control. To select homogeneous samples, match, or use statistical control, researchers must identify which variables to control. Second, these methods control only the specified characteristics, leaving others uncontrolled.

Although randomization is an excellent tool, it is not always feasible. It is better to use matching or statistical control than to ignore the problem of confounding variables.

CHARACTERISTICS OF GOOD DESIGN

A critical question in critiquing a quantitative study is whether the research design yielded valid evidence. Four key questions regarding research design, particularly in cause-probing studies, are as follows:

1. What is the strength of the evidence that a relationship between variables really exists?
2. If a relationship exists, what is the strength of the evidence that the independent variable (e.g., an intervention), rather than other factors, *caused* the outcome?
3. What is the strength of evidence that observed relationships are generalizable across people, settings, and time?
4. What are the theoretical constructs underlying the study variables, and are those constructs adequately captured?

These questions, respectively, correspond to four aspects of a study's **validity**: (1) statistical conclusion validity, (2) internal validity, (3) external validity, and (4) construct validity (Shadish et al., 2002).

Statistical Conclusion Validity

As noted previously, one criterion for establishing causality is a demonstrated relationship between the independent and dependent variable. Statistical tests are used to support inferences about whether such a relationship exists. We note here a few issues that can affect a study's **statistical conclusion validity**.

Statistical power, the capacity to detect true relationships, affects the validity of statistical conclusion. The most straightforward way to achieve statistical power is to use a large enough sample. With small samples, the analyses may fail to show that the independent variable and the outcome are related—*even when they are*. Power and sample size are discussed in Chapter 10.

Researchers can also enhance power by increasing differences on the independent variables (i.e., making the *cause* powerful) so as to maximize differences on the outcome (the effect). If the groups or treatments are not very different, the statistical analysis might not be sufficiently sensitive to detect effects that actually exist. Intervention fidelity can enhance the power of an intervention.

Thus, if you are critiquing a study in which outcomes for the groups being compared were not significantly different, one possibility is that the study had low statistical conclusion validity. The report might give clues about this possibility (e.g., too small a sample or substantial attrition) that should be taken into consideration in interpreting the results.

Internal Validity

Internal validity is the extent that the independent variable is assumed to cause the outcome. RCTs tend to have high internal validity because randomization enables researchers to rule out competing explanations for group differences. With quasiexperiments and correlational studies, there are competing explanations for what is causing the outcome, which are sometimes called **threats to validity**. Evidence hierarchies rank study designs mainly in terms of internal validity.

Threats to Validity

Temporal Ambiguity

In a causal relationship, the cause precedes the effect. In RCTs, researchers create the independent variable and then observe the outcome, so establishing a temporal sequence is not a problem. In correlational studies, however—especially ones using a cross-sectional design—it may be unclear whether the independent variable preceded the dependent variable, or vice versa, as illustrated in Figure 9.1.

Selection

The **selection threat (self-selection)** brings about biases due to pre-existing differences between groups. When people are not assigned randomly to groups, the groups being compared may not be equivalent; group differences in the outcome may be caused by extraneous factors rather than by the independent variable. Selection bias is the most challenging threat to the internal validity of studies not using an experimental design but can be partially addressed using control strategies described in the previous section.

History

The **history threat** is the occurrence of events concurrent with the independent variable that can affect the outcome. For example, suppose we were studying the effectiveness of a senior centre program to promote flu shots among the elderly. Now suppose a story about a flu epidemic was aired in the national media at about the same time. Our outcome variable, number of flu shots administered, is now influenced by at least two forces, and it would be hard to disentangle the two effects. In RCTs, history is not typically a threat because external events are as likely to affect one randomized group as another. The designs most likely to be affected by the history threat are one-group pretest–posttest designs and time-series designs.

Maturation

The **maturation threat** arises from processes occurring as a result of time (e.g., growth, fatigue) rather than the independent variable. For example, if we were studying the effect of an intervention for developmentally delayed children, our design would have to deal with the fact that progress would occur without an intervention. *Maturation* does not refer only to developmental changes but to any change that occurs as a function of time. Phenomena such as wound healing or postoperative recovery occur with little intervention, and so maturation may explain favourable posttreatment outcomes if the design does not include a comparison group. One-group pretest–posttest designs are especially vulnerable to the maturation threat.

Mortality/Attrition

Mortality is the threat that arises from attrition in groups being compared. If different kinds of people remain in the study in one group versus another, then these differences, rather than the independent variable, could account for group differences in outcomes. The most severely ill patients might drop out of an experimental condition because it is too demanding, for example. Attrition bias essentially is a selection bias that occurs after the study unfolds: Groups initially equivalent can lose comparability because of attrition, and differential group composition, rather than the independent variable, could be the "cause" of any group differences on outcomes.

 TIP If attrition is random (i.e., those dropping out of a study are similar to those remaining in it), then there would not be bias. However, attrition is rarely random. In general, the higher the rate of attrition, the greater the risk of bias. Biases are usually of concern if the rate exceeds 10% to 15%.

Internal Validity and Research Design

Quasiexperimental and correlational studies are especially susceptible to internal validity threats. These threats compete with the independent variable as a cause of the outcome. *The aim of a good quantitative research design is to rule out these competing explanations.* The control mechanisms previously described are strategies for improving internal validity—and thus for strengthening the quality of evidence.

An experimental design often, but not always, eliminates competing explanations. Experimental mortality is a particularly significant threat. Because researchers do different things with the groups, members may drop out of the study for different reasons. This is particularly likely to happen if the intervention is stressful or time-consuming or if the control condition is boring or disappointing. Participants remaining in a study may differ from those who left, abolishing the initial equivalence of the groups.

You should carefully consider possible rival explanations for study results, especially in non-RCT studies. When researchers do not have control over critical confounding variables, it is necessary to exercise caution in drawing conclusions about the evidence.

External Validity

External validity concerns inferences about whether relationships found for study participants might hold true for different people and settings. External validity is critical to evidence-based practice (EBP) because it is important to generalize evidence from controlled research settings to real-world practice settings.

External validity questions can take several different forms. For example, we may ask whether relationships observed with a study sample can be generalized to a larger population—for example, whether results about rates of postpartum depression in Saskatoon can be generalized to mothers in Prince Edward Island. Thus, one aspect of a study's external validity concerns sampling. If the sample is representative of the population, generalizing results to the population is safer (Chapter 10).

Other external validity questions are about generalizing to different types of people, settings, or situations. For example, can findings about a pain reduction treatment in Norway be generalized to people in Canada? New studies are often needed to answer questions about generalizability. An important concept here is *replication*. Multisite studies are powerful because generalizability of the results can be enhanced if the results have been replicated in several sites—particularly if the sites differ on important dimensions (e.g., size). Studies with a diverse sample of participants can assess whether results are replicated for various subgroups—for example, whether an intervention benefits men *and* women. Systematic reviews represent a crucial aid to external validity precisely because they explore consistency in results based on replications across time, space, people, and settings.

The competing demands for internal and external validity may create a dilemma. If a researcher exercises tight control to maximize internal validity, the setting may become too artificial to generalize to more naturalistic environments. Compromises are often necessary.

Construct Validity

Research involves constructs. Researchers conduct a study with specific exemplars of treatments, outcomes, settings, and people, but these are all representations for broad constructs. **Construct validity** involves making inferences from the particulars of the study to the higher order constructs they are intended to represent. If studies contain construct errors, the evidence could be misleading. One aspect of construct validity concerns the degree to which an intervention is a good representation of the construct that have the potential to cause beneficial outcomes. Lack of blinding undermines construct validity: Is it an intervention, or *awareness* of the intervention, that resulted in benefits? Another issue is whether the measures of the dependent variable are good operationalizations of constructs. This aspect of construct validity is discussed in Chapter 10.

CRITIQUING QUANTITATIVE RESEARCH DESIGNS

A key evaluative question is whether the research design enabled researchers to get good answers to the research question. This question has both substantive and methodologic components.

Substantively, the issue is whether the design matches the aims of the research. If the research purpose is descriptive or exploratory, an experimental design is not appropriate. If the researcher is searching to understand the full nature of a poorly understood phenomenon, a structured design that allows little flexibility might block insights (flexible designs are discussed in Chapter 11). We have discussed research control as a bias-reducing strategy, but too much control can introduce bias—for example, a researcher who applies tight controls over how phenomena are studied may run the risk of distorting their true nature.

Methodologically, the main design issue in quantitative studies is whether the research design provides the most valid, unbiased, and interpretable evidence possible. Indeed, there usually is no other aspect of a quantitative study that affects the quality of evidence as much as research design. Box 9.1 provides questions to assist you in evaluating research designs.

> **Box 9.1 Guidelines for Critiquing Research Design in a Quantitative Study**
>
> 1. Was the design experimental, quasiexperimental, or nonexperimental? What specific design was used? Was this a cause-probing study? Given the type of question (Therapy, Prognosis, etc.), was the most rigorous possible design used?
> 2. What type of comparison was called for in the research design? Was the comparison strategy effective in illuminating key relationships?
> 3. If the study involved an intervention, were the intervention and control conditions adequately described? Was blinding used, and if so, who was blinded? If not, is there a good rationale for failure to use blinding?
> 4. If the study was nonexperimental, why did the researcher opt not to intervene? If the study was cause-probing, which criteria for inferring causality were potentially compromised? Was a retrospective or prospective design used, and was such a design appropriate?
> 5. Was the study longitudinal or cross-sectional? Was the number and timing of data collection points appropriate?
> 6. What did the researcher do to control confounding participant characteristics, and were the procedures effective? What are the threats to the study's internal validity? Did the design enable the researcher to draw causal inferences about the relationship between the independent variable and the outcome?
> 7. What are the major limitations of the design used? Were these limitations acknowledged by the researcher and taken into account in interpreting results? What can be said about the study's external validity?

RESEARCH EXAMPLES WITH CRITICAL THINKING EXERCISES

This section presents examples of studies with different research designs. Read these summaries and then answer the critical thinking questions, referring to the full research report if necessary. Examples 1 and 2 are featured on the interactive *Critical Thinking Activity* on thePoint website. The critical thinking questions for Exercise 3 are based on the study that appears in its entirety in Appendix A of this book. Our comments for these questions are in the Student Resources section on thePoint.

EXAMPLE 1: A RANDOMIZED CONTROLLED CROSSOVER TRIAL

Study: Hydrocortisone cream to reduce perineal pain after vaginal birth: A randomized controlled trial (Manfre et al., 2015)

Statement of Purpose: The purpose of the study was to evaluate whether the use of hydrocortisone cream can decrease perineal pain in the immediate postpartum period.

Design and Treatment Conditions: The researchers used a randomized crossover design in which participants received three different methods for pain management at three sequential pain treatments after birth: two topical creams (corticosteroid and placebo) and a control treatment (no cream application). The placebo cream was a similar cetyl alcohol–based cream.

Method: A sample of 29 mothers who gave birth vaginally was randomly assigned to different orderings of the three conditions. The sample size was based on an analysis undertaken to ensure adequate statistical power. Mothers were first asked to rate their pain within 2 hours of admission to the postpartum unit. After the rating, the investigator applied the first randomly assigned treatment to a witch hazel pad and placed the pad on the perineum. Participants rated their pain again 30 to 60 minutes later. Following the initial application, the process was repeated every 6 hours for the second and third randomly assigned perineal treatment. The dependent variable was the change in perineal pain levels before and 30 to 60 minutes after application of the treatment. Both the participants and the investigators were blinded to cream type—a pharmacist prepared the study treatments and packaged them in sterile tubes. A total of 29 participants were enrolled in the study, with 27 completing all three treatments over a 12-hour period.

Key Findings: A significant reduction in pain was found after application of both the topical creams. The application of either hydrocortisone cream or placebo cream provided significantly better pain relief than no cream application. The average decline in pain was similar in the two cream groups: 6.7 points for the placebo cream and 4.8 with the hydrocortisone cream.

Critical Thinking Exercises

1. Answer the relevant questions from Box 9.1 regarding this study.
2. Also consider the following targeted questions:
   a. Could three-group design have been used in this study?
   b. Why might the two creams have been comparably effective in reducing pain?
3. If the results of this study are valid, what are some of the uses to which the findings might be put in clinical practice?

EXAMPLE 2: A QUASIEXPERIMENTAL DESIGN

Study: A study to promote breastfeeding in the Helsinki Metropolitan area in Finland (Hannula, Kaunonen, & Puukka, 2014).

Statement of Purpose: The purpose of the study was to test the effect of providing intensified support for breastfeeding during the perinatal period on the breastfeeding behaviour of women in Finland.

Treatment Groups: The women in the intervention group were offered a free, noncommercial web-based service that provided intensified support for parenthood, child care, and breastfeeding from the 20th gestation week until the child was 1 year old. The mothers were cared for by staff with specialized training who also provided individualized support. Women in the comparison group received usual care from midwifery and nursing professionals.

Method: The study was conducted in three public maternity hospitals in Helsinki. Because randomization was not possible, two of the hospitals implemented the intensified support services, and the third hospital served as the control. Women who were 18 to 21 weeks of gestation were recruited into the intervention group if they were expecting a singleton birth. Altogether, 705 women participated in the study, 431 were in the intervention group and 274 in the comparison group. Study participants completed questionnaires at hospital discharge or shortly afterward. The primary outcome in the study was whether or not the mother breastfed exclusively in the hospital. Secondary outcomes included the mothers' breastfeeding confidence, breastfeeding attitudes, and coping with breastfeeding.

Key Findings: The intervention and comparison group members were similar demographically in some respects (e.g., education, marital status), but several preintervention group differences were found. For example, patients in the intervention group were more likely to be primiparas and more likely to have participated in parenting education than women in the comparison group. To address this selection bias problem, these characteristics were controlled statistically. Women in the intervention group were significantly more likely to breastfeed exclusively at the time of the follow-up (76%) than those in the comparison group (66%). The authors concluded that intensive support helped the mothers to breastfeed exclusively.

Critical Thinking Exercises

1. Answer the relevant questions from Box 9.1 regarding this study.
2. Also consider the following targeted questions:
   a. Is this study prospective or retrospective?
   b. What other quasiexperimental designs could have been used in this study?
3. If the results of this study are valid, what are some of the uses to which the findings might be put in clinical practice?

EXAMPLE 3: NONEXPERIMENTAL STUDY IN APPENDIX A

● Read the method section of Swenson and colleagues' (2016) study ("Parents' use of praise and criticism in a sample of young children seeking mental health services") in Appendix A of this book.

Critical Thinking Exercises

1. Answer the relevant questions from Box 9.1 regarding this study.
2. Suggest modifications to the design of this study that might improve its external validity.

WANT TO KNOW MORE? ☀-

A wide variety of resources to enhance your learning and understanding of this chapter are available on thePoint.

● Interactive Critical Thinking Activity
● Chapter Supplement on Selected Experimental and Quasiexperimental Designs: Diagrams, Uses, and Drawbacks
● Answers to the Critical Thinking Exercises for Examples 3
● Internet Resources with useful websites for Chapter 9
● A Wolters Kluwer journal article on a topic related to this chapter

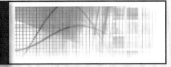

Summary Points

- The **research design** is the overall plan for answering research questions. In quantitative studies, the design designates whether there is an intervention, the nature of any comparisons, methods for controlling confounding variables, whether there will be blinding, and the timing and location of data collection.
- Therapy, Prognosis, and Etiology questions are cause-probing, and there is a hierarchy of designs for yielding best evidence for these questions.
- Key criteria for inferring causality include (1) a **cause** (independent variable) must precede an **effect** (outcome), (2) there must be a detectable relationship between a cause and an effect, and (3) the relationship between the two does not reflect the influence of a third (confounding) variable.
- A *counterfactual* is what would have happened to the same people simultaneously exposed *and* not exposed to a causal factor. The *effect* is the difference between the two. A good research design for cause-probing questions entails finding a good approximation to the idealized counterfactual.
- **Experiments** (or **randomized controlled trials [RCTs]**) involve an intervention (the researcher manipulates the independent variable by introducing an intervention), control (including the use of a **control group** that is not given the intervention), and **randomization** or **random assignment** (with participants allocated to experimental and control groups at random to make the groups comparable at the outset).
- RCTs are considered the gold standard because they come closer than any other design to meeting the criteria for inferring causal relationships.
- In **pretest–posttest designs**, data are collected both before the **intervention** (at **baseline**) and after it.
- In **crossover designs**, people are exposed to more than one experimental condition in random order and serve as their own controls.

- Crossover designs are inappropriate if there is a risk of *carryover effects*.
- The control group can undergo various conditions, including an alternative treatment, a **placebo** or pseudointervention, standard treatment ("usual care"), or a *wait-list* (*delayed treatment*) condition.
- **Quasiexperiments** (*trials without randomization*) involve an intervention but lack a comparison group or randomization. Strong quasiexperimental designs introduce controls to compensate for these missing components.
- **The nonequivalent control-group, pretest–posttest design** involves a **comparison group** that was not created through randomization and the collection of pretreatment data from both groups to assess initial group equivalence.
- In a **time-series design,** outcome data are collected over a period of time before and after the intervention, usually for a single group.
- **Nonexperimental** (*observational*) **studies** include **descriptive research**—studies that summarize the status of phenomena—and **correlational studies** that examine relationships among variables but involve no intervention.
- In **prospective (cohort) designs**, researchers begin with a possible cause and then subsequently collect data about outcomes.
- **Retrospective designs** (**case-control designs**) involve collecting data about an outcome in the present and then looking back in time for possible causes.
- Making causal inferences in correlational studies is risky; a basic research dictum is that *correlation does not prove causation*.
- **Cross-sectional designs** involve the collection of data at one time period, whereas **longitudinal designs** involve data collection at two or more times over an extended period. In nursing, longitudinal studies often are *follow-up studies* of clinical populations.
- Longitudinal studies are typically expensive, time-consuming, and subject to the risk of **attrition** (loss of participants over time) but yield valuable information about time-related phenomena.

- Quantitative researchers strive to control external factors that could affect study outcomes and subject characteristics that are extraneous to the research question.
- Researchers delineate the intervention in formal *protocols* that stipulate exactly what the treatment is. Careful researchers attend to *intervention fidelity*—whether the intervention was properly implemented and actually received.
- Techniques for controlling subject characteristics include **homogeneity** (restricting participants to reduce variability on confounding variables), **matching** (deliberately making groups comparable on some extraneous variables), statistical procedures, and randomization—the most effective method because it controls all possible confounding variables without researchers having to identify them.
- Study **validity** concerns the extent to which appropriate inferences can be made. **Threats to validity** are reasons that an inference could

be wrong. A key function of quantitative research design is to rule out validity threats.

- **Statistical conclusion validity** concerns the strength of evidence that a relationship exists between two variables. A threat to statistical conclusion validity is low **statistical power** (the ability to detect true relationships among variables).
- **Internal validity** concerns inferences that the outcomes were caused by the independent variable, rather than by extraneous factors. Threats to validity include temporal ambiguity (uncertainty about whether the presumed cause preceded the outcome), **selection** (pre-existing group differences), **history** (external events that could affect outcomes), **maturation** (changes due to the passage of time), and **mortality** (effects attributable to attrition).
- **External validity** concerns inferences about generalizability—whether findings hold true over variations in people, conditions, and settings.

REFERENCES

Austen, E. L., Beadle, J., Lukeman, S., et al. Using a Music Video Parody to Promote Breastfeeding and Increase Comfort Levels Among Young Adults. *Journal of Human Lactation, 33*(3), 560–569.

Chartrand J., Tourigny J., & MacCormick J. (2017). The effect of an educational pre-operative DVD on parents' and children's outcomes after a same-day surgery: a randomized controlled trial. *J Adv Nurs, 73*(3):599–611.

Dennis C. L., Merry L., & Gagnon A. J. (2017). Postpartum depression risk factors among recent refugee, asylum-seeking, non-refugee immigrant, and Canadian-born women: results from a prospective cohort study. *Soc Psychiatry Psychiatr Epidemiol, 52*(4):411–422.

Freeman S., Hirdes J. P., Stolee P., & Garcia J. (2016). A Cross-Sectional Examination of the Association Between Dyspnea and Distress as Experienced by Palliative Home Care Clients and Their Informal Caregivers. *Journal of Social Work in End-of-Life & Palliative Care, 12*(1–2), 82–103.

Hannula, L. S., Kaunonen, M., & Puukka, P. (2014). A study to promote breast feeding in the Helsinki Metropolitan area in Finland. *Midwifery, 30*, 696–704.

Jin C., Lobchuk M., Chernomas W., & Pooyania S. (2017). Examining Associations of Functional Deficits and Mood States With Empathic Responses of Stroke Family Caregivers. *Journal of Neuroscience Nursing, 49*(1), 12–14.

Kiddoo D., Sawatzky B., Bascu C. D., et al. (2015). Randomized Crossover Trial of Single Use Hydrophilic Coated vs Multiple Use Polyvinylchloride Catheters for Intermittent

Catheterization to Determine Incidence of Urinary Infection. *The Journal of Urology, 194*(1):174–179.

Lambert, S. D., McElduff, P., Girgis, A., et al. (2016). A pilot, multisite, randomized controlled trial of a self-directed coping skills training intervention for couples facing prostate cancer: accrual, retention, and data collection issues. *Support Care Cancer, 24*(2):711–722.

Lavoie-Tremblay M., O'Connor P., Biron A., et al. (2017). The Effects of the Transforming Care at the Bedside Program on Perceived Team Effectiveness and Patient Outcomes. *Health Care Manag (Frederick), 36*(1):10–20.

**Manfre, M., Adams, D., Callahan, G., et al. (2015). Hydrocortisone cream to reduce perineal pain after vaginal birth: A randomized controlled trial. *MCN: The American Journal of Maternal/Child Nursing, 40*, 306–312.

Marin, J. A., & Woo, K. Y. (2017). Clinical Characteristics of Mixed Arteriovenous Leg Ulcers: A Descriptive Study. *J Wound Ostomy Continence Nurs, 44*(1):41–47.

Markle-Reid M., Ploeg J., Fisher K., et al. (2016). The Aging, Community and Health Research Unit-Community Partnership Program for older adults with type 2 diabetes and multiple chronic conditions: a feasibility study. *Pilot and Feasibility Studies, 2*, 24.

Puts M. T. E., Sattar S., McWatters K., et al. (2017). Chemotherapy treatment decision-making experiences of older adults with cancer, their family members, oncologists and family physicians: a mixed methods study. *Supportive Care in Cancer, 25*(3), 879–886.

Shadish, W. R., Cook, T. D., & Campbell, D. T. (2002). *Experimental and quasi-experimental designs for generalized causal inference.* Boston, MA: Houghton Mifflin.

*Stavrinos, D., Garner, A., Franklin, C., et al. (2015). Distracted driving in teens with and without attention-deficit/hyperactivity disorder. *Journal of Pediatric Nursing, 30*, e183–e191.

Stern A., Mitsakakis N., Paulden M., et al. Pressure ulcer multidisciplinary teams via telemedicine: a pragmatic cluster randomized stepped wedge trial in long term care. *BMC Health Services Research, 14*, 83.

Stevens B. J., Yamada J., Promislow S., et al.; CIHR Team in Children's Pain. (2016). Pain assessment and management after a knowledge translation booster intervention. *Pediatrics, 138*(4). pii: e20153468

Swenson S., Ho G. W., Budhathoki C., et al. (2016). Parents' Use of Praise and Criticism in a Sample of Young Children Seeking Mental Health Services. *Journal of Pediatric Health Care, 30*(1), 49–56.

10 Sampling and Data Collection in Quantitative Studies

Learning Objectives

On completing this chapter, you will be able to:

- Distinguish between nonprobability and probability samples and compare their advantages and disadvantages
- Identify and describe several types of sampling designs in quantitative studies
- Evaluate the appropriateness of the sampling method and sample size used in a study
- Identify phenomena that lend themselves to self-reports, observation, and physiologic measurement
- Describe various approaches to collecting self-report data (e.g., interviews vs. questionnaires, composite scales)
- Describe methods of collecting and recording observational data
- Describe the major features and advantages of biophysiologic measures
- Critique a researcher's decisions regarding the data collection plan
- Describe approaches for assessing the reliability and validity of measures
- Define new terms in the chapter

Key Terms

- Biophysiologic measure
- Category system
- Checklist
- Closed-ended question
- Consecutive sampling
- Construct validity
- Content validity
- Convenience sampling
- Criterion validity
- Eligibility criteria
- Face validity
- Internal consistency
- Interrater reliability
- Interview schedule
- Likert scale
- Measurement
- Measurement property
- Non-probability sampling
- Observational methods
- Open-ended question
- Patient-reported outcome (PRO)
- Population
- Power analysis
- Probability sampling
- Psychometric assessment
- Purposive sampling
- Questionnaire
- Quota sampling
- Rating scale
- Reliability
- Response options
- Response rate
- Response set bias
- Sample
- Sample size
- Sampling bias
- Sampling plan
- Scale
- Self-report
- Simple random sampling
- Strata
- Stratified random sampling
- Systematic sampling
- Test–retest reliability
- Validity
- Visual analogue scale

This chapter covers two important research topics—how quantitative researchers select their study participants and how they collect data from them.

SAMPLING IN QUANTITATIVE RESEARCH

Researchers answer research questions using a sample of participants. In testing the effects of an intervention for pregnant women, nurse researchers reach conclusions without testing it with all pregnant women. Quantitative researchers develop a **sampling plan** that specifies in advance how participants will be selected and how many to include.

Basic Sampling Concepts

Let us begin by considering some terms associated with sampling.

Populations

A **population** ("P" in PICO questions) is the entire group of interest. For instance, if a researcher were studying Canadian nurses with specialized knowledge in perioperative nursing, the population could be defined as all registered nurses (RNs) in Canada who hold a Canadian Nurses Association certification in perioperative nursing. Other populations might be all patients who had cardiac surgery in Toronto General Hospital in 2016 or all Australian children younger than age 10 years with cystic fibrosis. Populations are not restricted to people. A population might be all patient records in Moncton City Hospital. A population is an entire aggregate of elements.

Researchers specify population characteristics through **eligibility criteria**. For example, consider the population of Canadian nursing students. Does the population include part-time students? Are RNs returning to school for a bachelor's degree included? Researchers establish criteria to determine whether a person qualifies as a member of the population (*inclusion* criteria) or should be excluded (*exclusion* criteria); for example, excluding patients who are severely ill.

> **Example of inclusion and exclusion criteria** • • • • • • • • • • • • • • • • • • •
> Stinson et al. (2016) studied the effectiveness of online peer mentoring programmes for adolescents with arthritis. To be eligible, adolescents had to be diagnosed with juvenile idiopathic arthritis, has access to Skype, and between the ages of 12 and 18 years. Children were excluded if they had cognitive impairment or psychiatric conditions, such as schizophrenia or bipolar disorder.

Quantitative researchers sample from an accessible population in the hope of generalizing to a target population. The *target population* is the entire population of interest. The *accessible population* is the portion of the target population that is accessible or available to the researcher. For example, a researcher's target population might be all diabetic patients in Canada, but, in reality, the population that is accessible might be diabetic patients treated by a particular health team.

Samples and Sampling

Sampling involves selecting a portion of the population to represent the population. A **sample** is a subset of population elements. In nursing research, the *elements* (basic units) are usually humans. Researchers work with samples rather than populations for practical reasons.

Information from samples can, however, lead to faulty conclusions. In quantitative studies, a criterion for judging a sample is its representativeness. A *representative sample* is one whose characteristics are closely matched with those of the population. Some sampling plans are more likely to yield biased samples than others. **Sampling bias** is the systematic overrepresentation or underrepresentation of a population segment in terms of key characteristics.

Strata

Populations consist of subpopulations, or **strata**. Strata are mutually exclusive segments of a population based on a specific characteristic. For instance, a population consisting of all RNs in Canada could be divided into two strata based on gender. Strata can be used in sample selection to enhance the sample's representativeness.

 TIP The sampling plan is usually discussed in a report's method section, sometimes in a subsection called "Sample" or "Study Participants." Sample characteristics (e.g., average age) are often described in the results section.

Sampling Designs in Quantitative Studies

The two broad classes of sampling designs in quantitative research are probability sampling and non-probability sampling.

Non-probability Sampling

In **non-probability sampling**, researchers select people into the study by non-random methods, and not everyone have the same chance to be included. Non-probability sampling is less likely than probability sampling to produce representative samples—and yet, *most* research samples in nursing and other disciplines are non-probability samples.

Convenience sampling entails selecting the most conveniently available people as participants. A nurse who distributes questionnaires about vitamin use to college students leaving the library is sampling by convenience, for example. The problem with convenience sampling is that people who are readily available might be atypical of the population. The price of convenience is the risk of bias. Convenience sampling is the weakest form of sampling, but it is also the most commonly used sampling method.

Example of a convenience sample •
Huang et al. (2016) studied the effects of risk factors and coping style on the quality of life and depressive symptoms of adults with type 2 diabetes. A convenience sample of 241 adults was recruited from a hospital metabolic outpatient department.

In **quota sampling**, researchers identify population strata and figure out how many people are needed from each stratum. By using information about the population, researchers can ensure that diverse segments are represented in the sample. For example, if the population is known to have 50% males and 50% females, then the sample should have similar percentages. Procedurally, quota sampling is similar to convenience sampling: Participants are a convenience sample from each stratum. Because of this fact, quota sampling shares some weaknesses of convenience sampling. Nevertheless, quota sampling is a big improvement over convenience sampling and does not require sophisticated skills or a lot of effort. Surprisingly, few researchers use this strategy.

Example of a quota sample •
Wang et al. (2015) described the protocol for a study of the effects of a health programme being implemented at a university in Singapore. The researchers plan to use a quota sample, stratifying participants based on the type of work they do (academic, administrative, support).

Consecutive sampling is a non-probability sampling method that involves recruiting *all* people from an accessible population over a specific time interval or for a specified sample size. For example, in a study of ventilator-associated pneumonia in intensive care unit (ICU) patients, a consecutive sample might consist of all eligible patients who were admitted to an ICU over a 6-month period. Or it might be the first 250 eligible patients admitted to the ICU, if 250 were the targeted sample size. Consecutive sampling is often the best possible choice when there is "rolling enrolment" into an accessible population.

Example of a consecutive sample •
Bryant, Phang, and Abrams (2015) compared radiographic reports of feeding tube placement with images generated by an electromagnetic feeding tube placement device. The sample consisted of 200 consecutive patients who had feeding tubes inserted.

Purposive sampling involves using researchers' knowledge about the population to handpick sample members. Researchers might decide purposely to select people presumed to be knowledgeable about the issues under study. This method can lead to bias but can be a useful approach when researchers want a sample of experts.

Example of purposive sampling •
Lalonde and McGillis Hall (2016) invited purposively sampled new nurses and their preceptors at the end of their preceptorship programme to explore the impact of preceptor characteristics (emotional intelligence, personality and cognitive intelligence) on new graduate nurses in terms of their turnover intent, job satisfaction, and role conflict and ambiguity.

 HOW-TO-TELL TIP How can you tell what type of sampling design was used in a quantitative study? If the report does not explicitly mention or describe the sampling design, it is usually safe to assume that a convenience sample was used.

Probability Sampling

Probability sampling involves random selection of elements from a population. With random sampling, each element in the population has an equal, independent chance of being selected. Random selection should not be (although it often is) confused with random assignment, which is a signature of an RCT. Random *assignment* to different treatment conditions has no impact on how participants in the RCT were selected.

Simple random sampling is the most basic probability sampling. In simple random sampling, researchers establish a *sampling frame*—a list of population elements. If nursing students at the University of Alberta were the population, a student roster would be the sampling frame. Elements in a sampling frame are numbered and then a table of random numbers or an online randomizer is used to draw a random sample of the desired size. Samples selected randomly are unlikely to be biased. There is no *guarantee* of a representative sample, but random selection guarantees that differences between the sample and the population are purely a function of chance. The probability of selecting a markedly atypical sample through random sampling is low and decreases as sample size increases.

Example of a simple random sample •
VanDenKerkhof et al. (2016) studied describe the epidemiology and symptoms of neuropathic pain in the community. Questionnaires were sent to a random sample of 8,000 households in the ten Canadian provinces.

In **stratified random sampling**, the population is first divided into two or more strata, from which elements are randomly selected. As with quota sampling, the aim of stratified sampling is to enhance representativeness.

Example of stratified random sampling •
Havaei, MacPhee, and Dahinten (2016) from the University of British Columbia compared emotional exhaustion and intention to leave health care between RNs and licensed practical nurses (LPNs). The researchers recruited a stratified, random sample of acute care nurses including RNs and LPNs.

 TIP Many large national studies use *multistage sampling,* in which large units are first randomly sampled (e.g., census tracts, hospitals), then smaller units are selected (e.g., individual people).

Systematic sampling involves the selection of every *k*th case from a list, such as every 10th person on a patient list. Systematic sampling can be done so that an essentially random sample is drawn. First, the size of the population is divided by the size of the desired sample to obtain the *sampling interval* (the fixed distance between selected cases). For instance, if we needed a sample of 50 from a population of 5,000, our sampling interval would be 100 (5,000 / 50 = 100). Every 100th case on a sampling frame would be sampled, with the first case selected randomly. If our random number were 73, the people corresponding to numbers 73, 173, 273, and so on, would be in the sample. Systematic sampling done in this manner is essentially the same as simple random sampling and is often convenient.

Example of a systematic sample •
Ridout et al. (2014) studied the incidence of failure to communicate vital information as patients progressed through the perioperative process. From a population of 1,858 patient records in a health care system meeting eligibility criteria, the researchers selected every 6th case, for a sample of 294 cases.

Evaluation of Non-probability and Probability Sampling

Probability sampling is the only viable method of obtaining representative samples. If all elements in a population have an equal chance of being selected, then the resulting sample is likely to do a good job of representing the population. Probability sampling also allows researchers to estimate the magnitude of *sampling error,* which is the difference between population values (e.g., the average age of the population) and sample values (e.g., the average age of the sample).

Non-probability samples are rarely representative of the population—some segment of the population is likely to be underrepresented. When there is sampling bias, there is a chance that the results could be misleading. Why, then, are non-probability samples used in most studies? Clearly, the advantage lies in their feasibility: Probability sampling is often impractical. Quantitative researchers using non-probability samples must be cautious about the inferences drawn from the data, and research consumers should be alert to possible sampling biases.

 TIP The quality of the sampling plan is of particular importance when the focus of the research is to obtain descriptive information about prevalence or average values for a population. National surveys almost always use probability samples. For studies whose purpose is primarily description, data from a probability sample is at the top of the evidence hierarchy for individual studies.

Sample Size in Quantitative Studies

Sample size—the number of study participants—is a major concern in quantitative research. There is no simple formula to determine what a sample size should be, but larger is usually better than smaller. When researchers calculate a percentage or an average using sample data, the purpose is to estimate a population value, and larger samples have less sampling error.

Researchers can estimate how large their samples should be for testing hypotheses through **power analysis**. An example can illustrate basic principles of power analysis. Suppose we were testing an intervention to help people quit smoking; smokers would be randomized to an intervention or a control group. How many people should be in the sample? When using power analysis, researchers must estimate how large the group difference will be (e.g., group differences in daily number of cigarettes smoked). The estimate might be based on prior research. When expected differences are large, a large sample is not needed to show group differences statistically, but large samples are necessary to detect small differences. In our example, if a small-to-moderate group difference in post-intervention smoking were expected, the sample size needed to test group differences in smoking, with standard statistical criteria, would be about 250 smokers (125 per group).

The risk of "getting it wrong" (statistical conclusion validity) increases when samples are too small: Researchers risk gathering data that will not support their hypotheses *even when those hypotheses are correct*. Large samples are not foolproof, though: With non-probability sampling, even a large sample cannot avoid bias. A good example illustrating this point is the failure of polls to accurately forecast the results of elections.

A large sample cannot correct for a faulty sampling design; nevertheless, a large non-probability sample is better than a small one. When critiquing quantitative studies, you must assess both the sample size and the sample selection method to judge how good the sample was.

 TIP The sampling plan is often one of the weakest aspects of quantitative studies. Most nursing studies use samples of convenience, and many are based on samples that are too small to provide an adequate test of the research hypotheses.

Critiquing Sampling Plans

In coming to conclusions about the quality of evidence, the sampling plan deserves careful examination. If the sample is seriously biased or too small, the findings may be misleading or just plain wrong.

Box 10.1 Guidelines for Critiquing Quantitative Sampling Plans

1. Was the population identified? Were eligibility criteria specified?
2. What type of sampling design was used? Was the sampling plan one that could be expected to yield a representative sample?
3. How many participants were in the sample? Was the sample size affected by high rates of refusals or attrition? Was the sample size large enough to support statistical conclusion validity? Was the sample size justified on the basis of a power analysis or other rationale?
4. Were key characteristics of the sample described (e.g., mean age, percentage of females)?
5. To whom can the study results reasonably be generalized?

In critiquing a description of a sampling plan, you should consider whether the researcher has adequately described the sampling strategy. Ideally, research reports should describe the following:

- The type of sampling approach used (e.g., convenience, consecutive, random)
- The population and eligibility criteria for sample selection
- The sample size, with a rationale
- A description of the sample's main characteristics (e.g., age, gender, clinical status, and so on)

A second issue is whether the researcher made good sampling decisions. An important question about a sampling plan in quantitative research is whether the sample is representative of the population. You will never know for sure, of course, but if the sampling strategy is weak or if the sample size is small, there is reason to suspect some bias.

Even with a rigorous sampling plan, the sample may be biased if not all people invited to participate in a study agree to do so. If certain subgroups in the population decline to participate, then a biased sample can result, even when probability sampling is used. Research reports ideally should provide information about **response rates** (i.e., the number of people participating in a study relative to the number of people sampled) and about possible *non-response bias*—differences between participants and those who declined to participate (also sometimes referred to as *response bias*). In a longitudinal study, attrition bias should be reported.

Your job as reviewer is to decide about the generalizability of the findings from the researcher's sample to the accessible population and a broader target population. If the sampling plan is flawed, it may be risky to generalize the findings at all without replicating the study with another sample.

Box 10.1 presents some guiding questions for critiquing the sampling plan of a quantitative research report.

DATA COLLECTION IN QUANTITATIVE RESEARCH

Phenomena in which researchers are interested must be translated into data for statistical analysis. This section discusses the challenging task of collecting quantitative research data.

Overview of Data Collection and Data Sources

Data collection methods vary along several dimensions. One issue is whether the researcher collects original data or uses existing data. Existing *records*, for example, are an important data source for nurse researchers. A wealth of clinical data gathered for non-research purposes can be fruitfully analysed to answer research questions.

Example of a study using records •
Woo et al. (2016) explored factors associated with pressure injuries across a spectrum of health care settings in Ontario. Data were obtained from the resident assessment instrument–minimum data-set, the health outcomes for better information and care (HOBIC) database, and the registered persons database.

Researchers most often collect new data. In developing a data collection plan, researchers must decide the type of data to gather. Three types have been frequently used by nurse researchers: self-reports, observations, and biophysiologic measures. **Self-report** data—also called **patient-reported outcome (PRO)** data—are participants' responses to researchers' questions, such as in an interview. In nursing studies, self-reports are the most common data collection approach. Direct observation of people's behaviours and characteristics can be used for certain questions. Nurses also use **biophysiologic measures** to assess important clinical variables.

Regardless of the type of data collected in a study, data collection methods vary along several dimensions, including structure, quantifiability, and objectivity. Data for quantitative studies tend to be quantifiable and structured, with the same information gathered from all participants in a comparable, prespecified way. Quantitative researchers generally strive for methods that are as objective as possible.

Self-Reports/Patient-Reported Outcomes

Structured self-report methods are used when researchers know in advance exactly what they need to know and can design appropriate questions to obtain the needed information. Structured self-report data are collected with a formal, written document—an *instrument*. The instrument is an **interview schedule** when the questions are asked orally face-to-face or by telephone, and a **questionnaire** when respondents complete the instrument themselves.

Question Form and Wording

In a totally structured instrument, respondents are asked to respond to the same questions in the same order. **Closed-ended (or *fixed-alternative*) questions** are ones in which the **response options** are prespecified. The options may range from a simple yes or no to complex expressions of opinion. Such questions ensure comparable responses and facilitate analysis. Some examples of closed-ended questions are presented in Table 10.1.

Some structured instruments, however, also include **open-ended questions**, which allow participants to respond to questions in their own words (e.g., Why did you stop smoking?). When open-ended questions are included in questionnaires, respondents must write out their responses. In interviews, the interviewer records responses verbatim.

Good closed-ended questions are more difficult to construct than open-ended ones but easier to analyse. Also, people may not compose lengthy written responses to open-ended questions in questionnaires. A major drawback of closed-ended questions is that researchers might omit potentially important responses. If respondents are verbally expressive and cooperative, open-ended questions allow for richer information than closed-ended questions. Finally, some respondents object to choosing from alternatives that do not reflect their opinions precisely.

In drafting questions for a structured instrument, researchers must carefully monitor the wording of each question for clarity, absence of bias, and (in questionnaires) reading level. Questions must be sequenced in a psychologically meaningful order that encourages

TABLE 10.1 Examples of Closed-Ended Questions

Question Type	Example
1. Dichotomous question	Have you ever been pregnant? 1. Yes 2. No
2. Multiple-choice question	How important is it to you to avoid a pregnancy at this time? 1. Extremely important 2. Very important 3. Somewhat important 4. Not important
3. Forced-choice question	Which statement most closely represents your point of view? 1. What happens to me is my own doing. 2. Sometimes I feel I don't have enough control over my life.
4. Rating question	On a scale from 0 to 10, where 0 means "extremely dissatisfied" and 10 means "extremely satisfied," how satisfied were you with the nursing care you received during your hospitalization?

cooperation and candour. Developing, pretesting, and refining a self-report instrument can take many months.

Interviews Versus Questionnaires

Researchers using structured self-reports must decide whether to use interviews or self-administered questionnaires. Questionnaires have the following advantages:

- Questionnaires are less costly and are advantageous for geographically dispersed samples. Internet questionnaires are especially economical and important means of gathering self-report data—although response rates to Internet questionnaires tend to be low.
- Questionnaires offer the possibility of anonymity, which may be crucial in obtaining sensitive information about certain opinions or traits.

Example of Internet questionnaires •
Ratanasiripong (2015) sent a web-based questionnaire to a convenience sample of 3,300 male college students attending a public university. The purpose of the study was to document the rate of human papillomavirus vaccination in college men and to examine factors associated with being vaccinated. Responses were received from 410 students.

Interviews are preferred to questionnaires because of the following advantages:

- Response rates tend to be high in face-to-face interviews. Respondents are less likely to refuse to talk to an interviewer than to ignore a questionnaire. Low response rates can lead to bias because people who chose to respond may not represent the original sample. In the Internet questionnaire study of college men (Ratanasiripong, 2015), the response rate was under 15%.
- Some people cannot fill out a questionnaire (e.g., young children). Interviews are feasible with most people.

Some advantages of face-to-face interviews also apply to telephone interviews. Long or complex instruments are not well suited to telephone administration, but for relatively brief instruments, telephone interviews combine relatively low costs with high response rates.

Example of telephone interviews •
Ganann et al. (2016) conducted telephone interviews with a sample of 519 immigrant women in Ontario 6 weeks, 6 months, and 1 year after childbirth to explore predictors of postpartum depression. A lack of social support was strongly associated with postpartum depression.

Scales

Social–psychological scales are often incorporated into questionnaires or interview schedules. A **scale** is a device that assigns a numeric score to people along a continuum, like a scale for measuring weight. Social–psychological scales differentiate people with different attitudes, perceptions, and psychological traits.

One method of differentiation is the **Likert scale**, which consists of several declarative statements (*items*) that express a viewpoint on a topic. Respondents are asked to indicate how much they agree or disagree with the statement. Table 10.2 presents a six-item Likert scale for measuring attitudes towards condom use. In this example, agreement with positively worded statements is assigned a higher score. The first statement is positively worded; agreement indicates a favourable attitude towards condom use. Because there are five response alternatives, a score of 5 would be given for *strongly agree*, 4 for *agree*, and so on. Responses of two hypothetical participants are shown by a check or an X, and their item scores are shown

TABLE 10.2 Example of a Likert Scale to Measure Attitudes Towards Using Condoms

Direction of Scoring[a]	Item	SA	A	?	D	SD	Person 1 (✓)	Person 2 (✗)
+	1. Using a condom shows you care about your partner.		✓			✗	4	1
–	2. My partner would be angry if I talked about using condoms.			✗	✓		5	3
–	3. I wouldn't enjoy sex as much if my partner and I used condoms.		✗		✓		4	2
+	4. Condoms are a good protection against AIDS and other sexually transmitted diseases.			✓	✗		3	2
+	5. My partner would respect me if I insisted on using condoms.	✓				✗	5	1
–	6. I would be too embarrassed to ask my partner about using a condom.		✗		✓		5	2
	Total score						26	11

Column groups: "Responses" spans SA, A, ?, D, SD; "Score" spans Person 1 (✓), Person 2 (✗).

[a]Researchers would not indicate the direction of scoring on a Likert scale administered to participants. The scoring direction is indicated in this table for illustrative purposes only.
SA, strongly agree; A, agree; ?, uncertain; D, disagree; SD, strongly disagree.

in the right-hand columns. Person 1, who agreed with the first statement, has a score of 4, whereas person 2, who strongly disagreed, got a score of 1. The second statement is negatively worded, and so scoring is reversed—a 1 is assigned for *strongly agree* and so forth. *Item reversals* ensure that a high score consistently reflects positive attitudes towards condom use.

A person's total score is the sum of item scores—hence, these scales are sometimes called *summated rating scales* or *composite scales*. In our example, person 1 has a more positive attitude towards condoms (total score = 26) than person 2 (total score = 11). Summing item scores makes it possible to discriminate among people with different opinions. Composite scales are often composed of two or more *subscales* that measure different aspects of a construct. Developing high-quality scales requires a lot of skill and effort.

Example of a Likert scale ·
Broadhurst in collaboration with the World Congress of Vascular Access (2017) developed an algorithm to aid assessment and management of central venous access devices (CVAD)–associated skin impairment (CASI). A sample of clinicians were asked to diagnose and describe their planned management for four case studies using the algorithm. Clinicians' confidence in making a diagnosis and formulating recommendations for management plans was measured using a five-point Likert scale: very confident, confident, somewhat confident, somewhat not confident, not at all confident.

Another type of scale is the **visual analogue scale** (VAS), which can be used to measure subjective experiences such as pain or fatigue. The VAS is a straight line, and the end anchors are labelled as the extreme limits of the sensation being measured (Fig. 10.1). People mark a point on the line corresponding to the amount of sensation experienced. Traditionally, a VAS line is 100 mm in length, which makes it easy to derive a score from 0 to 100 by measuring the distance from one end of the scale to the mark on the line.

Example of a visual analogue scale ·
Hu et al. (2015) tested the effects of earplugs, eye masks, and relaxing music on sleep quality in ICU patients. Sleep quality was measured using a 0 to 100 VAS.

Scales permit researchers to efficiently quantify subtle change in the intensity of individual characteristics. Scales can be administered either verbally or in writing and so can be used with most people. Scales are susceptible to several common problems; however, many of which are referred to as **response set biases**. The most important biases include the following:

- *Social desirability response set bias*—a tendency to misrepresent attitudes or traits by giving answers that are consistent with normal social views
- *Extreme response set bias*—a tendency to consistently express extreme attitudes (e.g., strongly agree), leading to distortions because extreme responses may be unrelated to the trait being measured
- *Acquiescence response set bias*—a tendency of some people to agree with statements regardless of their content (*yea-sayers*). The opposite tendency for other people (*nay-sayers*) to disagree with statements independently of the question content is less common.

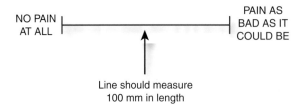

Line should measure
100 mm in length

Figure 10.1 Example of a visual analogue scale.

Researchers can reduce these biases by developing sensitively worded questions; creating a permissive, non-judgemental atmosphere; and guaranteeing the confidentiality of responses.

 TIP Other self-report approaches include vignettes and Q-sorts. *Vignettes* are brief descriptions of situations that allow respondents to describe their reactions. *Q-sorts* present participants with a set of cards on which statements are written. Participants are asked to sort the cards along a specified dimension, such as most helpful/least helpful. Vignettes and Q-sorts are described in the chapter supplement on the Point website.

Evaluation of Self-Report Methods

If researchers want to know how people feel or what they believe, the most direct approach is to ask them. Self-reports frequently provide information that would be difficult or impossible to gather by other means. Behaviours can be *observed* but only if people are willing to show them publicly and engage in them at the time of data collection.

Nevertheless, self-reports have some weaknesses. The most serious issue concerns the validity and accuracy of self-reports: How can we be sure that respondents feel or act the way they say they do? Investigators usually have no choice but to assume that most respondents have been frank. Yet, we all have a tendency to present ourselves in the best light, and this may conflict with the truth. When reading research reports, you should be alert to potential biases in self-reported data.

Observational Methods

For some research questions, direct observation of people's behaviour is an alternative to self-reports, especially in clinical settings. **Observational methods** can be used to gather such information as patients' conditions (e.g., their sleep–wake state), verbal communication (e.g., exchange of information at discharge), non-verbal communication (e.g., body language), activities (e.g., geriatric patients' self-grooming activities), and environmental conditions (e.g., noise levels).

In observational studies, researchers have some flexibility. For example, the observation can be focused on broadly defined events (e.g., patient mood swings) or on small, specific behaviours (e.g., facial expressions). Observations can be made through the human senses and then recorded manually, but they can also be done with equipment such as video recorders. Researchers do not always tell people they are being observed because awareness of being observed may cause people to behave atypically. Behavioural distortion due to the known presence of an observer is called *reactivity*.

Structured observation involves the use of formal instruments and protocols that guide the researchers in what to observe, how long to observe it, and how to record the data. Structured observation is not intended to capture a broad slice of life but rather to document specific behaviours, actions, and events. Structured observation requires the formulation of a system for accurately categorizing, recording, and encoding the observations.

 TIP Researchers often use structured observations when participants cannot be asked questions or cannot be expected to provide reliable answers. Many observational instruments are designed to capture the behaviours of infants, children, or people whose communication skills are impaired.

Methods of Structured Observation

The most common approach to making structured observations is to use a category system for classifying observed phenomena. A **category system** records events of interest that happen within a setting systematically.

Some category systems require that *all* observed behaviours in a specified domain (e.g., body positions) be classified. A contrasting technique is a system that only categorizes particular types of behaviour (which may or may not occur). For example, if we were studying children's aggressive behaviour, we might develop such categories as "strikes another child" or "throws objects." Some children may not exhibit aggressive actions. In this category system, many non-aggressive behaviours would not be classified.

Example of non-exhaustive categories •
Nilsen et al. (2014) conducted a study of nursing care quality that involved observations of communication between nurses and mechanically ventilated patients in ICU. Among many different types of observations made, observers recorded instances of positive and negative nurse behaviours, according to carefully defined criteria. Nurse behaviours were not categorized.

Category systems must have careful, explicit operational definitions of the behaviours and characteristics to be observed. Each category must be explained, giving observers clear-cut criteria for assessing the occurrence of the phenomenon (e.g. oral hygiene care).

Category systems are the basis for constructing a **checklist**—the instrument observers use to record observations. The checklist is usually formatted with a list of behaviours from the category system on the left and space for tallying the frequency or duration on the right. The task of the observer using an exhaustive category system is to place *all* observed behaviours in one category for each "unit" of behaviour (e.g., a time interval). With non-exhaustive category systems, categories of behaviours that may or may not be manifested by participants are listed. The observer watches for instances of these behaviours and records their occurrence.

Another approach to structured observations is to use a **rating scale**, an instrument that requires observers to rate phenomena along a descriptive continuum. The observer may be required to make ratings at intervals throughout the observation or to summarize an entire event after observation is completed. Rating scales can be used as an extension of checklists, in which the observer records not only the occurrence of some behaviour but also some qualitative aspect of it, such as its intensity. Although this approach yields a lot of information, it places an immense burden on observers.

Example of observational ratings •
Burk et al. (2014) sought to identify factors that would predict agitation in critically ill adults. Patients' degree of agitation was observed and measured using the Richmond Agitation–Sedation Scale, which requires ratings on a 10-point scale, from +4 (combative) to –5 (unarousable).

Observational Sampling

Researchers must decide when to apply their observational systems. Observational sampling methods are a means of obtaining representative examples of the behaviours being observed. One system is *time sampling*, which involves selecting time periods during which observations will occur. Time frames may be selected systematically (e.g., every 30 seconds at 2-minute intervals) or at random.

With *event sampling*, researchers select appropriate events to observe. Event sampling requires researchers to either know when events will occur (e.g., nursing shift changes) or wait for their occurrence. Event sampling is a good choice when events of interest are infrequent and may be missed if time sampling is used. When behaviours and events are relatively frequent, however, time sampling enhances the representativeness of the observed behaviours.

Example of event and time sampling •
Coker et al. (2017) conducted a study of oral hygiene care provided by nurses to older people hospitalized in Hamilton Health Sciences. Twenty-five RNs and RPNs were observed during 185 episodes of interaction with their assigned patients during their evening rounds. The patients received some type of oral hygiene intervention in 36% of encounters including denture care, brushing of natural teeth, cleansing the tongue and oral cavity; and moisturizing lips and oral tissues.

Evaluation of Observational Methods

Certain research questions are better suited to observation than to self-reports, such as when people cannot describe their own behaviours. This may be the case when people are unaware of their behaviour (e.g., stress-induced behaviour), when behaviours are emotion laden (e.g., grieving), or when people are not capable of reporting their actions (e.g., young children). Observational methods have an intrinsic appeal for directly capturing behaviours. Nurses are often in a position to watch people's behaviours and may, by training, be especially sensitive observers.

Shortcomings of observational methods include possible reactivity when the observer is conspicuous, and the vulnerability of observations to bias. For example, the observer's values and prejudices may lead to faulty inference. Observational biases probably cannot be eliminated, but they can be minimized through careful observer training and assessment.

Biophysiologic Measures

Clinical nursing studies involve biophysiologic instruments both for creating independent variables (e.g., a biofeedback intervention) and for measuring dependent variables. Our discussion focuses on the use of biophysiologic measures as dependent (outcome) variables.

Nurse researchers have used biophysiologic measures for a wide variety of purposes. Examples include studies of basic biophysiologic processes, explorations of the ways in which nursing actions and interventions affect physiologic outcomes, product or device assessments, studies to evaluate the accuracy of biophysiologic information gathered by nurses, and studies of the correlates of physiologic functioning in patients with health problems.

Both *in vivo* and *in vitro* measurements are used in research. *In vivo* measurements are those performed directly within or on living organisms, such as blood pressure and body temperature measurement. Technologic advances continue to improve the ability to measure biophysiologic phenomena accurately and conveniently. With *in vitro* measures, data are gathered from participants by extracting biophysiologic material from them and subjecting it to analysis by laboratory technicians. *In vitro* measures include chemical measures (e.g., the measurement of hormone levels), microbiologic measures (e.g., bacterial counts and identification), and cytologic or histologic measures (e.g., tissue biopsies). Nurse researchers also use *anthropomorphic measures*, such as the body mass index and waist circumference.

> **Example of a study with *in vivo* and *in vitro* measures** • • • • • • • • • • • • •
> Okoli, Kodet, and Robertson (2016) examined the physiologic responses of non-smokers to nicotine patch administration. The researchers measured heart rate, blood pressure, and serum nicotine levels at 0.5 hour, 1 hour, and 2 hours after applying a nicotine patch. Heart rate and blood pressure were considered *in vivo* measurements, whereas blood nicotine levels were *in vitro* data.

Biophysiologic measures offer a number of advantages to nurse researchers. They are relatively accurate and precise, especially compared to psychological measures, such as self-report measures of anxiety or pain. Also, biophysiologic measures are objective. Two nurses reading from the same spirometer output are likely to record identical tidal volume measurements, and two spirometers are likely to produce the same read-outs. Patients cannot easily distort measurements of biophysiologic functioning. Finally, biophysiologic instruments provide valid measures of targeted variables: Thermometers can be relied on to measure temperature and not blood volume. For non-biophysiologic measures, there are typically concerns about whether an instrument is really measuring the target concept.

Data Quality in Quantitative Research

In developing a data collection plan, researchers must strive for the highest possible quality data. One aspect of data quality concerns the procedures used to collect the data. For example, the people who collect and record the data must be properly trained and monitored to ensure that procedures are diligently followed. Another issue concerns the circumstances under which data were gathered. For example, it is important for researchers to ensure privacy and to create an atmosphere that encourages participants to be candid or behave naturally.

A crucial issue for data quality concerns the adequacy of the instruments or scales used to measure constructs. Researchers seek to enhance the quality of their data by selecting excellent *measures*. **Measurement** involves assigning numbers to represent the amount of an attribute present in a person or object. When a new measure of a construct (e.g., anxiety) is developed, instructions for assigning numerical values (*scores*) need to be established. The instructions must then be evaluated to see if they reflect values or numbers that truly and accurately correspond to different amounts of the targeted trait.

Measures that are not perfectly accurate yield measurements that contain some error. Many factors contribute to *measurement error*, including personal states (e.g., mood, fatigue), response set biases, and situational factors (e.g., temperature, lighting). In self-report measures, measurement errors can be affected by how questions are worded.

Careful researchers select measures that are known to be psychometrically sound. *Psychometrics* is the branch of psychology concerned with the theory and methods of psychological measurements. When a new measure is developed, the developers undertake a **psychometric assessment** to evaluate its **measurement properties**.

Psychometricians (and most nurse researchers) have traditionally focused on two measurement properties when assessing the quality of a measure: reliability and validity. In recent years, measurement experts in medicine also pay attention to the measurement of change (Polit & Yang, 2016). Here, we describe the two properties that you are most likely to encounter in reading articles in the nursing literature. Some of the methods used to assess these properties are described in the chapter on statistical analysis (Chapter 14).

Reliability

Reliability, broadly speaking, is the extent to which scores are free from measurement error. Reliability can also be defined as the extent to which scores for people *who have not changed* are the same for repeated measurements. In other words, reliability concerns consistency—the *absence* of variation—in measuring a stable attribute for an individual. In all types of assessments, reliability involves a *replication* to test whether scores for a stable trait remain the same.

In **test–retest reliability**, replication takes the form of administering a measure to the same people on two occasions (e.g., 1 week apart). The assumption is that for traits that have not changed, any differences in people's scores on the two testings are the result of measurement error. When score differences are small, reliability is high. This type of reliability is sometimes called *stability* or *reproducibility*—the extent to which similar scores can be reproduced on a repeated administration. Except for highly volatile constructs (e.g., mood), test–retest reliability can be assessed for most measures, including biophysiologic ones.

Measurement error occurs when a person is asked to make scoring judgements and provide the measurements. This is the situation for observational measures (e.g., ratings to measure agitation) and is also true for some biophysiologic measurements (e.g., skinfold measurement). In such situations, it is important to evaluate how reliably the measurements reflect attributes of the person being rated and not the attributes of the raters. The most typical approach is to undertake an **interrater (or *inter-observer*) reliability** assessment, which involves having two or more observers independently applying the measure to the same people to see if the scores are consistent across raters.

Another aspect of reliability is **internal consistency**. In responding to a self-report item, people are influenced not only by the underlying construct but also by idiosyncratic reactions to the words. By combining multiple items with different wordings, item irrelevancies are expected to cancel each other out. An instrument containing multiple items that produce similar measurement of the same trait has high internal consistency. For internal consistency, replication involves people's responses to multiple items during a single administration. Whereas other reliability estimates assess a measure's degree of consistency across time or raters, internal consistency captures consistency across items.

As we explain in Chapter 14, reliability coefficients are calculated to estimate how reliable a measure is. The coefficients normally range in value from 0.0 to 1.0, with higher values being especially desirable. Coefficients of .80 or higher are considered desirable. Researchers should select instruments with demonstrated reliability and should document this in their reports. Researchers undertaking a study do not undertake a full psychometric assessment of an existing measure, but they often do recompute internal consistency reliability coefficients with their data.

Example of internal consistency reliability •
Kennedy et al. (2015) developed and assessed a scale to measure nursing students' self-efficacy for practice competence. The 22-item scale had high internal consistency: The reliability coefficient was .92.

Validity

Validity is the degree that an instrument is actually measuring the construct it supposes to measure. When researchers develop a scale to measure *resilience*, they need to be sure that the resulting scores validly reflect this construct and not something else, such as self-efficacy or perseverance. Assessing the validity of abstract constructs requires a careful conceptualization of the construct—as well as a conceptualization of what the construct is *not*. Like reliability, validity has different aspects and assessment approaches. Four aspects of measurement validity are face validity, content validity, criterion validity, and construct validity.

Face validity refers to whether the instrument *looks* like it is measuring the target construct. Although face validity is not considered good evidence of validity, it is helpful for a measure to have face validity if other types of validity have also been demonstrated. Face validity is challenged if patients do not consider the scale is not asking the right questions that are relevant to their problems or situations.

Content validity may be defined as the extent that an instrument's content adequately captures the construct—that is, whether a composite instrument (e.g., a multi-item scale) has an appropriate sample of items to measure the construct. If the content of an instrument is a good reflection of a construct, then the instrument has a greater likelihood of achieving its measurement objectives. Content validity is usually assessed by having a panel of experts rate the scale items for relevance to the construct and comment on the need for additional items.

Criterion validity is the extent to which the scores on a measure are a replication of a "gold standard"—that is, a criterion considered an ideal measure of the construct. Not all measures can be validated using a criterion approach because there is not always a "gold standard." Two types of criterion validity exist. *Concurrent validity* is assessed when the measurements of the criterion and the focal instrument of interest occur at the same time. In such a situation, the hypothesis is that the focal measure is an adequate substitute for an established criterion. For example, scores on a scale to measure stress could be compared to wake-up salivary free cortisol levels (the criterion). In *predictive validity*, the focal measure is tested against a criterion that is measured in the future. Screening scales are often tested against some future criterion—namely, the occurrence of the phenomenon (e.g., a patient fall).

For many abstracts, unobservable human attributes (constructs), no gold standard criterion exists, and so other validation avenues must be considered. **Construct validity** is the degree to which a measure's scores represent the construct. Construct validity typically involves hypothesis testing, which follows a similar path: Hypotheses are developed about a relationship between scores on the focal measure and values on other constructs, data are collected to test the hypotheses, and then validity conclusions are reached based on the results of the hypothesis tests.

One widely used hypothesis testing approach to construct validity is sometimes called *known-groups validity*, which tests hypotheses about a measure's ability to discriminate between two or more groups known (or expected) to differ with regard to the construct of interest. For instance, in validating a measure of anxiety about the labour experience, the scores of primiparas and multiparas could be contrasted. On average, women who had never given birth would likely experience more anxiety than women who had already had children; one might question the validity of the instrument if such differences did not come about.

Example of known-groups validity ·
Lambert et al. (2014) explored the validity of the Appraisal of Caregiving Scale that was designed to evaluate stress associated with caregiving for someone with advanced cancer. Consistent with hypotheses, depressed caregivers had higher stress scores than non-depressed caregivers. Also, younger caregivers reported significantly higher scores on the General Stress subscale than older caregivers.

 TIP   Another aspect of construct validity is called cross-cultural validity, which is relevant for measures that have been translated or adapted for use with a different cultural group than that for the original instrument. *Cross-cultural validity* is the degree to which the components (e.g., items) of a translated or culturally adapted measure perform adequately and equivalently relative to their performance on the original instrument.

An instrument does not possess or lack validity; it is a question of degree. An instrument's validity is not proved, established, demonstrated, or verified but rather is supported to a greater or lesser extent by evidence. Researchers undertaking a study should select measures for which good validity information is available.

Critiquing Data Collection Methods

The goal of a data collection plan is to produce good data. Every decision researchers make about data collection methods and procedures can affect data quality, and hence the overall quality of the study.

It may, however, be difficult to critique data collection methods in studies reported in journals because researchers' descriptions are seldom detailed. However, researchers do have a responsibility to communicate basic information about their approach so that readers can assess the quality of evidence that the study yields. One important issue is the *mix* of data collection approaches. Triangulation of methods (e.g., self-report and observation) is often desirable.

Information about data quality (reliability and validity of the measures) should be provided in every quantitative research report. Ideally—especially for composite scales—the report should provide internal consistency coefficients based on data from the study itself, not just from previous research. Interrater or interobserver reliability is especially crucial for assessing data quality in observational studies. The values of the reliability coefficients should be sufficiently high to support confidence in the findings.

Validity is more difficult to document than reliability. At a minimum, researchers should defend their choice of existing measures based on validity information from the developers, and they should cite the relevant publication. Guidelines for critiquing data collection methods are presented in Box 10.2.

Box 10.2 Guidelines for Critiquing Quantitative Data Collection Plans

1. Did the researchers use the best method of capturing study phenomena (i.e., self-reports, observation, biophysiologic measures)? Was triangulation of methods used to advantage?
2. If self-report methods were used, did the researchers make good decisions about the specific methods used to solicit information (e.g., in-person interviews, Internet questionnaires, and so on)? Were composite scales used? If not, should they have been?
3. If observational methods were used, did the report adequately describe what the observations entailed and how observations were sampled? Were risks of observational bias addressed? Were biophysiologic measures used in the study, and was this appropriate?
4. Did the report provide adequate information about data collection procedures? Were data collectors properly trained?
5. Did the report offer evidence of the reliability of measures? Did the evidence come from the research sample itself, or is it based on other studies? If reliability was reported, which estimation method was used? Was the reliability sufficiently high?
6. Did the report offer evidence of the validity of the measures? If validity information was reported, which validity approach was used?
7. If there was no reliability or validity information, what conclusion can you reach about the quality of the data in the study?

RESEARCH EXAMPLES WITH CRITICAL THINKING EXERCISES

In this section, we describe the sampling and data collection plan of a quantitative nursing study. Read the summary and then answer the critical thinking questions that follow, referring to the full research report if necessary. Example 1 is featured on the interactive *Critical Thinking Activity* on thePoint website. The critical thinking questions for Example 2 are based on the study that appears in its entirety in Appendix A of this book. Our comments for these exercises are in the Student Resources section on thePoint. 🔆

EXAMPLE 1: SAMPLING AND DATA COLLECTION IN A QUANTITATIVE STUDY

Study: Insomnia symptoms are associated with abnormal endothelial function (Routledge et al., 2015) (Some information about the study was provided in Rask, Brigham, and Johns (2011).) 🔆

Purpose: The purpose of this study was to test the hypothesis that insomnia symptoms are associated with reduced endothelial function in working adults.

Design: The researchers used cross-sectional baseline data from a longitudinal study that involved the collection of extensive data from people enrolled in an Emory-Georgia Tech Predictive Health Institute study. The design for the study reported by Routledge and colleagues was descriptive correlational.

Sampling: The initial cohort of the study was a sample of full-time employees of a large university. The population of eligible employees was stratified by type of employees (faculty, exempt, and non-exempt employees). From the stratified sampling frame, every 10th employee was invited to participate in the research. About 30% of the solicited employees agreed to be contacted, and about 10% were ultimately enrolled. Additionally, about 10% of the sample was a convenience sample of workers from self-referral or health care provider referral. Specific criteria for enrolment included employees aged 18 years or older, with no hospitalization in the prior year except for accidents. Exclusion criteria included a history in the previous year of a severe psychosocial disorder, substance/drug abuse or alcoholism, current active malignant neoplasm, and any acute illness in the 2 weeks before baseline data collection. For the purpose of the Routledge et al. study, participants were excluded if they had a sleep apnea diagnosis or reported symptoms of sleep apnea. The sample for this study was 496 adults aged 19 to 82 years.

Data Collection: The overall study involved two baseline assessments, a 6-month assessment, and four annual assessments. Baseline measures used in Routledge et al. study included both self-report and biophysiologic measures. In terms of self-reports, participants completed an online questionnaire that asked questions about background characteristics (e.g., age, gender, smoking status). The questionnaire also included several composite scales to measure sleep quality (the Pittsburgh Sleep Quality Index), depression (the Beck Depression Inventory), and sleepiness (the Epworth Sleepiness Scale). Information from the sleep scales was used to categorize participants as being in an insomnia group or a "better sleepers" group. Anthropomorphic measurements (height and weight, body mass index) were obtained, blood pressure was measured, and a blood draw was completed and analysed for lipids. Finally, endothelial function was measured using brachial artery flow-mediated dilation (FMD) measures. FMD measurements were read by two ultrasound technicians. Information about the reliability and validity of the various measures was not provided.

Key Findings: In this sample, insomnia symptoms were reported by 40% of the participants. After controlling statistically for age and other variables, the researchers found that participants reporting insomnia symptoms had lower FMD than did participants reporting better sleep.

Critical Thinking Exercises

1. Answer the relevant questions from Box 10.1 regarding this study.
2. Answer the relevant questions from Box 10.2 regarding this study.
3. Are there variables in this study that could have been measured through observation but were not?
4. If the results of this study are valid and reliable, what might be some of the uses to which the findings could be put in clinical practice?

EXAMPLE 2: SAMPLING AND DATA COLLECTION IN THE STUDY IN APPENDIX A

- Read the method section of Swenson and colleagues' (2016) study ("Parents' use of praise and criticism in a sample of young children seeking mental health services") in Appendix A of this book.

Critical Thinking Exercises

1. Answer the relevant questions from Box 10.1 regarding this study.
2. Answer the relevant questions from Box 10.2 regarding this study.

WANT TO KNOW MORE?

A wide variety of resources to enhance your learning and understanding of this chapter are available on thePoint.

- Interactive Critical Thinking Activity
- Chapter Supplement on Vignettes and Q-Sorts
- Answers to the Critical Thinking Exercises for Example 2
- Internet Resources with useful websites for Chapter 10
- A Wolters Kluwer journal article on a topic related to this chapter

---

Summary Points

- **Sampling** is the process of selecting elements from a **population**, which is an entire aggregate of cases. An *element* is the basic unit of a population—usually humans in nursing research.

- **Eligibility criteria** (including both *inclusion criteria* and *exclusion criteria*) are used to define population characteristics.
- A key criterion in assessing a sample in a quantitative study is its *representativeness*—the extent to which the sample is similar to the population and avoids bias. **Sampling bias** is the systematic overrepresentation or underrepresentation of some segment of the population.

- **Nonprobability sampling** (in which elements are selected by non-random methods) includes convenience, quota, consecutive, and purposive sampling. Non-probability sampling is convenient and economical; a major disadvantage is its potential for bias.
- **Convenience sampling** uses the most readily available or convenient people.
- **Quota sampling** divides the population into homogeneous **strata** (subpopulations) to ensure representation of the subgroups in the sample; within each stratum, people are sampled by convenience.
- **Consecutive sampling** involves taking *all* of the people from an accessible population who meet the eligibility criteria over a specific time interval or for a specified sample size.
- In **purposive sampling**, participants are handpicked to be included in the sample based on the researcher's knowledge about the population.
- **Probability sampling** designs, which involve the random selection of elements from the population, yield more representative samples than nonprobability designs and permit estimates of the magnitude of *sampling error.*
- **Simple random sampling** involves the random selection of elements from a *sampling frame* that enumerates all the elements; **stratified random sampling** divides the population into homogeneous subgroups from which elements are selected at random.
- **Systematic sampling** is the selection of every *k*th case from a list. By dividing the population size by the desired sample size, the researcher establishes the *sampling interval,* which is the standard distance between the selected elements.
- In quantitative studies, researchers can use a **power analysis** to estimate **sample size** needs. Large samples are preferable because they enhance statistical conclusion validity and tend to be more representative, but even large samples do not *guarantee* representativeness.
- The three principal data collection methods for nurse researchers are self-reports, observations, and biophysiologic measures.
- **Self-reports**, which are also called **patient-reported outcomes** or PROs, involve directly

questioning study participants and are the most widely used method of collecting data for nursing studies.
- Structured self-reports for quantitative studies involve a formal **instrument**—a **questionnaire** or **interview schedule**—that may contain **open-ended questions** (which permit respondents to respond in their own words) and **closed-ended questions** (which offer respondents **response options** from which to choose).
- Questionnaires are less costly than interviews and offer the possibility of anonymity, but interviews yield higher response rates and are suitable for a wider variety of people.
- Social–psychological **scales** are self-report instruments for measuring such characteristics as attitudes and psychological attributes. **Likert scales** (*summated rating scales*) present respondents with a series of *items;* each item is scored (e.g., on a continuum from strongly agree to strongly disagree) and then summed into a composite score.
- A **visual analogue scale (VAS)** is used to measure subjective experiences (e.g., pain, fatigue) along a 100-mm line designating a bipolar continuum.
- Scales are versatile and powerful but are susceptible to **response set biases**—the tendency of some people to respond to items in characteristic ways, independently of item content.
- **Observational methods** are techniques for acquiring data through the direct observation of phenomena.
- Structured observations dictate what the observer should observe; they often involve **checklists**—instruments based on **category systems** for recording the appearance, frequency, or duration of behaviours or events. Observers may also use **rating scales** to rate phenomena along a dimension of interest (e.g., lethargic/energetic).
- Structured observations often involve a sampling plan (such as *time sampling* or *event sampling*) for selecting the behaviours, events, and conditions to be observed. Observational techniques are often essential, but observational biases can reduce data quality.

- Data may also be derived from **biophysiologic measures,** which include *in vivo* measurements (those performed within or on living organisms) and *in vitro* measurements (those performed outside the organism's body, such as blood tests). Biophysiologic measures have the advantage of being objective, accurate, and precise.
- In developing a data collection plan, the researcher must decide who will collect the data, how the data collectors will be trained, and what the circumstances for data collection will be.
- In quantitative studies, variables are measured. **Measurement** involves assigning numbers to represent the amount of an attribute present in a person, using a set of rules; researchers strive to use measures that have good rules that minimize *measurement errors.*
- Measures (and the quality of the data that the measures yield) can be evaluated in a **psychometric assessment** in terms of several **measurement properties,** most often reliability and validity.
- **Reliability** is the extent to which scores for people *who have not changed* are the same for repeated measurements. A reliable measure minimizes measurement error.
- Methods of assessing reliability include **test–retest reliability** (administering a measure twice in a short period to see if the measure yields consistent scores), **interrater reliability** (assessing whether two raters or observers independently assign similar scores), and **internal consistency** (assessing whether there is consistency across items in a composite scale in measuring a trait).
- Reliability is assessed statistically by computing coefficients that range from .00 to 1.00; higher values indicate greater reliability.
- **Validity** is the degree to which an instrument measures what it is supposed to measure.
- Aspects of validity include **face validity** (the extent to which a measure looks like it is measuring the target construct), **content validity** (in composite scales, the extent to which an instrument's content adequately captures the construct), **criterion validity** (the extent to which scores on a measure are a good reflection of a "gold standard"), and **construct validity** (the extent to which an instrument adequately measures the targeted construct, as assessed mainly by testing hypotheses).
- A measure's validity is not proved or established but rather is supported to a greater or lesser extent by evidence.

REFERENCES

Broadhurst D., Moureau N., Ullman A. J.; World Congress of Vascular Access (WoCoVA) Skin Impairment Management Advisory Panel. (2017). Management of Central Venous Access Device-Associated Skin Impairment: An Evidence-Based Algorithm. *Journal of Wound Ostomy & Continence Nursing, 44*(3), 211–220.

Bryant, V., Phang, J., & Abrams, K. (2015). Verifying placement of small-bore feeding tubes: Electromagnetic device images versus abdominal radiographs. *American Journal of Critical Care, 24*, 525–530.

Burk, R., Grap, M., Munro, C., Schubert, C., & Sessler, C. (2014). Predictors of agitation in the adult critically ill. *American Journal of Critical Care, 23*, 414–423.

Coker, E., Ploeg, J., Kaasalainen, S., & Carter, N. (2017). Observations of oral hygiene care interventions provided by nurses to hospitalized older people. *Geriatric Nursing, 38*(1), 17–21

Ganann R., Sword W., Thabane L., et al. (2016). Predictors of Postpartum Depression Among Immigrant Women in the Year After Childbirth. *Journal of Women's Health (Larchmt), 25*(2), 155–165.

Havaei, F., MacPhee, M., & Dahinten, V. S. (2016). RNs and LPNs: Emotional exhaustion and intention to leave. *Journal of Nursing Management, 24*(3), 393–399.

Hu, R., Jiang, X., Hegadoren, K., & Zhang, Y. (2015). Effects of earplugs and eye masks combined with relaxing music on sleep, melatonin and cortisol levels in ICU patients: A randomized controlled trial. *Critical Care, 19*, 115.

Huang, C. Y., Lai, H., Lu, Y., et al. (2016). Risk factors and coping style affect health outcomes in adults with type 2 diabetes. *Biological Research for Nursing, 18*, 82–89.

Kennedy, E., Murphy, G., Misener, R., & Alder, E. (2015). Development and psychometric assessment of the nursing competence self-efficacy scale. *Journal of Nursing Education, 54*, 550–558.

Lalonde M, & McGillis Hall L. (2016). Preceptor characteristics and the socialization outcomes of new graduate nurses during a preceptorship programme. *Nursing Open, 4*(1), 24–31.

Lambert S. D., Yoon H., Ellis K. R., & Northouse L. (2015). Measuring appraisal during advanced cancer: psychometric testing of the appraisal of caregiving scale. *Patient Education and Counseling, 98*(5), 633–639.

Nilsen, M., Sereika, S., Hoffman, L., Barnato, A., Donovan, H., & Happ, M. (2014). Nurse and patient interaction behaviors' effects on nursing care quality for mechanically ventilated older adults in the ICU. *Research in Gerontological Nursing, 7*, 113–125.

Okoli, C., Kodet, J., & Robertson, H. (2016). Behavioral and physiological responses to nicotine patch administration among nonsmokers based on acute and chronic secondhand tobacco smoke exposure. *Biological Research for Nursing, 18*, 60–67.

Polit, D. F. & Yang, F. M. (2016). *Measurement and the measurement of change: A primer for health professionals.* Philadelphia, PA: Wolters Kluwer.

Rask, K., Brigham, K., & Johns, M. (2011). Integrating comparative effectiveness research programs into predictive health: A unique role for academic health centers. *Academic Medicine, 86*, 718–723.

Ratanasiripong, N. T. (2015). Factors related to human papillomavirus (HPV) vaccination in college men. *Public Health Nursing, 32*, 645–653.

Ridout, J., Aucoin, J., Browning, A., Piedra, K., & Weeks, S. (2014). Does perioperative documentation transfer reliably? *Computers, Informatics, Nursing, 32*, 37–42.

Routledge, F., Dunbar, S., Higgins, M., et al. (2015). Insomnia symptoms are associated with abnormal endothelial function. *Journal of Cardiovascular Nursing.* Advance online publication.

Stinson J., Ahola Kohut S., Forgeron P., et al. (2016). The iPeer2Peer Program: A pilot randomized controlled trial in adolescents with juvenile idiopathic arthritis. *Pediatric Rheumatology Online Journal, 14*(1), 48. doi: 10.1186/s12969-016-0108-2.

VanDenKerkhof, E. G., Mann, E. G., Torrance, N., Smith, B. H., Johnson, A., & Gilron, I. (2016). An epidemiological study of neuropathic pain symptoms in Canadian adults. *Pain Research Management, 2016,* 9815750.

Wang, W., Zhang, H., Lopez, V., Wu, V., Poo, D., & Kowitlawakul, Y. (2015). Improving awareness, knowledge and heart-related lifestyle of coronary heart disease among working population through amHealth programme: Study protocol. *Journal of Advanced Nursing, 71,* 2200–2207.

Woo K. Y., Sears K., Almost J., et al. (2017). Exploration of pressure ulcer and related skin problems across the spectrum of health care settings in Ontario using administrative data. *International Wound Journal, 14*(1), 24–30.

*A link to this open-access article is provided in the Internet Resources section on thePoint website.

**This journal article is available on thePoint for this chapter.

11 Qualitative Designs and Approaches

Learning Objectives

On completing this chapter, you will be able to:

- Discuss the rationale for an emergent design in qualitative research and describe qualitative design features
- Identify the major research traditions for qualitative research and describe the domain of inquiry of each tradition
- Describe the main features and methods associated with ethnographic, phenomenologic, and grounded theory studies
- Describe key features of historical research, case studies, narrative analysis, and descriptive qualitative studies
- Discuss the goals and features of research with an ideologic perspective
- Define new terms in the chapter

Key Terms

- Basic social process (BSP)
- Bracketing
- Case study
- Constant comparison
- Constructivist grounded theory
- Core variable
- Critical ethnography
- Critical theory
- Descriptive phenomenology
- Descriptive qualitative study
- Emergent design
- Ethnonursing research
- Feminist research
- Grounded theory
- Hermeneutics
- Historical research
- Interpretive phenomenology
- Narrative analysis
- Participant observation
- Participatory action research (PAR)
- Reflexive journal

THE DESIGN OF QUALITATIVE STUDIES

Quantitative researchers develop a research design before collecting their data and rarely depart from that design once the study is underway: They design and *then* they do. In qualitative research, by contrast, the study design often changes during the project: Qualitative researchers design *as* they do. Qualitative studies use an **emergent design** that develops as researchers make ongoing decisions about their data needs based on what they have already learned. An emergent design indicates the researchers' intention to understand the realities and viewpoints of those under study—such information is not known at the beginning of the study.

Characteristics of Qualitative Research Design

Qualitative inquiry has been guided by different disciplines with distinct methods and approaches. However, some characteristics of qualitative research design are broadly applicable. In general, qualitative design:

- Is flexible to allow adjustment based on what is learned during data collection
- Involves triangulating various data collection strategies
- Tends to be holistic, striving for an understanding of the whole
- Requires researchers to become intensely involved and reflexive and can require a lot of time
- Benefits from ongoing data analysis to guide subsequent strategies

Although design decisions are not finalized in advance, qualitative researchers typically do require planning that supports their flexibility. For example, qualitative researchers make advance decisions with regard to their research tradition, the study site, a broad data collection strategy, and the equipment they will need in the field. Qualitative researchers plan for a variety of circumstances, but decisions about how to deal with them are made when the social context is better understood.

Qualitative Design Features

Some of the design features discussed in Chapter 9 apply to qualitative studies. To contrast quantitative and qualitative research design, we consider the elements identified in Table 9.1.

Intervention, Control, and Blinding

Qualitative research is almost always non-experimental—although a qualitative substudy may be embedded in an experiment (see Chapter 13). Qualitative researchers do not conceptualize their studies as having independent and dependent variables and rarely control the people or environment under study. Blinding is rarely used by qualitative researchers. The goal is to develop a rich understanding of a phenomenon as it exists and as it is constructed by individuals within their own context.

Comparisons

Qualitative researchers typically do not plan to make group comparisons because the intent is to thoroughly describe or explain a phenomenon, yet patterns emerging in the data sometimes suggest illuminating comparisons. Indeed, as Morse (2004) noted in an editorial in *Qualitative Health Research*, "All description requires comparisons" (p. 1323). In analysing qualitative data and in determining whether all categories are satisfactorily identified or saturated, there is a need to compare "this" to "that."

Example of qualitative comparisons •
Olsson et al. (2015) studied patients' decision making about undergoing transcatheter aortic valve implantation of severe aortic stenosis. They identified three distinct patterns of decision making in their sample of 24 patients, who were ambivalent about the treatment, obedient and willing to let others decide, or reconciled and accepting of the treatment.

Research Settings

Qualitative researchers usually collect their data in naturalistic settings. And, whereas quantitative researchers usually strive to collect data in one type of setting to maintain constancy of conditions (e.g., conducting all interviews in participants' homes), qualitative researchers may deliberately study phenomena in various natural contexts, especially in ethnographic research.

Time Frames

Qualitative research, like quantitative research, can be either cross-sectional, with one data collection point; or longitudinal, with multiple data collection points designed to observe the evolution of a phenomenon.

> **Example of a longitudinal qualitative study** ·
> Keller et al. (2015) explored the meaning and experience of mealtimes for families living with dementia in Southwest Ontario. Data were collected through in-depth interviews with 27 older persons with dementia and their family care partners annually over a 3-year period.

Causality and Qualitative Research

In evidence hierarchies that rank evidence according to its support for causal inferences (e.g., the one in Figure 2.1), qualitative research is often near the base, which has led some to criticize evidence-based initiatives. The issue of causality, which has been controversial throughout the history of science, is especially sensitive in qualitative research.

Some believe that causality is an inappropriate construct within the naturalistic paradigm. For example, Lincoln and Guba (1985) devoted an entire chapter of their book to a critique of causality and argued that it should be replaced with a concept that they called *mutual shaping*. According to their view, "Everything influences everything else, in the here and now" (p. 151).

Others, however, believe that qualitative methods are particularly well suited to understanding causal relationships. For example, Huberman and Miles (1994) argued that qualitative studies "can look directly and longitudinally at the local processes underlying a temporal series of events and states, showing how these led to specific outcomes, and ruling out rival hypotheses" (p. 434).

In attempting to not only describe but also to explain phenomena, qualitative researchers undertake in-depth studies to reveal patterns and processes suggesting causal interpretations. These interpretations can be (and often are) subjected to systematic testing using more controlled methods of inquiry.

QUALITATIVE RESEARCH TRADITIONS

There are a wide variety of qualitative approaches. One classification system involves describing qualitative research according to disciplinary traditions. These traditions vary in their conceptualization of what types of questions are important to ask and in the methods considered appropriate for answering them. Table 11.1 provides an overview of several such traditions, some of which we introduced previously. This section describes traditions that are common in nursing research.

Ethnography

Ethnography involves the description and interpretation of a culture and cultural behaviour. *Culture* refers to the way a group of people live—the patterns of human activity and the values and norms that give activity significance. Ethnographies typically involve extensive

TABLE 11.1 Overview of Qualitative Research Traditions

Discipline	Domain	Research Tradition	Area of Inquiry
Anthropology	Culture	Ethnography	Holistic view of a culture
Psychology/ Philosophy	Lived experience	Phenomenology Hermeneutics	Experiences of individuals within their life world Interpretations and meanings of individuals' experiences
Sociology	Social settings	Grounded theory	Social psychological and structural process within a social setting
History	Past behaviour, events, conditions	Historical analysis	Description/interpretation of historical events

fieldwork for the ethnographer to gather information and understand a culture. Because culture is not visible or tangible, it must be inferred from the words, actions, and products that belong to a group of people.

Ethnographic research sometimes concerns broadly defined cultures (e.g., the Maori culture of New Zealand) in what is sometimes called a *macroethnography*. However, ethnographies sometimes focus on more narrowly defined cultures in a *focused ethnography*. Focused ethnographies are studies of small units in a group or culture (e.g., the culture of an intensive care unit). An underlying assumption of the ethnographer is that every human group eventually develops a culture that shapes people's view of the world and their experiences.

Example of a focused ethnography •
Cable-Williams and Wilson (2017) used a focused ethnographic approach to study the awareness of impending death and initiation of a palliative approach to care for residents aged 85 years and older in Canadian long-term care facilities.

Ethnographers seek to learn from (rather than to study) members of a cultural group—to understand their worldview. Ethnographers distinguish "emic" and "etic" perspectives. An *emic perspective* refers to the way the members of the culture regard their world—the insiders' view. The emic is the local concepts or means of expression used by members of the group under study to characterize their experiences. The *etic perspective*, by contrast, is the outsiders' interpretation of the culture's experiences—the words and concepts they use to refer to the same phenomena. Ethnographers try to acquire an emic perspective of a culture and to uncover *tacit knowledge*—information about the culture that is so deeply embedded in cultural experiences that members do not talk about it or may not even be consciously aware of it.

Three broad types of information are usually sought by ethnographers: cultural behaviour (what members of the culture do), cultural artefacts (what members make and use), and cultural speech (what they say). Ethnographers rely on a wide variety of data sources, including observations, in-depth interviews, records, and other types of physical evidence (e.g., photographs, diaries). Ethnographers typically use a strategy called **participant observation** in order to observe the culture under study while participating in its activities. Ethnographers also enlist the help of *key informants* to help them understand and interpret the events and activities being observed.

Ethnographic research is time-consuming—months and even years of fieldwork may be required to learn about a culture. Ethnography requires a certain level of intimacy with members of the cultural group, and such intimacy can be developed only over time and by working with those members as active participants.

The products of ethnographies are rich, holistic descriptions and interpretations of the culture under study. Among health care researchers, ethnography provides access to the health beliefs and health practices of a culture. Ethnographic inquiry can thus help researchers understand behaviours that affect health and illness. Leininger (1985) coined the phrase **ethnonursing research**, which she defined as "the study and analysis of the local or indigenous people's viewpoints, beliefs, and practices about nursing care behavior and processes of designated cultures" (p. 38).

> **Example of an ethnographic study** •
> Kaposy et al. (2017) conducted an ethnographic study to identify ethical issues involving health care providers and clients from HIV clinics in Newfoundland and Labrador, and Manitoba. The key ethical issues were conflicts between client-autonomy and public health priorities, non-disclosure of HIV positive status, non-adherence to HIV treatment, the protection of confidentiality, barriers to treatment access, and negative social determinants of health and well-being.

Ethnographers are often, but not always, "outsiders" to the culture under study. A type of ethnography that involves self-scrutiny (including examination of groups or cultures to which researchers themselves belong) is called *autoethnography* or *insider research*. Autoethnography has several advantages, including ease of recruitment and the ability to get candid data based on pre-established trust. The drawback is that an "insider" may have biases about certain issues or may be so entrenched in the culture that valuable data get overlooked.

Phenomenology

Phenomenology is an approach to understanding people's everyday life experiences. Phenomenologic researchers ask: What is the *essence* of this phenomenon as experienced by these people, and what does it *mean*? Phenomenologists assume there is an *essence*—an essential structure—that can be understood, much as ethnographers assume that cultures exist. Essence is what makes a phenomenon what it is, and without which it would not be what it is. Phenomenologists investigate subjective phenomena and they believe critical truths about reality are grounded in people's lived experiences. The topics appropriate to phenomenology are fundamental to the life experiences of humans, such as the meaning of suffering or the quality of life with chronic pain.

In phenomenologic studies, the main data source is in-depth conversations. Through these conversations, researchers try to get into the informants' world and to have access to their experiences as lived. Phenomenologic studies involve a small number of participants—often 10 or fewer. For some phenomenologic researchers, the inquiry includes gathering information from informants as well as efforts to experience the phenomenon through participation, observation, and reflection. Phenomenologists share their insights in rich, vivid reports that describe key *themes*. The results section in a phenomenologic report should help readers "see" something in a different way that enriches their understanding of others' experiences.

Phenomenology has several variants and interpretations. The two main schools of thought are descriptive phenomenology and interpretive phenomenology (hermeneutics).

Descriptive Phenomenology

Descriptive phenomenology was developed first by Husserl, who was primarily interested in the question: *What do we know as persons?* Descriptive phenomenologists carefully portray ordinary conscious experience of everyday life—describing "things" as people experience them. These "things" include hearing, seeing, believing, feeling, remembering, deciding, and evaluating.

Descriptive phenomenologic studies often involve the following four steps: bracketing, intuiting, analysing, and describing. **Bracketing** refers to the process of identifying and withholding preconceived beliefs and opinions about the phenomenon under study. Researchers strive to bracket out presuppositions to confront the data in its pure form. Phenomenologic researchers (as well as other qualitative researchers) often maintain a **reflexive journal** in their efforts to bracket.

Intuiting is the second step in descriptive phenomenology. In this step, researchers maintain an openness to the meanings attributed to the phenomenon by those who have experienced it. Phenomenologic researchers then proceed to perform an analysis (i.e., extracting significant statements, categorizing, and making sense of essential meanings). Finally, the descriptive phase occurs when researchers come to understand and define the phenomenon.

Example of a descriptive phenomenologic study · · · · · · · · · · · · · · ·

Premji et al. (2017) from the University of Alberta used a descriptive phenomenologic approach in their study of mothers' experience of caring for their late preterm infants in the community. Overall, mothers report their lack of preparation to meet the special needs of their late preterm infants.

Interpretive Phenomenology

Heidegger, a student of Husserl, is the founder of **interpretive phenomenology**, or hermeneutics. Heidegger stressed interpreting and understanding—not just describing—human experience. He believed that lived experience is an interpretive process and argued that **hermeneutics** ("understanding") is a basic characteristic of human existence. (The term *hermeneutics* refers to the art and philosophy of interpreting the meaning of an object, such as a *text* or work of art). The goals of interpretive phenomenologic research are to enter another's world and to discover the understandings found there.

Gadamer, another interpretive phenomenologist, described the interpretive process as a circular relationship—the *hermeneutic circle*—where one understands the whole of a text (e.g., an interview transcript) in terms of its parts and the parts in terms of the whole. Researchers continually question the meanings of the text.

Heidegger believed it is impossible to bracket one's being-in-the-world, so bracketing does not occur in interpretive phenomenology. Hermeneutics accepts prior understanding on the part of the researcher. Interpretive phenomenologists ideally approach each interview text with openness—they must be open to hearing what it is the text is saying.

Interpretive phenomenologists, like descriptive phenomenologists, rely primarily on in-depth interviews with individuals who have experienced the phenomenon of interest, but they may go beyond a traditional approach to gathering and analysing data. For example, interpretive phenomenologists sometimes strengthen their understandings of the phenomenon through an analysis of supplementary texts, such as novels, poetry, or other artistic expressions—or they use such materials in their conversations with study participants.

Example of an interpretive phenomenologic study · · · · · · · · · · · · · · ·

LaDonna et al. (2016) used an interpretive phenomenologic approach in their exploration of the experience of caring for individuals with dysphagia and myotonic dystrophy.

Grounded Theory

Grounded theory has contributed to the development of many middle-range theories of phenomena relevant to nurses. Grounded theory was developed in the 1960s by two sociologists, Glaser and Strauss (1967), who were interested in *symbolic interaction* that focused on how people make sense of social interactions.

Grounded theory tries to account for people's actions from the perspective of those involved. Grounded theory researchers seek to identify a main concern or problem and then to understand the behaviour designed to resolve the issue—the **core variable**. One type of core variable is a **basic social process (BSP)**. Grounded theory researchers generate conceptual categories and integrate them into a substantive theory, grounded in the data.

Grounded Theory Methods

A study that truly follows Glaser and Strauss's (1967) instructions does not begin with a focused research problem. The problem and the process used to resolve it emerge from the data and are discovered during the study. In grounded theory research, data collection, data analysis, and sampling of participants occur simultaneously. The grounded theory process is recursive: Researchers collect data, categorize them, describe the emerging central phenomenon, and then recycle earlier steps.

A procedure called **constant comparison** is used to develop and refine theoretically relevant concepts and categories. Categories elicited from the data are constantly compared with data obtained earlier so that commonalities and variations can be detected. As data collection proceeds, the inquiry becomes increasingly focused on the emerging theory.

In-depth interviews and participant observation are common data sources in grounded theory studies, but existing documents and other data may also be used. Typically, a grounded theory study involves interviews with a sample of about 20 to 30 people.

Alternate Views of Grounded Theory

In 1990, Strauss and Corbin published a controversial book, *Basics of Qualitative Research: Techniques and Procedures for Developing Grounded Theory.* The purpose was to provide beginning grounded theory researchers with basic procedures for building a grounded theory.

Glaser, however, disagreed with some procedures advocated by Strauss (his original coauthor) and Corbin (a nurse researcher). Glaser (1992) believed that Strauss and Corbin (1998) developed a method that is not grounded theory but rather what he called "full conceptual description." According to Glaser, the purpose of grounded theory is to generate concepts and theories that explain and account for variation in behaviour in the substantive area under study. *Conceptual description,* by contrast, is aimed at describing the full range of behaviour of what is occurring in the substantive area.

Nurse researchers have conducted grounded theory studies using both the original Glaser and Strauss (1967) and the Strauss and Corbin (1998) approaches. They also use an approach called **constructivist grounded theory** (Charmaz, 2014). Charmaz (2014) regards Glaser and Strauss' grounded theory as having positivist roots. In Charmaz's approach, the developed grounded theory is seen as an interpretation. The data collected and analysed are acknowledged to be constructed from shared experiences and relationships between the researcher and the participants. Data and analyses are viewed as social constructions.

Example of a grounded theory study •
Hernandez et al. (2016) used Glaserian grounded theory to explore the experience of weight management in normal-weight individuals. Weight management was an ongoing process through five consciously and unconsciously used strategies.

Historical Research

Historical research is the systematic collection and critical evaluation of data relating to past occurrences. Historical research relies primarily on qualitative (narrative) data but can sometimes involve statistical analysis of quantitative data. Nurses have used historical research methods to examine a wide range of phenomena in both the recent and more distant past.

Data for historical research are usually in the form of written records: diaries, letters, newspapers, medical documents, and so forth. Non-written materials, such photographs and films, can be forms of historical data. In some cases, it is possible to conduct interviews with people who participated in historical events (e.g., nurses who served in recent wars).

Historical research is usually interpretive. Historical researchers try to describe what happened and also how and why it happened. Relationships between events and ideas, between people and organizations, are explored and interpreted within their historical context and within the context of new viewpoints about what is historically significant.

Example of historical research •
Vanderspank-Wright et al. (2015) explored the development of ICU nursing in Canada from 1960 to 2002 using a social history approach. The analysis was based on photographs, oral history interviews, documents and records, and professional literature published during those years.

OTHER TYPES OF QUALITATIVE RESEARCH

Qualitative studies often can be characterized and described in terms of the disciplinary research traditions discussed in the previous section. However, several other important types of qualitative research not associated with a particular discipline also deserve mention.

Case Studies

Case studies are in-depth investigations of a single entity or small number of entities. The entity may be an individual, family, institution, or other social unit. Case study researchers attempt to understand issues that are important to the focal entity.

In most studies, whether quantitative or qualitative, certain phenomena or variables are the core of the inquiry. In a case study, the *case* itself is at "center stage." The focus of case studies is typically on understanding *why* an individual thinks, behaves, or develops in a particular manner rather than on *what* his or her status or actions are. Exploratory research of this type may require study over a considerable period. Data are often collected not only about the person's present state but also about past experiences relevant to the problem being examined.

The greatest strength of case studies is the depth that is possible when a small number of entities are being investigated. Case study researchers can gain an intimate knowledge of a person's feelings, actions, and intentions. However, this same strength is a potential weakness: Researchers' familiarity with the case may make objectivity more difficult. Another limitation of case studies concerns generalizability: If researchers discover important relationships, it is difficult to know whether the same relationships would occur with others. However, case studies can play a role in challenging generalizations from other types of research.

Example of a case study •
McPherson et al. (2017) conducted an in-depth case study that focused on the development and evolution of a child health network in Eastern Nova Scotia that was developed in 1994. The data were obtained through interviews with 34 individuals representing network members, staff, and external partners. A total of 127 documents including meeting minutes, policy, and project reports were reviewed and analysed.

Narrative Analyses

Narrative analysis focuses on *story* as the object of inquiry to understand how individuals make sense of events in their lives. The underlying premise of narrative research is that people make sense of their world—and communicate these meanings effectively—by telling stories. Individuals construct stories when they wish to understand specific events and situations that require linking an inner world of thoughts to an external world of observable actions. Analysing stories includes *forms* of how the story is told in addition to its content. Narrative analysts ask, *Why did the story get told that way?* A number of structural approaches can be used to analyse stories, including ones based in literary analysis and linguistics.

Example of a narrative analysis •
Tobin, Murphy-Lawless, and Beck (2014) (including Beck, an author of this textbook) conducted a narrative analysis of asylum-seeking women's experience of childbirth in Ireland. Twenty-two mothers told their stories during in-depth interviews lasting from 40 to 90 minutes. Highlighted in their narratives was a lack of communication, connection, and culturally competent care.

Descriptive Qualitative Studies

Many qualitative studies claim no particular disciplinary or methodologic backgrounds. The researchers may simply indicate that they have conducted a qualitative study, a naturalistic inquiry, or a *content analysis* of qualitative data (i.e., an analysis of themes and patterns that emerge in the narrative content). Thus, some qualitative studies do not have a formal name or do not fit into the typology we have presented in this chapter. We refer to these as **descriptive qualitative studies**.

Descriptive qualitative studies tend to be diverse in their designs and methods and they are based on the general principles of constructivist inquiry. These studies are infrequently discussed in research methods textbooks.

 TIP The chapter supplement on thePoint website presents information on descriptive qualitative studies and studies that nurse researcher Sally Thorne (2013) called interpretive description.

Example of a descriptive qualitative study •
Dhaliwal et al. (2017) performed a descriptive qualitative study to explore the impact of financial barriers on patients' ability to self-manage their cardiovascular disease. The researchers conducted in-depth interviews with 13 patients in Alberta with heart disease.

Research with Ideologic Perspectives

Some qualitative researchers conduct inquiries within an ideologic framework to point out social problems or the needs of certain groups and to bring about change. These approaches represent important investigative avenues.

Critical Theory

Critical theory originated with a group of Marxist-oriented German scholars in the 1920s. Essentially, a critical researcher is concerned with a critique of society and with expecting new possibilities. Critical social science is action-oriented. Its aim is to make people aware of contradictions and disparities in social practices and become inspired to address them. Critical theory calls for inquiries that promote better self-knowledge and socio-political action.

Critical researchers often triangulate methods and emphasize multiple perspectives (e.g., alternative racial or social class perspectives) on problems. Critical researchers typically interact with participants in ways that emphasize participants' expertise.

Critical theory has been applied in several disciplines but has played an especially important role in ethnography. **Critical ethnography** focuses on raising consciousness in the hope of affecting social change. Critical ethnographers attempt to increase the political dimensions of cultural research and undermine oppressive systems.

Example of a critical ethnography •
Speechley et al. (2015) developed an "ethnodrama" to catalyse dialogue in home-based dementia care. The script was derived from a critical ethnographic study that followed people living with dementia, and their caregivers, over an 18-month period. Their script was designed to disseminate their research findings "in a way that catalyzes and fosters critical (actionable) dialogue" (p. 1551).

Feminist Research

Feminist research is similar to critical theory research, but the focus is on gender domination and discrimination within patriarchal societies. Similar to critical researchers, feminist researchers seek to establish collaborative and non-exploitative relationships with their informants and to conduct research that is transformative. Feminist investigators seek to understand how gender and a gendered social order have shaped women's lives. The aim is to facilitate change in ways relevant to ending women's unequal social position.

Feminist research methods typically include in-depth, interactive, and collaborative individual or group interviews that allow reciprocally educational opportunities. Feminists usually explore the meanings of the results with those participating in the study and to be self-reflective about what they themselves are learning.

Example of feminist research ·
Griscti et al. (2017) used a critical feminist lens in their study to explore power relations between nurses and patients with chronic disease when negotiating patient care in a hospitals. Eight patients from Nova Scotia discussed experiences when their voices were not heard.

Participatory Action Research

Participatory action research (PAR) is based on the view that the production of knowledge can be used to exert power. PAR investigators typically work with groups or communities that are vulnerable to the control or oppression of a dominant group.

The PAR tradition focuses on the powerlessness of the group under study. In PAR, investigators and participants collaborate in defining the problem, selecting research methods, analysing the data, and deciding how the findings will be used. The aim of PAR is to produce not only knowledge but also action, empowerment, and consciousness raising.

In PAR, the research methods are designed to facilitate processes of collaboration that can motivate and generate community solidarity. Thus, "data-gathering" strategies are not only the traditional methods of interview and observation but also may include storytelling, sociodrama, photography, and other activities designed to encourage people to find creative ways to explore their lives, tell their stories, and recognize their own strengths.

Example of participatory action research ·
Baird et al. (2015) used PAR to explore aboriginal women's experiences with gestational diabetes. Conversational interviews with nine Mi'kmaq women who experienced gestational diabetes mellitus were conducted, and talking circles were held.

CRITIQUING QUALITATIVE DESIGNS

Evaluating a qualitative design is often difficult. Qualitative researchers do not always document design decisions or describe the process to reach such decisions. Researchers often do, however, indicate whether the study was conducted within a specific qualitative tradition. This information helps us form opinions about the study design. For example, if a report indicated that the researcher conducted 2 months of fieldwork for an ethnographic study, you might suspect that insufficient time was spent in the field to obtain an emic perspective of the culture under study. Ethnographic studies may also be critiqued if their only source of information was from interviews rather than from a broader range of data sources, particularly observations.

In a grounded theory study, look for evidence about when the data were collected and analysed. If the researcher collected all the data before analysing any of it, you might question whether the constant comparative method was used correctly.

In critiquing a phenomenologic study, you should first determine if the study is descriptive or interpretive. This will help you to assess how closely the researcher kept to the basic principles of that qualitative research tradition. For example, in a descriptive phenomenologic study, did the researcher bracket? When critiquing a phenomenologic study, in addition to critiquing the methodology, you should also look at its power in capturing the meaning of the phenomena being studied.

> ### Box 11.1 Guidelines for Critiquing Qualitative Designs
>
> 1. Was the research tradition for the qualitative study identified? If none was identified, can one be inferred?
> 2. Is the research question congruent with a qualitative approach and with the specific research tradition? Are the data sources and research methods congruent with the research tradition?
> 3. How well was the research design described? Are design decisions explained and justified? Does it appear that the design emerged during data collection, allowing researchers to capitalize on early information?
> 4. Did the design lend itself to a thorough, in-depth examination of the focal phenomenon? Was there evidence of reflexivity? What design elements might have strengthened the study (e.g., a longitudinal perspective rather than a cross-sectional one)?
> 5. Was the study undertaken with an ideologic perspective? If so, is there evidence that ideologic goals were achieved? (e.g., Was there full collaboration between researchers and participants? Did the research have the power to be transformative?)

No matter what qualitative design is identified in a study, look to see if the researchers stayed true to a single qualitative tradition throughout the study or if they mixed qualitative traditions. For example, did the researcher state that grounded theory was used but then present results that described *themes* instead of generating a substantive theory?

The guidelines in Box 11.1 are designed to assist you in critiquing the designs of qualitative studies.

RESEARCH EXAMPLES WITH CRITICAL THINKING EXERCISES

This section presents examples of qualitative studies. Read these summaries and then answer the critical thinking questions, referring to the full research report if necessary. Example 1 is featured on the interactive *Critical Thinking Activity* on thePoint website. The critical thinking questions for Example 2 are based on the study that appears in its entirety in Appendix B of this book. Our comments for this exercise are in the Student Resources section on thePoint. ⚡

EXAMPLE 1: A GROUNDED THEORY STUDY

Study: The psychological process of breast cancer patients receiving initial chemotherapy (Chen et al., 2015) ⚡

Statement of Purpose: The purpose of the study was to generate a theory to describe the psychological stages of Taiwanese breast cancer patients going through initial chemotherapy.

Method: The researchers used Glaser's (1992) approach to grounded theory approach to understand women's psychological processes. Women were recruited from a teaching hospital in Southern Taiwan. Twenty breast cancer patients having finished their first round of chemotherapy were invited to participate in the study, and none refused. Participants were selected towards the end of the study on the basis of categories that emerged from the analysis of early data. In-depth interviews, lasting 30 to 60 minutes, were conducted in a quiet private room in the hospital by a nurse who had extensive knowledge about breast cancer chemotherapy. The interviewer asked broad questions, such as "What was on your mind before receiving chemotherapy?" and "How did the chemotherapy affect your life?" The interviewer was guided by the women's answers to ask more probing questions that could be linked to emergent concepts so as to reach theoretical saturation. The interviews were audiotaped and subsequently transcribed for analysis. Constant comparison was used in the analysis. The lead researcher maintained a reflective journal "to help with self-awareness."

Key Findings: The main concern in this study was the psychological aspects of going through chemotherapy. The analysis revealed a core category that the researchers called "rising from the ashes." The four stages of the psychological process were the (1) fear stage, (2) hardship stage, (3) adjustment stage, and (4) relaxation stage, when patients accepted the disease-related changes in their lives.

Critical Thinking Exercises

1. Answer the relevant questions from Box 11.1 regarding this study.
2. Also consider the following targeted questions:
   a. Was this study cross-sectional or longitudinal?
   b. Could this study have been undertaken as an ethnography? A phenomenologic inquiry?
3. If the results of this study are trustworthy, what are some of the uses to which the findings might be put in clinical practice?

EXAMPLE 2: PHENOMENOLOGIC STUDY IN APPENDIX B

● Read the method section of Beck and Watson's (2010) study ("Subsequent childbirth after a previous traumatic birth") in Appendix B of this book.

Critical Thinking Exercises

1. Answer the relevant questions from Box 11.1 regarding this study.
2. Also consider the following targeted questions:
   a. Was this study a descriptive or interpretive phenomenology?
   b. Could this study have been conducted as a grounded theory study? As an ethnographic study? Why or why not?
   c. Could this study have been conducted as a feminist inquiry? If yes, what might Beck have done differently?

WANT TO KNOW MORE?
A wide variety of resources to enhance your learning and understanding of this chapter are available on thePoint.

● Interactive Critical Thinking Activity
● Chapter Supplement on Qualitative Descriptive Studies
● Answer to the Critical Thinking Exercises for Example 2
● Internet Resources with useful websites for Chapter 11
● A Wolters Kluwer journal article on a topic related to this chapter

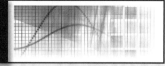

Summary Points

- Qualitative research involves an **emergent design** that develops in the field as the study unfolds. Qualitative studies can be either cross-sectional or longitudinal.
- Ethnography focuses on the culture of a group of people and relies on extensive fieldwork that usually includes **participant observation** and in-depth interviews with *key informants*. Ethnographers strive to acquire an *emic* (insider's) *perspective* of a culture rather than an *etic* (outsider's) *perspective*.
- Nurses sometimes refer to their ethnographic studies as **ethnonursing research.**
- Phenomenologists seek to discover the *essence* and *meaning* of a phenomenon as it is experienced by people, mainly through in-depth interviews with people who have had the relevant experience.
- In **descriptive phenomenology,** which seeks to describe lived experiences, researchers strive to **bracket** out preconceived views and to *intuit* the essence of the phenomenon by remaining open to meanings attributed to it by those who have experienced it.
- **Interpretive phenomenology (hermeneutics)** focuses on interpreting the meaning of experiences rather than just describing them.
- **Grounded theory** researchers try to account for people's actions by focusing on the main concern that their behaviour is designed to resolve. The manner in which people resolve this main concern is the **core variable**. A prominent type of core variable is called a **basic social process (BSP)** that explains the processes of resolving the problem.
- Grounded theory uses **constant comparison:** Categories elicited from the data are constantly compared with data obtained earlier.

- A controversy in grounded theory concerns whether to follow the original Glaser and Strauss (1967) procedures or to use procedures adapted by Strauss and Corbin (1998). Glaser argued that the latter approach does not result in *grounded theories* but rather in *conceptual descriptions.* More recently, Charmaz's **constructivist grounded theory** has emerged, emphasizing interpretive aspects in which the grounded theory is constructed from relationships between the researcher and participants.
- **Case studies** are intensive investigations of a single entity or a small number of entities, such as individuals, groups, families, or communities.
- **Narrative analysis** focuses on *story* in studies in which the purpose is to determine how individuals make sense of events in their lives.
- **Descriptive qualitative studies** are not embedded in a disciplinary tradition. Such studies may be referred to as qualitative studies, naturalistic inquiries, or qualitative content analyses.
- Research is sometimes conducted within an ideologic perspective. **Critical theory** is concerned with a critique of existing social structures; critical researchers conduct studies in collaboration with participants in an effort to foster self-knowledge and transformation. **Critical ethnography** uses the principles of critical theory in the study of cultures.
- **Feminist research,** like critical research, aims at being transformative, but the focus is on how gender domination and discrimination shape women's lives.
- **Participatory action research (PAR)** produces knowledge through close collaboration with groups that are vulnerable to control or oppression by a dominant culture; in PAR, a goal is to develop processes that can motivate people and generate community solidarity.

REFERENCES

Baird, M., Domian, E., Mulcahy, E., Mabior, R., Jemutai-Tanui, G., & Filippi, M. (2015). Creating a bridge of understanding between two worlds: Community-based collaborative-action research with Sudanese refugee women. *Public Health Nursing, 32,* 388–396.

Cable-Williams B, & Wilson DM. (2017). Dying and death within the culture of long-term care facilities in Canada. *International Journal of Older People Nursing, 12*(1). doi: 10.1111/opn.12125. Epub 2016 Jul 19.

Charmaz, K. (2014). *Constructing grounded theory* (2nd ed.). Thousand Oaks, CA: Sage.

**Chen, Y. C., Huang, H., Kao, C., Sun, C., Chiang, C., & Sun, F. (2015). The psychological process of breast cancer patients receiving initial chemotherapy. *Cancer Nursing, 39*(6), E17–E25.

Dhaliwal, K. K., King-Shier, K., Manns, B. J., Hemmelgarn, B. R., Stone, J. A., & Campbell, D. J. (2017). Exploring the impact of financial barriers on secondary prevention of heart disease. *BMC Cardiovascular Disorders, 17*(1), 61. doi: 10.1186/s12872-017-0495-4

Glaser, B. G. (1992). *Basics of grounded theory analysis: Emergence vs. forcing.* Mill Valley, CA: Sociology Press.

Glaser, B. G., & Strauss, A. L. (1967). *The discovery of grounded theory: Strategies for qualitative research.* Chicago, IL: Aldine.

Griscti, O., Aston, M., Warner, G., Martin-Misener, R., & McLeod, D. (2017). Power and resistance within the hospital's hierarchical system: The experiences of chronically ill patients. *Journal of Clinical Nursing, 26*(1–2), 238–247

Hernandez, C. A., Hernandez, D. A., Wellington, C. M., & Kidd, A. (2016). The experience of weight management in normal weight adults. *Applied Nursing Research, 32,* 289–295

Huberman, A. M., & Miles, M. (1994). Data management and analysis methods. In N. K. Denzin & Y. S. Lincoln (Eds.), *Handbook of qualitative research* (pp. 428–444). Thousand Oaks, CA: Sage.

Kaposy C., Greenspan N. R., Marshall Z., et al. (2017). Clinical ethics issues in HIV care in Canada: an institutional ethnographic study. *BMC Medical Ethics, 18*(1), 9.

Keller, H. H., Martin, L. S., Dupuis, S., Reimer, H., Genoe, R. (2015). Strategies to support engagement and continuity of activity during mealtimes for families living with dementia: A qualitative study. *BMC Geriatrics, 15,* 119.

LaDonna, K., Koopman, W., Ray, S., & Venance, S. (2016). Hard to swallow: A phenomenological exploration of the experience of caring for individuals with myotomic dystrophy and dysphagia. *Journal of Neuroscience Nursing, 48,* 42–51.

Leininger, M. M. (Ed.). (1985). *Qualitative research methods in nursing.* New York: Grune & Stratton.

Lincoln, Y. S., & Guba, E. G. (1985). *Naturalistic inquiry.* Newbury Park, CA: Sage.

McPherson, C., Ploeg, J., Edwards, N., Ciliska, D., & Sword, W. (2017). A catalyst for system change: a case study of child health network formation, evolution and sustainability in Canada. *BMC Health Services Research, 17*(1), 100. doi: 10.1186/s12913-017-2018-5.

Morse, J. M. (2004). Qualitative comparison: Appropriateness, equivalence, and fit. *Qualitative Health Research, 14*(10), 1323–1325.

Olsson, K., Näslund, U., Nillson, J., & Hörnsten, Å. (2015). Patients' decision making about undergoing transcatheter aortic valve implantation for severe aortic stenosis. *Journal of Cardiovascular Nursing.* Advance online publication.

Premji, S. S., Currie, G., Reilly, S., et al. (2017). A qualitative study: Mothers of late preterm infants relate their experiences of community-based care. *PLoS One, 12*(3), e0174419. doi: 10.1371/journal.pone.0174419. eCollection 2017.

Speechley, M., DeForge, R., Ward-Griffin, C., Marlatt, N., & Gutmanis, I. (2015). Creating an ethnodrama to catalyze dialogue in home-based dementia care. *Qualitative Health Research, 25,* 1551–1559.

Strauss, A., & Corbin, J. (1998). *Basics of qualitative research: Techniques and procedures for developing grounded theory* (2nd ed.). Thousand Oaks, CA: Sage.

Thorne, S. (2013). Interpretive description. In C. T. Beck (Ed.), *Routledge international handbook of qualitative nursing research* (pp. 295–306). New York: Routledge.

Tobin, C., Murphy-Lawless, J., & Beck, C. T. (2014). Childbirth in exile: Asylum seeking women's experience of childbirth in Ireland. *Midwifery, 30,* 831–838.

Vanderspank-Wright, B., Bourbonnais, F. F., Toman, C., & McPherson, C. (2015). A social construction of the development of ICU nursing in Canada, 1960 to 2002. *Canadian Journal of Critical Care Nursing, 26*(1), 19–24.

---

*A link to this open-access article is provided in the Internet Resources section on thePoint website.

**This journal article is available on thePoint for this chapter.

12 Sampling and Data Collection in Qualitative Studies

Learning Objectives

On completing this chapter, you will be able to:

- Describe the logic of sampling for qualitative studies
- Identify and describe several types of sampling in qualitative studies
- Evaluate the appropriateness of the sampling method and sample size used in a qualitative study
- Identify and describe methods of collecting unstructured self-report data
- Identify and describe methods of collecting and recording unstructured observational data
- Critique a qualitative researcher's decisions regarding the data collection plan
- Define new terms in the chapter

Key Terms

- Data saturation
- Diary
- Field notes
- Focus group interview
- Key informant
- Log
- Maximum variation sampling
- Participant observation
- Photo elicitation interview
- Photovoice
- Purposive (purposeful) sampling
- Semistructured interview
- Snowball sampling
- Theoretical sampling
- Topic guide
- Unstructured interview

This chapter covers two important aspects of qualitative studies—sampling (selecting good study participants) and data collection (gathering the right types and amount of information to address the research question).

SAMPLING IN QUALITATIVE RESEARCH

Qualitative studies typically use small nonprobability samples. Qualitative researchers are as concerned as quantitative researchers with the quality of their samples, but they use different considerations in selecting study participants.

The Logic of Qualitative Sampling

Quantitative researchers measure attributes and identify relationships in a population; they need a representative sample so that findings can be generalized. The aim of most qualitative studies is to discover *meaning* and to uncover multiple realities, not to generalize to a population.

Qualitative researchers ask such sampling questions as, Who would be an *information-rich* data source for my study? Whom should I talk to, or what should I observe, to maximize my understanding of the phenomenon? A first step in qualitative sampling is selecting settings with potential for information richness.

As the study progresses, new sampling questions emerge, such as, Who can I talk to or observe who would confirm, challenge, or enrich my understandings? As with the overall design, sampling design in qualitative studies is an emergent one that uses early information to guide subsequent action.

> **TIP** Like quantitative researchers, qualitative researchers often identify eligibility criteria for their studies. Although they do not specify an explicit population to whom results could be generalized, they do establish the kinds of people who are eligible to participate in their research.

Types of Qualitative Sampling

Qualitative researchers avoid random samples because they are not the best method of selecting people who are knowledgeable, articulate, reflective, and willing to talk at length with researchers. Qualitative researchers use various nonprobability sampling designs.

Convenience and Snowball Sampling

Qualitative researchers often begin with a *volunteer* (convenience) *sample.* Volunteer samples are often used when researchers want participants to come forward and identify themselves. For example, if we wanted to study the experiences of people with frequent nightmares, we might recruit them by placing a notice on a bulletin board or on the Internet. We would be less interested in obtaining a representative sample of people with nightmares than in recruiting a group with diverse nightmare experiences.

Sampling by convenience is efficient but is not a preferred approach. The aim in qualitative studies is to obtain the greatest possible information from a small number of people, and a convenience sample may not provide the most information-rich sources. However, a convenience sample may be an economical way to begin the sampling process.

Example of a convenience sample •
Vat et al. (2015) explored patients' reasons for returning to the emergency department after being discharged from an internal medicine unit. The convenience sample of eight patients was from a major teaching hospital in Montreal, Canada.

Qualitative researchers also use **snowball sampling** (or *network sampling*), asking early informants to make referrals. A weakness of this approach is that the final sample might be restricted to a small group of acquaintances. Also, the quality of the referrals may be affected by whether the referring sample member trusted the researcher and truly wanted to cooperate.

Example of a snowball sample •
The emergency department (ED) is a potentially confusing and harmful environment for older adults with dementia. Hunter et al. (2017) explored safety concerns from the perspective of health care professionals. A snowball process was used to recruit health care providers from two rural hospital EDs in two Canadian provinces.

Purposive Sampling

Qualitative sampling may begin with volunteer informants and may be supplemented with new participants through snowballing. Many qualitative researchers, however, select a **purposive (or purposeful) sampling** strategy to deliberately choose the cases or types of cases that will best contribute to the study.

Dozens of purposive sampling strategies have been identified (Patton, 2002), only some of which are mentioned here. Researchers do not necessarily refer to their sampling plans with Patton's labels; his classification shows the diverse strategies qualitative researchers have adopted to meet the conceptual needs of their research:

- **Maximum variation sampling** involves deliberately selecting cases with a wide range of variation on dimensions of interest.
- *Extreme (deviant) case sampling* provides opportunities for learning from the most unusual and extreme informants (e.g., outstanding successes and notable failures).
- *Typical case sampling* involves the selection of participants who illustrate or highlight what is typical or average.
- *Criterion sampling* involves studying cases who meet a predetermined criterion of importance.

Maximum variation sampling is often the sampling mode of choice in qualitative research because it is useful in showing the scope of a phenomenon and in identifying important patterns that cut across variations. Other strategies can also be useful, however, depending on the nature of the research question.

Example of maximum variation sampling • • • • • • • • • • • • • • • • • • •
Tobiano et al. (2016) studied patients' perceptions of participating in nursing care on medical wards. Maximum variation sampling was used to recruit patients who varied in terms of age, gender, and mobility status.

Sampling confirming and disconfirming cases is another purposive strategy used toward the end of data collection. As researchers analyze their data, emerging conceptualizations sometimes need to be checked. *Confirming cases* are additional cases that fit researchers' conceptualizations and strengthen credibility. *Disconfirming cases* are new cases that do not fit and serve to challenge researchers' interpretations. These "negative" cases may offer insights about how the original conceptualization needs to be revised.

   TIP   Some qualitative researchers call their sample *purposive* simply because they "purposely" selected people who experienced the phenomenon of interest. Exposure to the phenomenon is, however, an eligibility criterion. If the researcher then recruits *any* person with the desired experience, the sample is selected by convenience, not purposively. Purposive sampling implies an intent to choose *particular* exemplars or *types* of people who can best enhance the researcher's understanding of the phenomenon.

Theoretical Sampling

Theoretical sampling is a method used in grounded theory studies. Theoretical sampling involves decisions about where to find data to develop an emerging theory optimally. The basic question in theoretical sampling is: What types of people should the researcher turn to next, to further the development of the emerging conceptualization? Participants are selected for their theoretical relevance in developing emerging categories.

Example of a theoretical sampling •
Slatyer, Williams, and Michael (2015) used theoretical sampling in their grounded theory study of hospital nurses' perspective on caring for patients in severe pain. Early interviews and observations in a renal/hepatology unit provided data on caring for patients who had problems tolerating analgesic medications. The emerging category, labelled "medication ineffectiveness," guided the researchers to observe in an orthopedic ward where older patients continued to experience severe pain for months after hip surgery. This theoretical sampling led the researchers to notice differences in nurses' responses to patients with acute and chronic pain conditions. In turn, this prompted the researchers to sample in the eye/ear/plastic surgery ward where patients were treated for long-term pain.

Sample Size in Qualitative Research

Sample size in qualitative research is usually based on informational needs. **Data saturation** involves sampling until no new information is obtained and redundancy is achieved. The number of participants needed to reach saturation depends on various factors. For example, the broader the scope of the research question, the more participants will likely be needed. Data quality can affect sample size: If participants are insightful and can communicate effectively, saturation can be achieved with a relatively small sample. Also, a larger sample is likely to be needed with maximum variation sampling than with typical case sampling.

Example of saturation •
Van Rompaey et al. (2016) studied the patients' perception of a delirium in a Belgian intensive care unit (ICU). Adult patients in the ICU were interviewed at least 48 hours after the last positive score for delirium. Data collection continued until "data saturation was achieved after interviewing 30 patients" (p. 68).

 TIP Sample size adequacy in a qualitative study is difficult to evaluate because the main criterion is information redundancy, which consumers cannot assess. Some reports explicitly mention that saturation was achieved.

Sampling in the Three Main Qualitative Traditions

There are similarities among the main qualitative traditions with regard to sampling: Samples are small, nonrandom methods are used, and final sampling decisions take place during data collection. However, there are differences as well.

Sampling in Ethnography

Ethnographers often begin with a "big net" approach—they mingle and converse with many members of the culture. However, they usually rely heavily on a smaller number of **key informants**, who are knowledgeable about the culture and serve as the researcher's main link to the "inside." Ethnographers may use an initial framework to identify a pool of potential key informants. For example, an ethnographer might decide to recruit different types of key informants based on their *roles* (e.g., nurses, advocates). Once potential key informants are identified, primary considerations for final selection are their level of knowledge about the culture and their willingness to collaborate with the ethnographer in revealing and interpreting the culture.

Sampling in ethnography typically involves sampling *things* as well as people. For example, ethnographers make decisions about observing *events* and *activities*, about examining *records* and *artefacts*, and about exploring *places* that provide clues about the culture. Key informants often help ethnographers decide what to sample.

Example of an ethnographic sample •
In their ethnographic study, Michel et al. (2015) studied the meanings assigned to health care by nurses and long-lived elders in a health care setting in Brazil. The data collection, which involved observations and interviews, relied on the assistance of 20 key informants: 10 nursing professionals and 10 elders.

Sampling in Phenomenologic Studies

Phenomenologists tend to rely on very small samples of participants—typically 10 or fewer. Two principles guide the selection of a sample for a phenomenologic study: (1) All participants must have experienced the phenomenon, and (2) they must be able to articulate what it is like to have lived that experience. Phenomenologic researchers often want to explore the diversity of individual experiences, and so, they may specifically look for people with demographic or other differences who have shared a common experience.

Example of a sample in a phenomenologic study • • • • • • • • • • • • • • •
Pedersen et al. (2016) studied the meaning of weight changes among women treated for breast cancer. A purposive sample of 12 women being treated for breast cancer at a Danish university hospital was recruited. "Variations were sought regarding age, initial cancer treatment, type of surgery, and change in weight and waist" (p. 18).

Interpretive phenomenologists may, in addition to sampling people, sample artistic or literary sources. Experiential descriptions of a phenomenon may be selected from literature, such as poetry, novels, or autobiographies. These sources can help increase phenomenologists' insights into the phenomena under study.

Sampling in Grounded Theory Studies

Grounded theory research is typically done with samples of about 20 to 30 people using theoretical sampling. The goal in a grounded theory study is to select informants who can best contribute to the evolving theory. Sampling, data collection, data analysis, and theory construction occur at the same time, and so study participants are selected serially and contingently (i.e., contingent on the emerging conceptualization). Sampling might involve the following steps:

1. The researcher begins with a general notion of where and with whom to start. The first few cases may be selected by convenience.
2. Maximum variation sampling might be used next to gain insights into the range and complexity of the phenomenon.
3. The sample is continually adjusted: Emerging conceptualizations inform the theoretical sampling process.
4. Sampling continues until saturation is met.
5. Final sampling may include a search for confirming and disconfirming cases to test, refine, and strengthen the theory.

Box 12.1 Guidelines for Critiquing Qualitative Sampling Plans

1. Was the setting appropriate for addressing the research question, and was it adequately described?
2. What type of sampling strategy was used?
3. Were the eligibility criteria for the study specified? How were participants recruited into the study?
4. Given the information needs of the study—and, if applicable, its qualitative tradition—was the sampling approach effective?
5. Was the sample size adequate and appropriate? Did the researcher indicate that saturation had been achieved? Do the findings suggest a richly textured and comprehensive set of data without any apparent "holes" or thin areas?
6. Were key characteristics of the sample described (e.g., age, gender)? Was a rich description of participants and context provided, allowing for an assessment of the transferability of the findings?

Critiquing Qualitative Sampling Plans

Qualitative sampling plans can be evaluated in terms of their adequacy and appropriateness (Morse, 1991). *Adequacy* refers to the sufficiency and quality of the data. An adequate sample provides data without "thin" spots. When researchers have truly obtained saturation, informational adequacy has been achieved, and the resulting description or theory is rich and complete.

Appropriateness concerns the methods used to select a sample. An appropriate sample results from the selection of participants who can best supply information that meets the study's conceptual requirements. The sampling strategy must offer a full understanding of the phenomenon of interest. A sampling approach that excludes negative cases or that fails to include people with unusual experiences may not fully address the study's information needs.

Another important issue concerns the potential for transferability of the findings. The transferability of study findings depends on the similarity between the study sample and other people to whom the findings might be applied. Thus, in critiquing a report, you should assess whether the researcher provided an adequately *thick description* of the sample and the study context, so that someone interested in transferring the findings could make the correct decision. Further guidance in critiquing qualitative sampling decisions is presented in Box 12.1.

 TIP The issue of transferability within the context of broader models of generalizability is discussed in the supplement to this chapter on the book's website.

DATA COLLECTION IN QUALITATIVE STUDIES

In-depth interviews are the most common method of collecting qualitative data. Observation is used in some qualitative studies as well. Physiologic data are rarely collected in a constructivist inquiry. Table 12.1 compares the types of data and aspects of data collection used by researchers in the three main qualitative traditions. Ethnographers typically collect a wide array of data, with observation and interviews being the primary methods. Ethnographers also gather or examine products of the culture under study, such as documents, records, artefacts, photographs, and so on. Phenomenologists and grounded theory researchers rely primarily on in-depth interviews, although observation also plays a role in grounded theory studies.

TABLE 12.1 Comparison of Data Collection in Three Qualitative Traditions

Issue	Ethnography	Phenomenology	Grounded Theory
Types of data	Primarily observation and interviews, plus artefacts, documents, photographs, social network diagrams	Primarily in-depth interviews, sometimes diaries, other written materials	Primarily individual interviews, sometimes group interviews, observation, diaries, documents
Unit of data collection	Cultural system	Individuals	Individuals
Data collection points	Mainly longitudinal	Mainly cross-sectional	Cross-sectional or longitudinal
Length of time for data collection	Typically long, many months or years	Typically moderate	Typically moderate
Salient field issues	Gaining entrée, determining a role, learning how to participate, encouraging candour, loss of objectivity, premature exit, reflexivity	Bracketing one's views, building rapport, encouraging candour, listening while preparing what to ask next, keeping "on track," handling emotionality	Building rapport, encouraging candour, listening while preparing what to ask next, keeping "on track," handling emotionality

Qualitative Self-Report Techniques

Qualitative researchers do not have a set of questions that must be asked in a specific order and worded in a given way. Instead, they start with general questions and allow respondents to tell their stories or narratives in a naturalistic fashion. Qualitative interviews tend to be conversational. Interviewers encourage respondents to define the important dimensions of a phenomenon and to elaborate on what is relevant to them.

Types of Qualitative Self-Reports

Researchers use completely **unstructured interviews** when they have no preconceived view of the information to be gathered. Researchers begin by asking a *grand tour question* such as "What happened when you first learned that you had AIDS?" Subsequent questions are guided by initial responses. Ethnographic and phenomenologic studies often rely on unstructured interviews.

Semistructured (or *focused*) **interviews** are used when researchers have a list of topics or broad questions that must be covered in an interview. Interviewers use a written **topic guide** to ensure that all question areas are addressed. The interviewer's function is to encourage participants to talk freely about all the topics on the guide.

> **Example of a semistructured interview** •
> Udod et al. (2017) studied nurse managers' perceptions of their role stressors, coping strategies, and health-related outcomes. Semistructured interviews were conducted with 23 nurse managers. Findings suggest that managers experience tremendous role stress and their coping strategies may not be adequate.

Focus group interviews involve groups of about 5 to 10 people whose opinions and experiences are asked simultaneously. The interviewer (or *moderator*) guides the discussion using a topic guide. A group format is efficient and can generate a lot of dialogue, but not everyone is comfortable sharing their views or experiences in front of a group.

Example of focus group interviews •
Neville et al. (2015) explored perceptions of older lesbian, gay, and bisexual people among staff working in residential care homes. A total of 47 care workers from seven residential care facilities participated in seven focus groups. The topic guide included two vignettes highlighting the stories of two hypothetical gay/lesbian older people.

Personal **diaries** are a standard data source in historical research. It is also possible to generate new data for a study by asking participants to maintain a diary over a specified period. Diaries can be useful in providing an intimate description of a person's everyday life. The diaries may be completely unstructured; for example, individuals who had an organ transplantation could be asked to spend 15 minutes a day jotting down their thoughts. Frequently, however, people are asked to make diary entries regarding some specific aspect of their lives.

Example of diaries •
Curtis et al. (2014) explored responses to stress among Irish women with breast cancer. Thirty women with newly diagnosed breast cancer maintained diaries during their participation in a clinical trial. They were asked to write regularly about their experiences and feelings. A facilitator reminded them weekly about the diaries over a 5-week period but gave no further instructions.

Photo elicitation involves an interview guided using photographic images. This procedure, most often used in ethnographies and participatory action research, can help to promote a collaborative discussion. The photographs sometimes are ones that researchers have made of the participants' world, but photo elicitation can also be used with photos in participants' homes. Researchers have also used the technique of asking participants to take photographs themselves and then interpret them, a method sometimes called **photovoice**.

Example of a photovoice study •
Woodgate and Busolo (2017) used photovoice to explore adolescents' perspectives of cancer. Participants were provided with a disposable camera to take pictures of people, places, objects, or events that they feel represent cancer and cancer prevention. Fifty three adolescents provided 557 photos for analysis.

Gathering Qualitative Self-Report Data

Researchers gather narrative self-report data to construct a phenomenon that is consistent with that of participants. This goal requires researchers to overcome communication barriers and to enhance the flow of information. Although qualitative interviews are conversational, the conversations are purposeful ones that require preparation. For example, the wording of questions should reflect the participants' worldview and language. In addition to being good questioners, researchers must be good listeners. Only by attending carefully to what respondents are saying can in-depth interviewers develop useful follow-up questions.

Unstructured interviews are typically long, sometimes lasting an hour or more, and so an important issue is how to record such abundant information. Some researchers take notes during the interview, but this increase the risk of inaccurate recording. Most researchers record the interviews for later transcription. Although some respondents are self-conscious when their conversation is recorded, they typically forget about the presence of recording equipment after a few minutes.

TIP Although qualitative self-report data are often gathered in face-to-face interviews, they can also be collected in writing. Internet "interviews" are increasingly common.

Evaluation of Qualitative Self-Report Methods

In-depth interviews are a flexible approach to gathering data and, in many research contexts, offer distinct advantages. In clinical situations, for example, it is often appropriate to let people talk freely about their problems and concerns, allowing them to take the initiative in directing the flow of conversation. Unstructured self-reports may allow investigators to know what the basic issues or problems are, how sensitive or controversial the topic is, how individuals conceptualize and talk about the problems, and what range of opinions or behaviours exist relevant to the topic. In-depth interviews may also help elucidate the underlying meaning of a relationship, repeatedly observed in more structured research. On the other hand, qualitative methods are very time-consuming and demanding of researchers' skills in gathering, analyzing, and interpreting the resulting data.

Qualitative Observational Methods

Qualitative researchers sometimes collect loosely structured observational data, often as a supplement to self-report data. The aim of qualitative observation is to understand the behaviours and experiences of people in naturalistic settings. Skillful observation permits researchers to see the world as participants see it, to develop a rich understanding of the focal phenomena, and to grasp subtleties of cultural variation.

Unstructured observational data are often gathered through **participant observation**. Participant observers take part in the group under study by observing, asking questions, and recording information within the contexts and structures that are relevant to group members. Participant observation is characterized by prolonged periods of social interaction between researchers and participants. By assuming a participating role, observers often have insights that would have been missed by more passive or concealed observers.

TIP Not all qualitative observational research is *participant* observation (i.e., with observations occurring from *within* the group). Some unstructured observations involve watching and recording behaviours without the observers' active participation in activities. Be on the alert for the misuse of the term "participant observation." Some researchers use the term inappropriately to refer to all unstructured observations conducted in the field.

The Observer–Participant Role in Participant Observation

In participant observation, the role that observers play in the group is important because their social position determines what they are likely to see. The extent of the observers' actual participation in a group is best thought of as a continuum. At one extreme is complete immersion in the setting, with researchers assuming full participant status; at the other extreme is complete separation, with researchers as passive onlookers. Researchers may in some cases assume a fixed position on this continuum throughout the study, but often researchers' roles evolve toward increasing participation over the course of the fieldwork.

Observers must overcome two major hurdles in assuming a satisfactory role as participants. The first is to gain entrée into the social group under study; the second is to establish rapport and trust within that group. Without gaining entrée, the study cannot proceed; but without the trust of the group, the researcher will be restricted to "front stage" knowledge—information hidden and misrepresented by the group's protective pretenses. The goal of participant observers is to "get backstage"—to learn about the true realities of the group's experiences. On the other hand, being a fully participating member does not *necessarily* offer the best perspective for studying a phenomenon, just as being an actor in a play does not offer the most advantageous view of the performance.

Example of participant–observer roles •
Michaelsen (2012) studied nurses' relationships with patients they regarded as being difficult. Data were collected by means of participant observation and in-depth interviews over an 18-month period. Michaelsen conducted 18 observation sessions, lasting between 3 and 4 hours, of the nurses interacting with patients during home visits. She kept "a balance between being an 'insider' and an 'outsider,' between participation and observation" (p. 92).

Gathering Participant Observation Data

Participant observers typically place few restrictions on the nature of the data collected, but they often have a broad plan for types of information wanted. Planning an observed activity should take into consideration many relevant features, including the following:

1. *The physical setting*—"Where" questions. What are the main features of the setting?
2. *The participants*—"Who" questions. Who is present, and what are their characteristics?
3. *Activities*—"What" questions. What is going on? What are participants doing?
4. *Frequency and duration*—"When" questions. When did the activity begin and end? Is the activity a recurring one?
5. *Process*—"How" questions. How is the activity organized? How does it unfold?
6. *Outcomes*—"Why" questions. Why is the activity happening? What did not happen (especially, if it ought to have happened) and why?

Participant observers must decide how to sample events and select observational locations. They often use a combination of positioning approaches—staying in a single location to observe activities in that location (*single positioning*), moving around to observe behaviours from different locations (*multiple positioning*), or following a person around (*mobile positioning*).

Direct observation is usually supplemented with information from interviews. For example, key informants may be asked to describe what went on in a meeting the observer was unable to attend or to describe an event that occurred before the study began. In such cases, the informant functions as the observer's observer.

Recording Observations

The most common forms of record keeping for participant observation are logs and field notes, but photographs and videotapes may also be used. A **log** (or *field diary*) is a daily record of events and conversations. **Field notes** are broader and more interpretive. Field notes represent the observer's efforts to record information and to synthesize and understand the data.

Field notes serve multiple purposes. *Descriptive notes* are objective descriptions of events and conversations that were observed. *Reflective notes* document researchers' personal experiences, reflections, and progress in the field. For example, some notes document the observers' interpretive efforts; others are reminders about how subsequent observations should be made. Observers often record personal notes, including comments about their own feelings during the research process.

The success of participant observation depends on the quality of the logs and field notes. It is essential to record observations as quickly as possible, but participant observers cannot usually record information by openly carrying a clipboard or a recording device because this would compromise their role as ordinary participants. Observers must develop skills in making detailed mental notes that can later be written or recorded.

Evaluation of Unstructured Observational Methods

Qualitative observational methods, and especially participant observation, can provide a deeper understanding of human behaviours and social situations than is possible with structured methods. Participant observation is valuable for its ability to "get inside" a situation and appreciate its complexities. Participant observation is a good method for answering questions about phenomena that are difficult for insiders themselves to explain because these phenomena are taken for granted.

Like all research methods, however, participant observation faces potential problems. Observers may lose objectivity in sampling, viewing, and recording observations. Once they begin to participate in a group's activities, the possibility of emotional involvement becomes a concern. Researchers in their member role may fail to attend to key aspects of the situation or may develop a narrow view on issues of importance to the group. Finally, the success of participant observation depends on the observer's observational and interpersonal skills—skills that may be difficult to learn.

Critiquing Unstructured Data Collection

It is often difficult to critique the decisions that researchers made in collecting qualitative data because details about those decisions are seldom spelled out. In particular, there is often scant information about participant observation. It is common for a report to simply say that the researcher undertook participant observation, without descriptions of how much time

---

Box 12.2 Guidelines for Critiquing Data Collection Methods in Qualitative Studies

1. Given the research question and the characteristics of study participants, did the researcher use the best method of capturing study phenomena (i.e., self-reports, observation)? Should supplementary methods have been used to enrich the data available for analysis?
2. If self-report methods were used, did the researcher make good decisions about the specific method used to solicit information (e.g., unstructured interviews, focus group interviews, and so on)?
3. If a topic guide was used, did the report present examples of specific questions? Were the questions appropriate and comprehensive? Did the wording encourage rich responses?
4. Were interviews recorded and transcribed? If interviews were not recorded, what steps were taken to ensure data accuracy?
5. If observational methods were used, did the report adequately describe what the observations entailed? What did the researcher actually observe, in what types of setting did the observations occur, and how often and over how long a period were observations made?
6. What role did the researcher assume in terms of being an observer and a participant? Was this role appropriate?
7. How were observational data recorded? Did the recording method maximize data quality?

was spent in the field, what exactly was observed, how observations were recorded, and what level of participation was involved. Thus, one aspect of a critique is concentrated on how much information the article provided about the data collection methods. Even though space constraints in journals make it impossible for researchers to fully elaborate their methods, researchers have a responsibility to communicate basic information about their approach, so that readers can assess the quality of evidence. Researchers should provide examples of questions asked and types of observations made.

Triangulation of methods provides important opportunities for qualitative researchers to enhance the integrity of their data. Thus, an important issue to consider in evaluating unstructured data is whether the types and amount of data collected are sufficiently rich to support an in-depth, holistic understanding of the phenomena under study. Box 12.2 provides guidelines for critiquing the collection of unstructured data.

RESEARCH EXAMPLES WITH CRITICAL THINKING EXERCISES

In this section, we describe the sampling plans and data collection strategies used in a qualitative nursing study. Read the summary and then answer the critical thinking questions that follow, referring to the full research report if necessary. Example 1 is featured on the interactive *Critical Thinking Activity* on thePoint website. The critical thinking questions for Example 2 are based on the study that appears in its entirety in Appendix B of this book. Our comments for these exercises are in the Student Resources section on thePoint. ✴

EXAMPLE 1: SAMPLING AND DATA COLLECTION IN A QUALITATIVE STUDY

Study: Canadian adolescents' perspectives of cancer risk: A qualitative study (Woodgate, Safipour, & Tailor, 2015)

Statement of Purpose: The purpose of this study was to understand Canadian adolescents' perspectives of cancer and cancer prevention, including how they conceptualize and understand cancer risk.

Design: The researchers described their approach as ethnographic: "Exploring the shared understanding and perceptions of adolescents toward cancer and cancer risk lent itself to an ethnographic design using multiple data collection methods" (p. 686). Data were collected over a 3-year period.

Sampling Strategy: A purposive sample of 75 adolescents was recruited from four schools in a western Canadian province, with efforts to "maximize variation in demographic (e.g., age, gender, SES, urban/rural residency) and cancer experiences" (p. 686). Recruitment and analysis occurred concurrently, and recruitment ended when saturation was achieved. The study took place over a 3-year period. The sample included both males (27%) and females (73%), ranging in age from 11 to 19 years; 56% lived in an urban area, and about 30% had a family member with a history of cancer. The majority were described as "middle income" (72%) and of European descent (63%).

Data Collection: Data collection took place in the schools the youth attended. Two face-to-face interviews were planned for each adolescent, with the second one scheduled 4 to 5 weeks after the first. The second interview was intended to ensure "thick description" and to provide an opportunity for follow-up questions that helped to clarify issues identified in the initial interview. Each interview, lasting between 60 and 90 minutes, was digitally recorded and transcribed. For the first interview, the topic guide included general questions about cancer risk and prevention (e.g., "How do people get cancer?"). Photovoice methods were also introduced. The participants were given cameras and were asked to take pictures over a 4-week period of what they felt depicted cancer, cancer risks, and cancer prevention over a period of a month. Then, in the second interview, the adolescents were asked to describe what the photos meant to them. They were guided by such questions as "How does this [picture] relate to cancer?" (p. 688). Finally, four focus group interviews were conducted with adolescents who were previously interviewed "to complement existing findings and gather new group-based knowledge on cancer risks" (p. 688). Field notes were maintained to describe verbal and nonverbal behaviours of participants after both individual and focus group interviews.

Key Findings: The adolescents conceptualized cancer risk in terms of specific risk factors; lifestyle factors (e.g., smoking) were prominent. They rationalized risky health behaviours using a variety of cognitive strategies that helped to make cancer risks more acceptable to them. However, they did believe that it was possible for individuals to delay getting cancer by making the right choices.

Critical Thinking Exercises

1. Answer the relevant questions from Boxes 12.1 and 12.2 regarding this study.
2. Also consider the following targeted questions:
   a. Comment on the variation the researcher achieved in type of study participants.
   b. Comment on the researchers' overall data collection plan in terms of the amount of information gathered.
3. If the results of this study are valid and trustworthy, what might be some of the uses to which the findings could be put in clinical practice?

EXAMPLE 2: SAMPLING AND DATA COLLECTION IN THE STUDY IN APPENDIX B

● Read the method section of Beck and Watson's (2010) study ("Subsequent childbirth after a previous traumatic birth") in Appendix B of this book.

Critical Thinking Exercises

1. Answer the relevant questions from Boxes 12.1 and 12.2 regarding this study.
2. Also consider the following targeted questions, which may further sharpen your critical thinking skills and assist you in assessing aspects of the study's merit:
   a. Comment on the characteristics of the participants, given the purpose of the study.
   b. Do you think that Beck and Watson should have limited their sample to women from one country only? Provide a rationale for your answer.
   c. Could any of the variables in this study have been captured by observation? Should they have been?
   d. Did Beck and Watson's study involve a "grand tour" question?

WANT TO KNOW MORE? ✴

A wide variety of resources to enhance your learning and understanding of this chapter are available on thePoint.

- Interactive Critical Thinking Activity
- Chapter Supplement on Transferability and Generalizability
- Answer to the Critical Thinking Exercises for Example 2
- Internet Resources with useful websites for Chapter 12
- A Wolters Kluwer journal article on a topic related to this chapter

Summary Points

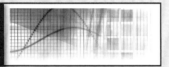

- Qualitative researchers typically select articulate and reflective informants with certain types of experience in an emergent way, capitalizing on early learning to guide subsequent sampling decisions.
- Qualitative researchers may start with convenience or **snowball sampling** but usually rely eventually on **purposive sampling** to guide them in selecting data sources that maximize information richness.
- One purposive strategy is **maximum variation sampling,** which entails purposely selecting diverse cases based on key traits. Another important strategy is *sampling confirming and disconfirming cases*—that is, selecting cases that enrich and challenge the researchers' conceptualizations.
- Samples in qualitative studies are typically small and based on information needs. A guiding principle is **data saturation,** which involves sampling to the point at which no new information is obtained and redundancy is achieved.
- Ethnographers make numerous sampling decisions, including not only *whom* to sample but *what* to sample (e.g., activities, events, documents, artefacts); decision making is often aided by their **key informants,** who serve as guides and interpreters of the culture.

- Phenomenologists typically work with a small sample of people (often 10 or fewer) who meet the criterion of having lived the experience under study.
- Grounded theory researchers typically use **theoretical sampling** in which sampling decisions are guided in an ongoing fashion by the emerging theory. Samples of about 20 to 30 people are typical.
- In-depth interviews are the most widely used method of collecting data for qualitative studies. Self-reports in qualitative studies include completely **unstructured interviews,** which are conversational discussions on the topic of interest; **semistructured** (or *focused*) **interviews,** using a broad **topic guide; focus group interviews,** which involve discussions with small groups; **diaries,** in which respondents are asked to maintain daily records about some aspects of their lives; and **photo elicitation interviews**, which are guided and stimulated by photographic images, sometimes using photos that participants themselves take (**photovoice**).
- In qualitative research, self-reports are often supplemented by direct observation in naturalistic settings. One type of unstructured observation is **participant observation,** in which the researcher gains entrée into a social group and participates to varying degrees in its functioning while making in-depth observations of activities and events. Maintaining **logs** of daily events and **field notes** of the experiences and interpretations are the major data collection methods.

REFERENCES

Beck C. T., & Watson S. (2010). Subsequent childbirth after a previous traumatic birth. *Nursing Research*, 59(4), 241–249.

**Curtis, R., Groarke, A., McSharry, J., & Kerin, M. (2014). Experience of breast cancer: Burden, benefit, or both? *Cancer Nursing*, 37, E21–E30.

Hunter, K. F., Parke, B., Babb, M., Forbes, D., & Strain, L. (2017). Balancing safety and harm for older adults with dementia in rural emergency departments: Healthcare professionals' perspectives. *Rural Remote Health*, 17(1), 4055. Epub 2017 Feb 9.

Michaelsen, J. J. (2012). Emotional distance to so-called difficult patients. *Scandinavian Journal of Caring Sciences*, 26, 90–97.

*Michel, T., Lenardt, M., Willig, M., & Alvarez, A. (2015). From real to ideal—the health (un)care of long-lived elders. *Revista Brasileira de Enfermagem*, 68, 343–349.

Morse, J. M. (1991). Strategies for sampling. In J. M. Morse (Ed.): *Qualitative nursing research: A contemporary dialogue*. Newbury Park, CA: Sage.

*Neville, S., Adams, J., Bellamy, G., Boyd, M., & George, N. (2015). Perceptions towards lesbian, gay and bisexual people in residential care facilities: A qualitative study. *International Journal of Older People Nursing*, 10, 73–81.

Patton, M. Q. (2002). *Qualitative research & evaluation methods* (3rd ed.). Thousand Oaks, CA: Sage.

Pedersen, B., Groenkjaer, M., Falkmer, U., Mark, E., & Delmar, C. (2016). "The ambiguous transforming body"—a phenomenological study of the meaning of weight changes among women treated for breast cancer. *International Journal of Nursing Studies*, 55, 15–25.

Slatyer, S., Williams, A. M., & Michael, R. (2015). Seeking empowerment to comfort patients in severe pain: A grounded theory study of the nurse's perspective. *International Journal of Nursing Studies*, 52, 229–239.

Tobiano, G., Bucknall, T., Marshall, A., Guinane, J., & Chaboyer, W. (2016). Patients' perceptions of participation in nursing care on medical wards. *Scandinavian Journal of Caring Sciences*, 30(2), 260–270.

Udod, S. A., Cummings, G., Care, W. D., & Jenkins, M. (2017). Impact of role stressors on the health of nurse managers: A Western Canadian context. *The Journal of Nursing Administration*, 47(3), 159–164.

Van Rompaey, B., Van Hoof, A., Van Bogaert, P., Timmermans, O., & Dilles, T. (2016). The patient's perception of a delirium: A qualitative research in a Belgian intensive care unit. *Intensive and Critical Care Nursing*, 32, 66–74.

Vat, M., Common, C., Laizner, A. M., Borduas, C., & Maheu, C. (2015). Reasons for returning to the emergency department following discharge from an internal medicine unit: Perspectives of patients and the liaison nurse clinician. *Journal of Clinical Nursing*, 24(23–24), 3605–3614.

Woodgate, R. L., & Busolo, D. S. (2017). Healthy Canadian adolescents' perspectives of cancer using metaphors: a qualitative study. *BMJ Open*, 7(1), e013958. doi: 10.1136/bmjopen-2016-013958.

*Woodgate, R. L., Safipour, J., & Tailor, K. (2015). Canadian adolescents' perspectives of cancer risk: A qualitative study. *Health Promotion International*, 30, 684–694.

*A link to this open-access article is provided in the Internet Resources section on the**Point** website.

This journal article is available on the Point** for this chapter.

13 Mixed Methods and Other Special Types of Research

Learning Objectives

On completing this chapter, you will be able to:

- Identify advantages of mixed methods research and describe specific applications
- Describe strategies and designs for conducting mixed methods research
- Identify the purposes and some of the distinguishing features of specific types of research (e.g., clinical trials, evaluations, outcomes research, surveys)
- Define new terms in the chapter

Key Terms

- Clinical trial
- Concurrent design
- Convergent design
- Delphi survey
- Economic (cost) analysis
- Evaluation research
- Explanatory design
- Exploratory design
- Health services research
- Intervention research
- Intervention theory
- Methodologic study
- Mixed methods research
- Nursing sensitive outcome
- Outcomes research
- Pragmatism
- Process analysis
- Quality improvement (QI)
- Secondary analysis
- Sequential design
- Surveys

In this final chapter on research designs, we explain several special types of research. We begin by discussing mixed methods research that combines quantitative and qualitative approaches.

MIXED METHODS RESEARCH

A growing trend in nursing research is the planned collection and integration of quantitative and qualitative data within a single study or coordinated clusters of studies. This section discusses the rationale for such **mixed methods research** and presents a few applications.

Rationale for Mixed Method Research

The dichotomy between quantitative and qualitative data represents a key methodologic distinction. Some argue that the paradigms associated with quantitative and qualitative research are incompatible. Most people, however, now believe that many areas of inquiry can be enriched by triangulating quantitative and qualitative data. The advantages of a mixed methods (MM) design include the following:

- *Complementarity.* Quantitative and qualitative approaches are complementary. By using MM, researchers can possibly avoid the limitations of a single approach.
- *Practicality.* Given the complexity of phenomena, it is practical to use methodologic tools that are best suited to addressing pressing research questions.
- *Enhanced validity.* When a hypothesis or model is supported by multiple and complementary types of data, researchers can be more confident about their inferences.

Perhaps the strongest argument for MM research, however, is that some questions *require* MM. **Pragmatism**, a paradigm often associated with MM research, confronts the "dictatorship of the research question" (Tashakkori & Teddlie, 2003, p. 21). Pragmatist researchers consider that it is the research question that should drive the design of the inquiry. They reject a forced choice between the traditional postpositivist and constructivist modes of inquiry.

Purposes and Applications of Mixed Methods Research

In MM research, along with an overarching goal, there are inevitably at least two research questions; each requires a different type of approach. For example, MM researchers may simultaneously ask exploratory (qualitative) questions and confirmatory (quantitative) questions. In an MM study, researchers can examine causal *effects* in a quantitative component but can shed light on causal *mechanisms* in a qualitative component.

Creswell and Plano Clark (2011) identified six types of research situations that are especially well suited to MM research:

1. The concepts are new and poorly understood, and there is a need for qualitative exploration before more formal, structured methods can be used.
2. Neither a qualitative nor a quantitative approach, by itself, is adequate in addressing the complexity of the research problem.
3. The findings from one approach can be greatly enhanced with a second source of data.
4. The quantitative results are puzzling and difficult to interpret, and qualitative data can help to explain the results.
5. A particular theoretical perspective might require both quantitative and qualitative data.
6. A multiphase project is needed to attain key objectives, such as the development and assessment of an intervention.

As this list suggests, MM research can be used in various situations. Some of the major applications include the following:

- *Instrument development.* Nurse researchers sometimes gather qualitative data as the basis for developing formal instruments—that is, for generating and wording the questions on quantitative scales that are subsequently subjected to rigorous testing.
- *Intervention development.* Qualitative research is also playing an important role in the development of promising nursing interventions that are then rigorously tested for efficacy.
- *Hypothesis generation.* In-depth qualitative studies provide rich insights about constructs or relationships among them. These insights then can be tested and confirmed with larger samples in quantitative studies.
- *Theory building and testing.* A theory gains acceptance if it endures testing by multiple methods. Theory that survived disconfirmation can provide a stronger context for the organization of clinical and intellectual work.

- *Explication.* Qualitative data are sometimes used to explain the *meaning* of quantitative descriptions or relationships. Quantitative methods can demonstrate that variables are systematically related but may fail to explain *why* they are related.

Example of explicating with qualitative data • • • • • • • • • • • • • • • • • • •
Edinburgh et al. (2015) undertook an MM study of the abuse experiences of 62 sexually exploited runaway adolescents seen at a Child Advocacy Centre. Quantitative data came from physical exams and responses to psychological scales. Qualitative data from forensic interviews were analyzed to explore the experience of sexual exploitation. On a scale to measure posttraumatic stress disorder (PTSD), nearly 80% of the youth had symptoms severe enough to meet *Diagnostic and Statistical Manual of Mental Disorders* (5th ed.; *DSM-IV*) criteria for PTSD. The in-depth interviews revealed how exploited youth were recruited and abused.

Mixed Method Designs and Strategies

In designing MM studies, researchers make many important decisions, which will be briefly described in the following sections.

Design Decisions and Notation

Two decisions in MM design concern sequencing and prioritization. There are three options for sequencing components of an MM study: Qualitative data are collected first, quantitative data are collected first, or both types are collected simultaneously. When the data are collected at the same time, the approach is **concurrent design**. The design is sequential when the two types of data are collected in phases. In well-conceived **sequential designs**, the analysis and interpretation in one phase informs the collection of data in the second.

In terms of prioritization, researchers usually decide which approach—quantitative or qualitative—to emphasize. One option is to give the two components (*strands*) equal attention. Usually, however, one approach is given priority. The distinction is sometimes referred to as *equal status* versus *dominant status*.

Janice Morse (1991), a prominent nurse researcher, made a major contribution to MM research by proposing a widely used notation system for sequencing and prioritization. In this system, priority is designated by uppercase and lowercase letters: QUAL/quan designates an MM study in which the dominant approach is qualitative, whereas QUAN/qual designates the reverse. If neither approach is dominant (i.e., both are equal), the notation is QUAL/QUAN. Sequencing is indicated by the symbols + or →. The arrow designates a sequential approach. For example, QUAN → qual is the notation for a primarily quantitative MM study in which qualitative data are collected in phase 2. When both approaches occur concurrently, a plus sign is used (e.g., QUAL + quan).

Specific Mixed Methods Designs

Numerous design typologies have been proposed by different MM methodologists. We illustrate a few basic designs described by Creswell (2015).

The purpose of the **convergent design** (sometimes called a *triangulation design*) is to obtain different, but complementary, data about the central phenomenon under study—i.e., to triangulate data sources. The goal of this design is to converge on "the truth" about a problem or phenomenon by allowing the limitations of one approach be offset by the strengths of the other. In this design, quantitative and qualitative data are collected simultaneously, with equal priority (QUAL + QUAN).

Example of a convergent design •
Wittenberg-Lyles et al. (2015) used a QUAL + QUAN design in their MM study that assessed the potential benefits of a secret Facebook group for bereaved hospice caregivers. Data were collected concurrently by means of posts and comments in the secret Facebook group and through standardized scales of anxiety and depression.

Explanatory designs are sequential designs with quantitative data collected in the first phase, followed by qualitative data collected in the second phase. Either the quantitative or the qualitative strand can be given a stronger priority: The design can be either QUAN → qual or quan → QUAL. In explanatory designs, qualitative data from the second phase are used to build on or explain the quantitative data from the initial phase. This design is especially suitable when results are complex and difficult to interpret.

Example of an explanatory design •
Kaasalainen in collaboration with the Ontario Nurse-Led Outreach Team (2015) studied the involvement of nurse practitioners (NPs) in activities related to preventing and managing fractures in nursing homes. This study used a sequential explanatory mixed methods design. Twelve NPs completed the online survey, which covered postfracture management, fracture risk assessment, and use of evidence-based guidelines. Following that, 11 NPs participated in a follow-up interview. Participants identified barriers to providing optimal care and improvement strategies such as access to on-site specialists and diagnostic imaging, communication, and education for staff and residents.

Exploratory designs are sequential MM designs, with qualitative data being collected first. The design highlights the need for initial in-depth exploration of a concept. Usually, the first phase focuses on exploration of a poorly understood phenomenon, and the second phase is focused on measuring it or classifying it. In an exploratory design, either the qualitative phase can be dominant (QUAL → quan) or the quantitative phase can be dominant (qual → QUAN).

Example of an exploratory design •
Vahabi and Lofters (2015) explored Muslim immigrant women's knowledge, beliefs, and attitudes about cervical cancer screening, cultural relevance, and acceptability of self-sampling for Pap test in Canada. Participants completed the study questionnaire that captured information, including their health status and health care utilization, cervical cancer screening practices, and attitudes toward HPV self-sampling. The women were then asked to participate in one of three focus groups.

 TIP Creswell and Plano Clark (2011) described a design called the *embedded design*—a term that is sometimes used in nursing studies. However, Creswell (2015) subsequently stopped referencing this design. An embedded design study collects one type of primary data and, at the same time, is supplemented or supported by another type of secondary data. Creswell now views embedding as an analytic strategy rather than as a design type.

Sampling and Data Collection in Mixed Methods Research

Sampling and data collection in MM studies are often a blend of approaches described in earlier chapters. A few special issues for an MM study merit brief discussion.

MM researchers can combine sampling designs in various ways. Sensible sampling strategy for the quantitative component is likely to enhance the generalizability of findings from the sample to a population. For the qualitative component, MM researchers usually adopt purposive sampling methods to select information-rich cases who are good informants about the phenomenon of interest. Sample sizes are also likely to be different in the quantitative and qualitative strands in ways one might expect—i.e., larger samples for the quantitative component. A unique sampling issue in MM studies concerns whether the same people will be in both the quantitative and qualitative strands. The best strategy depends on the study purpose and the research design, but using overlapping samples can be advantageous. Indeed, a particularly popular strategy is a *nested* approach in which a subset of participants from the quantitative strand is used in the qualitative strand.

Example of nested sampling •
Nguyen et al. (2016) explored the medical, service-related, and emotional reasons for emergency room visits of older cancer patients. They undertook a statistical analysis of administrative databases for 792 cancer patients aged 70 years or older. They conducted semistructured interviews with a subsample of 11 patients to better understand the experiences from the patients' perspective.

In terms of data collection, all of the data collection methods discussed previously can be creatively combined and triangulated in an MM study. Thus, possible sources of data include group and individual interviews, psychosocial scales, observations, biophysiologic measures, records, diaries, and so on. MM studies can involve *intramethod mixing* (e.g., structured and unstructured self-reports) and *intermethod mixing* (e.g., biophysiologic measures and unstructured observation). A fundamental issue concerns the methods' complementarity—that is, having the limitations of one method be balanced and offset by the strengths of the other.

 TIP One challenge in doing MM research concerns how best to analyze the quantitative and qualitative data. This may require an effort to merge results from the two strands and to develop interpretations and recommendations based on integrated understandings.

OTHER SPECIAL TYPES OF RESEARCH

The remainder of this chapter briefly describes types of research that vary by study purpose rather than by research design or tradition.

Intervention Research

In Chapter 9, we discussed randomized controlled trials (RCTs) and other experimental and quasi-experimental designs for testing the effects of interventions. In actuality, intervention research is often more complex than a simple experimental–control group comparison of outcomes—indeed, intervention research often relies on MM to develop, refine, test, and understand the intervention.

Different disciplines have developed their own approaches and terminology to discuss studies that involve intervention efforts. *Clinical trials* are associated with medical research, *evaluation research* is linked to the fields of education and public policy, and nurses are developing their own tradition of intervention research. We briefly describe these three approaches.

Clinical Trials

Clinical trials test clinical interventions. Clinical trials undertaken to evaluate an innovative therapy or drug are often designed in a series of phases:

- *Phase I* of the trial is designed to establish safety, tolerance, and dose with a simple design (e.g., one-group pretest–posttest). The focus is on developing the best treatment.
- *Phase II* is a pilot test of treatment effectiveness. Researchers see if the intervention is feasible and acceptable and holds promise. This phase is designed as a small-scale experiment or a quasi-experiment.
- *Phase III* is a full experimental test of the intervention—an RCT with random assignment to treatment conditions. The objective is to develop evidence about the treatment's *efficacy*—that is, whether the intervention is more efficacious than usual care or another alternative. When the term *clinical trial* is used, it often is referring to a phase III trial.
- *Phase IV* of clinical trials involves studies of the *effectiveness* of an intervention in the general population. The emphasis in effectiveness studies is on the external validity of an intervention that has demonstrated efficacy under controlled (but artificial) conditions.

Evaluation Research

Evaluation research focuses on developing useful information about a program or policy—information that decision makers need on whether to adopt, modify, or abandon the program.

Evaluations are undertaken to answer various questions. Questions about program effectiveness rely on experimental or quasi-experimental designs. Many evaluations are MM studies with distinct components.

For example, a **process analysis** is often undertaken to obtain descriptive information about the process to get a program implemented and how it actually functions. A process analysis addresses such questions as the following: What exactly *is* the treatment, and how does it differ from traditional practices? What are the barriers to successful program implementation? How do staff and clients feel about the intervention? Qualitative data play a big role in process analyses.

Evaluations may also include an **economic (or cost) analysis** to assess whether program benefits outweigh its monetary costs. Administrators make decisions about resource allocation for health services, not only on the basis of whether something "works" but also based on economic viability. Cost analyses are often done by researchers to evaluate program efficacy.

> **Example of an economic analysis** ·
> Lacny et al. (2016) compared the cost-effectiveness of a nurse practitioner–family physician model of care with family physician–only care in a Canadian nursing facility. The analysis showed a smaller increase in costs and emergency department transfers/person-month after the nurse practitioner–family physician model of care was implemented.

Nursing Intervention Research

Both clinical trials and evaluations involve *interventions*. However, the term **intervention research** is increasingly being used by nurse researchers to describe an approach distinguished by a distinctive *process* of planning, developing, and testing interventions—especially *complex interventions*. The common approach to design and evaluate interventions has been criticized for being simplistic and atheoretical. The recommended process involves an in-depth understanding of the problem and the target population; careful, collaborative planning with a diverse team; and the development or adoption of a theory to guide the inquiry.

Similar to clinical trials, nursing intervention research that involves the development of a complex intervention involves several phases: (1) basic developmental research, (2) pilot research, (3) efficacy research, and (4) effectiveness research.

Conceptualization, a major focus of the development phase, is supported through collaborative discussions, consultations with experts, critical literature reviews, and in-depth qualitative research to understand the problem. The construct validity of the intervention is enhanced through efforts to develop an **intervention theory** that clearly articulates what must be done to achieve desired outcomes. The intervention design, which emerges from the intervention theory, specifies what the clinical inputs should be. During the developmental phase, key *stakeholders*—people who have an interest in the intervention—are often identified and "brought on board." Stakeholders include potential beneficiaries of the intervention and their families, advocates and community leaders, and health care staff.

The second phase of nursing intervention research is a pilot test of the intervention. The central activities during the pilot test are to secure preliminary evidence of the intervention's benefits, to assess the feasibility of a rigorous test, and to refine the intervention theory and intervention protocols. The feasibility assessment should involve an analysis of factors that affected implementation during the pilot (e.g., recruitment, retention, and adherence problems). Qualitative research may be used to gain insight into how the intervention should be refined.

As in a classic clinical trial, the third phase involves a full experimental test of the intervention; the final phase focuses on effectiveness and utility in real-world clinical settings. This full model of intervention research is, at this point, more of an ideal than an actuality. For example, effectiveness studies in nursing research are rare. A few research teams have begun to implement portions of the model, and efforts are likely to expand.

Example of nursing intervention research • • • • • • • • • • • • • • • • • • •
Bergin et al. (2016) developed and pilot tested a complex nurse-led psychoeducational intervention to address the physical and psychological needs of women receiving radiotherapy for gynecologic cancer. The researchers developed the intervention based on relevant theory and consumer and expert consultations. Two theoretical perspectives informed intervention development: self-determination theory and a peer support theory. The intervention was pilot tested with six patients. The peer volunteers and nurse delivering the intervention maintained reflective diaries regarding feasibility and acceptability. The intervention is being formally tested in an RCT.

Health Services and Outcomes Research

Health services research is the broad interdisciplinary field that studies how organizational structures and processes, health technologies, social factors, and personal behaviours affect access to health care, the cost and quality of health care, and, ultimately, people's health and well-being. **Outcomes research**, a subset of health services research, aims to understand the end results of particular health care practices and to assess the effectiveness of health care services. Outcomes research represents a response to the increasing demand from policy makers and the public to justify care practices in terms of improved patient outcomes and costs.

Many nursing studies evaluate patient outcomes, but efforts to appraise the quality of nursing care—as distinct from care provided by the overall health care system—are less common. A major obstacle is attribution—that is, linking patient outcomes to specific nursing actions, distinct from those of other members of the health care team. It is also often difficult to ascertain a causal connection between outcomes and health care interventions because factors outside the health care system (e.g., patient characteristics) affect outcomes in complex ways.

Donabedian (1987), whose pioneering efforts created a framework for outcomes research, emphasized three factors in appraising quality in health care services: structure, process, and outcomes. The *structure* of care refers to broad organizational and administrative features. Nursing skill mix, the mix of health care professionals with various skills in an organization, is an example of a structural variable that is related to patient outcomes. *Processes* involve aspects of clinical management and decision making. *Outcomes* refer to specific clinical end results of patient care. Much progress has been made in identifying **nursing sensitive outcomes**—patient outcomes that improve if there is greater quantity or quality of nurses' care.

Several modifications to Donabedian's (1987) framework for appraising health care quality have been proposed, the most noteworthy of which is the Canadian National Nursing Quality Report (NNQR[C]) pilot project that was initiated by the Academy of Canadian Executive Nurses in collaboration with the Canadian Nurses Association, Health Canada (Office of Nursing Policy), Canada Health Infoway, and the Canadian Institute for Health Information (VanDeVelde-Coke et al., 2012). The goal of the NNQR(C) is to create a national set of structure, process, and outcome indicators to assist in evaluating the delivery of nursing services.

Outcomes research usually concentrates on studying linkages within such models rather than on testing the overall model. Some studies have examined the effect of health care structures on health care processes or outcomes, for example. Outcomes research in nursing often has focused on the process–patient–outcomes. Examples of nursing process variables include nursing actions; nurses' problem-solving and decision-making skills; clinical competence and leadership; and specific activities or interventions (e.g., communication, touch).

Example of outcomes research •
Rochefort, Rathwell, and Clarke (2016) studied the relationship between rationing of nursing care interventions (limiting or omitting interventions for particular patients) and patient outcomes in relation to parent and infant readiness for discharge and neonatal pain control in Quebec.

Survey Research

A **survey** obtains quantitative information about the prevalence, distribution, and interrelations of variables within a population. Political opinion polls are examples of surveys. Survey data are used primarily in correlational studies and are often used to gather information from nonclinical populations (e.g., college students, nurses).

Surveys obtain information about people's actions, knowledge, intentions, and opinions by self-report. Surveys, which primarily yield quantitative, may be cross-sectional or longitudinal. Any information that can be obtained by direct questioning can also be gathered in a survey, although surveys include mostly closed-ended questions.

Survey data can be collected in a number of ways, but the most reliable method is through personal interviews, in which interviewers meet in person with respondents to ask them questions. Personal interviews are expensive because they involve a lot of personnel time, but they provide high-quality data, and the refusal rate tends to be low. Telephone interviews are less costly, but when the interviewer is unknown, respondents may be uncooperative on the phone. Self-administered questionnaires (especially, those delivered over the Internet) are an economical approach to doing a survey but are not appropriate for surveying certain populations (e.g., the elderly, children) and tend to yield low response rates.

The greatest advantage of surveys is their flexibility and broadness of scope. Surveys can be used with many populations, can focus on a wide range of topics, and can be used for many purposes. The information obtained in most surveys, however, tends to be relatively superficial. Surveys rarely probe deeply into complexities of human behaviour and feelings. Survey research is better suited to extensive rather than intensive analysis.

Example of a survey •
Covell et al. (2017) conducted a survey of internationally educated nurses (IEN) in Canada. The purpose of the study was to explore the relationship between knowledge, professional experience, language proficiency, and IENs' workforce integration. More than 2,000 IEN completed an online survey.

Quality Improvement Studies

One further type of research-like endeavour is **quality improvement (QI)** projects. As discussed in Chapter 2, the purpose of QI is to improve practices and processes within a specific organization—not to generate knowledge that can be generalized beyond the specific context of the study. Nevertheless, there are similarities between QI, health care research, and evidence-based practice (EBP) projects. All three have a lot in common (e.g., the use of systematic methods of collecting and analyzing data to address a problem), but there are also differences.

A comparison chart describing the similarities and differences of the three types of efforts on over 20 dimensions has been prepared by Shirey et al. (2011). One dimension is "expectations for knowledge dissemination." In QI, the major expectation is that results would be disseminated internally—publication in a professional journal is not usually considered necessary. In EBP projects, knowledge dissemination is "increasingly becoming an expectation within facility in which EBP project undertaken and beyond that setting" (Shirey et al., 2011, p. 63). For research, widespread dissemination in accessible publications is the norm and often considered an obligation. A decade ago, publication in a professional journal was considered by many a criterion for classifying something as "research" rather than QI or EBP, but this is no longer the case. Many QI projects are described in professional journals.

The issue of how "generalizable" the knowledge gained from the project is another issue. Shirey and colleagues' (2011) chart states that knowledge from QI is not generalizable—it is specific to the organization where the QI is undertaken. However, some QI projects test improvements that could be effectively implemented in other institutions. Many nursing and health studies are done in local settings using convenience samples that provide little basis for generalization. Thus, one cannot necessarily distinguish QI and research based on whether the patients are from a specific clinical setting.

The field of QI has developed some distinctive methodologies and models for conducting inquiries. A frequently mentioned model is *Plan-Do-Study-Act* (PDSA), which is sometimes referred to as *Plan-Do-Check-Act* (PDCA). The PDSA cycle, part of the Institute for

Healthcare Improvement's Model for Improvement, was designed as a tool for accelerating QI. The steps in the cycle are:

1. Plan: Plan a change and develop a test or observation, including a plan for data collection.
2. Do: Try out the change on a small scale.
3. Study: Review and analyze the data, study the results, and identify what has been learned.
4. Act: Refine the change and take action based on the lessons learned from the test.

> **Example of a quality improvement study** • • • • • • • • • • • • • • • • • •
> Zimnicki (2015) used the PDCA model in a QI project involving the development of a flow chart for caring for patients undergoing planned ostomy surgery and an educational intervention to help staff nurses to perform preoperative stoma site marking and patient teaching.

A Few Other Types of Research

The majority of quantitative studies that nurse researchers have conducted are the types described thus far in this and earlier chapters. However, nurse researchers have pursued a few other specific types of research, as briefly described here. The supplement for this chapter on website provides more details about each type.

- **Secondary analysis**. Secondary analyses involve the use of existing data from a previous or ongoing study to test new hypotheses or answer questions that were not initially planned. Secondary analyses are often based on quantitative data from a large data set (e.g., from national surveys), but secondary analyses of data from qualitative studies have also been undertaken. The study in Appendix A of this book is a secondary analysis.
- **Delphi surveys**. Delphi surveys were developed as a tool for short-term forecasting. The technique involves a panel of experts who are asked to complete several rounds of questionnaires, focusing on their opinions about a topic of interest. Multiple rounds are used to achieve consensus.
- **Methodologic studies**. Nurse researchers have undertaken many methodologic studies, which focus on the development, validation, and assessment of methodologic tools or strategies (e.g., the psychometric testing of a new scale).

CRITIQUING STUDIES DESCRIBED IN THIS CHAPTER

It is difficult to provide guidance on critiquing the types of studies described in this chapter because they are so varied and because many fundamental methodologic issues require a critique of the overall design. Guidelines for critiquing design-related issues were presented in previous chapters.

You should, however, consider whether researchers took appropriate advantage of the possibilities of an MM design. Collecting both quantitative and qualitative data is not always necessary or practical, but in critiquing studies, you can consider whether the study would have been strengthened by triangulating different types of data. In studies in which MM were used, you should carefully consider whether the inclusion of both types of data was justified and whether the researcher really made use of both types of data to enhance knowledge on the research topic. Box 13.1 offers a few specific questions for critiquing the types of studies included in this chapter.

Box 13.1 Guidelines for Critiquing Studies Described in this Chapter

1. Was the study exclusively quantitative or exclusively qualitative? If so, could the study have been strengthened by incorporating both approaches?
2. If the study used an MM design, did the inclusion of both approaches contribute to enhanced validity? In what other ways (if any) did the inclusion of both types of data strengthen the study and further the aims of the research?
3. If the study used an MM approach, what was the design—how were the components sequenced, and which had priority? Was this approach appropriate?
4. If the study was a clinical trial or intervention study, was adequate attention paid to developing an appropriate intervention? Was there a well-conceived intervention theory that guided the endeavour? Was the intervention adequately pilot tested?
5. If the study was a clinical trial, evaluation, or intervention study, was there an effort to understand how the intervention was implemented (i.e., a process-type analysis)? Were the financial costs and benefits assessed? If not, should they have been?
6. If the study was outcomes research, which segments of the structure–process– outcomes model were examined? Would it have been desirable (and feasible) to expand the study to include other aspects? Do the findings suggest possible improvements to structures or processes that would be beneficial to patient outcomes?
7. If the study was a survey, was the most appropriate method used to collect the data (i.e., in-person interviews, telephone interviews, mail or Internet questionnaires)?

RESEARCH EXAMPLES WITH CRITICAL THINKING EXERCISES

The nursing literature abounds with studies of the types described in this chapter. Here we describe an important example. Read the summary and then answer the critical thinking questions that follow, referring to the full research report if necessary. Example 1 is featured on the interactive *Critical Thinking Activity* on thePoint website. The critical thinking questions for Example 2 are based on the study that appears in its entirety in Appendix D of this book. Our comments for this exercise are in the Student Resources section on thePoint.

EXAMPLE 1: MIXED METHODS STUDY WITH A SURVEY

Study: A mixed methods study of secondary traumatic stress in certified nurse-midwives: Shaken belief in the birth process (Beck, LoGiudice, & Gable, 2015).

Statement of Purpose: The purpose of this study was to examine secondary traumatic stress (STS) among certified nurse-midwives (CNMs) exposed to traumatized patients during childbirth. The research questions were: (1) What are the prevalence and severity of STS in CNMs exposed to traumatic birth? (2) Are CNMs' demographic characteristics related to STS? (3) What are the experiences of CNMs who attend at traumatic births? and (4) How do the quantitative and qualitative sets of results develop a more complete picture of STS in CNMs?

Methods: A convergent design (QUAL + QUAN) was used (i.e., independent strands of data were collected in a single phase). CNMs who had attended at least one traumatic birth were invited to participate in a survey. A total of 473 CNMs completed the quantitative portion—a questionnaire that included background questions and the 17-item STS Scale. Data for the qualitative strand, obtained from a nested sample of 246 survey participants, came from responses to the following: "Please describe in as much detail as you can remember your experience of attending one or more traumatic births. Please describe all of your thoughts, feelings, and perceptions until you have no more to write. If attending traumatic births has impacted your midwifery practice, please describe this impact" (p. 17).

Data Analysis and Integration: Statistical methods were used to answer research questions 1 and 2. Question 3 was addressed by means of a content analysis of the qualitative data on the CNMs' actual experiences. Themes were cross-tabulated with information about CNMs' characteristics and reported symptoms. The merged results were then integrated into an overall interpretation.

Key Findings: In this sample, 29% of the CNMs reported high-to-severe STS; 36% screened positive for PTSD due to attending traumatic births. Six themes were identified in the analysis of qualitative data (e.g., protecting my patients: agonizing sense of powerlessness and helplessness; shaken belief in the birth process: impacting midwifery practice). More than half the participants said that their practice had been impacted. Having both quantitative and qualitative data provided a richer, more complete picture of STS in CNMs. The quantitative results revealed the previously unknown high percentage of CNMs experiencing STS. The qualitative results, however, provided an insider's glimpse into what it is like for the CNMs to struggle with STS. For example, one highly rated item on the STS Scale was "I had trouble sleeping." Here is an excerpt from the qualitative data that brought this scale item to life: "The baby must have been dead for 5 days or so as the skin was peeling badly and blistered. Between the slime of the meconium and the skin issues it was hard to grip the head to help deliver the rest of the body. I felt like I was pulling off skin and worried I would pull off the head. For weeks I could not get pictures of that dead baby girl out of my mind. I had difficulty sleeping due to the nightmares" (p. 21).

Critical Thinking Exercises

1. Answer the relevant questions from Box 13.1 regarding this study.
2. Also consider the following targeted questions:
   a. What are the strengths and weaknesses of the sampling design in this study?
   b. What might be an advantage of using a sequential rather than a concurrent design in this study?
3. If the results of this study are valid, what are some of the uses to which the findings might be put in clinical practice?

EXAMPLE 2: MIXED METHODS STUDY IN APPENDIX D

- Read the report of the MM study by Sawyer and colleagues (2010) in Appendix D and then address the following suggested activities.

Critical Thinking Exercises

1. Answer questions 1 to 3 in Box 13.1 regarding this study.
2. Suppose that Sawyer and colleagues had only collected qualitative data. Comment on how this might have affected the results and the overall quality of the evidence. Then suppose they had collected all of their data

in a structured, quantitative manner. How might this have changed the results and affected the quality of the evidence?

3. If the results of this study are valid, what are some of the uses to which the findings might be put in clinical practice?

WANT TO KNOW MORE?

A wide variety of resources to enhance your learning and understanding of this chapter are available on thePoint.

- Interactive Critical Thinking Activity
- Chapter Supplement on Other Specific Types of Research
- Answer to the Critical Thinking Exercise for Example 2
- Internet Resources with useful websites for Chapter 13
- A Wolters Kluwer journal article on a topic related to this chapter

Summary Points

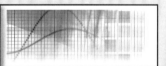

- For many research purposes, mixed method studies are advantageous. **Mixed methods research** involves the collection, analysis, and integration of both quantitative and qualitative data within a study or series of studies, often with an overarching goal of achieving both discovery and verification.

- Mixed methods (MM) research has numerous advantages, including the complementarity of quantitative and qualitative data and the practicality of using methods that best address a question. MM research has many applications, including the development and testing of instruments, theories, and interventions.

- The paradigm most often associated with MM research is **pragmatism**, which has as a major tenet "the dictatorship of the research question."

- Key decisions in designing an MM study involve how to sequence the components

and which strand (if either) will be given priority. In terms of sequencing, MM designs are either **concurrent** (both strands occurring in one simultaneous phase) or sequential (one strand occurring prior to and informing the second strand).

- Notation for MM research often designates priority—all capital letters for the dominant strand and all lowercase letters for the nondominant strand—and sequence. An arrow is used for **sequential designs**, and a "+" is used for concurrent designs. QUAL → quan, for example, is a sequential, qualitative-dominant design.

- Specific MM designs include the **convergent design** (QUAL + QUAN), **explanatory design** (e.g., QUAN → qual), and **exploratory design** (e.g., QUAL → quan).

- Sampling in MM studies can involve the same or different people in the different components. *Nesting* is a common sampling approach in which a subsample of the participants in one strand also participates in the other.

- Different disciplines have developed different approaches to (and terms for) efforts to evaluate interventions. **Clinical trials**, which are studies designed to assess the effectiveness of clinical interventions, often involve a series of phases. *Phase I* is designed to finalize features of the intervention. *Phase II* involves seeking preliminary evidence of efficacy and opportunities for refinements. *Phase III* is a full experimental test of treatment *efficacy*. In *Phase IV*, the researcher focuses primarily on generalized *effectiveness* and evidence about costs and benefits.

● **Evaluation research** assesses the effectiveness of a program, policy, or procedure to assist decision makers in choosing a course of action. Evaluations can answer a variety of questions. **Process analyses** describe the process by which a program gets implemented and how it functions in practice. **Economic (cost) analyses** seek to determine whether the monetary costs of a program are outweighed by benefits.

● **Nursing intervention research** is a term sometimes used to refer to a distinctive *process* of planning, developing, testing, and disseminating interventions. The construct validity of an emerging intervention is enhanced through efforts to develop an **intervention theory** that articulates what must be done to achieve desired outcomes.

● **Outcomes research** (a subset of **health services research**) is undertaken to document the quality and effectiveness of health care and nursing services. A model of health care quality encompasses several broad concepts, including *structure* (e.g., nursing skill mix), *process* (nursing interventions and actions), and *outcomes* (the specific end results of patient care in terms of patient functioning). Efforts have been made to identify **nursing sensitive outcomes**.

● **Survey research** examines people's characteristics, behaviours, intentions, and opinions by asking them to answer questions. Surveys can be administered through personal interviews, telephone interviews, or self-administered questionnaires.

● **Quality improvement (QI)** projects are designed to improve practices in a specific organization; they often use a model called *Plan-Do-Study-Act* (PDSA) or *Plan-Do-Check-Act* (PDCA).

REFERENCES

Beck, C. T., LoGiudice, J., & Gable, R. (2015). A mixed-methods study of secondary traumatic stress in certified nurse-midwives: Shaken belief in the birth process. *Journal of Midwifery & Women's Health, 60*, 16–23.

**Bergin, R., Grogan, S., Bernshaw, D., et al. (2016). Developing an evidence-based, nurse-led psychoeducational intervention with peer support in gynecologic oncology. *Cancer Nursing, 39*, E19–E30.

Covell, C. L., Primeau, M. D., Kilpatrick, K., & St-Pierre, I. (2017). Internationally educated nurses in Canada: Predictors of workforce integration. *Human Resources for Health, 15*(1), 26.

Creswell, J. W. (2015). *A concise introduction to mixed methods research*. Thousand Oaks, CA: Sage.

Creswell, J. W., & Plano Clark, V. L. (2011). *Designing and conducting mixed methods research* (2nd ed.). Thousand Oaks, CA: Sage.

Donabedian, A. (1987). Some basic issues in evaluating the quality of health care. In L. T. Rinke (Ed.). *Outcome measures in home care* (Vol. 1, pp. 3–28). New York: National League for Nursing.

*Edinburgh, L., Pape-Blabolil, J., Harpin, S., & Saewyc, E. (2015). Assessing exploitation experiences of girls and boys seen at a Child Advocacy Center. *Child Abuse & Neglect, 46*, 47–59.

Kaasalainen, S., Papaioannou, A., Burgess, J., & Van der Horst, M. L.. (2015). Exploring the nurse practitioner role in managing fractures in long-term care. *Clinical Nursing Research, 24*(6), 567–588.

Lacny, S., Zarrabi, M., Martin-Misener, R., et al. (2016). Cost-effectiveness of a nurse practitioner-family physician model of care in a nursing home: controlled before and after study. *Journal of Advanced Nursing, 72*(9), 2138–2152.

Morse, J. M. (1991). Approaches to qualitative-quantitative methodological triangulation. *Nursing Research, 40*, 120–123.

Nguyen, B., Tremblay, D., Mathieu, L., & Groleau, D. (2016). Mixed method exploration of the medical, service-related, and emotional reasons for emergency room visits of older cancer patients. *Supportive Care in Cancer, 24*, 2549–2556.

Rochefort, C. M., Rathwell, B. A., & Clarke, S. P. (2016). Rationing of nursing care interventions and its association with nurse-reported outcomes in the neonatal intensive care unit: A cross-sectional survey. *BMC Nursing, 15*, 46.

Shirey, M., Hauck, S., Embree, J., et al. (2011). Showcasing differences between quality improvement, evidence-based practice, and research. *The Journal of Continuing Education in Nursing, 42*, 57–68.

Tashakkori, A., & Teddlie, C. (2003). *Handbook of mixed methods in social & behavioral research* (2nd ed.). Thousand Oaks, CA: Sage.

Vahabi, M & Lofters, A. Muslim immigrant women's views on cervical cancer screening and HPV self-sampling in Ontario, Canada. *BMC Public Health, 16*(1), 868.

VanDeVelde-Coke, S., Doran, D., Grinspun, D., et al. (2012). Measuring outcomes of nursing care, improving the health of Canadians: NNQR (C), C-HOBIC and NQuIRE. *Canadian Journal of Nursing Leadership, 25*(2), 26–37.

Wittenberg-Lyles, E., Washington, K., Oliver, D. P., et al. (2015). "It is the 'starting over' part that is so hard": Using an online group to support hospice bereavement. *Palliative & Supportive Care, 13*, 351–357.

Zimnicki, K. M. (2015). Preoperative teaching and stoma marking in an inpatient population: A quality improvement process using a FOCUS-Plan-Do-Check-Act model. *Journal of Wound, Ostomy, and Continence Nursing, 42,* 165–169.

*A link to this open-access article is provided in the Internet Resources section on thePoint website.

**This journal article is available on thePoint for this chapter.

14 Statistical Analysis of Quantitative Data

Learning Objectives

On completing this chapter, you will be able to:

- Describe the four levels of measurement and identify which level was used for measuring specific variables
- Describe characteristics of frequency distributions and identify and interpret various descriptive statistics
- Describe the logic and purpose of parameter estimation and interpret confidence intervals
- Describe the logic and purpose of hypothesis testing and interpret p values
- Specify appropriate applications for t-tests, analysis of variance, chi-squared tests, and correlation coefficients and interpret the meaning of the calculated statistics
- Understand the results of simple statistical procedures described in a research report
- Identify several types of multivariate statistics and describe situations in which they could be used
- Identify indexes used in assessments of reliability and validity
- Define new terms in the chapter

Key Terms

- Absolute risk (AR)
- Absolute risk reduction (ARR)
- Alpha (α)
- Analysis of covariance (ANCOVA)
- Analysis of variance (ANOVA)
- Central tendency
- Chi-squared test
- Confidence interval (CI)
- Continuous variable
- Correlation
- Correlation coefficient
- Correlation matrix
- Crosstabs table
- d statistic
- Descriptive statistics
- Effect size
- F ratio
- Frequency distribution
- Hypothesis testing
- Inferential statistics
- Interval measurement
- Level of significance
- Logistic regression
- Mean
- Measurement level
- Median
- Mode
- Multiple correlation coefficient

(continued)

- Level of measurement
- Multiple regression
- Multivariate statistics
- N
- Negative relationship
- Nominal measurement
- Non-significant result (NS)
- Normal distribution
- Number needed to treat (NNT)
- Odds ratio (OR)

- Ordinal measurement
- p value
- Parameter
- Parameter estimation
- Pearson's r
- Positive relationship
- Predictor variable
- rR^2
- Range
- Ratio measurement
- Repeated measures ANOVA

- Skewed distribution
- Spearman's rho
- Standard deviation
- Statistic
- Statistical test
- Statistically significant
- Symmetric distribution
- Test statistic
- t-test
- Type I error
- Type II error
- Variability

Statistical analysis is used in quantitative research for three main purposes—to describe the data (e.g., what are the sample characteristics?); to test hypotheses (e.g., are patients more satisfied with care provided by nurse practitioners compared to physicians?); and to provide evidence regarding measurement properties of quantified variables (e.g., does a scale accurately and reliably measure pain in the neonates?) (Chapter 10). This chapter provides a brief overview of statistical procedures for these purposes. We begin, however, by explaining levels of measurement.

 TIP Although the thought of learning about statistics may be anxiety-provoking, consider Florence Nightingale's view of statistics: "To understand God's thoughts we must study statistics, for these are the measure of His purpose."

LEVELS OF MEASUREMENT

Statistical operations depend on a variable's **level of measurement**. There are four major levels of measurement.

Nominal measurement, the lowest level, involves using numbers simply to categorize characteristics or attributes. Gender is an example of a nominally measured variable (e.g., females = 1, males = 2). The numbers used in nominal measurement do not have quantitative meaning and cannot be treated mathematically. It makes no sense to compute a sample's average gender.

Ordinal measurement ranks people on an attribute. For example, consider this ordinal scheme to measure ability to perform activities of daily living (ADL): 1 = completely dependent, 2 = needs another person's assistance, 3 = needs mechanical assistance, and 4 = completely independent. The numbers indicate incremental ability to perform ADL independently, but they do not tell us how much greater one level is than another. As with nominal measures, the mathematic operations with ordinal-level data are restricted.

Interval measurement occurs when researchers can rank people on an attribute *and* specify the difference between them. Most psychological tests are interval-level measures. For example, an IQ test is an interval measure. The difference between a score of 140 and 120 is the same as the difference between 120 and 100. Many statistical procedures require interval data.

Ratio measurement is the highest level. Ratio scales, unlike interval scales, have a true meaningful zero and provide information about the absolute size of the attribute. Many physical measures, such as a person's weight, are ratio measures. It is meaningful to say that someone who weighs 200 pounds is twice as heavy as someone who weighs 100 pounds. Statistical procedures suitable for interval data are also appropriate for ratio-level data. Variables with interval and ratio measurements often are called **continuous variables**.

Example of different measurement levels •
Green and colleagues (2017) examined oncology nurses' attitudes towards and reported use of the Edmonton Symptom Assessment System in Canada. Sex and type of oncology nurse were measured as nominal-level variables. Years of practice in an oncology setting (0 to 5 years, 6 to 10 years, 11 to 15 years, 16 to 19 years, and 20+ years) was an ordinal measurement. Attitudes about symptom management were measured on interval-level scales. Other variables were measured on a ratio level (e.g., age, years of experience).

Researchers usually strive to use the highest levels of measurement possible because higher levels provide more information and allow powerful analyses.

    HOW-TO-TELL TIP   How can you tell a variable's measurement level? A variable is *nominal* if the values could be interchanged (e.g., 1 = male, 2 = female OR 1 = female, 2 = male). A variable is usually *ordinal* if there is a quantitative ordering of values AND if there are a small number of values (e.g., excellent, good, fair, poor). A variable is usually considered *interval* if it is measured with a composite scale or test. A variable is *ratio* level if it makes sense to say that one value is twice as much as another (e.g., 100 mg is twice as much as 50 mg).

DESCRIPTIVE STATISTICS

Statistical analysis enables researchers to make sense of numeric information. **Descriptive statistics** are used to summarize and describe data. When indexes such as averages and percentages are calculated with population data, they are **parameters**. A descriptive index from a sample is a **statistic**. Researchers use statistics to estimate parameters and make interpretations or inferences about the population.

Descriptively, data for a continuous variable can be described in terms of three characteristics: the distribution of values, central tendency, and variability.

Frequency Distributions

Data are organized to communicate useful information. Consider the 60 numbers in Table 14.1. Assume that these numbers are the scores of 60 preoperative patients on an anxiety scale. Visual inspection of these numbers provides little insight into patients' anxiety.

Frequency distributions impose order on numeric data. A **frequency distribution** is an arrangement of values from the lowest to highest, and a count or percentage of how many times each value occurred. A frequency distribution for the 60 anxiety scores (Table 14.2)

TABLE 14.1 Patients' Anxiety Scores

22	27	25	19	24	25	23	29	24	20	26	16	20	26	17
22	24	18	26	28	15	24	23	22	21	24	20	25	18	27
24	23	16	25	30	29	27	21	23	24	26	18	30	21	17
25	22	24	29	28	20	25	26	24	23	19	27	28	25	26

TABLE 14.2 Frequency Distribution of Patients' Anxiety Scores

Score	Frequency	Percentage (%)
15	1	1.7
16	2	3.3
17	2	3.3
18	3	5.0
19	2	3.3
20	4	6.7
21	3	5.0
22	4	6.7
23	5	8.3
24	9	15.0
25	7	11.7
26	6	10.0
27	4	6.7
28	3	5.0
29	3	5.0
30	2	3.3
N = 60		100.0%

makes it easy to see the highest and lowest scores, where scores clustered, and how many patients were in the sample (total sample size is designated as *N* in research reports).

Frequency data can be displayed graphically in a *frequency polygon* (Fig. 14.1). In such graphs, scores typically are on the horizontal line, and counts or percentages are on the vertical line. Distributions can be described by their shapes. **Symmetric distribution** occurs when the graph is cut in the middle and the two halves are mirror images of each other (Fig. 14.2). In an *asymmetric* or **skewed distribution**, the peak is off centre, and one

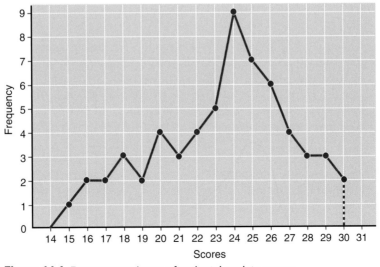

Figure 14.1 Frequency polygon of patients' anxiety scores.

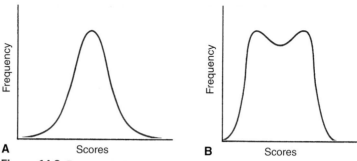

Figure 14.2 Examples of symmetric distributions.

tail is longer than the other. When the longer tail points to the right, the distribution has a *positive skew*, as in Figure 14.3A. Personal income is positively skewed: Most people have moderate incomes, with only a few people with high incomes at the distribution's right end. If the longer tail points to the left, the distribution has a *negative skew* (Fig. 14.3B). Age at death is negatively skewed: Most people are at the far right end of the distribution, with fewer people dying young.

Another aspect of a distribution's shape concerns how many peaks it has. A *unimodal distribution* has one peak (Fig. 14.2A), whereas a *multimodal distribution* has two or more peaks—two or more values of high frequency. A distribution with two peaks is *bimodal* (Fig. 14.2B).

A special distribution called the **normal distribution** (*a bell-shaped curve*) is symmetric, unimodal, and not very peaked (Fig. 14.2A). Many human attributes (e.g., height, intelligence) follow a normal distribution.

Central Tendency

Frequency distributions clarify patterns, but an overall summary often is desired. Researchers ask questions such as "What is the *average* daily calorie consumption of nursing home residents?" Such a question seeks a single number to summarize a distribution of calories. Indexes of **central tendency** indicate what is "typical." There are three indexes of central tendency: the mode, the median, and the mean.

- **Mode**: The mode is the number that occurs most frequently in a distribution. In the following distribution, the mode is 53:

$$50\ 51\ 51\ 52\ 53\ 53\ 53\ 53\ 54\ 55\ 56$$

The value of 53 occurred four times, more than any other number. The mode of the patients' anxiety scores in Table 14.2 was 24. The mode identifies the most "popular" value.

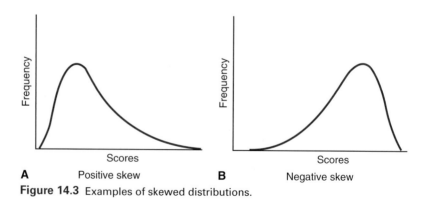

Figure 14.3 Examples of skewed distributions.

- **Median**: The median is the point in a distribution that divides scores in half. Consider the following set of values:

  2 2 3 3 4 5 6 7 8 9

The value that divides the cases in half is midway between 4 and 5; thus, 4.5 is the median. The median anxiety score is 24, the same as the mode. The median does not take into account individual values and is insensitive to extremes. In the given set of numbers, if the value of 9 were changed to 99, the median would remain 4.5.

- **Mean**: The mean equals the sum of all values divided by the number of participants—what we usually call the average. The mean of the patients' anxiety scores is 23.4 (1,405 ÷ 60). As another example, here are the weights of eight people:

  45 54 68 72 76 81 92 97

In this example, the mean is 73. Unlike the median, the mean is affected by the value of every score. If we exchanged the 97 kg person for one weighing 130 kg, the mean would increase from 73 to 77 kg. In research articles, the mean is often symbolized as M or $\bar{X}$ (e.g., $\bar{X} = 77$).

For continuous variables, the mean is usually reported. Of the three indexes, the mean is most stable: If repeated in a study with different samples that were drawn from the same population, the means would fluctuate less than the modes or medians. Because of its stability, the mean usually is the best estimate of a population central tendency. When a distribution is skewed, however, the median is preferred. For example, the median is a better central tendency index for income than the mean because income is positively skewed.

Variability

Two distributions with identical means could differ with respect to how spread out the data are—how different study participants are from one another on the attribute. This section describes the **variability** of distributions.

Consider the two distributions in Figure 14.4, which represent hypothetical scores for students from two schools on an IQ test. Both distributions have a mean of 100, but school A has a wider range of scores, with some below 70 and some above 130. In school B, there are few low or high scores. School A is more *heterogeneous* (i.e., more varied) than school B, and school B is more *homogeneous* than school A. Researchers compute an index of variability to show how much scores in a distribution differ from one another. Two common indexes are the range and standard deviation.

- **Range**: The range is the highest minus the lowest score in a distribution. In our anxiety score example, the range is 15 (30 − 15). In the distributions in Figure 14.4, the range for

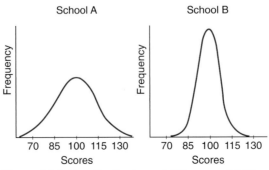

Figure 14.4 Two distributions of different variability.

school A is about 80 (140 − 60), whereas the range for school B is about 50 (125 − 75). The chief virtue of the range is ease of computation. Because it is based on only two scores, however, the range is unstable: from sample to sample drawn from a population, the range can fluctuate greatly.

● **Standard deviation**: The most widely used variability index is the standard deviation. Like the mean, the standard deviation is calculated based on every value in a distribution. The standard deviation summarizes the *average* amount of deviation of values from the mean.* In the anxiety scale example, the standard deviation is 3.725. In research reports, the standard deviation is often abbreviated as *SD*.

TIP *SD*s sometimes are shown in relation to the mean without a label. For example, the anxiety scores might be shown as *M* = 23.4 (3.7) or *M* = 23.4 ± 3.7, where 23.4 is the mean and 3.7 is the *SD*.

An *SD* is more difficult to interpret than the range. For the *SD* of anxiety scores, you might ask, 3.725 of *what*? What does the number mean? We can answer these questions from several angles. First, the *SD* is an index of how variable scores in a distribution are, and so if (for example) male and female patients had means of 23.0 on the anxiety scale, but their *SD*s were 7.0 and 3.0, respectively, it means that females were more homogeneous (i.e., their scores were more similar to one another).

The *SD* represents the *average* of deviations from the mean. The mean tells us the best value for summarizing an entire distribution, and an *SD* tells us how much, on average, the scores deviate from the mean. An *SD* can be interpreted as our degree of error when we use a mean to describe an entire sample.*

In normal and near-normal distributions, there are roughly three *SD*s above and below the mean. For a normal distribution with a mean of 50 and an *SD* of 10 (Fig. 14.5), a fixed percentage of cases fall within certain distances from the mean. Sixty-eight per cent of all cases fall within 1 *SD* above and below the mean. Thus, nearly 7 of 10 scores are between

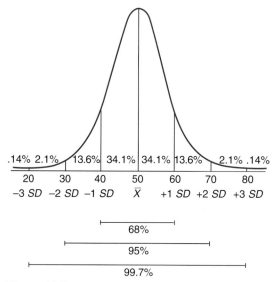

Figure 14.5 Standard deviations in a normal distribution.

---

*Formulas for computing the *SD* and other statistics discussed in this chapter are not shown in this textbook. The emphasis here is on helping you to understand statistical applications. Polit (2010) can be consulted for computation.

40 and 60. In a normal distribution, 95% of the scores fall within 2 *SD*s of the mean. Only a handful of cases—about 2% at each extreme—lie more than 2 *SD*s from the mean. Using this figure, we can see that a person with a score of 70 achieved a higher score than about 98% of the sample.

 TIP   Descriptive statistics (percentages, means, *SD*s) are most often used to describe sample characteristics and key research variables and to document methodologic features (e.g., response rates). They are seldom used to answer research questions—inferential statistics usually are used for this purpose.

Example of descriptive statistics •
Wilson and colleagues (2016) tested the effect of a nurse-led preoperative educational intervention on postsurgical pain-related interference in activities, pain, and nausea. They presented descriptive statistics about participants' characteristics. The mean age of the 73 participants in the intervention group was 67 years (*SD* = 8); 63% were female, 18% lived alone, and 53% had received postsecondary education. The mean rating of worst pain in the last 24 hours was 7 (*SD* = 2.4).

Bivariate Descriptive Statistics

So far, our discussion has focused on *univariate* (one-variable) *descriptive statistics*. *Bivariate* (two-variable) *descriptive statistics* describe relationships between two variables.

Cross-tabulations

A **crosstabs table** is a two-dimensional frequency distribution in which the frequencies of two variables are *cross-tabulated*. Suppose we had data on patients' sex and whether they were non-smokers, light smokers (<1 pack of cigarettes a day), or heavy smokers (≥1 pack a day). The question is whether men smoke more heavily than women, or vice versa (i.e., whether there is a *relationship* between smoking and sex). Fictitious data for this example are shown in Table 14.3. Six *cells* are created by placing one variable (sex) along one dimension and the other variable (smoking status) along the other dimension. Percentages are computed after subjects' data are allocated to the appropriate cells. The crosstab shows that women in this sample were more likely than men to be non-smokers (45.4% vs. 27.3%) and less likely to be heavy smokers (18.2% vs. 36.4%). Crosstabs are used with nominal data or ordinal data with few values. In this example, sex is nominal, and smoking, as operationalized, is ordinal (light or heavy).

TABLE 14.3 Crosstabs Table for Relationship Between Sex and Smoking Status

| | Sex | | | | | |
| | Women | | Men | | Total | |
Smoking Status	*n*	%	*n*	%	*n*	%
Non-smoker	10	45.4	6	27.3	16	36.4
Light smoker	8	36.4	8	36.4	16	36.4
Heavy smoker	4	18.2	8	36.4	12	27.3
TOTAL	22	100.0	22	100.0	44	100.0

Correlation

Relationships between two variables can be described by **correlation** methods. The correlation question is, To what extent are two variables related to each other? For example, to what degree are anxiety scores and blood pressure values related? This question can be answered by calculating a **correlation coefficient**, which describes *intensity* and *direction* of a relationship.

Two variables that are related are height and weight: Tall people tend to weigh more than short people. The relationship between height and weight would be a *perfect relationship* if the tallest person in a population was the heaviest, the second tallest person was the second heaviest, and so on. A correlation coefficient indicates the strength of a relationship. Possible values for a correlation coefficient range from −1.00 through 0.00 to +1.00. If height and weight were perfectly correlated, the correlation coefficient would be 1.00 (the actual correlation coefficient is approximately 0.50 to 0.60 for a general population). Height and weight have a **positive relationship** because greater height tends to be associated with greater weight.

When two variables are unrelated, the correlation coefficient is zero. One might anticipate that women's shoe size is unrelated to their intelligence. Women with large feet are as likely to perform well on IQ tests as those with small feet. The correlation coefficient summarizing such a relationship would be close to 0.00.

Correlation coefficients between 0.00 and −1.00 express a **negative (*inverse*) relationship**. When two variables are inversely related, higher values on one variable are associated with lower values in the second. For example, there is a negative correlation between depression and self-esteem. This means that, on average, people with *high* self-esteem tend to be *low* on depression. If the relationship were perfect (i.e., if the person with the highest self-esteem score had the lowest depression score and so on), then the correlation coefficient would be −1.00. In actuality, the relationship between depression and self-esteem is moderate—close to −.30 or −.40. Note that the higher the *absolute value* of the coefficient (i.e., the value disregarding the sign), the stronger the relationship. A correlation of −.50, for instance, is stronger than a correlation of +.30.

The most widely used correlation statistic is **Pearson's *r*** (the *product–moment correlation coefficient*), which is computed with continuous measures. For correlations between variables measured on an ordinal scale, researchers usually use an index called **Spearman's rho**. There are no guidelines on what should be interpreted as strong or weak correlations because it depends on the variables. If we measured patients' body temperature orally and rectally, an *r* of 0.70 between the two measurements would be low. For most psychosocial variables (e.g., stress and depression), however, an *r* of 0.70 would be high.

Correlation coefficients are often reported in tables displaying a two-dimensional **correlation matrix**, in which every variable is displayed in both a row and a column, and coefficients are displayed at the intersections. An example of a correlation matrix is presented at the end of this chapter.

> **Example of correlations** •
> Hall et al. (2017) investigated the relationships between parental sleep quality, fatigue, expectations and attitudes about infant sleep, and parental depression. They found the modest positive correlations between depression scores and parental fatigue ($r = 0.58$), sleep quality ($r = 0.46$), difficulties with sleep and feeding ($r = 0.23$), anger about infant sleep ($r = 0.34$), and difficulties setting sleep limits for infants ($r = 0.23$).

Describing Risk

The evidence-based practice (EBP) movement has made decision making based on research findings an important issue. Several descriptive indexes can be used to facilitate such decision

TABLE 14.4   Indexes of Risk and Association in a 2 × 2 Table

Exposure	Outcome		Total
	Undesirable Outcome	Desirable Outcome	
Yes, exposed (E) to intervention—experimentals (or, NOT exposed to a risk factor)	a	b	$a + b$
No, not exposed (NE) to intervention—controls (or, exposed to a risk factor)	c	d	$c + d$
TOTAL	$a + c$	$b + d$	$a + b + c + d$

Absolute risk, exposed group (AR_E) $= a / (a + b)$
Absolute risk, non-exposed group (AR_{NE}) $= c / (c + d)$
Absolute risk reduction (ARR) $= AR_{NE} - AR_E$

Odds ratio (OR) $= \dfrac{ad}{bc}$ OR $\dfrac{a / b}{c / d}$

Number needed to treat (NNT) $= \dfrac{1}{ARR}$

making. Many of these indexes involve calculating risk differences—for example, differences in risk before and after exposure to a beneficial intervention.

We focus on describing dichotomous outcomes (e.g., had a fall/did not have a fall) in relation to exposure or non-exposure to a beneficial treatment or protective factor. This situation results in a 2 × 2 crosstabs table with four cells. The four cells in the crosstabs table in Table 14.4 are labelled, so various indexes can be explained. *Cell a* is the number of cases with an undesirable outcome (e.g., a fall) in an intervention/protected group; *cell b* is the number with a desirable outcome (e.g., no fall) in an intervention/protected group; and *cells c* and *d* are the two outcome possibilities for a non-treated/unprotected group. We can now explain the meaning and calculation of some indexes of interest to clinicians.

Absolute Risk

Absolute risk can be computed for those exposed to an intervention/protective factor, and for those not exposed. **Absolute risk (AR)** is simply the proportion of people who experienced an undesirable outcome in each group. Suppose 200 smokers were randomly assigned to a smoking cessation intervention or to a control group (Table 14.5). The outcome is smoking status 3 months later. Here, the AR of continued smoking is 0.50 in the intervention group

TABLE 14.5   Hypothetical Data for Smoking Cessation Intervention Example, Risk Indexes

Exposure to Smoking Cessation Intervention	Outcome		Total
	Continued Smoking	Stopped Smoking	
Yes, exposed: E (Experimental group)	50 (a)	50 (b)	100
No, not exposed: NE (Control group)	80 (c)	20 (d)	100
TOTAL	130	70	200

Absolute risk $= 50/100$ $= 0.50$
Absolute risk, non-exposed group (AR_{NE}) $= 80/100$ $= 0.80$
Absolute risk reduction (ARR) $= 0.80 - 0.50 = 0.30$

Odds ratio (OR) $= \dfrac{(50/50)}{(80/20)}$ $= 0.25$

Number needed to treat (NNT) $= 1/0.30$ $= 3.33$

and 0.80 in the control group. Without the intervention, 20% of those in the experimental group would presumably have stopped smoking anyway, but the intervention boosted the rate to 50%.

Absolute Risk Reduction

The **absolute risk reduction (ARR)** index, a comparison of the two risks, is computed by subtracting the AR for the exposed group from the AR for the unexposed group. This index is the estimated proportion of people who would be spared the undesirable outcome through exposure to an intervention/protective factor. In our example, the value of ARR is 0.30: 30% of the control group subjects would presumably have stopped smoking if they had received the intervention, over and above the 20% who stopped without it.

Odds Ratio

The odds ratio is a widely reported risk index. The *odds*, in this context, are the proportion of people *with* the adverse outcome relative to those *without* it. In our example, the odds of continued smoking for the intervention group are 1.0:50 (those who continued smoking) divided by 50 (those who stopped). The odds for the control group are 80 divided by 20, or 4.0. The **odds ratio (OR)** is the ratio of these two odds—here, 0.25. The estimated odds of continuing to smoke are one-fourth as high among intervention group members as for control group members. Turned around, the estimated odds of continued smoking are four times higher among smokers who do not get the intervention as among those who do.

> **Example of odds ratios** ·
> Conway and colleagues (2016) examined risk factors for bacteremia associated with catheter-associated bacteriuria in acute care hospitals. Independent predictors of bacteremia were male sex (odds ratio, 2.76), treatment with immunosuppressants (odds ratio, 1.68), urinary tract procedure (odds ratio, 2.70), and catheter that remained in place after bacteriuria developed (odds ratio, 2.75). Patients with enterococcal bacteriuria were half as likely to become bacteremic as were patients with other pathogens in the urine (odds ratio, 0.46).

Number Needed to Treat

The **number needed to treat (NNT)** index estimates how many people would need to receive an intervention to prevent one undesirable outcome. NNT is computed by dividing 1 by the ARR. In our example, ARR = 0.30, and so NNT is 3.33. About three smokers would need to be exposed to the intervention to avoid one person's continued smoking. The NNT is valuable because it can be integrated with monetary information to show if an intervention is likely to be cost-effective.

 TIP   Another risk index is known as *relative risk* (RR). The RR is the estimated proportion of the original risk of an adverse outcome (in our example, continued smoking) that persists when people are exposed to the intervention. In our example, RR is 0.625 (0.50/0.80): The risk of continued smoking is estimated as 62.5% of what it would have been without the intervention.

INTRODUCTION TO INFERENTIAL STATISTICS

Descriptive statistics are useful for summarizing data, but researchers usually do more than describe. **Inferential statistics**, based on the *laws of probability*, provide a means for drawing inferences about a population, given data from a sample. Inferential statistics are used to test research hypotheses.

Sampling Distributions

Inferential statistics are based on the assumption of random sampling of cases from populations. Even with random sampling, however, sample characteristics are seldom identical to those of the population. Suppose we had a population of 100,000 nursing home residents whose mean score on a physical function (PF) test was 500 with an *SD* of 100. We do not know these parameters—assume we must estimate them based on scores from a random sample of 100 residents. It is unlikely that we would obtain a mean of exactly 500. Our sample mean might be, say, 505. If we drew a new random sample of 100 residents, the mean PF score might be 497. Sample statistics fluctuate and are unequal to the parameter because of *sampling error*. Researchers need a way to assess whether sample statistics are good estimates of population parameters.

To understand the logic of inferential statistics, we must perform a mental exercise. Consider drawing 5,000 consecutive samples of 100 residents per sample from the population of all residents. If we calculated a mean PF score each time, we could plot the distribution of these sample means, as shown in Figure 14.6. This distribution is a *sampling distribution of the mean*. A sampling distribution is theoretical: No one *actually* draws consecutive samples from a population and plots their means. Statisticians have shown that sampling distributions of means are normally distributed, and their mean equals the population mean. In our example, the mean of the sampling distribution is 500, the same as the population mean.

For a normally distributed sampling distribution of means, the probability is 95 out of 100 that a sample mean lies between +2 *SD* and −2 *SD* of the population mean. The *SD* of the sampling distribution—called the *standard error of the mean* (or SEM)—can be estimated

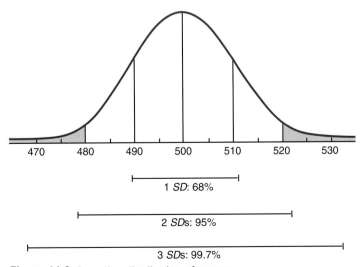

Figure 14.6 Sampling distribution of a mean.

using a formula that uses two pieces of information: the *SD* for the sample and sample size. In our example, the SEM is 10 (Fig. 14.6), which is the estimate of sampling error from one sample mean to another in an infinite number of samples of 100 residents.

We can now estimate the probability of drawing a sample with a certain mean. With a sample size of 100 and a population mean of 500, the chances are 95 out of 100 that a sample mean would fall between 480 and 520—2 *SD*s above and below the mean. Only 5 times out of 100 would the mean of a random sample of 100 residents be greater than 520 or less than 480.

The SEM is partly a function of sample size, so an increased sample size improves the accuracy of the estimate. If we used a sample of 400 residents to estimate the population mean, the SEM would be only 5. The probability would be 95 in 100 that a sample mean would be between 490 and 510. The chance of drawing a sample with a mean very different from that of the population is reduced as sample size increases.

You may wonder why you need to learn about these abstract statistical notions. Consider, though, that we are talking about the accuracy of researchers' results. As an intelligent consumer, you need to evaluate critically how believable research evidence is so that you can decide whether to incorporate it into your nursing practice.

Parameter Estimation

Statistical inference consists of two techniques: parameter estimation and hypothesis testing. **Parameter estimation** is used to estimate a population parameter—for example, a mean, a proportion, or a difference in means between two groups (e.g., smokers vs. non-smokers). *Point estimation* involves calculating a single statistic to estimate the parameter. In our example, if the mean PF score for a sample of 100 nursing home residents was 510, this would be the point estimate of the population mean.

Point estimates do not tell us about the estimate's margin of error. *Interval estimation* of a parameter provides a range of values that suggest a specified probability of finding the parameter. With interval estimation, researchers construct a **confidence interval (CI)** around the point estimate. The CI around a sample mean establishes a range of values for the population value and the probability of being right. By convention, researchers use either a 95% or a 99% CI.

 TIP CIs address a key EBP question for appraising evidence, as presented in Box 2.1: How *precise* is the estimate of effects?

As noted previously, 95% of the scores in a normal distribution lie within about 2 *SD*s (more precisely, 1.96 *SD*s) from the mean. In our example, if the point estimate for mean scores is 510 with an *SD* = 100, the SEM for a sample of 100 would be 10. We can build a 95% CI using this formula: 95% CI = $(\bar{X} \pm 1.96 \times \text{SEM})$. The confidence is 95% that the population mean lies between the values equal to 1.96 times the SEM, above and below the sample mean. In our example, with an SEM of 10, the 95% CI around the sample mean of 510 is between 490.4 and 529.6.

CIs reflect how much risk researchers are willing to take of being wrong. With a 95% CI, researchers risk being wrong 5 times out of 100. A 99% CI sets the risk at only 1% by allowing a wider range of possible values. In our example, the 99% CI around 510 is 484.2 to 535.8. With a lower risk of being wrong, precision is reduced. For a 95% interval, the CI range is about 39 points; for a 99% interval, the range about 52 points. The acceptable risk of error depends on the nature of the problem, but for most studies, a 95% CI is sufficient.

Example of confidence intervals around odds ratio • • • • • • • • • • • • • • •
Mann and colleagues (2017) compared pain self-efficacy between high users of health care (30 or more clinic visits or one or more emergency room visits) and low users.
     The high users were almost three times more likely than the low users to report low pain self-efficacy (OR ti 2.60, 95% CI [1.50–4.51]).

Hypothesis Testing

With statistical **hypothesis testing**, researchers use objective criteria to decide whether hypotheses should be accepted or rejected. Suppose we hypothesized that maternity patients who received online interactive breastfeeding support would breastfeed longer than mothers who did not. The mean number of days of breastfeeding is 131.5 for 25 intervention group mothers and 125.1 for 25 control group mothers. Should we conclude that our hypothesis has been supported? Group differences are in the predicted direction, but in another sample, the group means might be more similar. Two explanations for the observed outcome are possible: (1) The intervention was effective in encouraging breastfeeding or (2) the mean difference in this sample was due to chance (sampling error).

     The first explanation is the *research hypothesis*, and the second is the *null hypothesis*, which is that there is no relationship between the independent variable (the intervention) and the dependent variable (breastfeeding duration). Statistical hypothesis testing is a process of disproof. It cannot be demonstrated directly that the research hypothesis is correct. But it is possible to show that the null hypothesis has a high probability of being incorrect, and such evidence lends support to the research hypothesis. Hypothesis testing helps researchers to make objective decisions about whether results are likely to reflect chance differences or hypothesized effects. Researchers use **statistical tests** in the hopes of rejecting the null hypothesis.

     Null hypotheses are accepted or rejected based on sample data, but hypotheses are about population values. The interest in testing hypotheses, as in all statistical inference, is to use a sample to make inferences about a population.

Type I and Type II Errors

Researchers decide whether to accept or reject the null hypothesis by estimating how probable it is that observed group differences are due to chance. Without population data, it cannot be confirmed that the null hypothesis is or is not true. Researchers must be content to say that hypotheses are either *probably* true or *probably* false.

     Researchers can make two types of error: rejecting a true null hypothesis or accepting a false null hypothesis. Figure 14.7 summarizes possible outcomes of researchers' decisions. Researchers make a **Type I error** by rejecting a null hypothesis that is, in fact, true. For instance, if we decided that online support effectively promoted breastfeeding when, in fact, group differences were merely due to sampling error, we would be making a Type I error—a false-positive conclusion. If we decided that differences in breastfeeding were due to chance or sampling fluctuations when the intervention actually *did* have an effect, we would be making a **Type II error**—a false-negative conclusion.

Level of Significance

Researchers do not know when they have made an error in statistical decision making. However, they control the risk for a Type I error by selecting a **level of significance**, which is the probability of making a Type I error. The two most frequently used levels of significance (referred to as **alpha or α**) are 0.05 and 0.01. With a 0.05 significance level, we accept the

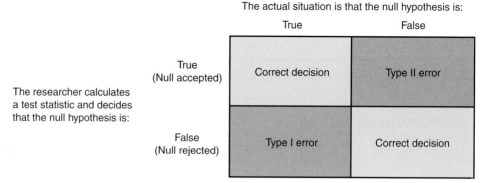

Figure 14.7 Outcomes of statistical decision making.

risk that out of 100 samples from a population, a true null hypothesis would be wrongly rejected five times. In 95 out of 100 cases, however, a true null hypothesis would be correctly accepted. With a 0.01 significance level, the risk of a Type I error is lower: In only 1 sample out of 100 would we wrongly reject the null. By convention, the minimal acceptable alpha level is 0.05.

 TIP   Levels of significance are analogous to the CI values described earlier—an alpha of 0.05 is analogous to the 95% CI, and an alpha of 0.01 is analogous to the 99% CI.

Researchers would like to reduce the risk of committing both types of error, but unfortunately, lowering the risk of a Type I error increases the risk of a Type II error. Researchers can reduce the risk of a Type II error, however, by increasing the sample size. The probability of committing a Type II error can be estimated through *power analysis*, the procedure we mentioned in Chapter 10 with regard to sample size. *Power* is the ability of a statistical test to detect true relationships. Researchers ideally use a sample size that gives them a minimum power of 0.80 and thus a risk for a Type II error of no more than 0.20.

 TIP   If a report indicates that a research hypothesis was not supported by the data, consider whether a Type II error might have occurred as a result of an inadequate sample size.

Tests of Statistical Significance

In hypothesis testing, researchers use study data to compute a **test statistic**. For every test statistic, there is a theoretical sampling distribution, similar to the sampling distribution of means. Hypothesis testing uses theoretical distributions to establish *probable* and *improbable* values for the test statistics, which are used to accept or reject the null hypothesis.

An example can illustrate this process. In our previous example of a physical functioning test for nursing home residents, suppose that there are population *norms*, which are values derived from large, representative samples. According to the norms, the mean PF score for nursing home residents is 500, which we take as the population mean. We recruit 100 nursing home residents to participate in an intervention to improve physical functioning. The null hypothesis is that those receiving the intervention have scores that are not different from those in the overall population—that is, 500—but the research hypothesis is that they will have higher scores. After the intervention, the mean PF score for the sample is 528. As we can see in Figure 14.6, a mean score of 528 is more than 2 *SD*s above the population mean—it is a value that is *improbable* if the null hypothesis is true. Thus, we accept the research hypothesis that the intervention resulted in higher physical functioning scores than those in the population.[†]

We would not be justified in saying that we had *proved* the research hypothesis because the possibility of a Type I error remains—but the possibility is less than 5 in 100. Researchers reporting the results of hypothesis tests state whether their findings are **statistically significant**.

The word *significant* does not mean important or meaningful. In statistics, the term *significant* means that results are not likely to have been due to chance at some specified level of probability. A **non-significant result (NS)** means that any observed difference or relationship could have been the result of a chance fluctuation.

Overview of Hypothesis Testing Procedures

In the next section, a few statistical tests are discussed. We emphasize applications and interpretations of statistical tests, not computations. Each statistical test can be used with specific kinds of data, but the overall hypothesis testing process is similar for all tests:

1. *Select a statistical test.* Researchers select a test based on factors such as the variables' levels of measurement.
2. *Specify the level of significance.* An α level of 0.05 is usually chosen.
3. *Compute a test statistic.* The value for a test statistic is calculated with study data.
4. *Determine degrees of freedom.* The term *degrees of freedom* (*df*) refers to the number of observations free to vary about a parameter. The concept is complex, but computing degrees of freedom is easy.
5. *Compare the test statistic to a theoretical value.* Theoretical distributions exist for all test statistics. The computed value of the test statistic is compared to a theoretical value to establish significance or non-significance.

When a computer is used for the analysis, as is almost always the case, researchers follow only the first step. The computer calculates the test statistic, degrees of freedom, and the actual probability that the relationship being tested is due to chance. For example, the printout may indicate that the probability (*p*) of an intervention group having a higher mean number of days of breastfeeding than a control group on the basis of chance alone is 0.025. This means that fewer than 3 times out of 100 (only 25 times out of 1,000) would a group difference of the size observed occur by chance. The computed ***p* value** is then compared with the desired alpha. In this example, if we had set the significance level to 0.05, the results would be significant because 0.025 is more stringent than 0.05. Any computed probability greater than 0.05 (e.g., 0.15) indicates a non-significant relationship (sometimes abbreviated *NS*), that is, one that could have occurred on the basis of chance in more than 5 out of 100 samples.

 TIP Most tests discussed in this chapter are *parametric tests*, which are ones that focus on population parameters and involve certain assumptions about variables in the analysis, notably the assumption that they are normally distributed in the population. *Non-parametric tests*, by contrast, do not estimate parameters and involve less restrictive assumptions about the distribution's shape.

[†]The design for our fictitious example is highly flawed, with several serious threats to internal validity. We used this example purely as a simple way to illustrate hypothesis testing.

BIVARIATE STATISTICAL TESTS

Researchers use a variety of statistical tests to make inferences about their hypotheses. Several frequently used bivariate tests are briefly described and illustrated.

t-Tests

Researchers frequently compare two groups of people on an outcome. A parametric test for testing differences in two group means is called a ***t*-test**.

Suppose we wanted to test the effect of early discharge of maternity patients on perceived maternal competence. We administer a scale of perceived maternal competence at discharge to 20 primiparas who had a vaginal delivery: 10 who remained in the hospital 25 to 48 hours (regular discharge group) and 10 who were discharged 24 hours or less after delivery (early discharge group). Data for this example are presented in Table 14.6. Mean scores for these two groups are 25.0 and 19.0, respectively. Are these differences *real* (i.e., do they exist in the population of early- and regular-discharge mothers?), or do group differences reflect chance fluctuations? The 20 scores vary from one mother to another, ranging from a low of 13 to a high of 30. Some variation reflects individual differences in maternal competence, some might result from participants' moods on a particular day, and so forth. The research question is whether a significant amount of the variation is associated with the independent variable—time of hospital discharge. The *t*-test allows us to make inferences about this question objectively.

The formula for calculating the *t* statistic uses group means, variability, and sample size. The computed value of *t* for the data in Table 14.6 is 2.86. Degrees of freedom here is the total sample size minus 2 ($df = 20 - 2 = 18$). For an α level of 0.05, the cut-off value for *t* with 18 degrees of freedom is 2.10. *This value is the upper limit to what is probable if the null hypothesis is true.* Thus, the calculated *t* of 2.86, which is larger than the theoretical value of *t*, is improbable (i.e., statistically significant). The primiparas discharged early had significantly lower perceived maternal competence than those who were not discharged early. In fewer than 5 out of 100 samples would a difference in means this large be found by chance. In fact, the actual *p* value is 0.011: Only in about 1 sample out of 100 would this size difference be found by chance.

The situation we just described requires an *independent groups t-test*: Mothers in the two groups were different people, independent of each other. There are situations for which this type of *t*-test is not appropriate. For example, if researchers would like to compare means for a single group of people measured before and after an intervention, a *paired t-test* (also called a *dependent groups t-test*) using a different formula will be used.

TABLE 14.6 Fictitious Data for *t*-Test Example: Scores on a Perceived Maternal Competence Scale

Regular Discharge Mothers		Early Discharge Mothers	
30	32	23	26
27	17	17	16
25	18	22	13
20	28	18	21
24	29	20	14
Mean = 25.0		Mean = 19.0	
t = 2.86, *df* = 18, *p* = 0.011.			

Example of *t*-tests •
Chartrand and colleagues (2016) from Ottawa examine the effect of an educational pre-operative DVD about surgery on parents' knowledge, participation, and anxiety and on children's distress, pain, analgesic requirements, and length of recovery after same-day surgery. They used independent groups *t*-tests to compare parents' participation behaviours and children's postoperative distress, pain, and recovery time in parents who were randomized to the educational intervention group versus those in the control group. They also used paired *t*-tests to assess differences in knowledge before and after the intervention within each group. Parents in the experimental group made greater use of cognitive strategies (e.g., positive reinforcement, distraction and relaxation) with their child in the recovery room than did parents in the control group.

Instead of *t*-tests, CIs can be constructed around the difference between two means. In the example in Table 14.6, we can construct CIs around the mean difference of 6.0 in maternal competence scores (25.0 − 19.0 = 6.0). For a 95% CI, the confidence limits are 1.6 and 10.4: We can be 95% confident that the difference between population means for early and regular discharge mothers lies between these values. With CI information, we can also see that the mean difference is significant at $p < 0.05$ *because the range does not include 0*. There is a 95% probability that the mean difference is not lower than 1.6, so this means that there is less than a 5% probability that there is no difference at all—therefore, the null hypothesis can be rejected.

Analysis of Variance

Analysis of variance (ANOVA) is used to test mean group differences of three or more groups. ANOVA sorts out the variability of an outcome variable into two components: variability due to the independent variable (e.g., experimental or control group status) and variability due to all other sources (e.g., individual differences). Variation *between* groups is compared with variation *within* groups to yield an **F ratio** statistic.

Suppose we were comparing the effectiveness of interventions to help people stop smoking. Group A smokers receive nurse counselling, Group B smokers receive a nicotine patch, and a control group (Group C) gets no intervention. The outcome is 1-day cigarette consumption 1 month after the intervention. Thirty smokers are randomly assigned to one of the three groups. The null hypothesis states that the population means for post-treatment cigarette smoking are the same for all three groups, and alternatively, the research hypothesis suggests a difference in population means between groups. Table 14.7 presents fictitious

TABLE 14.7 Fictitious Data for One-Way ANOVA Example: Number of Cigarettes Smoked in 1 Day Posttreatment

Group A Nurse Counselling		Group B Nicotine Patch		Group C Untreated Controls	
28	19	0	27	33	35
0	24	31	0	54	0
17	0	26	3	19	43
20	21	30	24	40	39
35	2	24	27	41	36
Mean$_A$ = 16.6		Mean$_B$ = 19.2		Mean$_C$ = 34.0	
$F = 4.98$, $df = 2, 27$, $p = 0.01$.					

data for the 30 participants. The mean numbers of post-treatment cigarettes consumed are 16.6, 19.2, and 34.0 for groups A, B, and C, respectively. These means are different, but are they significantly different—or do differences reflect random fluctuations?

An ANOVA applied to these data yields an *F*-ratio of 4.98. For $\alpha = 0.05$ and $df = 2$ and 27 (2 *df* between groups and 27 *df* within groups), the theoretical *F* value is 3.35. Because our obtained *F* value of 4.98 exceeds 3.35, we reject the null hypothesis that the population means are equal. The *actual* probability, as calculated by a computer, is 0.014. In only 14 samples out of 1,000 would group differences this great be obtained by chance alone.

ANOVA results support the hypothesis that different treatments were associated with different cigarette smoking, but we cannot tell from these results whether treatment A was significantly more effective than treatment B. Statistical analyses known as *post hoc tests* (or *multiple comparison procedures*) are used to find the significant differences between group means that resulted in the rejection of the overall null hypothesis.

A type of ANOVA known as **repeated-measures ANOVA (RM-ANOVA)** can be used when the means being compared are means at different points in time (e.g., mean blood pressure at 2, 4, and 6 hours after surgery). This is analogous to a paired *t*-test, extended to three or more points of data collection. When two or more groups are measured several times, an RM-ANOVA provides information about a main effect for time (Do the measures change significantly over time, irrespective of group?), a main effect for groups (Do the group means differ significantly, irrespective of time?), and an *interaction effect* (Do the groups differ more at certain times?).

Example of an ANOVA ·
Using data from the Alberta's Caring for Diabetes (ABCD) study, Johnson and co-researchers (2016) examined how diabetes-related distress and depressive symptoms (DS) may affect self-management behaviours in people living with type 2 diabetes.

One-way ANOVA was used to compare the four groups in terms of diabetes distress and depressive symptoms. Participants expressed moderate to severe levels of distress, and depressive symptoms were less adherent to dietary behaviours and were less physically active compared to those without distress and depressive symptoms ($p < 0.001$).

Chi-Squared Test

The **chi-squared (χ^2) test** is used to test hypotheses about differences in proportions, as in a crosstab. For example, suppose we were studying the effect of nursing instruction on patients' adherence with self-medication. Nurses implement a new instructional strategy with 50 patients, whereas 50 control group patients get usual care. The research hypothesis is that a higher proportion of people in the intervention than in the control condition will be adherent. Some fictitious data for this example are presented in Table 14.8, which shows that 60% of those in the intervention group were adherent, compared to 40% in the control group. But is this 20 percentage point difference statistically significant—i.e., likely to be "real"?

The value of the χ^2 statistic for the data in Table 14.8 is 4.00, which we can compare with the value from a theoretical chi-squared distribution. In this example, the theoretical value that must be exceeded to establish significance at the 0.05 level is 3.84. The obtained value of 4.00 is larger than would be expected by chance (the actual $p = 0.046$). We can conclude that a significantly larger proportion of experimental patients than control patients were adherent.

TABLE 14.8 Observed Frequencies for Chi-Squared Example: Rates of Compliance With Medications

	Group				Total
	Experimental		Control		
Patient Compliance	*n*	%	*n*	%	*n*
Compliant	30	60.0	20	40.0	50
Non-compliant	20	40.0	30	60.0	50
TOTAL	50	100.0	50	100.0	100

$\chi^2 = 4.0$, $df = 1$, $p = 0.046$.

Example of chi-squared test •
Wong and co-researchers (2017) explored occupational safety hazards experienced by nurses working in home care. They used chi-squared tests to explore the differences in the prevalence of safety hazards across four geographic settings: urban, suburban, town/small city, or rural. The five most recurrent occupational hazards experienced by HC nurses in Ontario were dangerous or aggressive pets (77.8%), winter or night driving conditions (77.5%), ergonomic issues (62.8%), exposure to oxygen equipment/tanks (53%), and environmental tobacco smoke exposure (44.8%). Nurses visiting patients in urban areas were more likely to have recurrent exposure to pest and unsafe neighbourhoods compared to nurses visiting patients in rural areas ($p < 0.01$).

As with means, we can construct CIs around the difference between two proportions. In our example, the group difference in proportion adherent was 0.20 (0.60 − 0.40 = 0.20). The 95% CI around 0.20 is 0.06 to 0.34. We can be 95% confident that the true population difference in adherence rates between the groups is between 6% and 34%. This interval does not include 0%, so we can be 95% confident that group differences are "real" in the population.

Correlation Coefficients

Pearson's *r* is both descriptive and inferential. As a descriptive statistic, *r* summarizes the magnitude and direction of a relationship between two variables. As an inferential statistic, *r* tests hypotheses about population correlations; the null hypothesis is that there is no relationship between two variables, i.e., that the population $r = 0.00$.

Suppose we were studying the relationship between patients' self-reported level of stress (higher scores indicate more stress) and the pH level of their saliva. With a sample of 50 patients, we find that $r = -0.29$. This value indicates a tendency for people with high stress to have lower pH levels than those with low stress. But is the *r* of −0.29 a random fluctuation observed only in this sample, or is the relationship significant? Degrees of freedom for correlation coefficients equal *N* minus 2 = 48 in this example. The theoretical value for *r* with $df = 48$ and $\alpha = 0.05$ is 0.28. Because the absolute value of the calculated *r* is 0.29, the null hypothesis is rejected: The relationship between patients' stress level and the acidity of their saliva is statistically significant.

Example of Pearson's *r* •
Lalonde and McGillis (2017) explore 45 new graduate nurses' perceptions of role conflict, role ambiguity, job satisfaction, and turnover intent at the end of their preceptorship program. New graduates' job dissatisfaction had a significant and strong relationship with role conflict ($r = 0.72$, $p < 0.001$) and moderate relationship with role ambiguity ($r = 0.43$, $p < 0.05$).

Effect-Size Indexes

Effect-size indexes are estimates of the magnitude of effects of an "I" (intervention) component on an "O" (outcome) component in PICO questions—an important issue in EBP (see Box 2.1). Effect-size information can be crucial because with large samples even miniscule effects can be statistically significant. *p* values tell you whether results are likely to be *real*, but effect sizes suggest whether they are important. Effect size plays an important role in meta-analyses.

It is beyond our scope to explain effect sizes in detail, but we offer an illustration. A frequently used effect-size index is the *d* **statistic**, which describes the magnitude of differences in two means, such as the difference between intervention and control group means on an outcome. Thus, *d* can be calculated to estimate effect size when *t*-tests are used. When *d* is zero, it means that there is no effect—the means of the two groups being compared are the same. By convention, a *d* of 0.20 or less is considered *small*, a *d* of 0.50 is considered *moderate*, and a *d* of 0.80 or greater is considered *large*.

Different effect-size indexes and interpretive conventions are associated with different situations. For example, the *r*-statistic can be interpreted directly as an effect-size index, as can the OR. The key point is that they provide information about how powerful the effect of an independent variable is on an outcome.

 TIP Researchers who conduct a *power analysis* to estimate how big a sample size they need to adequately test their hypotheses (i.e., to avoid a Type II error) must estimate in advance how large the effect size will be—usually based on prior research or a pilot study.

Example of calculated effect size •
Hevezi (2016) conducted a pilot study of a meditation intervention to reduce the stress associated with compassion fatigue among nurses, using a pretest–posttest design and paired *t*-tests. Effect-size indexes were also computed. For example, scores on a burnout scale declined significantly after the intervention (*t* = 3.58, *p* = 0.003), and the effect size was large: *d* = 0.92.

Guide to Bivariate Statistical Tests

The selection of a statistical test depends on several factors, such as number of groups and the levels of measurement of the research variables. To aid you in evaluating the appropriateness of statistical tests used by nurse researchers, Table 14.9 summarizes key features of the bivariate tests mentioned in this chapter.

 TIP Every time a report presents information about statistical tests such as those described in this section, it means that the researcher was testing hypotheses—whether those hypotheses were formally stated in the introduction or not.

MULTIVARIATE STATISTICAL ANALYSIS

We wish we could avoid discussing complex statistical methods in this introductory-level book. The fact is, however, that *most* quantitative nursing studies today rely on **multivariate statistics** that involve the analysis of three or more variables simultaneously. The increased use of sophisticated analytic methods has resulted in greater rigor in nursing

TABLE 14.9 Guide to Major Bivariate Statistical Tests

Name	Test Statistic	Purpose	Measurement Level Independent Variable	Measurement Level Dependent Variable
t-Test for independent groups	t	To test the difference between the means of two independent groups (e.g., experimental vs. control, men vs. women)	Nominal	Continuous[a]
t-Test for paired groups	t	To test the difference between the means of a paired group (e.g., pretest vs. posttest for the same people)	Nominal	Continuous[a]
Analysis of variance (ANOVA)	F	To test the difference among means of 3+ independent groups	Nominal	Continuous[a]
Repeated measures ANOVA	F	To test the difference among means of 3+ related groups, e.g., the same group over time, or to compare 2+ groups over time	Nominal	Continuous[a]
Pearson's correlation coefficient	r	To test the existence and strength of a relationship between two variables	Continuous[a]	Continuous[a]
Chi-squared test	χ^2	To test the difference in proportions in 2+ independent groups	Nominal (or ordinal, few categories)	Nominal (or ordinal, few categories)

[a]Continuous measures are on an interval- and ratio-level scale.

studies, but it can be challenging for those without statistical training to fully understand research reports.

Given the introductory nature of this book and the fact that many of you are not proficient with even basic statistical tests, we present only a brief description of three widely used multivariate statistics. The supplement to this chapter on thePoint website expands on this presentation.

Multiple Regression

Correlations enable researchers to make predictions. For example, if the correlation between secondary school grades and nursing school grades were 0.60, nursing school administrators could make predictions about applicants' performance in nursing school. Researchers can improve their prediction of an outcome by performing a **multiple regression** in which several independent variables are included in the analysis. As an example, we might predict infant birth weight (the outcome) from such variables as mothers' smoking, amount of prenatal care, and gestational period. In multiple regression, outcome variables are continuous variables. Independent variables (often called **predictor variables** in regression) are either continuous variables or dichotomous nominal-level variables, such as male/female.

The statistic used in multiple regression is the **multiple correlation coefficient**, symbolized as R. Unlike Pearson's r, R does not have negative values. R varies from 0.00 to 1.00, showing the *strength* of the relationship between several predictors and an outcome but not *direction*. Researchers can test whether R is statistically significant—i.e., different from 0.00. R, when squared, can be interpreted as the proportion of the variability in the outcome that is explained by the predictors. In predicting birth weight, if we achieved an R of 0.50 ($R^2 = 0.25$), we could say that the predictors accounted for one-fourth of the variation in birth weights. Three-fourths of the variation, however, resulted from factors not in the analysis. Researchers usually report multiple correlation results in terms of R^2 rather than R.

> **Example of multiple regression analysis** •
> Lovoie-Tremblay and her team from McGill University (2015) explored factors associated with nurse stress and work satisfaction among nurses practicing in an open-ward neonatal intensive care unit.
>
> In their multiple regression analysis, the researchers found that nurses reported greater work satisfaction when they had less than a university education, worked part-time, had greater support, felt the health care team was more effective at meeting patient and family needs and providing family-centred care, and experienced fewer environmental obstacles. These variables explained 29.4% of the variance in work satisfaction ($R^2 = 0.29$; $p < 0.001$).

Analysis of Covariance

Analysis of covariance (ANCOVA), which combines features of ANOVA and multiple regression, is used to control confounding variables to remove their effects statistically—that is, to "equalize" groups being compared. This approach is valuable in certain situations, like when a non-equivalent control group design is used. When control through randomization is lacking, ANCOVA offers the possibility of statistical control.

In ANCOVA, the confounding variables being controlled are called *covariates*. ANCOVA tests the significance of differences between group means on an outcome after removing the effect of covariates. ANCOVA produces F statistics to test the significance of group differences. ANCOVA is a powerful and useful analytic technique for controlling confounding influences on outcomes.

> **Example of ANCOVA** •
> Kapritsou and her research team (2016) studied the effect of early oral nutrition (during the first 24 hours of the day of surgery) in combination with ambulation and optimal pain control on oncology patients after major abdominal surgery. The postoperative outcomes included time to mobilization, length of intravenous fluid administration, postoperative hospitalization stay, and complications. In the ANCOVA, stress, pain, and related neuropeptidic responses (adrenocorticotropic hormone, cortisol, and neuropeptide Y) were the independent variables, and age, gender, and body mass index were the covariates.

Logistic Regression

Logistic regression analyses the relationships between multiple independent variables and a nominal-level outcome (e.g., compliant vs. non-compliant). It is similar to multiple regression, although it employs a different statistical estimation procedure. Logistic regression transforms the probability of an event occurring (e.g., that a woman will practise breast self-examination or not) into its *odds*. After further transformations, the analysis examines the relationship of the predictor variables to the transformed outcome variable. For each predictor, the logistic regression yields an *OR*, which is the factor by which the odds change for a unit change in the predictors after controlling other predictors. Logistic regression yields ORs for each predictor as well as CIs around the ORs.

Example of logistic regression •
TYemple and colleagues (2016) examined factors associated with the development of parastomal hernia based on survey result of 764 persons who were receiving services from the Manitoba Ostomy Program. The likelihood of having a parastomal hernia was significantly increased by a large stoma (OR = 1.9, p = 0.0057) and history of cancer (OR = 7.3, p = 0.0009).

MEASUREMENT STATISTICS

In Chapter 10, we described two measurement properties that represent key aspects of measurement quality—reliability and validity. When a new measure is developed, researchers undertake a psychometric assessment to estimate its reliability and validity. Such psychometric assessments rely on statistical analyses, using indexes that we briefly describe here. Researchers often report measurement statistics when they describe the measures they had chosen, to provide evidence that their data can be trusted.

Reliability Assessment

Reliability is the extent that scores on a measure are consistent across repeated measurements if the trait itself has not changed. In Chapter 10, we mentioned three major types of reliability, each of which relies on different statistical indexes: test–retest reliability, interrater reliability, and internal consistency reliability.

- Test–retest reliability, which concerns the stability of a measure, is assessed by making two separate measurements of the same people, often 1 to 2 weeks apart, and then testing the extent to which the two sets of scores are consistent. Some researchers use Pearson's r to correlate the scores at Time 1 with those at Time 2, but the preferred index for test–retest reliability is the **intraclass correlation coefficient (ICC)**, which can range in value from 0.00 and 1.00.
- Interrater reliability is used to assess the extent to which two independent raters or observers assign the same score in measuring an attribute. When the ratings are dichotomous classifications (e.g., presence vs. absence of infusion phlebitis), the preferred index is **Cohen's kappa**, whose values also range from 0.00 to 1.00. If the ratings are continuous scores, the ICC is usually used.
- Internal consistency reliability concerns the extent to which the various components of a multicomponent measure (e.g., items on a quality of life scale) are consistently measuring the same attribute. Internal consistency, a widely reported aspect of reliability, is estimated by an index called **coefficient alpha** (or Cronbach's alpha). If a psychosocial scale includes several subscales, coefficient alpha is usually computed for each subscale separately.

For all of these reliability indexes, the closer the value is to 1.00, the stronger is the evidence of good reliability. Although opinions about minimally acceptable values vary, values of 0.80 or higher are usually considered good. Researchers try to select measures with previously demonstrated high levels of reliability, but if they are using a multi-item scale, they usually compute coefficient alpha with their own data as well.

Validity Assessment

Validity is the degree to which an instrument is measuring what it is supposed to measure. Like reliability, validity has several aspects. Unlike reliability, however, it is challenging to establish a measure's validity. Validation is a process of evidence building, and typically, multiple forms of evidence are sought.

Content Validity

Content validity is relevant for complex measures, such as multi-item scales. The issue is whether the content of the items adequately reflects the construct of interest. Content validation usually relies on expert ratings of each item, and the ratings are used to compute an index called the *content validity index (CVI)*. A value of 0.90 or higher has been suggested as providing evidence of good content validity.

Criterion Validity

Criterion validity concerns the extent to which scores on a measure are consistent with an established "gold standard" criterion. The methods used to assess criterion validity depend on the level of measurement and the criterion.

When both the measurement and the criterion are continuous, researchers administer the two measures to a sample and then compute a Pearson's *r* between the two scores. Larger coefficients are desirable, but there is no threshold value that is considered a minimum. Usually, statistical significance is the standard for concluding that criterion validity is adequate.

If both the measure and the gold standard are dichotomous variables, researchers often apply methods of assessing *diagnostic accuracy*. **Sensitivity** is the ability of a measure to correctly identify a "case," that is, to correctly screen in or diagnose a condition. A measure's sensitivity provides the proportion of *true positives*. **Specificity** is the measure's ability to correctly identify non-cases; that is, to screen *out* those without the condition. Specificity is the proportion of *true negatives*.

To assess an instrument's sensitivity and specificity, researchers need to compare scores on the instrument with a highly reliable and valid criterion of "caseness." For example, if we wanted to test the validity of adolescents' self-reports about smoking (yes/no in past 24 hours), we could use urinary cotinine level, using a cut-off value for a positive test of ≥200 ng/mL, as the gold standard. Sensitivity would be calculated as the proportion of teenagers who said they smoked *and* who had high concentrations of cotinine, divided by all real smokers as indicated by the urine test. Specificity would be the proportion of teenagers who accurately reported they did not smoke, or the true negatives, divided by all *real* negatives. Both sensitivity and specificity can range from 0.00 to 1.00. It is difficult to set standards of acceptability for sensitivity and specificity, but both should be as high as possible.

When the focal measure is continuous and the gold standard is dichotomous, researchers often use a statistical tool called a *receiver operating characteristic (ROC) curve*. An ROC curve involves plotting each score on the focal measure against its sensitivity and specificity for correct classification based on a dichotomous criterion. A discussion of ROC curves is beyond the scope of this book, but interested readers can consult Polit and Yang (2016).

Construct Validity

Construct validity concerns the extent to which a measure is truly measuring the target construct and is often assessed using hypothesis testing procedures like those described in previous sections of this chapter. For example, a researcher might hypothesize that scores on a new measure of caregiver burden would correlate with scores on a depression scale based on the established relationship between caregiving and depression. Pearson's *r* would be used to test this hypothesis, and a significant correlation would provide some evidence of construct validity. For known groups' validity, which involves testing hypotheses about expected group differences on a new measure, an independent group's *t*-test could be used. Both bivariate and multivariate statistical tests are appropriate in assessments of a new measure's construct validity.

READING AND UNDERSTANDING STATISTICAL INFORMATION

Measurement statistics are most likely to be presented in the methods section of a report and are usually statistics reported previously by the instrument developer. Statistical *findings*, however, are communicated in the results section. Statistical information is described in the text and in tables (or, less frequently, in figures). This section offers assistance in reading and interpreting statistical information.

Tips on Reading Text With Statistical Information

Both descriptive and inferential statistics are reported in results sections. Descriptive statistics typically summarize sample characteristics. Information about the participants' background helps readers to draw conclusions about the people to whom the findings can be applied. Researchers may provide statistical information for evaluating biases. For example, when a quasi-experimental or case-control design has been used, researchers may test the equivalence of the groups being compared on baseline or background variables, using tests such as *t*-tests.

For hypothesis testing, the text of research articles usually provides the following information about statistical tests: (1) the test used, (2) the value of the calculated statistic, (3) degrees of freedom, and (4) level of statistical significance. Examples of how the results of various statistical tests might be reported in the text are shown in the following text.

1. *t*-test: $t = 1.68, df = 160, p = 0.09$
2. Chi-squared: $X^2 = 16.65, df = 2, p < 0.001$
3. Pearson's *r*: $r = 0.36, df = 100, p < 0.01$
4. ANOVA: $F = 0.18; df = 1, 69$, ns

The preferred approach is to report significance as the computed probability that the null hypothesis is correct, as in Example 1. In this case, the observed group mean differences could be found by chance in 9 out of 100 samples. This result is not statistically significant because the mean difference had an unacceptably high chance of being wrong. The probability level is sometimes reported simply as falling below or above the certain thresholds (Examples 2 and 3). These results are significant because the probability of obtaining such results by chance is less than 1 in 100. You must be careful to read the symbol following the *p* value correctly: The symbol < means *less than*. The symbol > means *greater than*—i.e., the results are not significant if the *p*-value is 0.05 or greater. When results do not achieve statistical significance at the desired level, researchers may simply indicate NS, as in Example 4.

Statistical information often is noted parenthetically in a sentence describing the findings, as in "Patients in the intervention group had a significantly lower rate of infection than those in the control group ($\chi^2 = 5.41, df = 1, p = 0.02$)." In reading research reports, the actual values of the test statistics (e.g., χ^2) are of no inherent interest. What is important is whether the statistical tests indicate that the research hypotheses were accepted as probably true (as demonstrated by significant results) or rejected as probably false (as demonstrated by NS).

Tips on Reading Statistical Tables

Tables allow researchers to condense a lot of statistical information and minimize redundancy. Consider, for example, putting information about dozens of correlation coefficients in the text.

Tables are efficient, but they may be daunting for novice readers partly because of the absence of standardization. There is no universally accepted format for presenting *t*-test results.

TABLE 14.10 Selected Demographic and Psychological Characteristics of Study Sample in Study on Finding Benefit From Prostate Cancer (N = 209)

Sample Characteristic	Frequency (n)	Percentage	Mean (SD)	Range
Relationship status				
In a relationship	160	76.63%		
Not in a relationship	48	23.4%		
Education level				
Secondary education	97	46.6%		
Higher/further education	111	53.1%		
Employment status				
Retired	153	73.2%		
Other	55	26.4%		
Age			72.0 (7.2)	53–92
Coping scale scores			43.9 (13.6)	28–112
Depression scale scores			2.8 (2.9)	0–21
Anxiety scale scores			3.5 (3.6)	0–21
Benefit finding scale score			36.2 (18.3)	17–85

Scales for measuring psychological characteristics are described in the report.
Adapted from Tables 1 and 2 of: Pascoe, E. C., & Edvardsson, D. (2016). Psychological characteristics and traits for finding benefit from prostate cancer: Correlates and predictors. *Cancer Nursing, 39*(6), 446–454.

We have a few suggestions for helping you to comprehend statistical tables. First, read the text and the tables simultaneously—the text may help you figure out what the table is communicating. Second, before trying to understand the numbers in a table, try to look for information from the accompanying words. Table titles and footnotes often present critical information. Table headings should be carefully scrutinized because they indicate what the variables in the analysis are (often listed as row labels in the first column, as in Table 14.10) and what statistical information is included (often specified as column headings). Third, you may find it helpful to consult the glossary of symbols on the inside back cover of this book to check the meaning of a statistical symbol. Not all symbols in this glossary were described in this chapter, so it may be necessary to refer to a statistics textbook, such as that of Polit (2010), for further information.

 TIP In tables, probability levels associated with significance tests are sometimes presented directly in the table, in a column labeled "*p*" (e.g., *p* = 0.03). However, researchers sometimes indicate significance levels in tables with asterisks placed next to the value of the test statistic. One asterisk usually signifies *p* < 0.05, two asterisks signify *p* < 0.01, and three asterisks signify *p* < 0.001 (there should be a key at the bottom of the table indicating what the asterisks mean). Thus, a table might show *t* = 3.00 in one column and *p* < 0.01 in another. Alternatively, the table might show *t* = 3.00**. The absence of an asterisk would signify an NS.

CRITIQUING QUANTITATIVE ANALYSES

It is often difficult to critique statistical analyses. We hope this chapter has helped to demystify statistics, but we recognize the limited scope of our coverage. It would be unreasonable to expect you to be adept at evaluating statistical analyses, but you can be on the lookout for certain things in reviewing research articles. Some specific guidelines are presented in Box 14.1.

Box 14.1 Guidelines for Critiquing Statistical Analyses

1. Did the descriptive statistics in the report sufficiently describe the major variables and background characteristics of the sample? Were appropriate descriptive statistics used—for example, was a mean presented when percentages would have been more informative?
2. Were statistical analyses undertaken to assess threats to the study's validity (e.g., to test for selection bias or attrition bias)?
3. Did the researchers report any inferential statistics? If inferential statistics were not used, should they have been?
4. Was information provided about both hypothesis testing and parameter estimation (i.e., confidence intervals)? Were effect sizes reported? Overall, did the reported statistics provide readers with sufficient information about the study results?
5. Were any multivariate procedures used? If not, should they have been used—for example, would the internal validity of the study be strengthened by statistically controlling confounding variables?
6. Were the selected statistical tests appropriate, given the level of measurement of the variables and the nature of the hypotheses?
7. Were the results of any statistical tests significant? What do the tests tell you about the plausibility of the research hypotheses? Were effects sizeable?
8. Were the results of any statistical tests non-significant? Is it possible that these reflect Type II errors? What factors might have undermined the study's statistical conclusion validity?
9. Was information about the reliability and validity of measures reported? Did the researchers use measures with good measurement properties?
10. Was there an appropriate amount of statistical information? Were findings clearly and logically organized? Were tables or figures used judiciously to summarize large amounts of statistical information? Are the tables clear, with good titles and row/column labels?

One aspect of the critique should focus on which analyses were reported. You should assess whether the statistical information adequately describes the sample and reports the results of statistical tests for all hypotheses. Another presentational issue concerns the researcher's judicious use of tables to summarize statistical information.

A thorough critique also addresses whether researchers used the appropriate statistics. Table 14.9 provides guidelines for some frequently used bivariate statistical tests. The major issues to consider are the number of independent and dependent variables, the levels of measurement of the research variables, and the number of groups (if any) being compared.

If researchers did not use a multivariate technique, you should consider whether the bivariate analysis adequately tests the relationship between the independent and dependent variables. For example, if a *t*-test or ANOVA was used, could the internal validity of the study have been enhanced through the statistical control of confounding variables, using ANCOVA? The answer will often be "yes."

Finally, you should pay attention to possible exaggerations or subjectivity in the reported results. Researchers should never claim that the data proved, verified, confirmed, or demonstrated that the hypotheses were correct or incorrect. Hypotheses should be described as being *supported* or *not supported*, *accepted* or *rejected*.

The main task for beginning consumers in reading a results section of a research report is to understand the meaning of the statistical tests. What do the quantitative results indicate about the researcher's hypothesis? How believable are the findings? The answer to such questions form the basis for interpreting the research results, a topic discussed in Chapter 15.

TABLE 14.11 Correlation Matrix for Selected Study Variables in Study on Finding Benefit from Prostate Cancer ($N = 209$)

Variable	1	2	3	4	5	6
1. Benefit finding score	1.00					
2. Education level	0.09	1.00				
3. Coping	0.59[b]	0.17[a]	1.00			
4. Depression score	0.17[b]	−0.04	0.33[b]	1.00		
5. Anxiety score	0.29[b]	0.01	0.45[b]	0.67[b]	1.00	
6. Age	−0.02	−0.12	−0.11	−0.12	−0.04	1.00

[a]$p < 0.05$. [b]$p < 0.01$.
Adapted from Table 3 of: Pascoe, E. C., & Edvardsson, D. (2016). Psychological characteristics and traits for finding benefit from prostate cancer: Correlates and predictors. *Cancer Nursing*, *39*(6), 446–454.

RESEARCH EXAMPLES WITH CRITICAL THINKING EXERCISES

In this section, we provide details about the analysis in a nursing study, followed by some questions to guide critical thinking. Read the summary and then answer the critical thinking questions that follow, referring to the full research report if necessary. Example 1 is featured on the interactive *Critical Thinking Activity* on thePoint website. The critical thinking questions for Example 2 are based on the study that appears in its entirety in Appendix A of this book. Our comments for these exercises are in the Student Resources section on thePoint.

EXAMPLE 1: DESCRIPTIVE AND INFERENTIAL STATISTICS

Study: Psychological characteristics and traits for finding benefit from prostate cancer: Correlates and predictors (Pascoe & Edvardsson, 2016).

Statement of Purpose: The purpose of this study was to explore the correlates and predictors of finding benefit from prostate cancer among men undergoing androgen deprivation therapy (ADT).

Methods: The researchers used a descriptive correlational design. They collected data from a sample of 209 men undergoing ADT in an acute tertiary hospital outpatient setting in Australia. Study participants completed self-report questionnaires that asked questions about demographic and clinical characteristics. The questionnaire also included several psychological scales, including scales to measure coping, anxiety, depression, and resilience. The researchers noted that a theoretical model of the coping process led them to select independent variables that comprise "psychological factors that may be influential to fostering or maintaining positive emotional states, which includes finding benefit" (p. 448). Participants completed the Benefit Finding Scale, a 17-item scale that asks about potential benefits of having experienced prostate cancer (e.g., "...has helped me take things as they come"). The researchers indicated that, in their sample of men, internal consistency for this scale was strong (coefficient alpha = 0.96). Good internal consistency was also found for the coping scale ($\alpha = 0.85$), the anxiety scale ($\alpha = 0.85$), the depression scale ($\alpha = 0.79$), and the resilience scale ($\alpha = 0.90$).

Descriptive Statistics: The researchers presented descriptive statistics (means, *SD*s, ranges, and percentages) to describe the characteristics of sample members, in terms of both demographic characteristics and scores on the psychological scales. Table 14.10 presents descriptive information for selected variables. The men in the sample ranged in age from 53 to 92 years, and their mean age was

72.0 years (±7.2). The typical participant was in a relationship (76.6%) and retired (73.2%). Just over half of the men had postsecondary education (53.1%). In terms of the participants' scores on the psychological scales, there was a good range of values, indicating adequate variability. Scores on the Benefit Finding Scale ranged from 17 to 85, which corresponds to the full range of possible scores.

Hypothesis Tests: The researchers used Pearson's r to test hypotheses that benefit finding for these men was correlated with various psychological characteristics. Table 14.11 presents a correlation matrix that shows the values of r for pairs of selected variables (the researchers' correlation matrix was more comprehensive). This table lists, on the left, six variables: Variable 1, scores on the Benefit Finding Scale (the dependent variable); Variable 2, education level; Variable 3, scores on the coping scale; Variable 4, scores on the depression scale; Variable 5, scores on the anxiety scale; and Variable 6, age. The correlation matrix shows, in Column 1, the correlation coefficient between benefit finding scores and all other variables. At the intersection of Row 1–Column 1, we find 1.00, which indicates that the scores are perfectly correlated with themselves. The next entry in Column 1 is the r between benefit finding scores and education level. The value of 0.09 indicates a very modest, positive relationship between these two variables—a relationship that was not statistically significant and so could be zero. The strongest correlation for the finding benefit scores was with scores on the coping scale, $r = 0.59$, $p < 0.01$.

Multivariate Analyses: The researchers found that six of their independent variables were significantly correlated with scores on the benefit finding scale. These six variables were entered into a multiple regression analysis. The R^2 for these six predictor variables was 0.38, $p < 0.001$. These variables explained 38% of the variance in finding benefit from prostate cancer. Self-reported coping made the largest contribution, suggesting that helping patients identify coping strategies might be valuable.

Critical Thinking Exercises

1. Answer the relevant questions from Box 14.1 regarding this study.
2. Also consider the following targeted questions:
   a. Using information from Table 14.11, with which variable was the men's educational level significantly correlated? What does the correlation indicate?
   b. What is the strongest correlation in Table 14.11? What is the weakest correlation in this table? What do the correlations indicate?
3. What might be some of the uses to which the findings could be put in clinical practice?

EXAMPLE 2: STATISTICAL ANALYSIS IN THE STUDY IN APPENDIX A

- Read the results section of Swenson and colleagues' (2016) study ("Parents' use of praise and criticism in a sample of young children seeking mental health services") in Appendix A of this book.

Critical Thinking Exercises

1. Answer the relevant questions from Box 14.1 regarding this study.
2. Also consider the following targeted questions:
   a. Looking at Table 14.1, what percentage of parents had graduated from college? What was the mean score (and the *SD*) of the parents on the CES-D depression scale?
   b. In Table 14.2, what percentage of parents reported that they "almost never" praised their child? And what percentage reported that they "almost never" criticized their child?
   c. In Table 14.4, what was the correlation coefficient between parents' self-reported use of criticism and their score on the depressive symptom scale? Was this correlation statistically significant?

WANT TO KNOW MORE?

A wide variety of resources to enhance your learning and understanding of this chapter are available on thePoint.

- Interactive Critical Thinking Activity
- Chapter Supplement on Multivariate Statistics
- Answer to the Critical Thinking Exercise for Example 2
- Internet Resources with useful websites for Chapter 14
- A Wolters Kluwer journal article on a topic related to this chapter

Summary Points

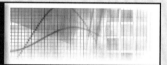

- There are four **levels of measurement**: (1) **nominal measurement**—the classification of attributes into mutually exclusive categories, (2) **ordinal measurement**—the ranking of people based on their relative standing on an attribute, (3) **interval measurement**—indicating not only people's rank order but also the distance between them, and (4) **ratio measurement**—distinguished from interval measurement by having a rational zero point. Interval- and ratio-level measures are often called **continuous**.

- **Descriptive statistics** are used to summarize and describe quantitative data.

- In **frequency distributions**, numeric values are ordered from the lowest to the highest, together with a count of the number (or percentage) of times each value was obtained.

- Data for a continuous variable can be completely described in terms of the shape of the distribution, central tendency, and variability.

- A distribution's shape can be **symmetric** or **skewed**, with one tail longer than the other; it can also be unimodal with one peak (i.e., one value of high frequency) or multimodal with more than one peak. A **normal distribution** (bell-shaped curve) is symmetric, unimodal, and not too peaked.

- Indexes of **central tendency** represent average or typical value of a set of scores. The

mode is the value that occurs most frequently, the **median** is the point above which and below which 50% of the cases fall, and the mean is the arithmetic average of all scores. The **mean** is the most stable index of central tendency.

- Indexes of **variability**—how spread out the data are—include the range and standard deviation. The **range** is the distance between the highest and lowest scores. The **standard deviation** (*SD*) indicates how much, on average, scores deviate from the mean.

- In a normal distribution, 95% of values lie within 2 *SD*s above and below the mean.

- A **crosstab table** is a two-dimensional frequency distribution in which the frequencies of two nominal- or ordinal-level variables are cross-tabulated.

- **Correlation coefficients** describe the direction and magnitude of a relationship between two variables and range from −1.00 (perfect **negative correlation**) through 0.00 to +1.00 (perfect **positive correlation**). The most frequently used correlation coefficient is **Pearson's *r***, used with continuous variables. **Spearman's rho** is usually the correlation coefficient used when variables are measured on an ordinal scale.

- Statistical indexes that describe the effects of exposure to risk factors or interventions provide useful information for clinical decisions. A widely reported risk index is the **OR**, which is the ratio of the odds for an exposed versus unexposed group, with the *odds* reflecting the proportion of people with an adverse outcome relative to those without it.

- **Inferential statistics**, based on laws of probability, allow researchers to make inferences about population **parameters** based on data from a sample.
- The *sampling distribution of the mean* is a theoretical distribution of the means of an infinite number of same-sized samples drawn from a population. Sampling distributions are the basis for inferential statistics.
- The *standard error of the mean (SEM)*—the *SD* of this theoretical distribution—indicates the degree of average error of a sample mean; the smaller the SEM, the more accurate are estimates of the population value.
- Statistical inference consists of two approaches: hypothesis testing and **parameter estimation** (estimating a population value).
- *Point estimation* provides a single value of a population estimate (e.g., a mean). *Interval estimation* provides a range of values—a **confidence interval (CI)**—between which the population value is expected to fall, at a specified probability. Most often, the 95% CI is reported, which indicates that there is a 95% probability that the true population value lies between the upper and lower confidence limits.
- **Hypothesis testing** through statistical tests enables researchers to make objective decisions about relationships between variables.
- The *null hypothesis* is that no relationship exists between variables; rejection of the null hypothesis lends support to the research hypothesis. In testing hypotheses, researchers compute a **test statistic** and then see if the statistic falls beyond a critical region on the theoretical distribution. The value of the test statistic indicates whether the null hypothesis is "improbable."
- A **Type I error** occurs if a null hypothesis is wrongly rejected (false positives). A **Type II error** occurs when a null hypothesis is wrongly accepted (false negatives).
- Researchers control the risk of making a Type I error by selecting a **level of significance** (or **alpha** level), which is the probability that such an error will occur. The 0.05 level (the conventional standard) means that in only 5 out of 100 samples would the null hypothesis be rejected when it should have been accepted.

- The probability of committing a Type II error is related to *power*, the ability of a statistical test to detect true relationships. The standard criterion for an acceptable level of power is 0.80. Power increases as sample size increases.
- Results from hypothesis tests are either significant or non-significant; **statistically significant** means that the obtained results are not likely to be due to chance fluctuations at a given probability (*p* **value**).
- Two common statistical tests are the *t*-test and **ANOVA**, both of which can be used to test the significance of the difference between group means; ANOVA is used when there are three or more groups. **RM-ANOVA** is used when data are collected at multiple time points.
- The **chi-squared test** is used to test hypotheses about group differences in proportions.
- Pearson's *r* can be used to test whether a correlation is significantly different from zero.
- **Effect-size** indexes (such as the *d* **statistic**) summarize the strength of the effect of an independent variable (e.g., an intervention) on an outcome variable.
- **Multivariate statistics** are used in nursing research to untangle complex relationships among three or more variables.
- **Multiple regression analysis** is a method for understanding the effect of two or more **predictor** (independent) **variables** on a continuous dependent variable. The squared **multiple correlation coefficient** (R^2) is an estimate of the proportion of variability in the outcome variable accounted for by the predictors.
- **ANCOVA** controls confounding variables (called *covariates*) before testing whether group mean differences are statistically significant.
- **Logistic regression** is used in lieu of multiple regression when the outcome is dichotomous.
- Statistics are also used in psychometric assessments to quantify a measure's reliability and validity.
- For test–retest reliability, the preferred index is the **ICC**. **Cohen's kappa** is used to estimate interrater reliability when the ratings of two

independent raters are dichotomous. The index used to estimate internal consistency reliability is **coefficient alpha**. Reliability coefficients of 0.80 or higher are desirable.

● In terms of content validity, expert ratings of scale items are used to compute *CVI*.

● Criterion validity is assessed with different statistical methods depending on the measurement level of the focal measure and the criterion. When both are dichotomous, sensitivity and specificity are usually calculated. **Sensitivity** is the instrument's ability to identify a case correctly (i.e., its rate of yielding true positives). **Specificity** is the instrument's ability to identify non-cases correctly (i.e., its rate of yielding true negatives).

● Construct validity is evaluated using hypothesis testing procedures, so statistical tests such as those described in this chapter (e.g., Pearson's *r*, *t*-tests) are appropriate.

REFERENCES

Chartrand J., Tourigny J., & MacCormick J. (2017). The effect of an educational pre-operative DVD on parents' and children's outcomes after a same-day surgery: a randomized controlled trial. *Journal of Advanced Nursing*, *73*(3), 599–611.

Conway L. J., Liu J., Harris A. D., & Larson E. L. (2016). Risk Factors for Bacteremia in Patients With Urinary Catheter-Associated Bacteriuria. *American Journal of Critical Care*, *26*(1), 43–52.

Green E., Yuen D., Chasen M., et al. (2017). Oncology Nurses' Attitudes Toward the Edmonton Symptom Assessment System: Results From a Large Cancer Care Ontario Study. *Oncology Nursing Forum*, *44*(1), 116–125.

Hall W. A., Moynihan M., Bhagat R., & Wooldridge J. (2017). Relationships between parental sleep quality, fatigue, cognitions about infant sleep, and parental depression pre and post-intervention for infant behavioral sleep problems. *BMC Pregnancy and Childbirth*, *17*(1), 104.

Hevezi, J. A. (2016). Evaluation of a meditation intervention to reduce the effects of stressors associated with compassion fatigue among nurses. *Journal of Holistic Nursing*, *34*(4), 343–350.

Johnson S. T., Al Sayah F., Mathe N., & Johnson J. A. (2016). The relationship of diabetes-related distress and depressive symptoms with physical activity and dietary behaviors in adults with type 2 diabetes: A cross-sectional study. *Journal of Diabetes and its Complications*, *30*(5), 967–970.

Lalonde M., & McGillis Hall L. (2016). Preceptor characteristics and the socialization outcomes of new graduate nurses during a preceptorship programme. *Nursing Open*, *4*(1), 24–31.

Mann E. G., Harrison M. B., LeFort S., & VanDenKerkhof E. G. (2017). What Are the Barriers and Facilitators for the Self-Management of Chronic Pain with and without Neuropathic Characteristics? *Pain Management Nursing*, *18*(5), 295–308.

**Pascoe, E. C., & Edvardsson, D. (2015). Psychological characteristics and traits for finding benefit from prostate cancer: Correlates and predictors. *Cancer Nursing*, 2016, *39*(6), 446–454.

Polit, D. F. (2010). *Statistics and data analysis for nursing research* (2nd ed.). Upper Saddle River, NJ: Pearson.

Polit, D. F., & Yang, F. (2016). *Measurement and the measurement of change*. Philadelphia, PA: Wolters Kluwer.

Temple B., Farley T., Popik K., et al. (2016). Prevalence of Parastomal Hernia and Factors Associated With Its Development. *Journal of Wound Ostomy & Continence Nursing*, *43*(5), 489–493.

Wilson R. A., Watt-Watson J., Hodnett E., & Tranmer J. (2016). A Randomized Controlled Trial of an Individualized Preoperative Education Intervention for Symptom Management After Total Knee Arthroplasty. *Orthopedic Nursing*, *35*(1), 20–29.

Wong M., Saari M., Patterson E., et al. (2017). Occupational hazards for home care nurses across the rural-to-urban gradient in Ontario, Canada. *Health & Social Care in the Community*, *25*(3), 1276–1286.

*A link to this open-access article is provided in the Internet Resources section on the**Point** website.

This journal article is available on the Point** for this chapter.

15 Interpretation and Clinical Significance in Quantitative Research

Learning Objectives

On completing this chapter, you will be able to:

● Describe dimensions for interpreting quantitative research results
● Describe the mindset conducive to a critical interpretation of research results
● Identify approaches to an assessment of the credibility of quantitative results and undertake such an assessment
● Distinguish statistical and clinical significance
● Identify some methods of drawing conclusions about clinical significance at the group and individual levels
● Critique researchers' interpretation of their results in a discussion section of a report
● Define new terms in the chapter

Key Terms

● Benchmark
● Change score
● Clinical significance
● CONSORT guidelines
● Minimal important change (MIC)
● Null hypothesis
● Research hypothesis
● Results

In this chapter, we consider approaches to interpreting researchers' statistical results, which require consideration of the various theoretical, methodological, and practical decisions that researchers make in undertaking a study. We also discuss an important but seldom discussed topic: clinical significance.

INTERPRETATION OF QUANTITATIVE RESULTS

Statistical **results** are summarized in the "Results" section of a research article. Researchers present their *interpretations* of the results in the "Discussion" section. Since researchers are seldom totally objective, you should develop your own interpretations.

Aspects of Interpretation

Interpreting study results involves attending to six different but overlapping considerations, which intersect with the "Questions for Appraising the Evidence" presented in Box 2.1:

● The credibility and accuracy of the results
● The precision of the estimate of effects
● The magnitude of effects and importance of the results

- The meaning of the results, especially about causality
- The generalizability of the results
- The implications of the results for nursing practice, theory development, or further research

Before discussing these considerations, we want to remind you about the role of inference in research thinking and interpretation.

Inference and Interpretation

An *inference* involves drawing conclusions based on limited information using logical reasoning. Interpreting research findings involves making multiple inferences. In research, virtually everything is a "stand-in" for something else. A sample is a representation of a population, a scale score is a proxy for the magnitude of an abstract attribute, and so on.

Research findings are meant to reflect "truth in the real world"—the findings are "stand-ins" for the true state of affairs (Fig. 15.1). Inferences about the real world are acceptable on condition that the researchers have selected appropriate proxies and have controlled sources of bias. This chapter offers several vantage points for assessing whether study findings really do reflect "truth in the real world."

The Interpretive Mindset

Evidence-based practice (EBP) involves integrating research evidence into clinical decision making. EBP encourages clinicians to think critically about clinical practice and to challenge the status quo when it conflicts with "best evidence." Interpreters of research are asked to think critically and demand high-quality evidence. Just as clinicians should ask, "What *evidence* is there that this intervention will be beneficial?" so must interpreters ask, "What *evidence* is there that the results are real and true"?

To be a good interpreter of research results, you can profit by starting with a sceptical ("show me") attitude and a null hypothesis. *The* null hypothesis *in interpretation is that the results are wrong and the evidence is flawed.* The "research hypothesis" is that the evidence reflects the truth. Interpreters decide whether the null hypothesis has merit by critically examining methodologic evidence. The greater the evidence that the researcher's design and methods were sound, the more likely that the null hypothesis can be rejected and the evidence is accepted to be accurate.

CREDIBILITY OF QUANTITATIVE RESULTS

A critical interpretive task is to assess whether the results are *right*. This corresponds to the first question in Box 2.1: "What is the quality of the evidence—that is, how rigorous and reliable is it?" If the results are not judged to be credible, the remaining interpretive issues (the meaning, magnitude, precision, generalizability, and implications of results) are unlikely to be relevant.

A credibility assessment requires a careful analysis of the study's methodologic and conceptual limitations and strengths. To come to a conclusion about whether the results closely approximate "truth in the real world," each aspect of the study—its design, sampling plan, data collection, and analyses—must be subjected to critical examination.

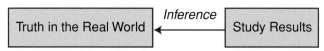

Figure 15.1 Inferences in interpreting research results.

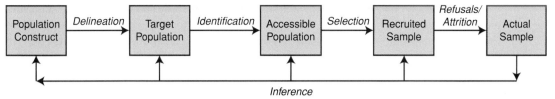

Figure 15.2 Inferences about populations: From final sample to the population.

There are various ways to approach the issue of credibility, including the use of the critiquing guidelines we have offered throughout this book and the overall critiquing protocol presented in Table 4.1. We share some additional perspectives in this section.

Proxies and Interpretation

Researchers begin with constructs and then devise ways to operationalize them. The constructs are linked to actual research strategies in a series of approximations; the results are more credible when better proxies are used. In this section, we illustrate successive proxies using sampling concepts to highlight the potential for inferential challenges.

When researchers formulate research questions, the population of interest is often abstract. For example, suppose we wanted to test the effectiveness of an intervention to increase physical activity in low-income women. Figure 15.2 shows the series of steps between the abstract population construct (low-income women) and actual study participants. Using data from the actual sample on the far right, the researcher would like to make inferences about the effectiveness of the intervention for a broader group, but each proxy along the way represents a potential problem for achieving the desired inference. In interpreting a study, readers must consider how *plausible* it is that the actual sample reflects the recruited sample, the accessible population, the target population, and the population construct.

Table 15.1 presents a description of a hypothetical scenario in which the researchers moved from the population construct (low-income women) to a sample of 161 participants

TABLE 15.1 Example of Successive Series of Proxies in Sampling

Element	Description	Possible Inferential Challenges
Population construct	Low-income women	
Target population	All women who receive public assistance (cash welfare) in the province of New Brunswick	Why only welfare recipients—why not the working poor? Why not those on disability? Why California?
Accessible population	All women who receive public assistance in Fredericton and who speak English or French	Why Fredericton? What about non-English/non-French speakers?
Recruited sample	A consecutive sample of 300 female welfare recipients (English or French speaking) who applied for benefits in January 2017 at two randomly selected welfare offices in Fredericton	Why only new applicants—what about women with long-term receipt? Why only two offices? Are these representative? Is January a typical month?
Actual sample	161 women from the recruited sample who fully participated in the study	Who refused to participate (or was too ill, etc.)? Who dropped out of the study?

(recent welfare recipients from two neighbourhoods in Fredericton). The table identifies questions that could be asked in drawing inferences about the study results. Answers to these questions would affect the interpretation of whether the intervention *really* is effective with low-income women—or only with recent welfare recipients in Fredericton who were cooperative.

Researchers make methodologic decisions that affect inferences, and these decisions must be examined. However, prospective participants' behaviour also needs to be considered. In our example, 300 women were recruited for the study, but only 161 provided data. The final sample of 161 almost surely would differ in important ways from the 139 who declined, and these differences affect the study evidence.

Fortunately, researchers are increasingly documenting participant flow in their studies—especially in intervention studies. Guidelines called the Consolidated Standards of Reporting Trials or **CONSORT guidelines** have been adopted by major medical and nursing journals to help readers track study participants. CONSORT flow charts, when available, should be scrutinized in interpreting study results. Figure 15.3 provides an example of such a flowchart

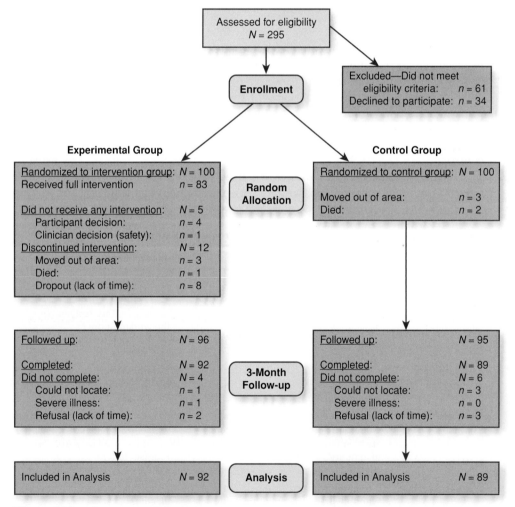

Figure 15.3 Example of CONSORT guidelines flowchart: Progression of participants in an intervention study.

for a randomized controlled trial (RCT). The chart shows that 295 people were assessed for eligibility, but 95 either did not meet eligibility criteria or refused to be in the study. Of the 200 study participants, half were randomized to the experimental group and the other half to the control group ($N = 100$ in each group). However, only 83 in the intervention group actually received the full intervention. At the 3-month follow-up, researchers attempted to obtain data from 96 people in the intervention group (everyone who did not move or die). They did get follow-up data from 92 in the intervention group, and these 92 comprised the analysis sample.

Credibility and Validity

Inference and validity are closely linked. To be careful interpreters, readers must search for evidence that the desired inferences are, in fact, valid. Part of this process involves considering alternative competing hypotheses about the credibility and meaning of the results.

In Chapter 9, we discussed four types of validity that relate to the credibility of study results: statistical conclusion validity, internal validity, external validity, and construct validity. We use our sampling example (Fig. 15.2 and Table 15.1) to demonstrate the relevance of methodologic decisions to all four types of validity—and hence to inferences about study results.

In our example, the population construct is *low-income women*, which was translated into population eligibility criteria for New Brunswick social assistance program recipients. Yet, there are alternative operationalizations of the population construct (e.g., New Brunswick women living below the official poverty level). Construct validity involves inferences from the particulars of the study to higher order and abstract constructs. So it is fair to ask: Do the eligibility criteria adequately capture the population construct, low-income women?

Statistical conclusion validity—the extent to which correct inferences can be made about the existence of "real" group differences—is also affected by sampling decisions. Ideally, researchers would do a power analysis at the beginning to estimate how large a sample they need. In our example, let us assume (based on previous research) that the effect size for the exercise intervention would be small to moderate, with $d = .40$. For a power of .80, with risk of a Type I error set at .05, we would need a sample of about 200 participants. The actual sample of 161 yields a nearly 30% risk of a Type II error (i.e., wrongly concluding that the intervention was not successful).

External validity—the generalizability of the results—is affected by sampling. To whom would it be fair to generalize the results in this example—to the population construct of low-income women? To all welfare recipients in New Brunswick? To all new welfare recipients in Moncton who speak English or French? Inferences about the extent to which the study results correspond to "truth in the real world" must take sampling decisions and sampling problems (e.g., recruitment difficulties) into account.

Finally, the study's internal validity (the extent to which a causal inference can be made) is also affected by sample composition. In this example, attrition would be a concern. Were those in the intervention group more likely (or less likely) than those in the control group to drop out of the study? If so, any observed differences in outcomes could be caused by individual differences in the groups (e.g., differences in motivation) rather than by the intervention itself.

Methodologic decisions and the careful implementation of those decisions—whether they be about sampling, intervention design, measurement, research design, or analysis—inevitably affect the rigor of a study. And all of them can affect the four types of validity and hence the interpretation of the results.

TABLE 15.2 Selected List of Major Biases or Errors in Quantitative Studies in Four Research Domains

Research Design	Sampling	Measurement	Analysis
Expectation bias	Sampling error	Social desirability bias	Type I error
Hawthorne effect	Volunteer bias	Acquiescence bias	Type II error
Contamination of treatments	Non-response bias	Naysayers bias	
Carryover effects		Extreme response bias	
Non-compliance bias		Recall/memory bias	
Selection bias		Reactivity	
Attrition bias		Observer biases	
History bias			

Credibility and Bias

A researcher's job is to translate abstract constructs into appropriate proxies. Another major effort is to eliminate, reduce, or control biases—or, as a last resort, to detect and understand them. As a reader of research reports, your job is to look for biases and to consider them into your assessment about the credibility of the results.

Biases create distortions and undermine researchers' efforts to reveal "truth in the real world." Biases are pervasive and virtually inevitable. It is important to consider what types of bias might be present and how extensive, sizeable, and systematic they are. We have discussed many types of bias in this book—some reflect design inadequacies (e.g., selection bias), others reflect recruitment problems (non-response bias), and others relate to measurement (social desirability). Table 15.2 presents biases and errors mentioned in this book. This table is meant to serve as a reminder of some of the problems to consider in interpreting study results.

 TIP The supplement to this chapter on thePoint website includes a longer list of biases, including some not described in this book; we offer definitions for all biases listed. Different disciplines, and different writers, use different names for the same or similar biases. The actual names are unimportant—but it is important to reflect on how different forces can distort results and affect inferences.

Credibility and Corroboration

Earlier, we noted that research interpreters should seek evidence to reject the "null hypothesis" that research results are wrong. The potential to discredit this null hypothesis depends on the quality of the proxies that stand in for abstractions, effort to rule out biases, and corroboration for the results.

Corroboration can come from internal and external sources, and the concept of *replication* is an important one in both cases. Interpretations are aided by considering prior research on the topic, for example. Interpreters can examine whether the study results are similar to those of other studies. Consistency across studies tends to discredit the "null hypothesis" of erroneous results.

Researchers may have opportunities for replication themselves. For example, in multisite studies, if the results are similar across sites, this suggests that something "real" is occurring. Triangulation can be another form of replication. We are strong advocates of mixed-methods studies (see Chapter 13). When findings from the analysis of qualitative data are consistent with the results of statistical analyses, internal corroboration can be especially powerful and persuasive.

OTHER ASPECTS OF INTERPRETATION

If an assessment leads you to accept that the results of a study are probably "real," you have made important progress in interpreting the study findings. Other interpretive tasks depend on a conclusion that the results are likely credible.

Precision of the Results

Results from statistical hypothesis tests indicate whether a relationship or group difference is probably "real." A p value in hypothesis testing offers information that is important (whether the null hypothesis is probably false) but incomplete. Confidence intervals (CIs), by contrast, communicate information about how precise the study results are. Dr. David Sackett (2000), a founding father of the EBP movement, and his colleagues said this about CIs: "P values on their own are…not informative…. By contrast, CIs indicate the strength of evidence about quantities of direct interest, such as treatment benefit. They are thus of particular relevance to practitioners of evidence-based medicine" (p. 232). It seems likely that nurse researchers will increasingly report CI information in the years ahead because of its value for interpreting study results and assessing their utility for nursing practice.

Magnitude of Effects and Importance

In quantitative studies, results that support the researcher's hypotheses are described as *significant*. A careful analysis of study results involves evaluating whether, in addition to being statistically significant, the effects are large and clinically important.

Attaining statistical significance does not necessarily mean that the results are meaningful to nurses and clients. Statistical significance indicates that the results are unlikely to be due to chance—not that they are important. With large samples, even modest relationships are statistically significant. For instance, with a sample of 500, a correlation coefficient of 0.10 is significant at the 0.05 level, but a relationship this weak may have little practical relevance. This issue concerns an important EBP question (Box 2.1): "What *is* the evidence—what is the magnitude of effects?" Estimating the magnitude and importance of effects is relevant to the issue of clinical significance, a topic we discuss later in this chapter.

The Meaning of Quantitative Results

In quantitative studies, researchers and consumers must interpret statistical results in the form of p values, effect sizes, and CIs. Questions about the meaning of statistical results often reflect a desire to draw the conclusion about causal connections. Interpreting what descriptive results mean is not typically a challenge. For example, suppose we found that, among patients undergoing electroconvulsive therapy (ECT), the percentage who experiences an ECT-induced headache is 59.4% (95% CI [56.3, 63.1]). This result is directly interpretable. But if we found that headache prevalence is significantly lower in a cryotherapy intervention group than among patients given acetaminophen, we would need to interpret what the results mean. In particular, we need to interpret whether it is plausible that cryotherapy *caused* the reduced prevalence of headaches. In this section, we discuss the interpretation of research outcomes within a hypothesis testing context, with an emphasis on causal interpretations.

Interpreting Hypothesized Results

Interpreting statistical results is easiest when hypotheses are supported (i.e., when there are *positive results*). Researchers have already considered prior findings and theory in developing hypotheses. Nevertheless, a few limitations should be kept in mind.

It is important to avoid the temptation of going beyond the data to explain what results mean. For example, suppose we hypothesized that pregnant women's anxiety levels about childbearing are correlated with the number of children they have. The data reveal a significant negative relationship between anxiety levels and parity ($r =-0.40$). We interpret this to mean that increased experience with childbirth results in decreased anxiety. Is this conclusion supported by the data? The conclusion appears logical, but in fact, there is nothing in the data that leads to this interpretation. An important—indeed, critical—research principle is that *correlation does not prove causation*. The finding that two variables are related offers no evidence suggesting which of the two variables—if either—caused the other. In our example, perhaps causality runs in the opposite direction (i.e., a woman's anxiety level influences how many children she bears). Or maybe a third variable, such as the woman's relationship with her husband, influences both anxiety and number of children. Inferring causality is especially difficult in studies that have not used an experimental design.

Empirical evidence supporting research hypotheses does not provide a direct *proof* of the truth. Hypothesis testing is probabilistic. There is always a possibility that observed relationships resulted from chance—that is, that a Type I error has occurred. Researchers must be cautious about their results and about interpretations of them. Thus, even when the results are in line with expectations, researchers should draw conclusions with restraint.

Example of corroboration of a hypothesis • • • • • • • • • • • • • • • • • • •
Houck et al. (2011) studied factors associated with self-concept in 145 children with attention-deficit hyperactivity disorder (ADHD). They hypothesized that behaviour problems in these children would be associated with less favourable self-concept, and they found that internalizing behaviour problems were significantly predictive of lower self-concept scores. In their discussion, they stated that "age and internalizing behaviors were found to negatively influence the child's self-concept" (p. 245).

This study is a good example to discuss the challenges of interpreting findings in correlational studies. The researchers' interpretation was that behaviour problems *influenced* ("caused") low self-concept. This conclusion is supported by earlier research, yet there is nothing in the data that would rule out the possibility that a child's self-concept *influenced* their behaviour or that some other factor influenced both behaviour and self-concept. The researchers' interpretation is plausible, but their cross-sectional design makes it difficult to rule out other explanations. A major threat to the internal validity of the inference in this study is temporal ambiguity.

Interpreting Non-significant Results

Non-significant results pose interpretative challenges. Statistical tests are designed to disconfirm the null hypothesis. Failure to reject a null hypothesis can occur for many reasons, and the real reason may be hard to figure out.

The null hypothesis *could* actually be true, accurately reflecting the absence of a relationship among research variables. On the other hand, the null hypothesis could be false.

Retention of a false null hypothesis (a Type II error) can result from such methodologic problems as poor internal validity, an abnormal sample, a weak statistical procedure, or unreliable measures. In particular, failure to reject null hypotheses is often a consequence of insufficient power, usually reflecting too small a sample size.

It is important to recognize that a null hypothesis that is not rejected does not confirm the *absence* of relationships among variables. *Non-significant results provide no evidence of the truth or the falsity of the hypothesis.*

Because statistical procedures are designed to reject null hypotheses, they are not well suited for testing *actual* research hypotheses about the absence of relationships or about equivalence between groups. However, sometimes this is exactly what researchers want to do, especially in clinical situations in which the goal is to test whether one practice is as effective as another but perhaps less painful or costly. When the actual research hypothesis is null (e.g., a prediction of *no* group difference), additional strategies must be used to provide supporting evidence. It is useful to compute effect sizes or CIs to illustrate that the risk of a Type II error was small.

Example of support for a hypothesized nonsignificant result · · · · · · · · · ·
Thiessen et al. (2016) conducted a trial to test the hypothesis that maternal and neonatal outcomes were similar for low-risk births attended by registered midwives, obstetricians/gynaecologists, or family practice physicians in Winnipeg, Manitoba. A total of 83,774 births were reviewed. Analyses showed that midwives (0.13 [0.10–0.16]) and family practice physicians (0.44 [0.40–0.48]) had lower odds of caesarean delivery than OB/GYN–attended births. There were no significant differences in clinical outcomes between midwifery care and care provided by family practice physicians.

Interpreting Unhypothesized Significant Results

Unhypothesized significant results can occur in two situations. The first involves exploring relationships that were not considered during the design of the study. For example, in examining correlations among research variables, a researcher might notice that two variables that were not central to the research questions were nevertheless significantly correlated—and interesting.

Example of a serendipitous significant finding · · · · · · · · · · · · · · · · · ·
Latendresse and Ruiz (2011) studied the relationship between chronic maternal stress and preterm birth. They reported an unexpected finding that maternal use of selective serotonin reuptake inhibitors (SSRIs) was associated with a 12-fold increase in preterm births.

The second situation is more puzzling and happens infrequently: obtaining results *opposite* to those hypothesized. For instance, a researcher might hypothesize that individualized teaching about AIDS risks is more effective than group instruction, but the results might indicate that the group method was significantly better. Although this might seem disconcerting, research should not be undertaken to corroborate predictions but rather to arrive at truth. There is no such thing as a study whose results "came out wrong" if they reflect the truth. When significant findings are opposite to what was hypothesized, the interpretation should involve comparisons with other research, a consideration of alternate theories, and a critical scrutiny of the research methods.

Example of a significant result contrary to hypothesis • • • • • • • • • • • • •
Dotson et al. (2014), who tested hypotheses about nurse retention with a sample of 861 registered nurses (RNs), predicted that higher levels of altruism would be associated with stronger intentions to stay in nursing; however, the opposite was found. They speculated that this might mean that some nurses "are no longer experiencing the fulfillment of their altruistic desires in the field of nursing" (p. 115).

In summary, interpreting the meaning of research results is a demanding task, but it offers the possibility of intellectual rewards. Interpreters must play the role of scientific detectives, trying to make pieces of the puzzle fit together to get a coherent picture.

Generalizability of the Results

Researchers typically seek evidence that can be used by others. If a new nursing intervention is found to be successful, others might want to adopt it. Therefore, another interpretive question is whether the intervention will "work" or whether the relationships will "hold" in other settings, with other people. Part of the interpretive process involves asking the question, "To what groups, environments, and conditions can the results reasonably be applied?"

Implications of the Results

Once you have reached conclusions about the credibility, precision, importance, meaning, and generalizability of the results, you are ready to think about their implications. You might consider the implications of the findings with respect to future research: What should other researchers in this area do—what is the right "next step"? You are most likely to consider the implications for nursing practice: How should the results be used by nurses in their practice?

All of the interpretive dimensions we have discussed are critical in evidence-based nursing practice. With regard to generalizability, it may not be enough to ask a broad question about to whom the results could apply—you need to ask: Are these results relevant to *my* particular clinical situation? Of course, if you have concluded that the results have limited credibility or importance, they may be of little utility to your practice.

CLINICAL SIGNIFICANCE

It has long been recognized that statistical hypothesis testing provides limited information for interpretation purposes. In particular, attaining statistical significance does not address the question of whether a finding is clinically meaningful or relevant. With a large enough sample, a trivial relationship can be statistically significant. Broadly speaking, we define **clinical significance** as the practical importance of research results in terms of whether they have undisputable, real effects on the daily lives of patients or on the health care decisions made on their behalf.

In fields other than nursing, notably in medicine and psychotherapy, recent attention has been paid to defining clinical significance and developing ways to operationalize it. There has been no consensus on either front, but a few conceptual and statistical solutions are being used with some regularity. In this section, we provide a brief overview of recent advances in defining and operationalizing clinical significance; further information is available in Polit and Yang (2016).

In statistical hypothesis testing, consensus was reached decades ago that a p value of 0.05 would be the standard for statistical significance. It is unlikely that a uniform standard will ever be adopted for clinical significance because of its complexity. For example, in some cases, *no change* over time could be clinically significant if it means that a group with a progressive disease has not deteriorated. In other cases, clinical significance is associated with improvements. Another issue concerns is whose *perspective* on clinical significance is relevant. Sometimes clinicians' perspectives are key because of implications for health management (e.g., regarding cholesterol levels). For other outcomes, the patient's view is what matters (e.g., about quality of life). Two other issues concern whether clinical significance is for group-level findings or about individual patients and whether clinical significance is attached to point-in-time outcomes or to change scores. Most recent work is about the clinical significance of **change scores** for individual patients (e.g., a change from a baseline measurement to a follow-up measurement). We begin, however, with a brief discussion of group-level clinical significance.

Clinical Significance at the Group Level

Many studies concern group-level comparisons. For example, one-group pretest–posttest designs involve comparing a group at two or more points in time to examine whether or not a change in outcomes has occurred. In RCTs and case-control studies, the central comparison is about average differences for different groups of people. Group-level clinical significance (which is sometimes called *practical significance*) typically involves using statistical information other than *p* values to draw conclusions about the usefulness of research findings. The most widely used statistics for this purpose are effect size (ES) indexes, CIs, and number needed to treat (NNT).

ES indexes summarize the magnitude of a change or a relationship and thus provide insights into how a group, *on average*, might benefit from a treatment. In most cases, a clinically significant finding at the group level means that the ES is sufficiently large to have relevance for patients. CIs are also useful tools for understanding clinical significance; CIs provide the most plausible range of values, at a given level of confidence, for the unknown population parameter. Some researchers promote NNTs as useful indicators of clinical significance because the information is relatively easy to understand. For example, if the NNT for an important outcome is found to be 2.0, only two patients have to receive a particular treatment in order for one patient to benefit. If the NNT is 10.0, however, 9 patients out of 10 receiving the treatment would get no benefit.

With any of these group-level indexes, researchers should designate in advance what would constitute clinical significance—just as they would establish an alpha value for statistical significance. For example, would an ES of 0.20 (for the *d* index described in Chapter 14) be considered clinically significant? A *d* of 0.20 has been described as a "small" effect, but sometimes, small improvements can have clinical relevance. Claims about attainment of clinical significance for groups should be based on defensible criteria.

> **Example of clinical significance at the group level** · · · · · · · · · · · · · · · · ·
> Despriee and Langeland (2016) tested the effect of 30% sucrose compared with a placebo (water) on relieving pain during the immunization of 15-month-old children. The mean group difference of 15 fewer seconds of crying among infants in the intervention group was statistically significant. The large ES led the researchers to conclude that the improvement was also clinically significant.

Clinical Significance at the Individual Level

Clinicians usually are not interested in what happens in a *group* of people—they are concerned with individual patients. As noted in Chapter 2, a key goal in EBP is to personalize "best evidence" into decisions for a specific patient's needs, within a particular clinical context.

Efforts to come to conclusions about clinical significance at the individual level can be directly linked to EBP goals.

Dozens of approaches to defining and operationalizing clinical significance at the individual level have been developed, but they share one thing in common: They involve establishing a **benchmark** (or *threshold*) that corresponds to the score value on a measure (or the value of a change score) that suggests clinical significance. With an established benchmark, each person in a study can be classified as having or not having a score or change score that is clinically significant.

Conceptual Definitions of Clinical Significance

Numerous definitions of clinical significance can be found in the health literature, most of which concern changes in measures of patient outcomes (e.g., a score at Time 1 subtracted from a score at Time 2). One approach to conceptualizing clinical significance dominates medical fields. In a paper cited hundreds of times in the medical literature, Jaeschke, Singer, and Guyatt (1989) offered the following definition: "The minimal clinically important difference (MCID) can be defined as the smallest difference in score in the domain of interest which patients perceive as beneficial and which would mandate, in the absence of troublesome side effects and excessive cost, a change in the patient's management" (p. 408). Although these researchers referred to the conceptual threshold for clinical significance as a minimal clinically important *difference* (MCID), we follow an influential group of measurement experts in using the term **minimal important change (MIC)** because the focus is on individual change scores, not differences between groups.

Operationalizing Clinical Significance: Establishing the Minimal Important Change Benchmark

The Jaeschke et al. (1989) definition regarding change score benchmarks has inspired researchers to go in many different directions to quantify it. Broadly speaking, the MIC benchmark is usually operationalized as a value for the amount of change in score points on a measure that an individual patient must achieve to be considered as having a clinically important change.

A traditional approach to setting a benchmark for health outcomes is to obtain input from a panel of health care experts—sometimes called a *consensus panel*. For example, a consensus panel convened in 2005 to establish the clinical significance of changes in self-reported pain intensity (e.g., on a visual analogue scale) established the benchmark as a 30% reduction in pain.

Another approach is to undertake a study to determine what patients themselves think is a minimally important change on a focal measure. The developers of many new multi-item scales now make efforts to estimate the MIC as part of the psychometric assessment of their instrument. Calculating an MIC using this type of approach requires a careful research design with a large sample of people and their scores on the instrument are expected to change over time.

A third approach to defining the MIC is based on the distributional characteristics of a measure. Most often, the MIC using this approach is set to a threshold of 0.5 *SDs*—that is, one-half a standard deviation (*SD*) on a distribution of baseline scores. For example, if the baseline *SD* for a scale were 6.0, then the MIC using the 0.5 *SD* criterion would be 3.0. This value, like any MIC, can be used as the benchmark to classify individual patients as having or not having experienced clinically meaningful change.

Many researchers have used the MIC to interpret group-level findings. The MIC is, however, an index of *individual* change, not group differences. Experts have warned that it is inappropriate to interpret mean differences in relation to the MIC. For example, if the MIC on an important outcome has been established as 4.0, this value should not be used to interpret the clinical significance of the mean difference between two groups. If the mean group difference were found to be 3.0, for instance, it would be wrong to conclude that the results were not clinically significant. A mean difference of 3.0 suggests that a sizeable percentage of participants *did* achieve a clinically meaningful benefit—an improvement of 4 points or more.

MIC thresholds can be used to calculate rates of clinical significance for individual study participants. Once the MIC is known, researchers can classify all people in a study to indicate whether they have attained or not attained the threshold. Then, researchers can compare the percentage of people who "responded" at clinically important levels in the study groups (e.g., those in the intervention and those in the control group). Such a *responder analysis* is easy to understand and has strong implications for EBP.

Example of a responder analysis ·
Lima et al. (2015) examined blood pressure responses to walking and resistance exercise in patients with peripheral artery disease. The researchers used a previously established MIC of a 4 mm Hg decrease in diastolic or systolic blood pressure to classify participants. Chi-squared analysis and *t*-tests were used to compare the clinical characteristics of responders (those who benefited at clinically significant levels from exercise) and non-responders.

CRITIQUING INTERPRETATIONS

Researchers offer an interpretation of their findings and discuss what the findings might imply for nursing in the discussion section of research articles. When critiquing a study, your own interpretation can be contrasted against those of the researchers.

A good discussion section should point out study limitations. Researchers are in the best position to detect and assess sampling deficiencies, practical constraints, data quality problems, and so on, and it is a professional responsibility to alert readers to these difficulties. Also, when researchers acknowledge methodologic shortcomings, readers know that these limitations were considered in interpreting the results. Of course, researchers are unlikely to note all relevant limitations. Your task as reviewer is to develop your own interpretation and assessment of methodologic problems, challenge conclusions that do not appear to be warranted, and consider how the study's evidence could have been enhanced.

You should also carefully scrutinize causal interpretations, especially in non-experimental studies. Sometimes, even the titles of reports suggest a potentially inappropriate causal inference. If the title of a non-experimental study includes terms like "the effect of … " or "the impact of …, " this may signal the need for critical scrutiny of the researcher's inferences.

In addition to comparing your interpretation with that of the researchers, your critique should also draw conclusions about the stated implications of the study. Some researchers make grandiose claims or offer unfounded recommendations on the basis of modest results.

Our discussion of clinical significance is a new topic in this edition of our book. The conceptualization and operationalization of clinical significance have not received much attention in nursing, and so studies that do not mention clinical significance should not be faulted for this omission. We hope that nurse researchers will pay more attention to this issue in the years ahead.

Some guidelines for evaluating researchers' interpretation are offered in Box 15.1.

Box 15.1 Guidelines for Critiquing Interpretations/Discussions in Quantitative Research Reports

Interpretation of the Findings
1. Were all the important results discussed?
2. Did the researchers discuss any study limitations and their possible effects on the credibility of the findings? Did the interpretations take limitations into account?
3. What types of evidence were offered in support of the interpretation, and was that evidence persuasive? Were results interpreted in light of findings from other studies?
4. Did the researchers make any unjustifiable causal inferences? Were alternative explanations for the findings considered? Were the rationales for rejecting these alternatives convincing?
5. Did the interpretation take into account the precision of the results and/or the magnitude of effects?
6. Did the researchers draw any unwarranted conclusions about the generalizability of the results?

Implications of the Findings and Recommendations
7. Did the researchers discuss the study's implications for clinical practice or future nursing research? Did they make specific recommendations?
8. If yes, are the stated implications appropriate, given the study's limitations and the magnitude of the effects as well as evidence from other studies? Are there important implications that the report neglected to include?

Clinical Significance
9. Did the researchers mention or assess clinical significance? Did they make a distinction between statistical and clinical significance?
10. If clinical significance was examined, was it assessed in terms of group-level information (e.g., effect sizes) or individual-level results? If the latter, how was clinical significance operationalized?

RESEARCH EXAMPLES WITH CRITICAL THINKING EXERCISES

In this section, we provide details about the interpretive portion of a quantitative study. Read the summary and then answer the critical thinking questions that follow, referring to the full research report if necessary. Example 1 is featured on the interactive *Critical Thinking Activity* on thePoint website. The critical thinking questions for Examples 2 and 3 are based on the studies that appear in their entirety in Appendices A and C of this book. Our comments for Example 2 are in the Student Resources section on thePoint.

EXAMPLE 1: INTERPRETATION IN A QUANTITATIVE STUDY

Study: Neurobehavioural effects of aspartame consumption (Lindseth et al., 2014)

Statement of Purpose: The purpose of this study was to examine the effects of consuming diets with higher amounts of aspartame (25 mg/kg body weight/day) versus lower amounts of aspartame (10 mg/kg body weight/day) on neurobehavioural outcomes.

Method: The researchers used a randomized crossover design to assess the effects of aspartame amounts. Study participants were 28 healthy adults, university students, who consumed study-prepared diets. Participants were randomized to orderings of the aspartame protocol (i.e., some received the high-aspartame diet first; others received the low amount first). Participants were blinded to which diet they were receiving, and data collectors were also blinded. They consumed one of the diets for an 8-day period, followed by a 2-week washout period. Then, they consumed the alternative diet for another 8 days. At the end of each 8-day session, measurements were made for neurobehavioural outcomes, including cognition (working memory and spatial visualization), depression, and mood (irritability).

Analyses: Within-subjects tests (paired *t*-tests, repeated-measures analysis of variance [ANOVA]) were used to test the statistical significance of differences in outcomes for the two dietary protocols, with alpha set at 0.05. In terms of clinical significance, a participant was considered to have a clinically significant neurobehavioural effect if his or her score was 2+ *SD*s outside the mean score for normal functioning based on norms for each measure. Thus, change scores for participants were not computed. Rather, each score was assessed for crossing the benchmark value for a normative state—a criterion that has been frequently used in trials of psychotherapeutic interventions.

Results: Statistically significant differences, favouring the low-aspartame diet, were observed for three neurobehavioural outcomes: spatial orientation, depression, and irritability. Despite the fact that the participants were healthy adult students, a few of them experienced clinically significant outcomes in the high-aspartame condition. For example, two participants had clinically significant cognitive impairment (two with working memory deficits and two others with spatial orientation impairment) after 8 days of consuming the high-aspartame diet. Three other participants (different from the four with cognitive impairment) had clinically relevant levels of depression at the end of the high-aspartame condition. None of the participants' scores was clinically significant after 8 days on the low-aspartame diet.

Discussion: The researchers devoted a large portion of their discussion section to the issue of *corroboration*, which we mentioned in connection with effects to interpret the credibility of study results. They pointed out ways in which their findings were consistent with (or diverged from) other studies on the effects of aspartame. In keeping with the researchers' use of a strong experimental design, they concluded that there was a causal relationship between high amounts of aspartame consumption and negative neurobehavioural effects: "A high dose of aspartame caused more irritability and depression than a low-aspartame dose consumed by the same participants, supporting earlier study findings by Walton et al. (1993)" (p. 191). The researchers also commented on the clinical significance findings: "Additionally, three participants in our study scored in the clinically depressed category while consuming the high-aspartame diet, despite no previous histories of depression" (p. 191). The researchers concluded their discussion section with remarks about the limitations of their study, which included problems of generalizability: "Limitations of our study included the small homogeneous sample, which may make it difficult to apply our conclusions to other study populations. Also, our sample size of 28 participants resulted in statistical power of .72, which is on the lower end of the acceptable range. A washout period before the baseline assessments and using food diaries during the between-treatment washout period to verify that aspartame was not consumed would have strengthened the design" (p. 191).

Critical Thinking Exercises

1. Answer the relevant questions from Box 15.1 regarding this study. (We encourage you to read the report in its entirety, especially the discussion, to answer these questions.)
2. Also consider the following targeted questions:
   a. Is the statistical conclusion about this study appropriate?
   b. Would this study benefit from the inclusion of a CONSORT-type flow chart?
3. How could these findings be used in clinical practice?

EXAMPLE 2: DISCUSSION SECTION IN THE STUDY IN APPENDIX A

● Read the "Discussion" section of Swenson and colleagues' (2016) study ("Parents' use of praise and criticism in a sample of young children seeking mental health services") in Appendix A of this book.

Critical Thinking Exercises

1. Answer the relevant questions from Box 15.1 regarding this study.
2. Also consider the following targeted questions:
   a. Was a CONSORT-type flow chart used in this study? If not, was information about participant flow provided in the text?
   b. Can you think of any limitations of this study that the researchers did not mention?

EXAMPLE 3: QUANTITATIVE STUDY IN APPENDIX C

● Read Wilson and colleagues' (2016) study ("A randomized controlled trial of an individualized preoperative education intervention for symptom management after total knee arthroplasty") in Appendix C, then address the following suggested activities or questions.

Critical Thinking Exercises

1. Before reading our critique, which accompanies the full report, write your own critique or prepare a list of what you think are the study's major strengths and weaknesses. Pay particular attention to validity threats and bias, then contrast your critique with ours. Remember that you (or your instructor) do not necessarily have to agree with all of the points made in our critique, and you may identify strengths and weaknesses that we overlooked. You may find the broad critiquing guidelines in Table 4.1 helpful.
2. Write a short summary of how credible, important, and generalizable you find the study results to be. Your summary should conclude with your interpretation of what the results mean and what their implications are for nursing practice. Contrast your summary with the discussion section in the report itself.
3. In selecting studies to include with this textbook, we deliberately chose a study with many strengths. In the following questions, we offer some "pretend" scenarios in which the researchers for the study in Appendix C made different methodologic decisions than the ones they in fact did make. Write a paragraph or two critiquing these "pretend" decisions, pointing out how these alternatives would have affected the rigor of the study and the inferences that could be made.
   a. Pretend that the researchers had been unable to randomize subjects to treatments. The design, in other words, would be a non-equivalent control group quasi-experiment.
   b. Pretend that 143 participants were randomized (this is actually what did happen) but that only 80 participants remained in the study at Time 3.

WANT TO KNOW MORE? >=

A wide variety of resources to enhance your learning and understanding of this chapter are available on thePoint.

- Interactive Critical Thinking Activity
- Chapter Supplement on Research Biases
- Answer to the Critical Thinking Exercise for Examples 2 and 3
- Internet Resources with useful websites for Chapter 15
- A Wolters Kluwer journal article on a topic related to this chapter

Summary Points

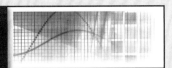

- The interpretation of quantitative research **results** (the outcomes of the statistical analyses) typically involves consideration of (1) the credibility of the results, (2) precision of estimates of effects, (3) magnitude of effects, (4) underlying meaning, (5) generalizability, and (6) implications for future research and nursing practice.
- The particulars of the study—especially the methodologic decisions made by researchers—affect the inferences that can be made about the correspondence between study results and "truth in the real world."
- A cautious outlook is appropriate in drawing conclusions about the credibility and meaning of study results.
- An assessment of a study's credibility can involve various approaches, one of which involves an evaluation of the degree of congruence between abstract constructs or idealized methods on the one hand and the proxies actually used on the other.
- Credibility assessments also involve an assessment of study rigor through an analysis of validity threats and biases that could undermine the accuracy of the results.
- Corroboration (replication) of results, through either internal or external sources, is another approach in a credibility assessment.

- Researchers can facilitate interpretations by carefully documenting methodologic decisions and the outcomes of those decisions (e.g., by using the **CONSORT guidelines** to document participant flow).
- Broadly speaking, **clinical significance** refers to the practical importance of research results—that is, whether the effects are genuine and palpable in the daily lives of patients or in the management of their health. Clinical significance has not received great attention in nursing research.
- Clinical significance for group-level results is often inferred on the basis of such statistics as effect size indexes, confidence intervals, and number needed to treat. However, clinical significance is most often discussed in terms of effects for individual patients—especially whether they have achieved a clinically meaningful change.
- Definitions and operationalizations of clinical significance for individuals typically involve a **benchmark** or threshold to designate a meaningful amount of change. This benchmark is often called a **MIC**, which is a value for the amount of change score points on a measure that an individual patient must achieve to be classified as having a clinically important change.
- MICs cannot legitimately be used to interpret group means or differences in means. However, the MIC can be used to ascertain

whether each person in a sample has or has not achieved a change greater than the MIC and then a *responder analysis* can be undertaken to compare the percentage of people meeting the threshold in different study groups.

● In their discussions of study results, researchers should themselves point out known study limitations, but readers should draw their own conclusions about the rigor of the study and about the plausibility of alternative explanations for the results.

REFERENCES

Despriee, Å., & Langeland, E. (2016). The effect of sucrose as pain relief/comfort during immunisation of 15-month-old children in health care centres: A randomised controlled trial. *Journal of Clinical Nursing, 25*, 372–380.

**Dotson, M. J., Dave, D., Cazier, J., & Spaulding, T. (2014). An empirical analysis of nurse retention: What keeps RNs in nursing? *The Journal of Nursing Administration, 44*, 111–116.

Houck, G., Kendall, J., Miller, A., Morrell, P., & Wiebe, G. (2011). Self-concept in children and adolescents with attention deficit hyperactivity disorder. *Journal of Pediatric Nursing, 26*, 239–247.

Jaeschke, R., Singer, J., & Guyatt, G. H. (1989). Measurement of health status: Ascertaining the minimal clinically important difference. *Controlled Clinical Trials, 10*, 407–415.

Latendresse, G., & Ruiz, R. (2011). Maternal corticotropin-releasing hormone and the use of selective serotonin reuptake inhibitors independently predict the occurrence of preterm birth. *Journal of Midwifery & Women's Health, 56*, 118–126.

Lima, A., Miranda, A., Correia, M., et al. (2015). Individual blood pressure responses to walking and resistance exercise in peripheral artery disease patients: Are the mean values describing what is happening? *Journal of Vascular Nursing, 33*, 150–156.

Lindseth, G. N., Coolahan, S., Petros, T., & Lindseth, P. (2014). Neurobehavioral effects of aspartame consumption. *Research in Nursing & Health, 37*, 185–193.

Polit, D. F., & Yang, F. M. (2016). Measurement and the measurement of change. Philadelphia, PA: Wolters Kluwer.

Sackett, D. L., Straus, S., Richardson, W., Rosenberg, W., & Haynes, R. (2000). Evidence-based medicine: How to practice and teach EBM (2nd ed.). Edinburgh: Churchill Livingstone.

Thiessen K., Nickel N., Prior H. J., et al. (2016). Maternity Outcomes in Manitoba Women: A Comparison between Midwifery-led Care and Physician-led Care at Birth. *Birth, 43*(2), 108–115.

*A link to this open-access article is provided in the Internet Resources section on the Point website.

**This journal article is available on the Point for this chapter.

16 Analysis of Qualitative Data

Learning Objectives

On completing this chapter, you will be able to:

- Describe activities that qualitative researchers perform to manage and organize their data
- Discuss the procedures used to analyze qualitative data, including both general procedures and those used in ethnographic, phenomenologic, and grounded theory research
- Assess the adequacy of researchers' descriptions of their analytic procedures and evaluate the suitability of those procedures
- Define new terms in the chapter

Key Terms

- Axial coding
- Basic social process (BSP)
- Central category
- Constant comparison
- Core category
- Domain
- Emergent fit
- Focused coding
- Hermeneutic circle
- Metaphor
- Open coding
- Paradigm case
- Qualitative content analysis
- Selective coding
- Substantive coding
- Taxonomy
- Theme
- Theoretical coding

Qualitative data are derived from narrative materials, such as transcripts from audiotaped interviews or participant observers' field notes. This chapter describes methods for analyzing such qualitative data.

INTRODUCTION TO QUALITATIVE ANALYSIS

Qualitative data analysis is challenging, for several reasons. First, there are no universal rules for analyzing qualitative data. A second challenge is the huge amount of work required. Qualitative analysts must organize and make sense of hundreds or even thousands of pages of narrative materials. Qualitative researchers typically examine their data carefully, often reviewing the data over and over in a search for understanding. Also, doing qualitative analysis requires creativity and strong inductive skills (inducing universals from particulars). A qualitative analyst must be skillful in identifying patterns and putting them together into an integrated whole.

Another challenge comes in reducing data for reporting purposes. Quantitative results can often be summarized in a few tables. Qualitative researchers, by contrast, must balance the need to be concise with the need to maintain the richness of their data.

 TIP Qualitative analyses are more difficult to *do* than quantitative ones, but qualitative findings are easier to understand than quantitative ones because the stories are told in everyday language. Qualitative analyses are often hard to critique, however, because readers cannot know if researchers adequately captured thematic patterns in the data.

QUALITATIVE DATA MANAGEMENT AND ORGANIZATION

Qualitative analysis is supported by several tasks that help to organize and manage the mass of narrative data.

Developing a Coding Scheme

Qualitative researchers begin their analysis by developing a method to classify and index their data. Researchers must be able to get to parts of the data without having repeatedly to reread the entire data set.

The usual procedure is to create a *coding scheme*, based on a careful review of actual data, and then code data according to the categories in the coding scheme. Developing a high-quality coding scheme involves a thorough reading of the data, with an eye to identifying underlying concepts. The nature of the codes may vary in level of detail, as well as in level of abstraction.

Researchers often use codes that are fairly concrete to describe and differentiate various types of actions or events, for example. In developing a coding scheme, related concepts are grouped together to facilitate the coding process.

Example of a descriptive coding scheme •
Ersek and Jablonski (2014) studied safety concerns in rural emergency department (ED) for older adults with dementia. Twelve interdisciplinary health care providers with experience working or consulting in the participating EDs participated in the interviews.
    The interviews were audio-recorded and transcribed. Data from individual transcripts were coded into broad categories, such as characteristics of physical environment such as department atmosphere, equipment, and space design.

Many studies, such as those designed to develop a theory, are more likely to involve the development of abstract, conceptual coding categories. In creating abstract categories, researchers break the data into segments, closely examine them, and compare them to other segments to uncover the meaning of those phenomena. The researcher asks questions such as the following about discrete statements: What is this? What is going on? What else is like this? What is this distinct from?

Important concepts that emerge from examining the data are then given a label. These names are abstractions, but the labels usually explicitly state the nature of the material—and are often provocative.

Example of an abstract coding scheme •
Box 16.1 shows the category scheme developed by Beck and Watson (2010) to code data from their interviews on childbirth after a previous traumatic birth (the full study is

in Appendix B). The coding scheme includes major thematic categories with subcodes. For example, an excerpt that described how a mother viewed this subsequent birth as healing because she felt respected during this subsequent labour and delivery would be coded 3A; the category is labelled "Treated with respect."

Coding Qualitative Data

After a coding scheme has been developed, the data are read in their entirety and coded into categories—a task that is not easy. Researchers may have difficulty deciding the most appropriate code, for example. It sometimes takes several readings of the material.

Also, researchers often discover during coding that the initial coding system was incomplete. Categories may emerge that were not initially identified. When this happens, it is risky to assume that the category was absent in previously coded materials. A concept might not be identified as important until it has appeared several times. In such a case, it would be necessary to reread all previously coded material to check if the new code should be applied.

Box 16.1 Beck and Watson's (2010) Coding Scheme for the Subsequent Childbirth After a Previous Traumatic Birth

Theme 1: Riding the Turbulent Wave of Panic During Pregnancy
A. Reactions to learning of pregnancy
B. Denial during the first trimester
C. Heightened state of anxiety
D. Panic attacks as delivery date gets closer
E. Feeling numb toward the baby

Theme 2: Strategizing: Attempts to Reclaim Their Body and Complete the Journey to Motherhood
A. Spending time nurturing self by exercising, going to yoga classes, and swimming
B. Keeping a journal throughout pregnancy
C. Turning to doulas for support during labour
D. Reading avidly to understand the birth process
E. Engaging in birth art exercises
F. Opening up to health care providers about their previous birth trauma
G. Sharing with partners about their fears
H. Learned relaxation techniques

Theme 3: Bringing Reverence to the Birthing Process and Empowering Women
A. Treated with respect
B. Pain relief taken seriously
C. Communicated with labour and delivery staff
D. Reclaimed their body
E. Strong sense of control
F. Birth plan honoured by labour and delivery staff
G. Mourned what they missed out with prior birth
H. Healing subsequent birth but it can never change the past

Theme 4: Still Elusive: The Longed for Healing Birth Experience
A. Failed again as a woman
B. Better than first traumatic birth but not healing
C. Hopes of a healing home birth dashed

Excerpt	Codes
"After 3 months of denying the fact that I was going to have to go through birth again, I decided that I would treat my next labour and delivery as a healing and empowering experience. I wanted to get myself as physically ready for labour as possible, so I focused on getting my body strong and my mind strong, too. I took antenatal yoga which helped me bond with my unborn son. I did stretching exercises and put an exercise plan in place. We hired a doula so I would have more support this time around in labour. I read many books and kept a journal, so I could be fully informed about my choices for labour and delivery. I learned relaxation techniques to help me with all the anxiety I felt throughout the 9 long months of my pregnancy."	1B 2A 2C 2B, 2D 1C, 2H

Figure 16.1 Coded excerpt from Beck and Watson's (2010) study on subsequent childbirth after a previous traumatic birth.

Narrative materials usually are not linear. For example, paragraphs from transcribed interviews may contain elements relating to three or four different categories.

Example of a multitopic segment •
Figure 16.1 shows an example of a multitopic segment of an interview from Beck and Watson's (2010) subsequent childbirth after a previous traumatic birth study. The codes in the margin represent codes from the scheme in Box 16.1.

Methods of Organizing Qualitative Data

Before the advent of software for qualitative data management, analysts used *conceptual files* to organize their data. This approach involves creating a physical file for each category and then cutting out and inserting all the materials relating to that category into the file. Researchers then retrieve the content on a particular topic by reviewing the applicable file folder.

Creating conceptual files is a difficult, labour-intensive task, particularly when segments of the narratives have multiple codes. For example, in Figure 16.1, seven copies of the paragraph would be needed, corresponding to the seven codes that were used. Researchers must also provide enough context that the cut-up material can be understood, and so it is often necessary to include material preceding or following the relevant material.

Computer-assisted qualitative data analysis software (CAQDAS) removes the work of cutting and pasting pages of narrative material. These programs permit an entire data set to be entered and coded; text corresponding to specified codes can then be retrieved for analysis. The software can also be used to examine relationships between codes. Computer programs offer many advantages for managing qualitative data, but some people prefer manual methods because they allow researchers to get closer to the data. Other people refuse to turn an intellectual process into a technologic activity. Despite concerns, many researchers have switched to computerized data management because it frees up their time and permits them to devote more attention to conceptual issues.

ANALYTIC PROCEDURES

Data *management* in qualitative research is reductionist in nature: It involves converting masses of data into smaller, more manageable segments. By contrast, qualitative data *analysis* is constructionist: It involves putting segments together into meaningful conceptual patterns. Various approaches to qualitative data analysis exist, but some elements are common to several of them.

A General Analytic Overview

The analysis of qualitative materials often begins with a search for broad categories or themes. In their review of how the term *theme* is used among qualitative researchers, DeSantis and Ugarriza (2000) offered this definition: "A **theme** is an abstract entity that brings meaning and identity to a current experience and its variant manifestations. As such, a theme captures and unifies the nature or basis of the experience into a meaningful whole" (p. 362).

Themes emerge from the data. They may develop within categories of data (i.e., within categories of the coding scheme) but may also cut across them. The search for themes involves not only discovering commonalities across participants but also seeking variation. Themes are never universal. Researchers must pay attention to the nature of themes and their patterns. Does the theme apply only to certain types of people or in certain contexts? At certain periods? In other words, qualitative analysts must be sensitive to *relationships* within the data.

 TIP Qualitative researchers often use major themes as subheadings in the "Results" section of their reports. For example, in their analysis of interviews with indigenous primary caregivers, elders, and program workers about the experiences of engaging indigenous families in a community-based early childhood program in British Columbia, Canada. Gerlach and coresearchers (2017) identified three main themes: (i) overcoming mistrust; (ii) "being willing to move a step forward"; and (iii) resisting what's taken for granted.

Researchers' search for themes and patterns in the data can sometimes be facilitated by devices that enable them to chart the development of behaviours and processes. For example, for qualitative studies that focus on dynamic experiences (e.g., decision making), flow charts or timelines can be used to highlight time sequences or major decision points.

Some qualitative researchers use metaphors as an analytic strategy. A **metaphor** uses figurative language to create a visual, symbolic comparison. Metaphors can be expressive tools for qualitative analysts, but they can run the risk of "supplanting creative insight with hackneyed cliché masquerading as profundity" (Thorne & Darbyshire, 2005, p. 1111).

Example of a metaphor •
Denise-Larocque and colleagues from McGill University (2017) studied nurses' perceptions with respect to caring for parents of children with medical complexity in the pediatric intensive care unit. The researchers captured the nature of the main theme with the metaphor "Thrown to the wolves."

A further analytic step involves validation. In this phase, the concern is whether the themes accurately represent the participants' perspectives. Several validation procedures are discussed in Chapter 17.

In the final analysis stage, researchers attempt to put the thematic pieces together. The various themes are integrated to provide an overall structure (such as a theory or full description) to the data. Successful integration demands creativity and intellectual rigour.

 TIP Although relatively few qualitative researchers make formal efforts to quantify features of their data, be alert to quantitative implications when you read a qualitative report. Qualitative researchers routinely use words like "some," "most," or "many" in characterizing participants' experiences and actions, which implies some level of quantification.

Qualitative Content Analysis

In the remainder of this section, we discuss analytic procedures used by ethnographers, phenomenologists, and grounded theory researchers. Qualitative researchers who conduct descriptive qualitative studies may, however, simply say that they performed a content analysis. **Qualitative content analysis** involves analyzing the content of narrative data to identify prominent themes and patterns among the themes. Qualitative content analysis involves breaking down data into smaller *units*, coding and naming the units according to the content they represent, and grouping coded material based on shared concepts. The literature on content analysis often refers to *meaning units*. A meaning unit, essentially, is the smallest segment of a text that contains a recognizable piece of information.

Content analysts often make the distinction between manifest and latent content. *Manifest content* is what the text actually says. In purely descriptive studies, qualitative researchers may focus mainly on summarizing the manifest content communicated in the text. Often, however, content analysts also analyze what the text talks *about*, which involves interpretation of the meaning of its *latent content*. Interpretations vary in depth and level of abstraction and are usually the basis for themes.

Example of a content analysis ·
Schmidt and colleagues (2016) did a content analysis of semistructured interviews with 10 older adults aged 69 to 94 in rural Saskatchewan, Canada. The purpose of the study was to understand the contributing factors to physical activity engagement among older adults in rural areas. Seven overarching themes emerged, including maintaining health, social hour, volunteer opportunities, accessible and safe, aging, concerned family, and fear of falling.

Ethnographic Analysis

Analysis typically begins the moment ethnographers set foot in the field. Ethnographers are continually looking for *patterns* in the behaviour and thoughts of participants, comparing one pattern against another, and analyzing many patterns simultaneously. As they analyze patterns of everyday life, ethnographers acquire a deeper understanding of the culture being studied. Maps, flow charts, and organizational charts are also useful tools to show the data being collected. Matrices (two-dimensional displays) can also help to highlight a comparison graphically, cross-reference categories, and discover emerging patterns.

Spradley's (1979) research sequence is sometimes used for ethnographic data analyses. His 12-step sequence included strategies for both data collection and data analysis. In Spradley's method, there are four levels of data analysis: *domain analysis*, *taxonomic analysis*, *componential analysis*, and *theme analysis*. **Domains** are broad categories that represent units of cultural knowledge. During this first level of analysis, ethnographers identify relational patterns among terms in the domains that are used by members of the culture. The ethnographer focuses on the cultural meaning of terms and symbols (objects and events) used in a culture and their interrelationships.

In *taxonomic analysis*, the second level in Spradley's (1979) data analytic method, ethnographers decide how many domains the analysis will include. Will only one or two domains be analyzed in depth, or will several domains be studied less intensively? After making this decision, a **taxonomy**—a system of classifying and organizing terms—is developed to illustrate the internal organization of a domain.

In *componential analysis*, multiple relationships among terms in the domains are examined. The ethnographer analyzes data for similarities and differences among cultural terms in a domain. Finally, in *theme analysis*, cultural themes are uncovered. Domains are connected in cultural themes, which help to provide a holistic view of the culture being studied. The discovery of cultural meaning is the outcome.

Example using Spradley's method •
Michel et al. (2015) studied the meanings assigned to health care by long-lived elders and nurses in a health care setting. They used Spradley's (1979) method of ethnographic analysis and identified and analyzed six domains. The overarching cultural theme that emerged was the real to the ideal—the health (un)care of long-lived elders.

Other approaches to ethnographic analysis have been developed. For example, as described in McFarland and Wehbe-Alamah (2015), Leininger's ethnographers follow a four-phase ethnonursing data analysis guide. In the first phase, ethnographers collect, describe, and record data. The second phase involves identifying and categorizing descriptors. In phase 3, data are analyzed to discover repetitive patterns in their context. The fourth and final phase involves abstracting major themes and presenting findings.

Example using Leininger's method •
Raymond and Omeri (2015) studied the culture care for Mauritian immigrant childbearing families living in Australia. Using Leininger's four phases of ethnonursing inquiry, the researchers identified five dominant themes: care as extended family and friendship support, care as best professional and/or folk practices, self-care as responsibility, care as enabling and empowerment, and care as maintenance of a hygienic and supportive environment.

Phenomenologic Analysis

Schools of phenomenology have developed different approaches to data analysis. Three frequently used methods for descriptive phenomenology are the methods of Colaizzi (1978), Giorgi (1985), and van Kaam (1966), all of whom are from the *phenomenologic psychological approach of* phenomenology, based on Husserl's philosophy.

The basic outcome of all three methods is the description of the essential nature of an experience, often through the identification of essential themes. Some important differences among these three approaches exist. Colaizzi's (1978) method, for example, is the only one that calls for a validation of results by querying study participants. Giorgi's (1985) view is that it is inappropriate either to return to participants to validate findings or to use external judges to review the analysis. Van Kaam's (1966) method requires that intersubjective agreement be reached with other expert judges.

Figure 16.2 provides an illustration of the steps involved in Colaizzi's (1978) data analysis approach, which is the most widely used of the three approaches by nurse researchers.

Example of a study using Colaizzi's method •
Patchell and colleagues (2015) explored the experience of pregnancy and childbirth during an intimate partner's military deployment. Transcribed interviews with four women in Canadian military families were analyzed using Colaizzi's (1978) method. The overarching themes were "being by myself," physically alone or in a world that did not understand their experience, and "believing in us," the possibility of having a child, of a partner's return, and of becoming a family. Other sub-themes emerged: working it out time wise, longing for togetherness, appreciating technology, protecting us, knowing that somebody is there, and homecoming.

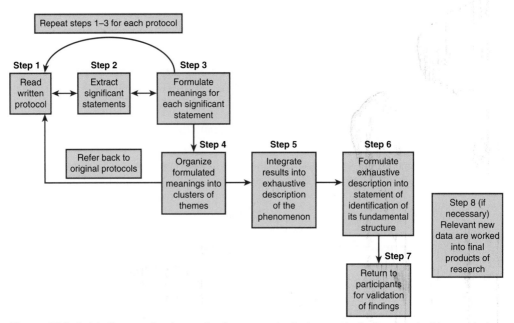

Figure 16.2 Colaizzi's procedural steps in phenomenologic data analysis. Reprinted with permission from Beck, C. T. (2009). The arm: There is no escaping the reality for mothers of children with obstetric brachial plexus injuries. *Nursing Research, 58,* 237–245.

Phenomenologists from the *Utrecht School,* such as van Manen (1997), combine characteristics of descriptive and interpretive phenomenology. Van Manen's approach involves six activities: (1) turning to the nature of the lived experience, (2) exploring the experience as we live it, (3) reflecting on essential themes, (4) describing the phenomenon through the art of writing and rewriting, (5) maintaining a strong relation to the phenomenon, and (6) balancing the research context by considering parts and whole. According to van Manen, thematic aspects of experience can be uncovered from participants' descriptions of the experience by three methods: the holistic, selective, or detailed approach. In the *holistic approach,* researchers view the text as a whole and try to capture its meanings. In the *selective* (or highlighting) *approach,* researchers pull out statements that seem essential to the experience under study. In the *detailed* (or line-by-line) *approach,* researchers analyze every sentence. Once themes have been identified, they become the objects of interpretation through follow-up interviews with participants. Through this process, essential themes are discovered.

Example of a study using van Manen's method ·

Wilkins (2015) conducted a study to understand the lived experiences of people who had cancer multiple times. Participants were asked to take a photograph of whatever represented their experiences and talk about what it has been like to have had cancer multiple times. Thematic statements were isolated using van Manen's (1997) methods. Preliminary analyses suggest that the essence of having cancer multiple times is best described as an "unwanted encore."

In addition to identifying themes from participants' descriptions, van Manen (1997) also recommended thematic descriptions from artistic sources. Van Manen urged qualitative researchers to keep in mind that literature, painting, photographs, and other art forms can provide rich experiential data that can increase insight into the essential meaning of the experience being studied.

A third school of phenomenology is an interpretive approach called Heideggerian hermeneutics. Key to analyzing data in a hermeneutic study is the notion of the **hermeneutic circle**. The circle signifies a methodologic process that involves a continual movement between the parts and the whole of the text being analyzed. Gadamer (1975) stressed that, to interpret a text, researchers cannot separate themselves from the meanings of the text and must try to understand possibilities that the text can tell.

Benner (1994) offered an analytic approach for hermeneutic analysis that involves three interrelated processes: the search for paradigm cases, thematic analysis, and analysis of exemplars. **Paradigm cases** are "strong instances of concerns or ways of being in the world" (Benner, 1994, p. 113). Paradigm cases are used early in the analytic process as a strategy for gaining understanding. Thematic analysis is done to compare and contrast similarities across cases. Finally, paradigm cases and thematic analysis can be enhanced by *exemplars* that clarify aspects of a paradigm case or theme. Paradigm cases and exemplars presented in research reports allow readers to play a role in validation of the results by deciding whether the cases support the researchers' conclusions.

Example using Benner's hermeneutical analysis • • • • • • • • • • • • • • • • •
Solomon and Hansen (2015) conducted an interpretive phenomenologic study of the unique lived experience of a dying patient and her family members. The researchers used Benner's (1994) approach in their analysis, which included paradigm cases, thematic analysis, and exemplars. Exemplars included "Driving her own course" and "Not being a burden."

Grounded Theory Analysis

Grounded theory methods emerged in the 1960s when two sociologists, Glaser (1967) and Strauss (1998), were studying dying in hospitals. The two co-originators eventually split and developed divergent approaches, which have been called the "Glaserian" and "Straussian" versions of grounded theory. A third analytic approach by Charmaz (2014), constructivist grounded theory, has also emerged.

Glaser and Strauss' Grounded Theory Method

Grounded theory in all three analytic systems uses **constant comparison**, a method that involves comparing elements present in one data source (e.g., in one interview) with those in another. The process continues until the content of all sources has been compared so that commonalities are identified. The concept of fit is an important element in Glaserian grounded theory analysis. *Fit* has to do with how closely the emerging concepts fit with the incidents they are representing—which depends on how thoroughly constant comparison was done.

Coding in the Glaserian approach is used to identify patterns in the data. Coding helps the researcher to discover the basic problem the participants face. The substance of the topic under study is conceptualized through two types of **substantive codes**: open and selective. **Open coding**, used in the first stage of constant comparison, captures what is going on in the data. Open codes may be the actual words participants used. Through open coding, data are broken down, and their similarities and differences are examined.

There are three levels of open coding that vary in degree of abstraction. *Level I codes* (or *in vivo codes*) are derived directly from the language of the substantive area. They create rich images and "grab." Table 16.1 presents five level I codes and illustrative interview excerpts from Beck's (2002) grounded theory study on mothering twins.

TABLE 16.1 Collapsing Level I Codes into the Level II Code of "Reaping the Blessings" (Beck, 2002)

Excerpt	Level I Code
I enjoy just watching the twins interact so much, especially now that they are mobile. They are not walking yet but they are crawling. I will tell you they are already playing. Like one will go around the corner and kind of peek around and they play hide and seek. They crawl after each other.	Enjoying Twins
With twins it's amazing. She was sick and she had a fever. He was the one acting sick. She didn't seem like she was sick at all. He was. We watched him for like 6 to 8 hours. We gave her the medicine and he started calming down. Like WOW! That is so weird. 'Cause you read about it but it's like, Oh come on! It's really neat to see.	Amazing
These days it's really neat 'cause you go to the store or you go out and people are like, "Oh, they are twins, how nice." And I say, "Yeah they are. Look, look at my kids."	Getting Attention
I just feel blessed to have two. I just feel like I am twice as lucky as a mom who has one baby. I mean that's the best part. It's just that instead of having one baby to watch grow and change and develop and become a toddler and school-age child, you have two.	Feeling Blessed
It's very exciting. It's interesting and it's fun to see them and how the twin bond really is. There really is a twin bond. You read about it and you hear about it, but until you experience it, you just don't understand. One time they were both crying and they were fed. They were changed and burped. There was nothing wrong. I couldn't figure out what was wrong. So I said to myself, "I am just going to put them together and close the door." I put them in my bed together, and they patty-caked their hands and put their noses together and just looked at each other and went right to sleep.	Twin Bonding

As researchers constantly compare new level I codes with previously identified ones, they condense them into broader *level II codes*. For example, in Table 16.1, Beck's (2002) five level I codes were collapsed into a single level II code, "Reaping the Blessings." *Level III codes* (or theoretical constructs) are the most abstract. Collapsing level II codes aids in identifying constructs.

   TIP   Additional material relating to Beck's (2002) twin study is presented in the supplement to this chapter on the book's website.

Open coding ends when the core category is discovered and then selective coding begins. The **core category** (or *core variable*) is a pattern of behaviour that is relevant and/or problematic for study participants. In **selective coding**, researchers code only those data that are related to the core category. One kind of core category is a **basic social process (BSP)** that evolves over time in two or more phases. All BSPs are core categories, but not all core categories have to be BSPs.

Glaser (1978) provided criteria to help researchers decide on a core category: It must be central, meaning that it is related to many categories; it must reoccur frequently in the data; it relates meaningfully and easily to other categories; and it has clear and grabbing implications for formal theory.

Theoretical codes provide insights into how substantive codes relate to each other. Theoretical codes help grounded theorists to put the broken pieces of data back together again. Glaser (1978) proposed 18 families of theoretical codes that researchers can use to conceptualize how substantive codes relate to each other (although he subsequently expanded possibilities in 2005). Four examples of his families of theoretical codes include the following:

- Process: stages, phases, passages, transitions
- Strategy: tactics, techniques, manoeuvring
- Cutting point: boundaries, critical junctures, turning points
- The six Cs: causes, contexts, contingencies, consequences, covariances, and conditions

Throughout coding and analysis, grounded theory analysts document their ideas about the data and emerging conceptual scheme in *memos*. Memos encourage researchers to reflect on and describe patterns in the data, relationships between categories, and emergent conceptualizations.

The product of a typical Glaserian grounded theory analysis is a theoretical model to explain a pattern of behaviour that is relevant for study participants. Once the basic problem emerges, the grounded theorist goes on to discover the process these participants experience in coping with or resolving this problem.

Example of Glaser and Strauss' grounded theory analysis • • • • • • • • • • •

Figure 16.3 presents Beck's (2002) model from a study in which "Releasing the Pause Button" was conceptualized as the core category and process through which mothers of twins progressed as they tried to resume their lives after giving birth. The process involves four phases: Draining Power, Pausing Own Life, Striving to Reset, and Resuming Own Life. Beck used 10 coding families in her theoretical coding for the study. The family *cutting point* offers an illustration. Three months seemed to be a turning point for mothers when life started to be more manageable. Here is an excerpt from an interview that Beck coded as a cutting point: "Three months came around and the twins sort of slept through the night and it made a huge, huge difference."

Glaser and Strauss cautioned against consulting the literature before a framework is stabilized, but they also saw the benefit of examining other work. Glaser (1978) discussed the development of grounded theories through the process of **emergent fit** to prevent certain established theories from being "respected little islands of knowledge" (p. 148). As he noted, generating grounded theory does not necessarily require discovering all new categories or ignoring ones previously identified in the literature. Through constant comparison,

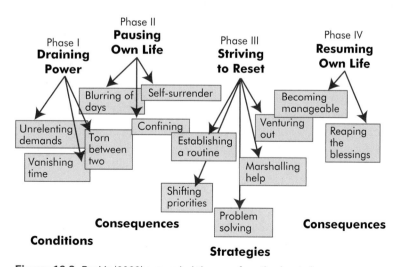

Figure 16.3 Beck's (2002) grounded theory of mothering twins.

TABLE 16.2 Comparison of Glaser's and Corbin and Strauss' Methods

	Glaser	Corbin and Strauss
Initial data analysis	Breaking down and conceptualizing data involves comparison of incident to incident so patterns emerge	Breaking down and conceptualizing data includes taking apart a single sentence, observation, and incident
Types of coding	Open, selective, theoretical	Open and axial
Connections between categories	18 coding families plus theoretical codes from many different fields of study	Paradigm (conditions, actions–interactions, and consequences or outcomes) and the conditional/consequential matrix
Outcome	Emergent theory (discovery)	Conceptual description (verification)

researchers can compare concepts emerging from the data with similar concepts discussed in existing theory or research to evaluate which parts have emergent fit with the developing theory.

Strauss and Corbin's Approach

The Strauss and Corbin approach to grounded theory analysis, most recently described in Corbin and Strauss (2015), differs from the original Glaser and Strauss method with regard to method, processes, and outcomes. Table 16.2 summarizes major analytic differences between these two grounded theory analysis methods.

Glaser (1978) stressed that to generate a grounded theory, the basic problem must be discovered from the data. The theory is, from the very start, grounded in the data rather than starting with a preconceived problem. Strauss and Corbin, however, argued that the research itself is only one of four possible sources of a research problem. Research problems can, for example, come from the literature or a researcher's personal and professional experience.

The Corbin and Strauss (2015) method involves two types of coding: open and axial coding. In *open coding*, data are broken down into parts and concepts identified based on interpreted meaning of the raw data. In **axial coding**, the analyst codes for context. Here, the analyst is "locating and linking action–interaction within a framework of subconcepts that give it meaning and enable it to explain what interactions are occurring and why and what consequences, real or anticipated, are happening" (Corbin & Strauss, 2015, p. 156). The *paradigm* is used as an analytic strategy to help integrate structure and process. The basic components of the paradigm include conditions, actions–interactions, and consequences or outcomes. Corbin and Strauss suggested the conditional/consequential matrix as an analytic strategy for considering the range of possible conditions and consequences that can enter into the context.

The first step in integrating the findings is to decide on the **central category** (sometimes called the *core category*), which is the main theme of the research. The outcome of the Strauss and Corbin approach is a full conceptual description. The original grounded theory method, by contrast, generates a theory that explains how a basic social problem emerged from the data is processed in a social setting.

Example of Strauss and Corbin grounded theory analysis • • • • • • • • • • •
Lawler, Begley, and Lalor (2015) sought to understand the process of transitioning to motherhood for women with a disability. Data from interviews with 22 women were analyzed using Strauss and Corbin's method of open and axial coding: "The data were

broken down, examined, compared, conceptualized, and categorized so that the data could be interpreted, concepts and categories selected. Once the categories and subcategories were sufficiently reinforced the data were reconstructed in different ways through the linking of categories and subcategories.... Categories were then integrated to refine the evolving theory" (p. 1675).

Constructivist Grounded Theory Approach

The constructivist approach to grounded theory is in some ways similar to a Glaserian approach. According to Charmaz (2014), in constructivist grounded theory, the "coding generates the bones of your analysis. Theoretical integration will assemble these bones into a working skeleton" (p. 113). Charmaz offered guidelines for word-by-word, line-by-line, and incident-to-incident coding. Unlike Glaser and Strauss' grounded theory approach in which theory is discovered from data separate from the researcher, Charmaz's position is that researchers build grounded theories from their past and current involvements and interactions with individuals and research practices.

Charmaz (2014) distinguished *initial coding* and **focused coding**. In initial coding, the pieces of data (e.g., words, lines, segments, incidents) are studied so the researcher can learn what the participants view as problematic. In focused coding, the analysis is directed toward identifying the most significant initial codes, which are then theoretically coded.

Example of constructivist grounded theory analysis • • • • • • • • • • • • • • •
Giles, de Lacey, and Muir-Cochrane (2016) used constructivist methods to develop a grounded theory of family presence during resuscitation, which they called "The Social Construction of Conditional Permission." Their article provides an excellent, detailed description of their methods, tracing the construction of the core category ("conditional permission") from initial and focused codes through to the final substantive grounded theory. This article is available on thePoint website.

 TIP Grounded theory researchers often present conceptual maps or models, such as the one in Figure 16.2, to summarize their results, especially when the central phenomenon is a dynamic or evolving process.

CRITIQUING QUALITATIVE ANALYSIS

Evaluating a qualitative analysis is not easy to do. Readers do not have access to the information they would need to assess whether researchers exercised good judgment and critical insight in coding the narrative materials, developing a thematic analysis, and integrating materials into a meaningful whole. Researchers are seldom able to include more than a handful of examples of actual data in a journal article. Moreover, the process they used to inductively abstract meaning from the data is difficult to describe and illustrate.

A major focus of a critique of qualitative analyses is whether the researchers have adequately documented the analytic process. The report should provide information about the approach used to analyze the data. For example, a report for a grounded theory study should indicate whether the researchers used the Glaser and Strauss, Corbin and Strauss (2015), or constructivist method.

Another possible critique of qualitative analyses is whether the researchers have used one approach consistently and have been faithful to the integrity of its procedures. Thus, for

---

Box 16.2 Guidelines for Critiquing Qualitative Analyses

1. Was the data analysis approach appropriate for the research design or tradition?
2. Was the category scheme described? If so, does the scheme appear logical and complete?
3. Did the report adequately describe the process by which the actual analysis was performed? Did the report indicate whose approach to data analysis was used (e.g., Glaserian, Straussian, or constructivist in grounded theory studies)?
4. What major themes or processes emerged? Were relevant excerpts from the data provided, and do the themes or categories appear to capture the meaning of the narratives—that is, does it appear that the researcher adequately interpreted the data and conceptualized the themes? Is the analysis parsimonious—could two or more themes be collapsed into a broader and, perhaps, more useful conceptualization?
5. Was a conceptual map, model, or diagram effectively displayed to communicate important processes?
6. Was the context of the phenomenon adequately described? Did the report give you a clear picture of the social or emotional world of study participants?
7. Did the analysis yield a meaningful and insightful picture of the phenomenon under study? Is the resulting theory or description trivial or obvious?

---

example, if researchers say they are using the Glaserian approach to grounded theory analysis, they should not also include elements from the Strauss and Corbin method. An even more serious problem occurs when, as sometimes happens, the researchers "muddle" traditions. For example, researchers who describe their study as a grounded theory study should not present *themes* because grounded theory analysis does not yield themes. Researchers who attempt to blend elements from two traditions may not have a clear grasp of the analytic precepts of either one. For example, a researcher who claims to have undertaken an ethnography using a grounded theory approach to analysis may not be well informed about the underlying goals and philosophies of these two traditions.

Some further guidelines that may be helpful in evaluating qualitative analyses are presented in Box 16.2.

RESEARCH EXAMPLES WITH CRITICAL THINKING EXERCISES

This section describes the analytic procedures used in a qualitative study. Read the summary and then answer the critical thinking questions that follow, referring to the full research report if necessary. Example 1 is featured on the interactive *Critical Thinking Activity* on thePoint website. The critical thinking questions for Example 2 are based on the study that appears in its entirety in Appendix B of this book. Our comments for this exercise are in the Student Resources section on thePoint. ⚙

EXAMPLE 1: A CONSTRUCTIVIST GROUNDED THEORY ANALYSIS

Study: Care transition experiences of spousal caregivers: From a geriatric rehabilitation unit to home (Byrne, Orange, & Ward-Griffin 2011).

Statement of Purpose: The purpose of this study was to develop a theory about caregivers' transition processes and experiences during their spouses' return home from a geriatric rehabilitation unit (GRU).

Method: This grounded theory study involved in-depth interviews with 18 older adult spousal caregivers. Most of the caregivers were interviewed on three occasions: 48 hours prior to discharge from a 36-bed GRU in a Canadian long-term care hospital, 2 weeks postdischarge, and 1 month postdischarge. In addition to the interviews, which lasted between 35 and 120 minutes, the researchers made observations of interactions between spouses and care recipients.

Analysis: Analysis began with line-by-line coding by the first author. All authors contributed to focused coding, followed by theoretical coding. They used constant comparison throughout the coding and analysis process and provided a good example: "In the early stages of data collection and analysis, we noticed that caregivers continually used the phrase 'I don't know,' and thus an open code by this name was created.... As data collection and analysis proceeded, we engaged in focused coding using the term *knowing/not knowing* to reflect these instances" (p. 1374). The researchers illustrated with an interview excerpt how they came to understand that knowing/not knowing was part of the process of *navigating*. The researchers also noted that "Moving from line-by-line coding to focused coding was not a linear process. As we engaged with the data, we returned to the data collected to explore new ideas and conceptualization of codes" (p. 1375).

Key Findings: The basic problem the caregivers faced was "fluctuating needs," including the physical, emotional, social, and medical needs of the caregivers and their spouses. The researchers developed a theoretical framework in which *reconciling in response to fluctuating needs* emerged as the basic social process. Reconciling encompassed three subprocesses: navigating, safekeeping, and repositioning. The context that shaped reconciling was a trajectory of prior care transitions and intertwined life events.

Critical Thinking Exercises

1. Answer the relevant questions from Box 16.2 regarding this study.
2. Also consider the following targeted questions:
   a. Is the researcher's decision to use both interview data and observations appropriate?
   b. The authors wrote that "to foster theoretical sensitivity, memos focused on actions and processes, and gradually incorporated relevant literature (e.g., theoretical perspectives on transition)" (p. 1375). What does this statement reveal?
3. What might be some of the uses to which the findings could be put in clinical practice?

EXAMPLE 2: A PHENOMENOLOGIC ANALYSIS IN APPENDIX B

- Read the method and results sections of Beck and Watson's (2010) phenomenologic study ("Subsequent childbirth after a previous traumatic birth") in Appendix B of this book.

Critical Thinking Exercises

1. Answer the relevant questions from Box 16.2 regarding this study.
2. Also consider the following targeted questions:
   a. What is the amount of data that had to be analyzed in this study?
   b. Refer to Table 2 in the article, which presents a list of 10 significant statements made by participants. In Colaizzi's approach, the next step is to construct *formulated meanings* from the significant statements. What are your own *formulated meanings* of one or two of these significant statements?

WANT TO KNOW MORE?

A wide variety of resources to enhance your learning and understanding of this chapter are available on thePoint.

- Interactive Critical Thinking Activity
- Chapter Supplement on a Glaserian Grounded Theory Study: Illustrative Materials
- Answer to the Critical Thinking Exercise for Example 2
- Internet Resources with useful websites for Chapter 16
- A Wolters Kluwer journal article on a topic related to this chapter

Summary Points

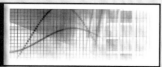

- Qualitative analysis is a challenging, labour-intensive activity, with few fixed rules.
- A first step in analyzing qualitative data is to organize and index the materials for easy retrieval, typically by coding the content of the data according to a *coding scheme* that involves devising descriptive or abstract categories.
- Traditionally, researchers have organized their data by developing *conceptual files*, which are physical files in which coded excerpts of data for specific categories are placed. Now, however, computer software (CAQDAS) is widely used to perform basic indexing functions and to facilitate data analysis.
- The actual analysis of data begins with a search for patterns and **themes**, which involves the discovery not only of commonalities across participants but also of natural variation in the data. Some qualitative analysts use *metaphors* or figurative comparisons to evoke a visual and symbolic analogy. In a final step, analysts try to weave the thematic strands together into an integrated picture of the phenomenon under investigation.
- Researchers whose goal is qualitative description often say they used **qualitative content analysis** as their analytic method. Content analysis can vary in terms of an emphasis on *manifest content* or *latent content*.

- In ethnographies, analysis begins as the researcher enters the field. One analytic approach is Spradley's method, which involves four levels of analysis: *domain analysis* (identifying **domains** or units of cultural knowledge), *taxonomic analysis* (selecting key domains and constructing **taxonomies**), *componential analysis* (comparing and contrasting terms in a domain), and a *theme analysis* (to uncover cultural themes).
- There are numerous approaches to phenomenologic analysis, including the descriptive methods of Colaizzi, Giorgi, and van Kaam, in which the goal is to find common patterns of experiences shared by particular instances.
- In van Manen's approach, which involves efforts to grasp the essential meaning of the experience being studied, researchers search for themes, using a *holistic approach* (viewing text as a whole), a *selective approach* (pulling out key statements and phrases), or a *detailed approach* (analyzing every sentence).
- Central to analyzing data in a hermeneutic study is the notion of the **hermeneutic circle**, which signifies a process in which there is continual movement between the parts and the whole of the text under analysis.
- Benner's approach consists of three processes: searching for **paradigm cases**, thematic analysis, and analysis of *exemplars*.
- Grounded theory uses the **constant comparative** method of data analysis, a method that involves comparing elements present in one data source (e.g., in one interview) with those in another. *Fit* has to do with how

closely concepts fit with incidents they represent, which is related to how thoroughly constant comparison was done.

- One grounded theory approach is the Glaser and Strauss (Glaserian) method, in which there are two broad types of codes: **substantive codes** (in which the empirical substance of the topic is conceptualized) and **theoretical codes** (in which the relationships among the substantive codes are conceptualized).
- Substantive coding involves **open coding** to capture what is going on in the data and then **selective coding**, in which only variables relating to a core category are coded. The **core category**, a behaviour pattern that has relevance for participants, is sometimes a **basic social process (BSP)** that involves an evolutionary process of coping or adaptation.
- In the Glaserian method, open codes begin with *level I (in vivo) codes*, which are collapsed into a higher level of abstraction in *level II codes*. Level II codes are then used to formulate *level III codes*, which are theoretical constructs. Through constant comparison, the researcher compares concepts emerging from the data with similar concepts from existing theory or research to see which parts have **emergent fit** with the theory being generated.
- Strauss and Corbin's method is an alternative grounded theory method whose outcome is a full preconceived conceptual description. This approach to grounded theory analysis involves two types of coding: open (in which categories are generated) and **axial coding** (where categories are linked with subcategories and integrated).
- In Charmaz's constructivist grounded theory, coding can be word-by-word, line-by-line, or incident-by-incident. Initial coding leads to **focused coding,** which is then followed by theoretical coding.

REFERENCES

Beck, C. T. (2002). Releasing the pause button: Mothering twins during the first year of life. *Qualitative Health Research, 12,* 593–608.

Beck, C. T., & Watson, S. (2010). Subsequent childbirth after a previous traumatic birth. *Nursing Research, 59,* 241–249.

Benner, P. (1994). The tradition and skill of interpretive phenomenology in studying health, illness, and caring practices. In P. Benner (Ed.). *Interpretive phenomenology: Embodiment, caring, and ethics in health and illness* (pp. 99–128). Thousand Oaks, CA: Sage.

Byrne, K., Orange, J., & Ward-Griffin, C. (2011). Care transition experiences of spousal caregivers: From a geriatric rehabilitation unit to home. *Qualitative Health Research, 21,* 1371–1387.

Charmaz, K. (2014). *Constructing grounded theory* (2nd ed.). Thousand Oaks, CA: Sage.

Colaizzi, P. (1978). Psychological research as the phenomenologist views it. In R. Valle & M. King (Eds.). *Existential-phenomenological alternatives for psychology* (pp. 48–71). New York: Oxford University Press.

Corbin, J., & Strauss, A. (2015). *Basics of qualitative research: Techniques and procedures for developing grounded theory.* Thousand Oaks, CA: Sage.

Denis-Larocque G., Williams K., St-Sauveur I., et al. (2017). Nurses' perceptions of caring for parents of children with chronic medical complexity in the pediatric intensive care unit. *Intensive and Critical Care Nursing,* pii: S0964-3397(16)30070-2.

DeSantis, L., & Ugarriza, D. N. (2000). The concept of theme as used in qualitative nursing research. *Western Journal of Nursing Research, 22,* 351–372.

*Ersek, M., & Jablonski, A. (2014). A mixed-methods approach to investigating the adoption of evidence-based pain practices in nursing homes. *Journal of Gerontological Nursing, 40,* 52–60.

Gadamer, H. G. (1975). *Truth and method (G. Borden & J. Cumming, Trans.).* London, United Kingdom: Sheed & Ward.

Gerlach A. J., Browne A. J., & Greenwood M. (2017). Engaging Indigenous families in a community-based Indigenous early childhood programme in British Columbia, Canada: A cultural safety perspective. *Health & Social Care in the Community, 25*(6), 1763–1773.

**Giles, T. M., de Lacey, S., & Muir-Cochrane, E. (2016). Coding, constant comparisons, and core categories: A worked example for novice constructivist grounded theorists. *Advances in Nursing Science, 39,* E29–E44.

Giorgi, A. (1985). *Phenomenology and psychological research.* Pittsburgh, PA: Duquesne University Press.

Glaser, B. G. (1978). *Theoretical sensitivity.* Mill Valley, CA: Sociology Press.

Glaser, B. G., & Strauss, A. L. (1967). The discovery of grounded theory: Strategies for qualitative research. Chicago: Aldine Pub. Co.

Lawler, D., Begley, C., & Lalor, J. (2015). (Re)constructing myself: The process of transition to motherhood for women with a disability. *Journal of Advanced Nursing, 71,* 1672–1683.

McFarland, M. R., & Wehbe-Alamah, H. B. (2015). *Leininger's culture care diversity and universality: A worldwide nursing theory.* Burlington, MA: Jones & Bartlett.

*Michel, T., Lenardt, M., Willig, M., & Alvarez, A. (2015). From real to ideal—the health (un)care of long-lived elders. *Revista Brasileira de Enfermagem, 68,* 343–349.

Patchell et al. (2015). Being by myself and believing in us: the experience of pregnancy and childbirth during an intimate partner's military deployment. *Journal of Military, Veteran and Family Health*, *2*(1), 19–27.

Raymond, L. M., & Omeri, A. (2015). Transcultural midwifery: Culture care for Mauritian immigrant childbearing families living in New South Wales, Australia. In M. R. McFarland & H. B. Wehbe-Alamah (Eds.). *Leininger's culture care diversity and universality: A worldwide nursing theory* (pp. 183–254). Burlington, MA: Jones & Bartlett.

Solomon, D., & Hansen, L. (2015). Living through the end: The phenomenon of dying at home. *Palliative & Supportive Care*, *13*, 125–134.

Spradley, J. P. (1979). *The ethnographic interview*. Belmont, CA: Wadsworth, Cengage Learning.

Strauss A., & Corbin J. (1998). Basics of Qualitative Research – Techniques and Procedures for Developing Grounded Theory, second edition, London, Sage Publications.

Thorne, S., & Darbyshire, P. (2005). Land mines in the field: A modest proposal for improving the craft of qualitative health research. *Qualitative Health Research*, *15*, 1105–1113.

van Kaam, A. (1966). *Existential foundations of psychology*. Pittsburgh, PA: Duquesne University Press.

van Manen, M. (1997). *Researching lived experience: Human science for an action sensitive pedagogy* (2nd ed.). Ontario, Canada: The Althouse Press.

*A link to this open-access article is provided in the Internet Resources section on the**Point** website.

This journal article is available on the Point** for this chapter.

Trustworthiness and Integrity in Qualitative Research

Learning Objectives

On completing this chapter, you will be able to:

● Discuss some controversies relating to the issue of quality in qualitative research
● Identify the quality criteria proposed in two frameworks for evaluating quality and integrity in qualitative research
● Discuss strategies for enhancing quality in qualitative research
● Describe different dimensions relating to the interpretation of qualitative results
● Define new terms in the chapter

Key Terms

● Audit trail
● Authenticity
● Confirmability
● Credibility
● Data triangulation
● Dependability
● Disconfirming evidence
● Inquiry audit

● Investigator triangulation
● Member check
● Method triangulation
● Negative case analysis
● Peer debriefing
● Persistent observation
● Prolonged engagement

● Reflexivity
● Researcher credibility
● Thick description
● Transferability
● Triangulation
● Trustworthiness

Integrity in qualitative research is a critical issue for both those doing the research and those considering the use of qualitative evidence.

PERSPECTIVES ON QUALITY IN QUALITATIVE RESEARCH

Qualitative researchers agree on the importance of doing high-quality research, yet defining "high quality" has been controversial. We offer a brief overview of the arguments of the debate.

Debates About Rigour and Validity

One contentious issue concerns use of the terms *rigour* and *validity*—terms some people avoid because they are associated with the positivist paradigm. For these critics, the concept of rigour is by its nature a term that does not fit into an interpretive paradigm that values insight and creativity.

Others disagree with those opposing the term *validity*. Morse (2015), for example, has argued that qualitative researchers should return to the terminology of the social sciences—that is, rigour, reliability, validity, and generalizability.

This complex debate has given rise to a variety of positions. At one extreme are those who think that validity is an appropriate quality criterion in both quantitative and qualitative studies, although qualitative researchers use different methods to achieve it. At the opposite extreme are those who criticize the "absurdity" of validity. A widely adopted stance is what has been called a *parallel perspective*. This position was proposed by Lincoln and Guba (1985), who created standards for the **trustworthiness** of qualitative research that parallel the standards of reliability and validity in quantitative research.

Generic Versus Specific Standards

Another controversy concerns whether there should be a generic set of quality standards or whether specific standards are needed for different qualitative traditions. Some writers believe that research conducted within different qualitative traditions must address different concerns and that techniques for enhancing research integrity vary. Thus, different standards have been proposed for specific forms of qualitative inquiry, such as grounded theory, phenomenology, ethnography, and critical research. Some writers believe, however, that some quality criteria are fairly universal within the constructivist paradigm. For example, Whittemore, Chase, and Mandle (2001) prepared a synthesis of criteria that they viewed as essential to all qualitative inquiry.

Terminology Proliferation and Confusion

The result of these controversies is that there is no common vocabulary for quality criteria in qualitative research. While terms such as *truth value*, *goodness*, *integrity*, and *trustworthiness* are commonly used, each proposed term has been challenged by some critics. With regard to actual *criteria* for evaluating quality in qualitative research, dozens have been suggested but consensus is lacking.

Given the lack of consensus and the heated arguments supporting and contesting various frameworks, it is difficult to provide guidance about quality standards. We present information about *criteria* from the Lincoln and Guba (1985) framework in the next section. (Criteria from another framework are described in the supplement to this chapter on thePoint website.) We then describe *strategies* that researchers use to strengthen integrity in qualitative research. These strategies should provide guidance for considering whether a qualitative study is sufficiently rigorous, trustworthy, insightful, or valid.

LINCOLN AND GUBA'S FRAMEWORK OF QUALITY CRITERIA

The criteria often viewed as the "gold standard" for qualitative research are those outlined by Lincoln and Guba (1985). These researchers suggested four criteria for developing the trustworthiness of a qualitative inquiry: credibility, dependability, confirmability, and transferability. These criteria represent parallels to the positivists' criteria of internal validity, reliability, objectivity, and external validity, respectively. In later writings, responding to criticisms and to their own evolving views, a fifth criterion more distinctively aligned with the constructivist paradigm was added: authenticity (Guba & Lincoln, 1994).

Credibility

Credibility refers to confidence in the truth value of the data and interpretations of them. Qualitative researchers must try to establish confidence in the truth of the findings for the particular participants and contexts in the research. Lincoln and Guba (1985) pointed out that credibility involves two aspects: first, carrying out the study in a way that enhances the believability of the findings; and second, taking steps to *demonstrate* credibility to readers. Credibility is a crucial criterion in qualitative research that has been proposed in several quality frameworks.

Dependability

Dependability refers to the stability (reliability) of data over time and over conditions. The dependability question is: Would the study findings be repeated if the inquiry were replicated with the same (or similar) participants in the same (or similar) context? Credibility cannot be attained without dependability, just as validity in quantitative research cannot be achieved without reliability.

Confirmability

Confirmability refers to objectivity—the potential for similar conclusions between two or more independent people about the data's accuracy, relevance, or meaning. This criterion is concerned with establishing that the data represent the information participants provided and that the interpretations of those data are not imagined by the researcher. For this criterion to be achieved, the findings must reflect the participants' voice and the conditions of the inquiry and not the researcher's biases.

Transferability

Transferability, analogous to generalizability, is the extent that qualitative findings can be applied in other settings or groups. Lincoln and Guba (1985) noted that the investigator's responsibility is to provide sufficient descriptive data that readers can evaluate the applicability of the data to other contexts: "Thus the naturalist cannot specify the external validity of an inquiry; he or she can provide only the thick description necessary to enable someone interested in making a transfer to reach a conclusion about whether transfer can be contemplated as a possibility" (p. 316).

Authenticity

Authenticity refers to the extent to which researchers fairly and faithfully show a range of different realities. Authenticity is demonstrated when a report conveys the feeling tone (awareness of pleasant and unpleasant feelings) of participants' lives as they are lived. A text that has authenticity allows readers to enter the experience of lives being described and develop a heightened sensitivity to the concerns that are relevant to the participants. Readers are better able to understand the lives being described with some sense of the mood, experience, language, and context of those lives.

STRATEGIES TO ENHANCE QUALITY IN QUALITATIVE INQUIRY

This section describes some of the strategies that qualitative researchers can use to establish integrity in their studies. We hope this description will prompt you to carefully assess the steps researchers did or not take to improve quality.

We have not organized strategies according to the five criteria just described (e.g., strategies researchers use to enhance *credibility*) because many strategies simultaneously address multiple criteria. Instead, we have organized strategies by phase of the study—data

TABLE 17.1 Quality-Enhancement Strategies in Relation to Lincoln and Guba's Quality Criteria for Qualitative Inquiry

Strategy	Credibility	Dependability	Confirmability	Transferability	Authenticity
Throughout the Inquiry					
Reflexivity/reflexive journaling	X				X
Careful documentation, decision trail		X	X		
Data Generation					
Prolonged engagement	X				X
Persistent observation	X				X
Comprehensive field notes	X			X	
Audio recording and verbatim transcription	X				X
Triangulation (data, method)	X	X			
Saturation of data	X			X	
Member checking	X	X			
Data Coding/Analysis					
Transcription rigour/data cleaning	X				
Intercoder checks	X		X		
Triangulation (investigator)	X	X	X		
Search for disconfirming evidence/negative case analysis	X				
Peer review/debriefing	X		X		
Inquiry audit		X	X		
Presentation of Findings					
Documentation of quality-enhancement efforts	X			X	
Thick, vivid description				X	X
Impactful, evocative writing					X
Documentation of researcher credentials, background	X				
Documentation of reflexivity	X				

generation, coding and analysis, and report preparation. Table 17.1 indicates how various quality-enhancement strategies map onto Lincoln and Guba's (1985) criteria.

Quality-Enhancement Strategies During Data Collection

Some of the strategies used by qualitative researchers are difficult to recognize in a report. For example, intensive listening during an interview, careful probing to obtain rich and comprehensive data, and taking pains to gain participants' trust are all strategies to enhance data quality that cannot easily be communicated in a report. In this section, we focus on some strategies that can be described to readers to increase their confidence in the integrity of the study results.

Prolonged Engagement and Persistent Observation

An important step in establishing integrity in qualitative studies is **prolonged engagement**—the investment of sufficient time collecting data to have an in-depth understanding of the culture, language, or views of the people or group under study; to test for misinformation; and to ensure saturation of important categories. Prolonged engagement is also important for building trust with informants, which in turn makes it more likely that useful and rich information will be obtained.

Example of prolonged engagement ·
Woodgate and colleagues (2015) conducted an ethnographic study to understand the experiences of parenting children with complex care needs.

It was noted that "measures including prolonged engagement with participants and data, careful line-by-line analysis of the transcripts, and detailed memo writing were in place to enhance the methodological rigour of the study" (p. 4).

High-quality data collection in qualitative studies also involves **persistent observation** or the researchers' focus on the characteristics or aspects of a situation that are relevant to the phenomena being studied. As Lincoln and Guba (1985) noted, "If prolonged engagement provides scope, persistent observation provides depth" (p. 304).

Example of persistent observation ·
Nortvedt et al. (2016) conducted a qualitative study of 14 immigrant women on long-term sick leave during their rehabilitation in Norway. In addition to interviews, the first author conducted participant observation during two rehabilitation courses at an outpatient clinic. Each course occurred over 10 days for 10 weeks each. The total number of hours of observation of these immigrant women was 45 hours.

Reflexivity Strategies

Reflexivity involves awareness that the researcher as an individual brings to the inquiry a unique background, set of values, and a professional identity that can affect the research process. Reflexivity involves attending continually to the researcher's effect on the collection, analysis, and interpretation of data.

The most widely used strategy for maintaining reflexivity is to maintain a reflexive journal or diary. Reflexive notes can be used to record, in an ongoing fashion, thoughts about how previous experiences and readings about the phenomenon are affecting the inquiry. Through self-interrogation and reflection, researchers seek to be well positioned to probe deeply and to grasp the experience, process, or culture under study through the lens of participants.

 TIP Researchers sometimes begin a study by being interviewed themselves with regard to the phenomenon under study. Of course, this approach is possible only if the researcher has experienced that phenomenon.

Data and Method Triangulation

Triangulation refers to the use of multiple ways to learn about the truth. The aim of triangulation is to "overcome the intrinsic bias that comes from single-method, single-observer, and single-theory studies" (Denzin, 1989, p. 313). Triangulation can also help to capture a more complete, contextualized picture of the phenomenon under study. Denzin (1989) identified four types of triangulation (data triangulation, investigator triangulation, method triangulation, and theory triangulation), and other types have been proposed. Two types are relevant to data collection.

Data triangulation involves the use of multiple data sources for the purpose of validating conclusions. There are three types of data triangulation: time, space, and person. *Time triangulation* involves collecting data on the same phenomenon or about the same people at different points in time (e.g., at different times of the year). This concept is similar to test–retest reliability assessment—the point is not to study a phenomenon longitudinally to assess change but to establish the stability of the phenomenon across time. *Space triangulation* involves collecting data on the same phenomenon in multiple sites to test for cross-site consistency. Finally, *person triangulation* involves collecting data from different types or levels of people (e.g., patients, health care staff) with the aim of validating data through multiple perspectives on the phenomenon.

Example of person and space triangulation

Woo and his team (2017) undertook a qualitative study to understand the experience of receiving wound care in the community. They interviewed 16 patients who were affected with different types of chronic wounds including pressure injuries, venous leg ulcers, and diabetic foot ulcers. Nine patients were treated by multidisciplinary wound care teams from two different clinics and seven patients received standard care from home-care nurses alone. In addition, 12 clinicians from various professional backgrounds including nursing, medicine, podiatry, and management were interviewed to look for consistencies in the wound care experiences and compare their perspectives through person triangulation. There are four overarching themes: wound care expertise is required across health care sectors, psychosocial needs of patients with chronic wounds are key barriers to treatment concordance, structured training, and a well-coordinated multidisciplinary team approach.

Method triangulation involves using multiple methods of data collection. In qualitative studies, researchers often use a rich mix of unstructured data collection methods (e.g., interviews, observations, documents) to develop a comprehensive understanding of a phenomenon. Diverse data collection methods provide an opportunity to evaluate that the description of the phenomenon is consistent and coherent.

Example of method triangulation

Wright and an interprofessional research team (2015) studied caregivers' experiences of end-of-life delirium. Data collection methods included 15 months of participant observation over 80 field visits, including day, evening, and night shifts; 28 semi-structured interviews with hospice caregivers (nurses, physicians, volunteers, administrators); and document analysis.

Comprehensive and Vivid Recording of Information

In addition to taking steps to record interview data accurately (e.g., via careful transcriptions of recorded interviews), researchers ideally prepare field notes that are rich with descriptions of what transpired in the field—even if interviews are the only source of data.

Some researchers specifically develop an **audit trail**—a systematic collection of materials that would allow an independent auditor to draw conclusions about the data. An audit trail might include the raw data (e.g., interview transcripts), methodologic and reflexive notes, topic guides, and data reconstruction products (e.g., drafts of the final report). Similarly, the maintenance of a *decision trail* that communicates the researcher's decision rules for categorizing data and making analytic inferences is a useful way to enhance the dependability of the study. When researchers share some decision trail information in their reports, readers can better evaluate the soundness of the decisions.

Example of an audit trail •
Manuel and Brunger (2016) used a grounded theory approach to examine the experience of living with an implantable cardioverter defibrillator (ICD) for arrhythmogenic right ventricular cardiomyopathy in the province of Newfoundland and Labrador. An audit trail and memos were used to enhance credibility, identify any potential bias, and recognize variations in the data. Participants' perceptions about ICD were influenced by four themes: accepting that the ICD is needed to survive, anticipating and understanding why the ICD fired, drawing on social support, and living with everyday challenges.

Member Checking

In a **member check**, researchers give participants feedback about emerging interpretations and then seek participants' reactions. The argument is that participants should have an opportunity to assess and validate whether the researchers' interpretations are good representations of their realities. Member checking can be carried out as data are being collected (e.g., through probing to ensure that interviewers have properly interpreted participants' meanings) and more formally after data have been analyzed in follow-up interviews.

Despite the potential that member checking has for enhancing credibility, it has potential drawbacks. For example, member checks can lead to erroneous conclusions if participants share a common façade or a desire to "cover up." Also, some participants might agree with researchers' interpretations out of politeness or in the belief that researchers are "smarter" than they are. Thorne and Darbyshire (2005) cautioned against what they called *adulatory validity*, "a mutual stroking ritual that satisfies the agendas of both researcher and researched" (p. 1110). They noted that member checking tends to describe participants in favourable terms.

Few strategies for enhancing data quality are as controversial as member checking. Nevertheless, it is a strategy that has the potential to enhance credibility if it is done in a manner that encourages candour and critical appraisal by participants.

Example of member checking •
Martin and colleagues (2016) conducted a qualitative study to explore the feasibility of a community-based participatory HIV-prevention intervention within a Canadian men's correctional facility. Twelve men from a medium-security federal correctional facility participated in the study. Eight participants were serving life sentences, three were Aboriginal and their education levels ranged from below grade 8 to 11 years of post-secondary education. The researcher met with participants to "member check" the preliminary findings. Four themes emerged: educational preferences for content, delivery and diversity of education, stigma and fear, and social capital and future action.

Strategies Relating to Coding and Analysis

Excellent qualitative inquiry is likely to involve the simultaneous collection and analysis of data, and so, several of the strategies described earlier also contribute to analytic integrity. Member checking, for example, can occur in an ongoing fashion as part of the data collection process but typically also involves participants' review of preliminary analysis. In this section, we introduce a few additional quality-enhancement strategies associated with the coding, analysis, and interpretation of qualitative data.

Investigator Triangulation

Investigator triangulation refers to the use of two or more researchers to make data collection, coding, and analysis decisions. The underlying premise is that through collaboration, investigators can reduce the possibility of biased decisions and idiosyncratic interpretations.

Conceptually, investigator triangulation is analogous to interrater reliability in quantitative studies and is a strategy that is often used in coding qualitative data. Some researchers take formal steps to compare two or more independent category schemes or independent coding decisions.

> **Example of independent coding** •
> Dosani and coresearchers (2016) studied the experiences of mothers and the perceptions of public health nurses (PHNs) about breastfeeding late preterm infants in Calgary, Alberta, Canada. In-depth interviews were conducted with 11 mothers and 10 public health nurses. Initial coding of the verbatim transcripts was undertaken by two researchers independently. Three themes emerged from the interviews with the mothers: significant difficulty with breastfeeding, failing to recognize the infant's feeding distress and disorganized behaviour, and the parental stress caused by the multiple feeding issues.

Collaboration can also be used at the analysis stage. If investigators bring to the analysis task a complementary blend of skills and expertise, the analysis and interpretation can potentially benefit from divergent perspectives. In Dosani et al.'s (2016) study of breastfeeding late preterm infants, emerging themes were discussed and debated among the team.

Searching for Disconfirming Evidence and Competing Explanations

A powerful verification procedure involves a systematic search for data that will challenge a categorization or explanation that has emerged early in the analysis. The search for **disconfirming evidence** occurs through purposive or theoretical sampling methods. Clearly, this strategy depends on concurrent data collection and data analysis: Researchers cannot look for disconfirming data unless they have a sense of what they need to know.

> **Example of searching for disconfirming evidence** • • • • • • • • • • • • • • • •
> Slaughter and her research group (2017) conducted a focus group study to examine the perception of having a health care aide (HCA) designated to remind, guide, and encourage fellow HCAs to carry out specific care practices with residents of long-term care. A convenience sample of 24 HCAs from five residential care facilities in western Canada participated in the study. One of the research assistants with no previous experience in health care was assigned to critically search for disconfirming evidence during the analysis. Confirmability of the study was enhanced by discussions leading to consensus about the themes. Ideas to optimize the role including: effective implementation strategies, perceptions of the role, role credibility, and a supportive context.

Lincoln and Guba (1985) discussed the related activity of **negative case analysis**. This strategy (sometimes called *deviant case analysis*) is a process by which researchers search for cases that appear to disconfirm earlier hypotheses and then revise their interpretations as necessary. The goal of this procedure is to continuously refine a hypothesis or theory until it accounts for *all* cases.

Example of a negative case analysis •
Begley et al. (2015) studied whether clinical specialists in Ireland were fulfilling role expectations in terms of involvement with research and evidence-based practice (EBP) activities. After collecting interview and observational data, the team came together to develop themes. The team searched for examples of negative cases "that might disprove, or validate, emerging findings" (p. 104).

Peer Review and Debriefing

Peer debriefing involves external validation, often in face-to-face sessions with peers to review aspects of the inquiry. Peer debriefing exposes researchers to the searching questions of others who are experienced in either the methods of constructivist inquiry, the phenomenon being studied, or both.

In a peer review or debriefing session, researchers might present written or oral summaries of the data that have been gathered, categories and themes that are emerging, and researchers' interpretations of the data. In some cases, taped interviews might be played. Among the questions that peer debriefers might address are the following:

● Do the gathered data adequately describe the phenomenon? Have all important themes or categories been identified?
● If there are important oversights, what strategies might correct this problem?
● Are there any apparent errors of fact or possible errors of interpretation?
● Is there evidence of researcher bias?
● Are the themes and interpretations fitting together into a clear, useful, and creative conceptualization of the phenomenon?

Example of peer review •
Browne and colleagues (2016) conducted an ethnographic study to identify the key dimensions of equity-oriented health services for marginalized populations. A total of 114 patients and staff participated in the interviews. Coding categories and themes were assessed through regular meetings and discussions with the indigenous community advisory committee including leaders in indigenous health services, patient representatives, and people recognized as indigenous elders. These stakeholders confirmed that the identified themes reflected their experiences and interpretations. Four key dimensions of equity-oriented health services are foundational to supporting the health and well-being of indigenous people: inequity-responsive care, culturally safe care, trauma- and violence-informed care, and contextually tailored care.

Inquiry Audits

A similar, but more formal, approach is to undertake an **inquiry audit**, a procedure that involves a scrutiny of the actual data and relevant supporting documents by an external reviewer. Such an audit requires careful documentation of all aspects of the inquiry. Once the *audit trail* materials are assembled, the inquiry auditor proceeds to audit, in a fashion analogous to a financial audit, the trustworthiness of the data and the meanings attached to them. Such audits are a good tool for persuading others that qualitative data are worthy of confidence. Relatively few comprehensive inquiry audits have been reported in the literature, but some studies report partial audits.

Example of an inquiry audit •
Rotegård, Fagermoen, and Ruland (2012) studied cancer patients' experiences and perceptions of their personal strengths through their illness and recovery in four focus group interviews with 26 participants. A partial audit was undertaken by having an external researcher review a sample of transcripts and interpretations.

Strategies Relating to Presentation

This section describes some aspects of the qualitative report itself that can help to persuade readers of the high quality of the inquiry.

Thick and Contextualized Description

Thick description refers to a rich, thorough, and vivid description of the research context, the study participants, and events and experiences observed during the inquiry. Transferability cannot occur unless investigators provide sufficient information for judging contextual similarity. Lucid and textured descriptions, with the judicious inclusion of verbatim quotes from study participants, also contribute to the authenticity of a qualitative study.

    TIP   Sandelowski (2004) cautioned as follows: "...the phrase *thick description* likely ought not to appear in write-ups of qualitative research at all, as it is among those qualitative research words that should be seen but not written" (p. 215).

In high-quality qualitative studies, descriptions typically go beyond a faithful representation of information. Powerful description is moving and has the capacity for emotional impact. Qualitative researchers must be careful, however, not to misrepresent their findings by sharing only the most emotional stories. Thorne and Darbyshire (2005) cautioned against what they called *lachrymal validity*, a criterion based on whether the report can cause readers to cry. At the same time, they noted the opposite problem with reports that are "bloodless." Bloodless findings are characterized by a tendency of some researchers to "play it safe in writing up the research, reporting the obvious … [and] failing to apply any inductive analytic spin to the sequence, structure, or form of the findings" (p. 1109).

Researcher Credibility

Another aspect of credibility is **researcher credibility**. In qualitative studies, researchers *are* the data-collecting instruments—as well as creators of the analytic process—and so, their qualifications, experience, and reflexivity are relevant in establishing confidence in the data. Patton (2002) has argued that trustworthiness is enhanced if the report contains information about the researchers, including information about credentials and any personal connections the researchers had to the people, topic, or community under study. For example, it is relevant for a reader of a report on the coping mechanisms of AIDS patients to know that the researcher is HIV-positive. Researcher credibility is also enhanced when reports describe the researchers' efforts to be reflexive.

Example of researcher credibility •
Woodgate and Busolo (2017) conducted an ethnographic study of healthy adolescents' perspectives of cancer using metaphors. Data were collected through individual open-ended interviews, the Photovoice method, and focus groups. The principal researcher

was a professor with extensive experience in qualitative research and arts-based methods, including Photovoice. She was the Canadian Institutes of Health Research Applied Chair in Reproductive, Child and Youth Health Services and Policy Research.

INTERPRETATION OF QUALITATIVE FINDINGS

It is difficult to describe the interpretive process in qualitative studies, but there is considerable agreement that the ability to "make meaning" from qualitative texts depends on whether researchers are immersed in and close to the data. Incubation is the process of living the data for researchers to understand their meanings, find essential patterns, and draw insightful conclusions. Another ingredient in interpretation and meaning making is researchers' self-awareness and the ability to reflect on their own worldview—that is, reflexivity. Creativity also plays an important role in uncovering meaning in the data. Researchers need to spend sufficient time to get the inspiration and insight that comes with making meaning beyond the facts.

For *readers* of qualitative reports, interpretation is affected by having limited access to the data and no opportunity to "live" the data. Researchers are selective in the amount and types of information to include in their reports. Nevertheless, you should try to consider some of the same interpretive dimensions for qualitative studies as for quantitative ones (see Chapter 15).

The Credibility of Qualitative Results

As with quantitative reports, you should consider whether the results of a qualitative inquiry are believable. It is reasonable to expect authors of qualitative reports to provide *evidence* of the credibility of the findings. Because consumers view only a portion of the data, they must rely on researchers' efforts to support findings through such strategies as peer debriefings, member checks, audits, triangulation, and negative case analysis. They must also rely on researchers' honesty in acknowledging known limitations.

In considering the believability of qualitative results, you need to decide if there is convincing evidence to buy into the researchers' conceptualization. It is also appropriate to consider whether the conceptualization is consistent with your own clinical insights.

The Meaning of Qualitative Results

The researcher's interpretation and analysis of qualitative data occur virtually simultaneously in a repetitive process. Unlike quantitative analyses, the meaning of the data flows directly from qualitative analysis. Efforts to validate the analysis will also help support interpretations. Nevertheless, careful qualitative researchers hold their interpretations up for closer scrutiny—self-scrutiny as well as review by external reviewers.

 TIP Interpretation in qualitative studies sometimes yields hypotheses that can be tested in more controlled quantitative studies. Qualitative studies are well suited to generating causal hypotheses but not to testing them.

The Importance of Qualitative Results

Qualitative research is especially productive when it is used to describe and explain poorly understood phenomena. However, the phenomenon must be one that benefits scrutiny.

You should also consider whether the findings themselves are minor. Perhaps the topic is worthwhile, but you may feel after reading a report that nothing has been learned beyond what is everyday knowledge—this can happen when the data are "thin" or when the conceptualization is shallow. Readers, like researchers, want to be inspired when they read about the lives of clients and their families. Qualitative researchers often attach catchy labels to their themes, but you should ask yourself whether the labels have really portrayed an insightful construct.

The Transferability of Qualitative Results

Qualitative researchers do not aim for generalizability, but the possible application of the results to other settings is important to EBP. Thus, in interpreting qualitative results, you should consider how transferable the findings are. In what types of settings and contexts would you expect the phenomena under study unfold in a similar fashion? Of course, to make such an assessment, the researchers must have described the participants and context in sufficient detail. Because qualitative studies are context-bound, it is only through a careful analysis of the key features of the study context that transferability can be assessed.

The Implications of Qualitative Results

If the findings are judged to be believable and important and if you are satisfied with the interpretation of the results, you can begin to consider what the implications of the findings might be. First, you can consider implications for further research: Should a similar study be undertaken in a different setting? Has an important construct been identified that benefits the development of a formal measuring instrument? Do the results suggest hypotheses that could be tested through controlled quantitative research? Second, do the findings have implications for nursing practice? For example, could the health care needs of a subculture (e.g., the homeless) be addressed more effectively as a result of the study? Finally, do the findings shed light on fundamental processes that could play a role in nursing theories?

CRITIQUING INTEGRITY AND INTERPRETATIONS IN QUALITATIVE STUDIES

For qualitative research to be judged trustworthy, investigators must earn the trust of their readers. In a world that is conscious about the quality of research evidence, qualitative researchers need to be proactive in doing high-quality research and persuading others that they were successful.

Demonstrating integrity to others involves providing a good description of the quality-enhancement activities that were undertaken. Yet many qualitative reports do not provide much information about efforts to ensure that the study is strong with respect to trustworthiness. Just as clinicians seek *evidence* for clinical decisions, research consumers need evidence that findings are valid. Researchers should include enough information about their quality-enhancement strategies for readers to draw conclusions about study quality.

Part of the difficulty that qualitative researchers face in demonstrating trustworthiness is that page constraints in journals impose conflicting demands. It takes a precious amount of space to present quality-enhancement strategies adequately and convincingly. Using space for such documentation means that there is less space for the thick description of context and rich verbatim accounts that support authenticity and vividness. Qualitative research is often characterized by the need for critical compromises. It is well to keep such compromises in mind in critiquing qualitative research reports.

> **Box 17.1 Guidelines for Evaluating Trustworthiness and Integrity in Qualitative Studies**
>
> 1. Did the report discuss efforts to enhance or evaluate the quality of the data and the overall inquiry? If so, was the description sufficiently detailed and clear? If not, was there other information that allowed you to draw inferences about the quality of the data, the analysis, and the interpretations?
> 2. Which specific techniques (if any) did the researcher use to enhance the trustworthiness and integrity of the inquiry? What quality-enhancement strategies were *not* used? Would additional strategies have strengthened your confidence in the study and its evidence?
> 3. Did the researcher adequately represent the multiple realities of those being studied? Do the findings seem *authentic*?
> 4. Given the efforts to enhance data quality, what can you conclude about the study's validity/integrity/rigour/trustworthiness?
> 5. Did the report discuss any study limitations and their possible effects on the credibility of the results or on interpretations of the data? Were results interpreted in light of findings from other studies?
> 6. Did the researchers discuss the study's implications for clinical practice or future research? Were the implications well grounded in the study evidence and in evidence from earlier research?

An important point in thinking about quality in qualitative inquiry is that attention needs to be paid to both "art" and "science" and to interpretation and description. Creativity and insightfulness need to be attained but not at the expense of soundness, and the quest for soundness cannot sacrifice inspiration or else the results are likely to be "perfectly healthy but dead" (Morse, 2006, p. 6). Good qualitative work is both descriptively accurate and explicit and interpretively rich and innovative. Some guidelines that may be helpful in evaluating qualitative methods and analyses are presented in Box 17.1.

RESEARCH EXAMPLES WITH CRITICAL THINKING EXERCISES

This section describes quality-enhancement efforts in a grounded theory study—a study that was also described in Chapter 11. Read the summary and then answer the critical thinking questions that follow, referring to the full research report if necessary. Example 1 is featured on the interactive *Critical Thinking Activity* on thePoint website. The critical thinking questions for Example 2 are based on the study that appears in its entirety in Appendix B of this book. Our comments for these exercises are in the Student Resources section on thePoint.

EXAMPLE 1: TRUSTWORTHINESS IN A GROUNDED THEORY STUDY

Study: The psychological process of breast cancer patients receiving initial chemotherapy (Chen et al., 2016)

Statement of Purpose: The purpose of this study was to explore patients' suffering and adverse effects during the process of receiving the first course of chemotherapy for breast cancer.

Method: The researchers used Glaser's grounded theory methods. Twenty Taiwanese women, ranging in age from 39 to 62 years, were interviewed within 6 months of completing the first course of chemotherapy. Purposive sampling was used initially, and then theoretical sampling was used to select additional participants until categories were saturated. The interviews included such broad questions as the following: During chemotherapy, what was on your mind? How did the chemotherapy affect your life? The audio-recorded interviews were transcribed for analysis.

Quality Enhancement Strategies: The researchers' report provided good detail about efforts to enhance the trustworthiness of their study, as described in a subsection of their "Method" section labelled "Rigour." The researchers noted that the lead investigator participated in the care of the women during their hospitalization and during follow-up visits, thereby contributing to prolonged engagement—and to the development of a good therapeutic relationship. The researcher continued to observe the verbal and nonverbal expressions of these patients during follow-up visits; this strategy was described as persistent observation but could also be considered data triangulation if the analysis was informed by both the interview data and the informal observations. Three experts were invited to review and discuss the emerging conceptualization (peer debriefing). Two study participants reviewed the findings in a member check effort. The lead researcher also maintained a reflexive journal that guided her during data collection. During the interviews, the questioning was informed by ongoing data analysis so that questions were linked to emergent categories to achieve saturation. The report also included explicit statements about the researchers' credentials and experience, thus supporting researcher credibility. In terms of thick description, the researchers provided many vivid excerpts from the interviews. Moreover, they provided a table that described each individual participant in terms of age, marital status, religion, occupation, breast cancer stage, and type of chemotherapy.

Key Findings: The researchers concluded that the core category was "Rising from the ashes." Four categories represented four stages of the psychological process experienced by these patients: the fear stage, the hardship stage, the adjustment stage, and the relaxation stage. The authors noted that each stage is likely to occur repeatedly.

Critical Thinking Exercises

1. Answer the relevant questions from Box 17.1 regarding this study.
2. Also consider the following targeted questions:
    a. Which quality-enhancement strategy used by Chen et al. gave you the *most* confidence in the integrity and trustworthiness of their study? Why?
    b. Think of an additional type of triangulation that the researchers could have used in their study. How could this have been operationalized?
3. What might be some of the uses to which the findings could be put in clinical practice?

EXAMPLE 2: TRUSTWORTHINESS IN THE PHENOMENOLOGIC STUDY IN APPENDIX B

● Read the method and results sections of Beck and Watson's (2010) phenomenologic study ("Subsequent childbirth after a previous traumatic birth") in Appendix B of this book.

Critical Thinking Exercises

1. Answer the relevant questions from Box 17.1 regarding this study.
2. Also consider the following targeted questions:
    a. What are one or two ways in which triangulation could have been used in this study?
    b. Which quality-enhancement strategy used by Beck and Watson gave you the most confidence in the integrity and trustworthiness of their study? Why?

WANT TO KNOW MORE?
A wide variety of resources to enhance your learning and understanding of this chapter are available on thePoint.

- Interactive Critical Thinking Activity
- Chapter Supplement on Whittemore and Colleagues' Framework of Quality Criteria in Qualitative Research
- Answer to the Critical Thinking Exercise for Example 2
- Internet Resources with useful websites for Chapter 17
- A Wolters Kluwer journal article on a topic related to this chapter

Summary Points

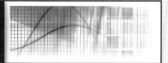

- One of several controversies regarding *quality* in qualitative studies involves terminology. Some argue that *rigour* and *validity* are quantitative terms that are not suitable as goals in qualitative inquiry, but others believe these terms are appropriate. Other controversies involve what criteria to use as indicators of integrity and whether there should be generic or study-specific criteria.
- Lincoln and Guba proposed one framework for evaluating **trustworthiness** in qualitative inquiries in terms of five criteria: credibility, dependability, confirmability, transferability, and authenticity.
- **Credibility**, which refers to confidence in the truth value of the findings, has been viewed as the qualitative equivalent of internal validity. **Dependability**, the stability of data over time and over conditions, is somewhat analogous to reliability in quantitative studies. **Confirmability** refers to the objectivity of the data. **Transferability**, the analogue of external validity, is the extent to which findings can be transferred to other settings or groups. **Authenticity** is the extent to which researchers faithfully show a range of different realities and convey the feeling tone of lives as they are lived.

- Strategies for enhancing quality during qualitative data collection include **prolonged engagement**, which strives for adequate scope of data coverage; **persistent observation**, which is aimed at achieving adequate depth; comprehensive recording of information (including maintenance of an **audit trail**); triangulation; and **member checks** (asking study participants to review and react to emerging conceptualizations).
- **Triangulation** is the process of using multiple referents to draw conclusions about what constitutes the truth. This includes **data triangulation** (using multiple data sources to validate conclusions) and **method triangulation** (using multiple methods to collect data about the same phenomenon).
- Strategies for enhancing quality during the coding and analysis of qualitative data include **investigator triangulation** (independent coding and analysis of data by two or more researchers), searching for **disconfirming evidence**, searching for rival explanations and undertaking a **negative case analysis** (revising interpretations to account for cases that appear to disconfirm early conclusions), external validation through **peer debriefings** (exposing the inquiry to the searching questions of peers), and launching an **inquiry audit** (a formal scrutiny of audit trail documents by an independent auditor).
- Strategies that can be used to convince report readers of the high quality of qualitative

inquiries include using **thick description** to vividly portray contextualized information about study participants and the focal phenomenon and making efforts to be transparent about researcher credentials and reflexivity so that **researcher credibility** can be established.

- Interpretation in qualitative research involves "making meaning"—a process that is difficult to describe or critique. Yet interpretations in qualitative inquiry need to be reviewed in terms of credibility, importance, transferability, and implications.

REFERENCES

Beck, C. T., & Watson, S. (2010). Subsequent childbirth after a previous traumatic birth. *Nursing Research*, *59*, 241–249.

Begley, C., Elliott, N., Lalor, J., & Higgins, A. (2015). Perceived outcomes of research and audit activities of clinical specialists in Ireland. *Clinical Nurse Specialist*, *29*, 100–111.

Browne A. J., Varcoe C., Lavoie J., et al. (2016). Enhancing health care equity with Indigenous populations: evidence-based strategies from an ethnographic study. *BMC Health Services Research*, *16*(1), 544.

Chen, Y. C., Huang, H., Kao, C., Sun, C., Chiang, C., & Sun, F. (2016). The psychological process of breast cancer patients receiving initial chemotherapy: Rising from the ashes. *Cancer Nursing*, *39*(6), E36–E44.

Denzin, N. K. (1989). *The research act: A theoretical introduction to sociological methods* (3rd ed.). Upper Saddle River, NJ: Prentice Hall.

Dosani A., Hemraj J., Premji S. S., et al. (2017). Breastfeeding the late preterm infant: experiences of mothers and perceptions of public health nurses. *International Breastfeeding Journal*, *12*, 23.

Guba, E., & Lincoln, Y. (1994). Competing paradigms in qualitative research. In N. Denzin & Y. Lincoln (Eds.). *Handbook of qualitative research* (pp. 105–117). Thousand Oaks, CA: Sage.

Lincoln, Y. S., & Guba, E. G. (1985). Naturalistic inquiry. Newbury Park, CA: Sage.

Manuel A., & Brunger F. (2016). Embodying a New Meaning of Being At Risk: Living With an Implantable Cardioverter Defibrillator for Arrhythmogenic Right Ventricular Cardiomyopathy. *Global Qualitative Nursing Research*, *3*:2333393616674810. doi: 10.1177/2333393616674810. eCollection 2016 Jan-Dec.

Martin R. E., Turner R., Howett L., et al. (2016). Twelve Committed Men: the feasibility of a community-based participatory HIV-prevention intervention within a Canadian men's correctional facility. *Global Health Promotion*, pii: 1757975916659045.

Morse, J. M. (2006). Insight, inference, evidence, and verification: Creating a legitimate discipline. *International Journal of Qualitative Methods*, *5*, 93–100. Retrieved from http://www.ualberta.ca/ijqm/

Morse, J. M. (2015). Critical analysis of strategies for determining rigor in qualitative inquiry. *Qualitative Health Research*, *25*, 1212–1222.

Nortvedt, L., Lohne, V., Kumar, B. N., & Hansen, H. P. (2016). A lonely life–A qualitative study of immigrant women on long-term sick leave in Norway. *International Journal of Nursing Studies*, *54*, 54–64.

Patton, M. Q. (2002). *Qualitative research & evaluation methods* (3rd ed.). Thousand Oaks, CA: Sage.

Rotegård, A., Fagermoen, M., & Ruland, C. (2012). Cancer patients' experiences of their personal strengths through illness and recovery. *Cancer Nursing*, *35*, E8–E17.

Sandelowski, M. (2004). Counting cats in Zanzibar. *Research in Nursing & Health*, *27*, 215–216.

Slaughter S. E., Bampton E., Erin D. F., et al. (2017). Knowledge translation interventions to sustain direct care provider behaviour change in long-term care: A process evaluation. *Journal of Evaluation in Clinical Practice*. doi: 10.1111/jep.12784.

Thorne, S., & Darbyshire, P. (2005). Land mines in the field: A modest proposal for improving the craft of qualitative health research. *Qualitative Health Research*, *15*, 1105–1113.

Whittemore, R., Chase, S. K., & Mandle, C. L. (2001). Validity in qualitative research. *Qualitative Health Research*, *11*, 522–537.

Woo K. Y., Wong J., Rice K., et al. (2017). Patients' and clinicians' experiences of wound care in Canada: a descriptive qualitative study. *Journal of Wound Care*, *26*(Sup7):S4–S13.

Woodgate R. L., & Busolo D. S. (2017). Healthy Canadian adolescents' perspectives of cancer using metaphors: a qualitative study. *BMJ Open*, *7*(1), e013958.

Woodgate R. L., Edwards M., Ripat J. D., et al. (2015). Intense parenting: a qualitative study detailing the experiences of parenting children with complex care needs. *BMC Pediatrics*, *15*, 197.

Wright D. K., Brajtman S., Cragg B., & Macdonald M. E. (2015). Delirium as letting go: An ethnographic analysis of hospice care and family moral experience. *Palliative Medicine*, *29*(10), 959–966.

*A link to this open-access article is provided in the Internet Resources section on thePoint website.

**This journal article is available on thePoint for this chapter. ✂

18 Systematic Reviews: Meta-Analysis and Metasynthesis

Learning Objectives

On completing this chapter, you will be able to:

- Discuss alternative approaches to integrating research evidence, and advantages to using systematic methods
- Describe key decisions and steps in doing a meta-analysis and metasynthesis
- Critique key aspects of a written systematic review
- Define new terms in the chapter

Key Terms

- Effect size index
- Forest plot
- Frequency effect size
- Intensity effect size
- Manifest effect size
- Meta-analysis
- Meta-ethnography
- Meta-summary
- Metasynthesis
- Primary study
- Publication bias
- Statistical heterogeneity
- Subgroup analysis
- Systematic review

In Chapter 7, we described major steps in conducting a literature review. This chapter also discusses reviews of existing evidence but focuses on systematic reviews, especially those in the form of *meta-analyses* and *metasyntheses*. Systematic reviews, a cornerstone of evidence-based practice (EBP), are inquiries that follow many of the same rules as those for **primary studies** (i.e., original research investigations). This chapter provides guidance in helping you to understand and evaluate systematic research integration.

RESEARCH INTEGRATION AND SYNTHESIS

A **systematic review** integrates research evidence about a specific research question using careful sampling and data collection procedures that are spelled out in advance. The review process is disciplined and transparent, so that readers of a systematic review can assess the integrity of the conclusions.

Twenty years ago, systematic reviews usually involved narrative integration using non-statistical methods to synthesize research findings. Narrative systematic reviews continue to be published, but meta-analytic techniques that use statistical integration are widely used. Most reviews in the Cochrane Collaboration, for example, are meta-analyses. Statistical integration, however, is sometimes inappropriate, as we shall see.

Qualitative researchers have also developed techniques to integrate findings across studies. Many terms exist for such activities (e.g., *meta-study*, *meta-ethnography*), but the one that has emerged as the top term is *metasynthesis*.

The field of research integration is expanding steadily. This chapter provides a brief introduction to this important and complex topic.

META-ANALYSIS

Meta-analyses of randomized controlled trials (RCTs) are at the top of traditional evidence hierarchies (see Fig. 2.1). The essence of a **meta-analysis** is that findings from each study are used to compute a common index, an *effect size*. Effect size values are averaged across studies, providing information about the relationship between variables across multiple studies.

Advantages of Meta-Analyses

Meta-analysis offers a simple advantage as an integration method: *objectivity*. It is difficult to draw objective conclusions about a body of evidence using narrative methods when results are inconsistent, as they often are. Narrative reviewers make subjective decisions about how much weight to give findings from different studies, and so different reviewers may reach different conclusions in reviewing the same studies. Meta-analysts make decisions that are explicit and open to examination. The integration itself also is objective because it uses statistical formulas. Readers of a meta-analysis can be confident that another analyst using the same data set and analytic decisions would come to the same conclusions.

Another advantage of meta-analysis is *power* (i.e., the probability of detecting a true relationship between variables; see Chapter 14). By combining effects across multiple studies, power is increased. In a meta-analysis, it is possible to conclude that a relationship is real (e.g., an intervention is effective), even when several small studies produced nonsignificant findings. In a narrative review, 10 nonsignificant findings would almost surely be interpreted as lack of evidence of a true effect, which could be the wrong conclusion.

Despite these advantages, meta-analysis is not always appropriate. Indiscriminate use has led critics to warn against potential abuses.

Criteria for Using Meta-Analytic Techniques in a Systematic Review

Reviewers need to decide whether statistical integration is suitable. A basic criterion is that the research question should be almost identical across studies. This means that the independent and dependent variables and the study populations are sufficiently similar for integration. The variables may be operationalized differently. A nurse-led intervention to promote healthy diets among diabetics could be a 4-week clinic-based program in one study and a 6-week home-based intervention in another, for example. However, a study of the effects of a 1-hour lecture to discourage eating "junk food" among overweight adolescents would be a poor candidate to include in this meta-analysis. This is frequently referred to as the "apples and oranges" or "fruit" problem. Meta-analyses should not be about *fruit*—that is, a broad category—but rather about "apples," or, even better, "Granny Smith apples."

Another criterion relates to whether a sufficient knowledge base is available for statistical integration. If there are only a few studies or if all of the studies are poorly designed, it usually would not make sense to compute an "average" effect.

One other issue is about the consistency of the evidence. When the same hypothesis has been tested in multiple studies and the results are highly conflicting, meta-analysis is likely not appropriate. As an extreme example, if half the studies testing an intervention found benefits for those in the intervention group but the other half found benefits for the controls, it would be misleading to compute an average effect. In this situation, it would be better to do an in-depth narrative analysis of *why* the results are conflicting.

Example of inability to conduct a meta-analysis • • • • • • • • • • • • • • • •
Hoben and her team from the University of Alberta (2017) undertook a systematic review of strategies designed to prevent/overcome residents' responsive behaviours to oral care or enable/motivate residents to perform their own oral care in nursing homes. They were not able to statistically pool results of included studies for meta-analysis due to insufficient number of studies with similar designs, methods, and outcomes. They conducted a narrative synthesis of the included studies.

Steps in a Meta-Analysis

We begin by describing major steps in a meta-analysis so that you can appreciate and evaluate the decisions a meta-analyst makes that affect the quality of the review.

Problem Formulation

A systematic review begins with a problem statement and a research question or hypothesis. Questions for a meta-analysis are usually narrow, focusing, for example, on a particular type of intervention and specific outcomes. The careful definition of key constructs is critical for deciding whether a primary study qualifies for the synthesis.

Example of a question from a meta-analysis • • • • • • • • • • • • • • • • • • •
Harrison and colleagues (2017) conducted a meta-analysis that addressed the question of whether sweet solutions were more effective than placebo or no treatment for analgesia in neonates. The clinical question was established using the PICO framework (see Chapter 2). The **p**opulation was neonates. The **i**ntervention was use of sweet solutions, and the **c**omparison was placebo solutions (e.g., water) or no treatment. **O**utcomes included pain reduction.

A strategy that is gaining momentum is to undertake a *scoping review* to refine the specific question for a systematic review. A scoping review is a preliminary investigation that clarifies the range and nature of the evidence base using flexible procedures. Such scoping reviews can suggest strategies for a full systematic review and can also indicate whether statistical integration (a meta-analysis) is feasible.

The Design of a Meta-Analysis

Sampling is an important design issue. In a systematic review, the sample consists of the primary studies that have addressed the research question. The eligibility criteria must be stated. Substantively, the criteria specify the population (P) and the variables (I, C, and O). For example, if the reviewer is integrating findings about the effectiveness of an intervention, which outcomes *must* the researchers have studied? With regard to the population, will (for example) certain age groups be excluded? The criteria might also specify that only studies that used a randomized design will be included. On practical grounds, reports not written in English might be excluded. Another decision is whether to include both published and unpublished reports.

Example of sampling criteria •
Parker and coresearchers (2017) published a meta-analysis to examine strategies associated with successful peripheral intravenous catheterization on the first attempt in
adult emergency department patients and inpatients. Primary studies had to be RCTs
involving inpatients or patients from emergency department 18 years of age or greater
and reported PIVC first attempt success or number of skin punctures. Trials were
excluded if they were not reported in English.

Researchers sometimes use study quality as a sampling criterion. Screening out studies
of lower quality can occur indirectly if the meta-analyst excludes studies that did not use
a randomized design. More directly, each potential primary study can be rated for quality
and excluded if the quality score falls below a threshold. Alternatives to dealing with study
quality are discussed in a later section. Evaluations of study quality are part of the integration
process, and analysts need to decide how to assess quality and what to do with assessment
information.

Another design issue concerns the **statistical heterogeneity** of results in the primary
studies. For each study, meta-analysts compute an index to summarize the strength of relationship between an independent variable and a dependent variable. Just as there is inevitably variation *within* studies (not all people in a study have identical scores on outcomes),
so there is inevitably variation in effects *across* studies. If the results are highly variable (e.g.,
results are conflicting across studies), a meta-analysis may be inappropriate, but if the results
are moderately variable, researchers can explore why this might be so. For example, the
effects of an intervention might be systematically different for men and women. Researchers
often plan for *subgroup analyses* during the design phase of the project.

The Search for Evidence in the Literature

Many standard methods of searching the literature were described in Chapter 7. Reviewers
must decide whether their review will cover published and unpublished findings. There is
some disagreement about whether reviewers should limit their sample to published studies
or should cast as wide a net as possible and include *grey literature*—that is, documents produced by all levels of government, academia, business, and industry in electronic or printed
formats that are not controlled by commercial publishers. Some people restrict their sample to reports in peer-reviewed journals, arguing that the peer review system is a desirable
screen for evidence worthy of consideration.

Excluding nonpublished findings, however, runs the risk of biased results. **Publication bias** is the tendency for published studies to systematically overrepresent statistically significant findings. This bias is widespread: Authors may refrain from submitting
manuscripts with nonsignificant results, reviewers and editors tend to reject such reports
when they are submitted, and users of evidence may ignore the findings if they are published. The exclusion of grey literature in a meta-analysis can lead to the overestimation
of effects.

Meta-analysts can use various search strategies to locate grey literature in addition to
the usual methods for a literature review. These include contacting key researchers in the
field to see if they have done studies (or know of studies) that have not been published and
reviewing abstracts from conference proceedings.

 TIP There are statistical procedures to detect and correct for publication biases, but
opinions vary about their utility. A brief explanation of methods for assessing publication bias is included in the Supplement to this chapter on theVault.

Example of a search strategy from a systematic review • • • • • • • • • • • •
Guillaumie and colleagues (2016) did a meta-analysis of the effect of mindfulness-based interventions on registered nurses and nursing students. Their search strategy included a search of five electronic databases (Medline, Embase, PsycINFO, Cochrane Library, and The Cumulative Index to Nursing and Allied Health Literature (CINAHL)), previous literature reviews and the bibliographies of identified studies were checked manually. There is sufficient evidence to support the use of mindfulness interventions to improve nurses' mental health.

Evaluations of Study Quality

In systematic reviews, the evidence from primary studies needs to be evaluated to assess how much confidence to place in the findings. Rigorous studies should be given more weight than weaker ones in coming to conclusions about a body of evidence. In meta-analyses, evaluations of study quality sometimes involve overall ratings of evidence quality on a multi-item scale. Hundreds of rating scales exist, but the use of such scales has been criticized. Quality criteria vary from instrument to instrument, and the result is that study quality can be rated differently with different assessment scales—or by different raters using the same scale. Also, when an overall scale score is used, the meaning of the scores often is not transparent to users of the review.

The *Cochrane Handbook* (Higgins & Green, 2008) recommends a domain-based evaluation—that is, a *component approach*, as opposed to a *scale approach*. Individual design elements are coded separately for each study. So, for example, a researcher might code for whether randomization was used, whether participants were blinded, the extent of attrition from the study, and so on.

Quality assessments of primary studies, regardless of approach, should be done by two or more qualified individuals. If there are disagreements between the raters, there should be a discussion until a consensus has been reached or until another rater helps to resolve the difference.

Example of a quality assessment •
Johnston et al. (2017) completed a Cochrane review of RCTs testing the effects of skin-to-skin care or "kangaroo care" for procedural pain in neonates. They used the Cochrane domain approach to capture elements of trial quality. The first two authors completed assessments, and disagreements were resolved by discussion. Skin-to-skin care appears to be effective and safe for a single painful procedure, as evidenced by reduction in pain measured by both physiologic and behavioural indicators.

Extraction and Encoding of Data for Analysis

The next step in a meta-analysis is to extract and record relevant information about the findings, methods, and study characteristics. The goal is to create a data set for statistical analysis.

Basic source information must be recorded (e.g., year of publication, country where data were collected). Important methodologic features include sample size, whether participants were randomized to treatments, whether blinding was used, rates of attrition, and length of follow-up. Characteristics of participants must be encoded as well (e.g., their mean age). Finally, information about findings must be extracted. Reviewers must either calculate effect sizes (discussed in the next section) or must record sufficient statistical information that computer software can compute them.

As with other decisions, extraction and coding of information should be completed by two or more people, at least for a portion of the studies in the sample. This allows for an assessment of interrater agreement, which should be sufficiently high to persuade readers of the review that the data are accurate.

Example of intercoder agreement $\cdots\cdots\cdots\cdots\cdots\cdots\cdots\cdots\cdots\cdots\cdots$
Chiu et al. (2016) completed a meta-analysis of the effects of community-based hip fracture rehabilitation interventions for older adults with cognitive impairment. Two reviewers independently extracted data from each of the included studies using a standardized spreadsheet developed by the research team. Disagreements were resolved until consensus was reached. Posthospital discharge interventions including inpatient and outpatient physiotherapy, family education, and a discharge assessment may improve various physical function outcomes, mobility, and activities of daily living for older adults with cognitive impairment following a hip fracture.

Calculation of Effects

Meta-analyses depend on the calculation of an **effect size index** that is represented by a single number—the relationship between the independent and outcome variable in each study. Effects are captured differently depending on the measurement level of variables. The three most common scenarios for meta-analysis involve comparisons of two groups such as an intervention versus a control group on a continuous outcome (e.g., blood pressure), comparisons of two groups on a dichotomous outcome (e.g., stopped smoking vs. continued smoking), or correlations between two continuous variables (e.g., between blood pressure and anxiety scores).

The first scenario, comparison of two group means, is especially common. When the outcomes across studies are on identical scales (e.g., all outcomes are measures of weight in kilograms), the effect is captured by simply subtracting the mean for one group from the mean for the other. For example, if the mean postintervention weight in an intervention group was 80 kg and that for a control group was 88 kg, the effect would be −8. Typically, however, outcomes are measured on different scales (e.g., different scales to measure pain). Mean differences across studies cannot in such situations be combined and averaged; researchers need an index that is neutral to the original metric. Cohen's d, the effect size index most often used, transforms all effects into standard deviation units (see Chapter 14). If d were computed to be 0.50, it means that the group mean for one group was one-half a standard deviation higher than the mean for the other group—regardless of the original measurement scale.

 TIP The term *effect size* is widely used for d in the nursing literature, but the term usually used for Cochrane reviews is *standardized mean difference* or SMD.

When the outcomes in the primary studies are dichotomies, meta-analysts usually use the odds ratio (OR) or the relative risk (RR) index. In nonexperimental studies, a common effect size statistic is Pearson's r, which indicates the strength and direction of effect.

Data Analysis

After an effect size is computed for each study, a pooled effect estimate is computed as a *weighted average* of the individual effects. The bigger the weight given to any study, the more that study will contribute to the weighted average. A widely used approach is to give more weight to studies with larger samples.

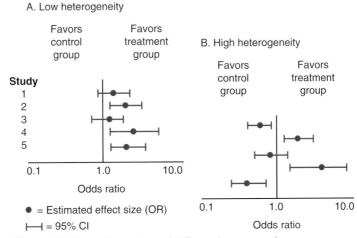

Figure 18.1 Two forest plots of different heterogeneity.

An important decision concerns how to deal with the heterogeneity of findings—that is, differences from one study to another in the strength and direction of effects. Statistical heterogeneity should be formally tested, and meta-analysts should report their results.

Visual inspection of heterogeneity usually relies on the construction of **forest plots**, which are often included in meta-analytic reports. A forest plot graphs the effect size for each study, together with the 95% confidence interval (CI) around each estimate. Figure 18.1 illustrates forest plots for studies with low heterogeneity (panel A) and those with high heterogeneity (panel B). In panel A, all five effect size estimates (here, odds ratios) favour the intervention group. The CI information indicates the intervention effect is statistically significant (does not encompass 1.0) for studies 2, 4, and 5. In panel B, by contrast, the results are "all over the map." Two studies favour the control group at significant levels (studies 1 and 5), and two favour the treatment group (studies 2 and 4). Meta-analysis is not appropriate for the situation in panel B.

 TIP Heterogeneity affects not only whether a meta-analysis is appropriate but also which statistical model should be used in the analysis. When findings are similar, the researchers may use a *fixed effects model*. When results are more varied, it is better to use a *random effects model*.

Some meta-analysts seek to understand *why* effect size estimates vary across studies. Differences could be the result of clinical characteristics. For example, in intervention studies, variation in effects could be related to whether the intervention agents were nurses or other health care professionals, or variation in results could be explained by differences in participant characteristics (e.g., patients in different age groups). One strategy for exploring systematic differences in effect size is to do **subgroup analyses**. Such analyses (sometimes called *moderator* analyses) involve splitting the sample into distinct categorical groups—for example, based on gender. Effects for studies with all-male (or predominantly male) samples could be compared to those for studies with all or predominantly female samples.

Example of a subgroup analysis •
Peirson and colleagues (2016) did a meta-analysis of interventions for prevention and treatment of tobacco smoking in school-aged children and adolescents. Prespecified subgroup analyses based on baseline age (5 to 12 years, 13 to 18 years), baseline smoking status (never, former, regular [daily or weekly], occasional), intervention intensity

(high [e.g., ≥ two meetings with a health professional of any length or one long session, such as a half-day or full-day workshop], low [e.g., one brief meeting with a health professional or provision of written materials]), and study risk of bias rating (high, unclear, low) were conducted to evaluate potential differences in intervention effect. They found greater intervention benefits for regular smokers relative to controls (RR 2.06; 95% CI 1.40, 3.04) than for experimental or occasional smokers relative to controls (RR 0.91; 95% CI 0.65, 1.29).

Another analytic issue is about study quality. There are several strategies for dealing with study quality in a meta-analysis. One, as previously noted, is to establish a quality threshold for sampling studies (e.g., omitting studies with a low-quality score). A second strategy is to undertake analyses to evaluate whether excluding lower quality studies changes the results (this is called a *sensitivity analysis*). Another approach is to use quality as the basis for a subgroup analysis. For example, do randomized designs yield different average effect size estimates than quasi-experimental designs? A mix of strategies is probably a sensible approach to dealing with differences in study quality.

METASYNTHESES

Integration of qualitative findings is a growing and evolving field with few standardized procedures. This section provides a brief overview of some major issues.

Metasynthesis Defined

Terminology relating to qualitative integration is diverse and complex. Thorne and four other leading thinkers on qualitative integration (2004) used the term **metasynthesis** as an umbrella term, broadly representing "a family of methodologic approaches to developing new knowledge based on rigorous analysis of existing qualitative research findings" (p. 1343).

Many writers on this topic are fairly clear about what a metasynthesis is *not*. Metasynthesis is not a literature review—that is, a summary of research findings—nor is it a concept analysis. Schreiber, Crooks, and Stern (1997) offered a definition that has often been used for what metasynthesis *is*, "…the bringing together and breaking down of findings, examining them, discovering the essential features and, in some way, combining phenomena into a transformed whole" (p. 314). Metasyntheses are more than the sum of their parts—they offer new insights and interpretations of findings. Most methods of qualitative synthesis involve a transformational process.

Metasynthesis has had its share of controversies, especially about whether to integrate studies based on different research traditions. Some researchers have argued against combining studies from different theoretical perspectives, but others advocate for full integration across traditions and methods. Which path to follow is likely to depend on several factors, including the focus of the inquiry and the nature of the available evidence.

Steps in a Metasynthesis

Many of the steps in a metasynthesis are similar to ones we described for meta-analysis, and so some details will not be repeated here. However, we point out some distinctive issues relating to qualitative integration.

Problem Formulation

In metasynthesis, researchers begin with a research question or focus of investigation, and a key issue concerns the scope of the inquiry. Finfgeld (2003) recommended a strategy that balances breadth and utility. She advised that the scope be broad enough to fully capture the phenomenon of interest but focused enough to yield findings that are meaningful to clinicians, other researchers, and public policy makers.

Example of a statement of purpose in a metasynthesis • • • • • • • • • • • • •
Duggleby and colleagues (2017) stated that the objective of their synthesis was "To (a) explore the transition experience of family caregivers caring for persons with advanced cancer living in the community, (b) describe potential triggers for transitions, (c) identify what influences this experience, and (d) develop a conceptual framework of their transition experience."

The Design of a Metasynthesis

Like a meta-analysis, a metasynthesis requires advance planning. Having a team of at least two researchers to design and implement the study is often advantageous because of the subjective nature of interpretation. Just as in a primary study, the design of a qualitative metasynthesis should involve efforts to enhance integrity, and investigator triangulation is one such strategy.

 TIP Meta-analyses often are undertaken by researchers who did not do one of the primary studies in the review. Metasyntheses, by contrast, are often done by researchers whose area of interest has led them to do both original studies and metasyntheses on the same topic. Prior work in an area offers advantages in terms of researchers' ability to grasp subtle differences and to think abstractly about a topic, but a disadvantage may be some bias toward one's own work.

Metasynthesists must make up-front sampling decisions. For example, they decide on whether to include only findings from peer-reviewed journals. One advantage of including alternative sources, in addition to wanting a more inclusive sample, is that journal articles have page constraints. Finfgeld (2003) noted that in her metasynthesis on *courage*, she used dissertations even when a peer-reviewed journal article was available from the same study because the dissertation had richer information. Another sampling decision, as previously noted, involves whether to search for studies about a phenomenon in multiple qualitative traditions. Finally, a researcher may decide to exclude studies when they are not adequately supported with direct quotes from participants.

Example of sampling decisions •
Duggleby et al. (2015) conducted a metasynthesis of studies exploring the end-of-life experiences of indigenous peoples. They searched for relevant studies from all qualitative traditions published between 1993 and 2013. Seventeen studies and one film met the inclusion criteria. The selected studies represent a wide range of methodologies: six phenomenologies, four descriptive/content/thematic analyses, three participatory/community action research studies, two grounded-theory studies, one case study, one mixed-methods study, and one ethnography.

The Search for Data in the Literature

It is generally more difficult to find qualitative than quantitative studies using mainstream approaches such as searching electronic databases. For example, "qualitative" became an MeSH (medical subject heading) term in MEDLINE in 2003, but it is not safe to assume that all qualitative studies (e.g., ethnographies) are coded as qualitative.

TIP Sample sizes in nursing metasyntheses are highly variable, ranging from 5 or fewer studies to over 100. Sample size is likely to vary depending on scope of the inquiry, the extent of prior research, and type of metasynthesis undertaken. As with primary studies, one guideline for sampling adequacy is whether categories in the metasynthesis are saturated.

Evaluations of Study Quality

Formal evaluations of primary study quality are increasingly being undertaken by metasynthesists, in some cases simply to describe the sample of studies in the review but in other cases to make sampling decisions. Many nurse researchers use the 10-question assessment tool from the Critical Appraisal Skills Programme (CASP) of the Centre for Evidence-Based Medicine in the United Kingdom (a link is on thePoint).

Not everyone agrees that study quality should be a criterion for study inclusion. Some have argued that a flawed study does not necessarily invalidate the rich data from those studies. Noblit and Hare (1988), whose meta-ethnographic approach is widely used by nurse researchers, advocated including all relevant studies but also suggested giving more weight to higher quality studies. Another application of assessments in a metasynthesis is to explore whether interpretations are changed when low-quality studies are removed.

Extraction of Data for Analysis

Information about various features of the study need to be abstracted and coded. Metasynthesists record features of the data source (e.g., year of publication), characteristics of the sample (e.g., mean age), and methodologic features (e.g., research tradition). Most important, information about the study findings must be extracted and recorded—typically the key themes, metaphors, or categories from each study.

As Sandelowski and Barroso (2002) have noted, however, *finding* the findings is not always easy. Qualitative researchers combine data with interpretation and findings from other studies with their own. Noblit and Hare (1988) advised that, just as primary study researchers must read and reread their data before they can proceed with a meaningful analysis, metasynthesists must read the primary studies multiple times to fully grasp the categories or metaphors being described.

Data Analysis and Interpretation

Strategies for metasynthesis vary most markedly at the analysis stage. We briefly describe two approaches. Regardless of approach, metasynthesis is a complex interpretive task that involves "carefully peeling away the surface layers of studies to find their hearts and souls in a way that does the least damage to them" (Sandelowski, Docherty, & Emden, 1997, p. 370).

The Noblit and Hare Approach

Noblit and Hare (1988), whose approach is called **meta-ethnography**, argued that integration should be interpretive and not aggregative—that is, that the synthesis should focus on making interpretations rather than descriptions. Their approach includes seven phases that overlap and repeat as the metasynthesis progresses. The first three phases occur before the analysis: (1) deciding on the phenomenon, (2) deciding which studies are relevant for the synthesis, and (3) reading and rereading each study. Phases 4 through 6 concern the analysis.

- *Phase 4*: Deciding how the studies are related. In this phase, the researcher lists the key metaphors (or themes/concepts) in each study and their relation to each other. Studies can be related in three ways: *reciprocal* (directly comparable), *refutational* (in opposition to each other), or in a *line of argument* rather than reciprocal or refutational.

- *Phase 5*: Translating the qualitative studies into one another. Noblit and Hare noted that "translations are especially unique syntheses because they protect the particular, respect holism, and enable comparison. An adequate translation maintains the central metaphors and/or concepts of each account in their relation to other key metaphors or concepts in that account" (p. 28).
- *Phase 6*: Synthesizing translations. Here, the challenge for the researcher is to make a whole into more than its individual parts.

The final phase in the Noblit and Hare approach involves writing up the synthesis.

Example of Noblit and Hare's approach •
Voldbjerg et al. (2016) used Noblit and Hare's (1988) approach in their meta-ethnography of 17 studies on newly graduated nurses' use of knowledge sources. The metasynthesis revealed a line of argument among the report findings underscoring progression in knowledge use among newly graduated nurses.

The Sandelowski and Barroso Approach

Sandelowski and Barroso (2007) dichotomized integration efforts based on level of synthesis and interpretation in the primary studies. Studies are called summaries if they provide descriptive outlines of the qualitative data, usually with lists and frequencies of themes. Syntheses, by contrast, are more interpretive and involve conceptual or metaphorical reframing. Sandelowski and Barroso have argued that only syntheses should be used in a metasynthesis.

Both summaries and syntheses can, however, be used in a **meta-summary**, which can develop into a metasynthesis. Sandelowski and Barroso (2007) provided an example of a meta-summary using studies of mothering within the context of HIV infection. The first step, extracting findings, resulted in almost 800 sentences from 45 reports and represented a comprehensive inventory of findings. The 800 sentences were then reduced to 93 thematic statements or abstracted findings.

The next step involved calculating **manifest effect sizes** (i.e., effect sizes calculated from the manifest content pertaining to mothering in the context of HIV, as represented in the 93 abstracted findings). (Qualitative effect sizes are not to be confused with effects in a meta-analysis.) Two types of effect size can be created. A **frequency effect size**, indicating the *magnitude* of the findings, is the number of reports that contain a given finding, divided by all reports (excluding those with duplicated findings from the same data). For example, Sandelowski and Barroso (2007) calculated an overall frequency effect size of 60% for the finding of mothers' struggle about disclosing their HIV status to their children. In other words, 60% of the 45 primary studies had a finding of this nature.

An **intensity effect size** indicates the concentration of findings *within* each report. It is calculated by computing the number of different findings in a given report divided by the total number of findings in all reports. As an example, one primary study in Sandelowski and Barroso's (2007) meta-summary had 29 out of the 93 total findings, for an intensity effect size of 31%.

Metasyntheses can build upon meta-summaries but require findings that are more interpretive (i.e., from studies characterized as syntheses). The purpose of a metasynthesis is not to summarize but to offer new interpretations of qualitative findings. Such interpretive integrations require metasynthesists to piece the individual syntheses together to build a new consistent explanation of a target event or experience.

Example of Sandelowski and Barroso's approach • • • • • • • • • • • • • •
In the previous example of study conducted by Duggleby et al. (2015) to explore the end-of-life experiences of indigenous peoples, Sandelowski and Barroso's methodology for synthesizing qualitative research was used. Reciprocal translation was then used to integrate the metasynthesis findings using general concepts in the literature. The findings of 18 qualitative studies were synthesized into the overarching theme of "preparing the spirit" for transition to the next. "Preparing the spirit" occurred within the context of "where we come from." Processes involved in "preparing the spirit" were healing, connecting, and protecting; through these processes, "what I want at the end of life" was realized.

TIP The emergence of mixed methods research (see Chapter 13) has given rise to interest in systematic reviews that integrate findings from a broad range of studies and methodologies. Such reviews (which have been called *mixed methods review*, *mixed research synthesis*, and *systematic mixed studies reviews*) use disciplined and auditable procedures to integrate and synthesize findings from quantitative, qualitative, and mixed methods studies.

CRITIQUING SYSTEMATIC REVIEWS

Reports for systematic reviews, including meta-analyses and metasyntheses, typically follow a similar format as for a primary study report. The format usually includes an introduction, method section, results section, discussion, and full citations for the entire sample of studies in the review (often identified separately from other citations by using asterisks).

The method section is especially important. Readers of the review need to assess the validity of the findings, so methodologic and statistical strategies and their rationales should be adequately described. For example, if reviewers of quantitative studies decided that a meta-analysis was not justified, the rationale for this decision should be made clear. Tables and figures typically play a key role in reports of systematic reviews. For meta-analyses, forest plots are often presented, showing effect size and 95% CI information for each study and for the overall pooled result. A table showing the characteristics of studies in the review is often included.

Metasynthesis reports are similar to meta-analytic reports, except that the results section contains the new interpretations rather than quantitative findings. When a meta-summary has been done, however, the meta-findings are typically summarized in a table. The method section of a metasynthesis report should contain a detailed description of the sampling criteria, the search procedures, and efforts made to enhance the integrity and rigour of the integration.

A thorough discussion section is crucial in systematic reviews. The discussion should include the reviewers' assessment about the strengths and limitations of the body of evidence, suggestions on further research needed to improve the evidence base, and the implications of the review for clinicians. The review should also discuss the consistency of findings across studies and provide an interpretation of why there might be inconsistency.

Like all studies, systematic reviews should be critiqued before the findings are considered trustworthy and clinically relevant. Box 18.1 offers guidelines for evaluating systematic reviews. Although these guidelines are fairly broad, not all questions apply equally well to all types of systematic reviews. In particular, we have distinguished questions about analysis separately for meta-analyses and metasyntheses. The list of questions in Box 18.1 is not necessarily comprehensive. Supplementary questions might be needed for particular types of review.

Box 18.1 Guidelines for Critiquing Systematic Reviews

The Problem
- Did the report state the research problem and/or research questions? Is the scope of the project appropriate? Was the approach to integration described, and was the approach appropriate?

Search Strategy
- Did the report describe criteria for selecting primary studies, and are the criteria defensible?
- Were the databases used by the reviewers identified, and are they appropriate and comprehensive? Were key words identified?
- Did the reviewers use supplementary efforts to identify relevant studies?

The Sample
- Did the search strategy yield a good sample of studies?
- If an original report was lacking key information, did reviewers attempt to contact the original researchers for additional information?

Quality Appraisal
- Did the reviewers appraise the quality of the primary studies? Did they use a well-defined set of criteria or a validated quality appraisal scale?
- Did two or more people do the appraisals, and was interrater agreement reported?
- Was quality information used effectively in selecting studies or analyzing results?

Data Extraction
- Was adequate information extracted about the study design, sample characteristics, and study findings?
- Were steps taken to enhance the integrity of the dataset (e.g., Were two or more people used to extract and record information for analysis)?

Data Analysis—General
- Did the reviewers explain their method of pooling and integrating the data?
- Were tables, figures, and text used effectively to summarize findings?

Data Analysis—Quantitative
- If a meta-analysis was not performed, was there adequate justification for using narrative integration? If a meta-analysis *was* performed, was this justifiable?
- For meta-analyses, did the report describe how effect sizes were computed?
- Was heterogeneity of effects assessed? Was the decision to use a random effects model versus a fixed effects model sound? Were subgroup analyses undertaken, or was the absence of subgroup analyses justified?

Data Analysis—Qualitative
- In a metasynthesis, did the reviewers describe the techniques they used to compare the findings of each study, and did they explain their method of interpreting their data?
- If a meta-summary was done, was effect size information presented effectively?
- In a metasynthesis, did the synthesis achieve a fuller understanding of the phenomenon to advance knowledge? Was a sufficient amount of data included to support interpretations?

Conclusions
- Did the reviewers draw reasonable conclusions about their results and about the quality of evidence relating to the research question?
- Were limitations of the review/synthesis noted?
- Were implications for nursing and health care practice and further research clearly stated?

☐ All systematic reviews
☐ Systematic reviews of quantitative studies
☐ Metasyntheses

RESEARCH EXAMPLES WITH CRITICAL THINKING EXERCISES

We conclude this chapter with a description of two systematic reviews, a meta-analysis and a metasynthesis. Read the summaries and then answer the critical thinking questions that follow, referring to the full research report if necessary. Examples 1 and 2 are featured on the interactive *Critical Thinking Activity* on thePoint website. ⋇

EXAMPLE 1: A META-ANALYSIS

Study: Medication adherence interventions that target subjects with adherence problems: Systematic review and meta-analysis (Conn et al., 2016)

Purpose: The purpose of the meta-analysis was to integrate research evidence concerning the effectiveness of interventions designed to increase medication adherence among patients with adherence problems.

Eligibility Criteria: A primary study was considered eligible for the meta-analysis if it met the following criteria: (1) the study involved an intervention to increase medication adherence in adult patients recruited specifically because they had problems with adherence to prescription medications and (2) sufficient information for computing the effect size (*d*) was available. The studies included both published and nonpublished reports. There were no restrictions based on publication date, sample size, or research design.

Search Strategy: A search was undertaken in 13 bibliographic databases. Numerous search terms were used, including the MeSH terms *patient compliance* (before 2009) and *medication adherence* (after 2008). Additional search methods were used, including ancestry searching, searches in research registries and conference proceedings, and hand searching in 57 journals. Two research specialists assessed each potential study for eligibility.

Sample: The analysis was based on a sample of 53 eligible studies. Initially, 3,216 reports with medication adherence interventions were identified in the electronic search, but most were excluded because of failure to report adherence outcomes or failure to target patients with adherence problems. The sample of 53 studies involved 8,423 individual participants.

Quality Appraisal: Study quality was not assessed using a formal scale, but design features were coded (e.g., randomization, blinding of data collectors). Two reviewers independently coded all data. Discrepancies were discussed to achieve 100% agreement.

Data Extraction: A formal extraction protocol was developed for data extraction. The data that were abstracted included information about study source, study design, participant characteristics, intervention features, and outcome data.

Effect Size Calculation: Cohen's *d* was used as the effect size index. If a report did not provide sufficient information for calculating the effect size, authors were contacted to obtain the information.

Statistical Analyses: The researchers found evidence of significant statistical heterogeneity and used a random effects model for their main analysis, in which the effect sizes were weighted by the study sample size. Subgroup analyses were conducted to evaluate the extent to which heterogeneity of effects was related to characteristics of the study participants, study design and methods, and the interventions themselves. Publication bias was also assessed.

Key Findings: The overall effect size for treatment versus control group subjects was 0.30, a modest but significant effect favouring those who had received the intervention. Significantly larger effects were found for interventions delivered face-to-face rather than by telephone or e-mail (0.41 vs. 0.18) and for interventions incorporating prompts to take medications compared to those lacking medication prompts (0.57 vs. 0.22). The researchers found evidence of statistically significant publication bias.

Discussion: The researchers concluded that interventions for patients with a history of adherence problems can result in modest but significant improvements in medication taking and that face-to-face interventions may be especially effective.

Critical Thinking Exercises

1. Answer the relevant questions from Box 18.1 regarding this study.

2. What might be some of the uses to which the findings could be put in clinical practice?

EXAMPLE 2: A METASYNTHESIS

Study: Older people's experiences of care in nursing homes: A metasynthesis (Vaismoradi et al., 2016)

Purpose: The purpose of this metasynthesis was to synthesize qualitative studies on older person's experiences of being cared for in nursing homes.

Eligibility Criteria: A study was included if it (1) was a peer-reviewed qualitative study in the caring sciences, (2) examined the experiences of older persons being cared for in nursing homes, (3) involved study participants whose cognitive status was sufficiently intact, and (4) was published in an online scientific journal. The researchers placed no limits based on publication date, country of origin, or research tradition.

Search Strategy: A search of several electronic databases was undertaken (CINAHL, MEDLINE, Scopus, Ovid, Wiley Online Library, and ScienceDirect). Key search terms included "older," "nursing home," combined with "experience," "nurse," and "qualitative." An ancestry search was also conducted, using the reference lists of eligible studies, plus a hand search in journals that publish relevant studies on the topic.

Sample: The report presented a flow chart showing the researchers' sampling decisions. Of the 12,952 citations initially identified by title, 299 abstracts were screened, and then 79 full papers were examined for eligibility; 70 were excluded based on quality. A total of seven papers were included in the analysis. The combined sample of participants in the primary studies included 128 older people in 24 nursing homes in five different countries: Sweden, Canada, Taiwan, Norway, and Spain.

Quality Appraisal: The researchers used an existing quality appraisal tool called the Consolidated criteria for reporting qualitative research (COREQ) 32-item checklist. The four authors did independent quality reviews, but they ultimately decided not to use a scoring system. Instead, they discussed the quality of each study and came to consensus on whether or not to exclude it.

Data Analysis: The analysis was based on Noblit and Hare's meta-ethnographic approach. The four researchers independently read and reread each of the seven articles. The researchers decided that the studies were reciprocal and then proceeded to extract the key metaphors from each study. Next, the key metaphors from each study were translated into the other six studies.

Key Findings: One overarching theme of "retaining the meaning of being alive" was discovered. Then three main themes were identified: (1) confrontation of needs, (2) participation in living, and (3) adjustment. Each of these main themes had several subthemes, which were illustrated in a schematic model of older people's experiences of being cared for in nursing homes. As an example, the first theme of *confrontation of needs* encompassed two subthemes: presentation of expectations and meeting organizational demands.

Discussion: The researchers concluded that their findings revealed the institutional nature of nursing homes which restricts older person's decision making. The researchers described some important implications of their findings for nursing policy makers, in terms of developing a caring environment of holistic care.

Critical Thinking Exercises

1. Answer the relevant questions from Box 18.1 regarding this study.
2. Do you think the researchers should have included non–peer-reviewed studies in their review? Why or why not?
3. What might be some of the uses to which the findings could be put in clinical practice?

WANT TO KNOW MORE? ☀

A wide variety of resources to enhance your learning and understanding of this chapter are available on thePoint.

- Interactive Critical Thinking Activity
- Chapter Supplement on Publication Bias in Meta-Analyses
- Answer to the Critical Thinking Exercise for Examples 1 and 2
- Internet Resources with useful websites for Chapter 18
- A Wolters Kluwer journal article on a topic related to this chapter

---

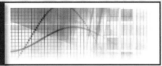

Summary Points

- EBP relies on rigorous integration of research evidence on a topic through **systematic reviews**.
- Systematic reviews of quantitative studies often involve statistical integration of findings in a **meta-analysis**, a procedure whose advantages include objectivity and enhanced power. Yet, meta-analysis is not appropriate for broad questions or when findings are substantially inconsistent.
- The steps in both quantitative and qualitative integration are similar and involve formulating the problem, designing the study (including establishing sampling criteria), searching the literature for a sample of **primary studies**, evaluating study quality, extracting and encoding data for analysis, analyzing the data, and reporting the findings.
- There is no consensus on whether integrations should include the *grey literature*—that is, unpublished reports. In meta-analyses, a concern is that **publication bias** stemming from the underrepresentation of nonsignificant findings in published reports can lead to overestimates of effects.
- In meta-analysis, findings from primary studies are represented by an **effect size index** that quantifies the magnitude and direction of relationship between the independent and dependent variables. The most common effect size indexes in nursing are

d (the *standardized mean difference*), the odds ratio, and correlation coefficients.

● Effects from individual studies are pooled to yield an estimate of the population effect size by calculating a weighted average of effects, usually giving greater weight to studies with larger samples.

● **Statistical heterogeneity** (diversity in effects across studies) is a major issue in meta-analysis and affects decisions about which statistical model to use and whether a meta-analysis is justified. Heterogeneity can be examined visually using a **forest plot**.

● Heterogeneity can be explored through **subgroup analyses**, the purpose of which is to see whether effects systematically vary as a function of clinical or methodologic characteristics.

● Quality assessments (which may involve formal quantitative ratings of methodologic rigour) are sometimes used to exclude weak studies from reviews, but they can also be used to differentially weight studies or to evaluate whether including or excluding weaker studies changes conclusions.

● **Metasyntheses** are more than just summaries of prior qualitative findings; they involve a discovery of essential features of a body of findings and a transformation that yields new interpretations.

● Numerous approaches to metasynthesis (and many terms related to qualitative integration) have been proposed. Metasynthesists grapple with such issues as whether to combine findings from different research traditions and whether to exclude poor-quality studies.

● One approach to qualitative integration called **meta-ethnography** was proposed by Noblit and Hare; this approach involves listing key themes or metaphors across studies and then translating them into each other.

● A **meta-summary**, a method developed by Sandelowski and Barroso, involves listing abstracted findings from the primary studies and calculating **manifest effect sizes**. A **frequency effect size** is the percentage of reports that contain a given finding. An **intensity effect size** indicates the percentage of all findings that are contained in any given report.

● In the Sandelowski and Barroso approach, a meta-summary can lay the foundation for a metasynthesis, which can use a variety of qualitative approaches to analysis and interpretations.

REFERENCES

Chiu, H., Shyu, Y., Chang, P., & Tsai, P. (2016). Effects of acupuncture on menopause-related symptoms in breast cancer survivors: A meta-analysis of randomized controlled trials. *Cancer Nursing, 39,* 228–237.

Conn, V., Ruppar, T., Enriquez, M., & Cooper, P. (2016). Medication adherence interventions that target subjects with adherence problems: Systematic review and meta-analysis. *Research in Social and Administrative Pharmacy, 12,* 218–246.

Duggleby W., Kuchera S., MacLeod R., et al. (2015). Indigenous people's experiences at the end of life. *Palliative & Supportive Care, 13*(6), 1721–1733.

Duggleby W., Tycholiz J., Holtslander L., et al. (2017). A metasynthesis study of family caregivers' transition experiences caring for community-dwelling persons with advanced cancer at the end of life. *Palliative Medicine, 31*(7), 602–616.

Finfgeld, D. (2003). Metasynthesis: The state of the art–so far. *Qualitative Health Research, 13,* 893–904.

Guillaumie L., Boiral O., & Champagne J. (2017). A mixed-methods systematic review of the effects of mindfulness on nurses. *Journal of Advanced Nursing, 73*(5), 1017–1034.

Harrison D., Larocque C., Bueno M., et al. (2017). Sweet Solutions to Reduce Procedural Pain in Neonates: A Meta-analysis. *Pediatrics, 139*(1), pii, e20160955.

Hoben M., Kent A., Kobagi N., et al. (2017). Effective strategies to motivate nursing home residents in oral care and to prevent or reduce responsive behaviors in oral care: A systematic review. *PLoS One, 12*(6), e0178913.

Higgins, J., & Green, S. (2008). *Cochrane handbook for systematic reviews of interventions.* Chichester, UK: Wiley.

Johnston C., Campbell-Yeo M., Disher T., et al. (2017). Skin-to-skin care for procedural pain in neonates. *The Cochrane Database of Systematic Reviews, 2,* CD008435.

Noblit, G., & Hare, R. D. (1988). *Meta-ethnography: Synthesizing qualitative studies.* Newbury Park, CA: Sage.

Parker S. I. A., Benzies K. M., & Hayden K. A. (2017). A systematic review: effectiveness of pediatric peripheral intravenous catheterization strategies. *Journal of Advanced Nursing, 73*(7), 1570–1582.

Peirson L., Ali M. U., Kenny M., et al. (2016). Interventions for prevention and treatment of tobacco smoking in school-aged children and adolescents: A systematic review and meta-analysis. *Preventive Medicine, 85,* 20–31.

Sandelowski, M., & Barroso, J. (2002). Finding the findings in qualitative studies. *Journal of Nursing Scholarship, 34,* 213–219.

Sandelowski, M., & Barroso, J. (2007). *Handbook for synthesizing qualitative research.* New York: Springer.

Sandelowski, M., Docherty, S., & Emden, C. (1997). Qualitative metasynthesis: Issues and techniques. *Research in Nursing & Health, 20,* 365–371.

Schreiber, R., Crooks, D., & Stern, P. N. (1997). Qualitative meta-analysis. In J. M. Morse (Ed.). *Completing a qualitative project: Details and dialogue* (pp. 311–326). Thousand Oaks, CA: Sage.

Thorne, S., Jensen, L., Kearney, M., Noblit, G., & Sandelowski, M. (2004). Qualitative metasynthesis: Reflections on methodological orientation and ideological agenda. *Qualitative Health Research, 14,* 1342–1365.

Vaismoradi, M., Wang, I. L., Turunen, H., & Bondas, T. (2016). Older people's experiences of care in nursing homes: A meta-synthesis. *International Nursing Review, 63,* 111–121.

Voldbjerg, S., Grønkjaer, M., Sørensen, E., & Hall, E. (2016). Newly graduated nurses' use of knowledge sources: A meta-ethnography. *Journal of Advanced Nursing, 72*(8), 1751–1765.

*A link to this open-access article is provided in the Internet Resources section on thePoint website.

**This journal article is available on thePoint for this chapter.

Journal of Pediatric Health Care. 2016 Jan-Feb; 30(1): 49–56

Parents' Use of Praise and Criticism in a Sample of Young Children Seeking Mental Health Services

Stephanie Swenson, BSN, RN, Grace W. K. Ho, PhD, RN, Chakra Budhathoki, PhD, Harolyn M. E. Belcher, MD, MHS, Sharon Tucker, PhD, RN, FAAN, Kellie Miller, & Deborah Gross, DNSc, RN, FAAN

Stephanie Swenson, Registered Nurse, Children's National Medical Center, Washington, DC.

Grace W. K. Ho, Morton and Jane Blaustein Postdoctoral Fellow in Mental Health & Psychiatric Nursing, School of Nursing, Johns Hopkins University, Baltimore, MD.

Chakra Budhathoki, Assistant Professor, School of Nursing, Johns Hopkins University, Baltimore, MD.

Harolyn M.E. Belcher, Director of Research, Center for Child and Family Traumatic Stress at Kennedy Krieger Institute, and Associate Professor of Pediatrics, Johns Hopkins School of Medicine, Baltimore, MD.

Sharon Tucker, Director of Nursing Research, Evidence-Based Practice & Quality, University of Iowa Hospitals & Clinics, Iowa City, IA.

Kellie Miller, Research Coordinator, School of Nursing, Johns Hopkins University, Baltimore, MD.

Deborah Gross, Leonard and Helen Stulman Professor in Mental Health & Psychiatric Nursing, School of Nursing, Johns Hopkins University, Baltimore, MD.

This study was conducted as part of the first author's research honours project while she was a student at Johns Hopkins University School of Nursing. Data are from a larger study supported by a grant from the National Institute for Nursing Research (R01 NR012444) to Drs. Gross and Belcher.

Conflicts of interest: None to report.

Correspondence: Stephanie Swenson, BSN, RN, c/o Deborah Gross, DNSc, RN, FAAN, School of Nursing, Johns Hopkins University, Ste 531, 525 N Wolfe St, Baltimore, MD 21205; e-mail: stephswenson@gmail.com.

0891-5245/$36.00

Published online October 30, 2015.

http://dx.doi.org/10.1016/j.pedhc.2015.09.010

ABSTRACT

Parents' use of praise and criticism are common indicators of parent-child interaction quality and are intervention targets for mental health treatment. Clinicians and researchers often rely on parents' self-reports of parenting behaviour, although studies about the correlation of parents' self-reports and actual behaviour are rare. We examined the concordance between parents' self-reports of praise and criticism of their children and observed use of these behaviours during a brief parent-child play session. Parent self-report and observational data were collected from 128 parent-child dyads referred for child mental health treatment. Most parents reported praising their children often and criticizing their children rarely. However, parents were observed to criticize their children nearly three times more often than they praised them. Self-reported and observed praise were positively correlated ($r_s = 0.32$, $p < .01$), whereas self-reported and observed criticisms were negatively correlated ($r_s = -0.21, p < .05$). Parents' tendencies to overestimate their use of praise and underestimate their use of criticism are discussed. J Pediatr Health Care. (2016) 30, 49-56.

KEY WORDS

Parenting, young children, praise, critical statements, parent self-report

Parents are a powerful source of feedback in shaping their young children's behaviour and sense of self. It is within these earliest relationships that children first begin to acquire a sense of themselves as capable, competent, and loved (Bohlin, Hagekull, & Rydell, 2000; Bowlby, 1988; Cassidy, 1988). Two common sources of parental feedback used to shape young children's behaviour and self-esteem are *praise* (i.e., positive statements designed to reinforce desirable behaviours in children or communicate pleasure with the child) and *criticism* (i.e., negative statements designed to stop or change children's undesirable behaviour or communicate displeasure with the child).

> Parents are a powerful source of feedback in shaping their young children's behaviour and sense of self.

Praise from parents has been used as a marker of positive parenting behaviours in numerous studies (Breitenstein et al., 2012; Chorpita, Caleiden, & Weisz, 2005; Wahler & Meginnis, 1997). Praise is often accompanied by other parenting behaviours indicative of parental warmth, responsiveness, and nurturance (Furlong et al., 2013). Although the question of whether excessive use of praise can negatively influence children's intrinsic motivation has been debated (Owens, Slep, & Heyman, 2012), substantial research now shows that praise, used strategically, can boost children's feelings of competence and confidence. Therefore, praise remains an important indicator of positive parenting behaviour (Brummelman, Thomaes, Orobio de Castro, Overbeek, & Bushman, 2014; Cimpian, 2010; Henderlong & Lepper, 2002; Mueller & Dweck, 1998; Zentall & Morris, 2010).

Parents may use critical statements to express disapproval with their children's behaviour or attitude. However, using criticism can undermine their self-esteem, lead to greater child defiance and aggression, and increase the likelihood of their developing behavioural problems (Barnett & Scaramella, 2013; Lorber & Egeland, 2011; Tung, Li, & Lee, 2012; Webster-Stratton & Hammond, 1998). Thus, contrary to parents' expectations, using critical statements to shape child behaviour actually may be counterproductive. In clinical studies of young children in mental health treatment, parents who directed more critical statements at their children were also more likely to drop out of treatment (Fernandez & Eyberg, 2009).

Given their salience in child development research, parent training interventions have been designed to increase parents' use of praise and reduce their use of criticisms with their children (Breitenstein et al., 2012; Brotman et al., 2009; Eyberg et al., 2001; Gross et al., 2009). In clinical practice and research, parents' use of praise and criticism is often assessed using parent self-report. However, some investigators have questioned the accuracy of using self-reports to measure actual parenting behaviours, particularly when those behaviours are susceptible to recall or social desirability biases (Morsbach & Prinz, 2006). These biases may be particularly heightened in a child mental health population,

where parents might be highly sensitive to feeling "blamed" for their child's illness or to the stigma of engaging the mental health system (Meltzer, Ford, Goodman, & Vostanis, 2011; Angold, et al., 1998).

This study examines the extent to which parents' self-reports of praise and criticism are reflected in their observed behaviour in a sample of parents of preschool children referred for mental health treatment. We also explore whether two indicators of parents' tendency to hold negative attributions about themselves and their children, depressive symptoms and perceptions of their children as being more behaviourally difficult, moderate the relationship between self-report and observed use of praise and critical statements. Consistent with cognitive attribution theory, depressed parents may develop biases that their children's misbehaviour is intentional and within their control, leading them to be less positive and more critical in their interactions (Dix, Ruble, Grusec, & Nixon, 1986; Leung & Slep, 2006; Scott & Dadds, 2009).

Using a descriptive, cross-sectional design, we posed the following research questions:

- What is the relationship between parents' self-reported and observed use of praise based on (a) frequency and (b) the proportion of statements to their child that are praise during a 15-minute free play session?
- What is the relationship between parents' self-reported and observed use of criticism based on (a) number and (b) the proportion of statements to their child that are criticisms during a 15-minute free play session?
- Do parents' depressive symptoms moderate the association between their self-reported and observed use of praise and critical statements?
- Do parents' perception of the severity of their children's behaviour problems affect the association between their self-reported and observed used of praise and critical statements?

The goals of this study are to (a) understand the extent to which parents' self-reported use of praise and criticism accurately reflect the appraisals of their observed behaviour and (b) offer guidance to practitioners on how to address these two important parenting practices in pediatric primary care with parents of young children at risk for mental health problems.

METHODS

This study is a secondary analysis of baseline parent-report and observation data collected as part of a larger clinical trial comparing two evidence-based parent training programs. The larger clinical trial was conducted in an urban mental health clinic serving low-income families with preschool children (Gross et al., 2014) and was approved by the Johns Hopkins University Medical Institutions Institutional Review Board.

Sampling Design

Data were drawn from a convenience sample of 128 parents seeking treatment at an urban child mental health clinic serving families of young children, birth to 5 years old, who were recruited into the larger clinical trial. Approximately 80% of the clinic population is African American or multiracial, and more than 95% of families receive Medicaid. Criteria for inclusion were that the parent is (a) the biological or adoptive parent or legal guardian for a 2- to 5-year-old child and (b) seeking mental health treatment for their child's behaviour problems. Parents were excluded if they had a severe mental illness, substance use disorder, or cognitive impairment that would interfere with their child's treatment. Children were excluded if they were actively suicidal or psychotic, had a diagnosis of autism or pervasive developmental disorder, or had a congenital or genetic anomaly that would interfere with treatment. Parents who met the inclusion criteria and consented to participate in the clinical trial completed a set of baseline measures and were video recorded with their child during a 15-minute free-play session (see the Procedures section).

Variables and Measures

Self-reported praise and criticism

Parents' self-reported use of praise and criticism was measured using two survey items from the Parenting Questionnaire (Gross, Fogg, Garvey, & Julion, 2004; McCabe, Clark, & Barnett, 1999), a 40-item Likert-type measure of parent discipline strategies. One item asks parents to circle the frequency with which they praise their child along a 5-point scale of 1 (*almost never*) to 5 (*very often*). Another item asks parents to circle the frequency with which they criticize their child, using the same 5-point scale of 1 (*almost never*) to 5 (*very often*).

Parent depressive symptoms

The 20-item Center for Epidemiologic Studies Depression Scale–Revised (CESD-R) was used to measure parent depressive symptoms. This version of the CESD was created to better reflect the range of symptoms indicative of major depression (Eaton, Muntaner, Smith, Tien, & Ybarra, 2004). Validity of the CESD-R has been supported by confirmatory factor analysis and positive correlations with other measures of depression and anxiety (Van Dam & Earleywine, 2011). Higher scores are indicative of more depressive symptoms; a score of 16 or higher indicates depressive symptomatology within the clinical range. The Cronbach α for the CESD-R in this sample was 0.92.

Child behaviour problems

Parents' reports of their child's behaviour problems were measured using the Child Behavior Checklist for ages 1½ to 5 years (CBCL; Achenbach & Rescorla, 2000).

The CBCL measures two dimensions of child behaviour problems: externalizing behaviour (e.g., aggression, noncompliance, and inattention) and internalizing behaviour (e.g., anxiety, depression, and withdrawal). Parents rate their child's behaviour problems on a scale of 0 (behaviour is not true) to 2 (behaviour is very true or often true); higher scores are indicative of more behaviour problems. In the current study, only externalizing behaviour problems were examined because these behaviours tend to be more aversive to parents. The CBCL externalizing scale contains 24 items, and scores range from 0 to 48. Standardized T scores are used to identify children with externalizing behaviour problems in the borderline clinical (93rd percentile) and clinical (98th percentile) range. In low-income racial and ethnic minority populations, α reliabilities for the externalizing scale range from 0.88 to 0.91 (Gross et al., 2006), and validity has been supported (Gross et al., 2007; Sivan, Ridge, Gross, Richardson, & Cowell, 2008).

Observed use of praise and criticism

Frequencies of observed praise and criticism were measured from 15-minute video recorded parent-child free play interactions using a modified version of the Dyadic Parent-Child Interaction Coding System (DPICS; Eyberg & Robinson, 1992). The DPICS measures frequencies of select observed parent and child verbalizations and behaviour. Observed parentv erbalizations collected in this study include numbers of critical statements, encouraging statements, praise statements, and commands. Parents' use of praise and criticism were estimated in two ways; (a) the *frequency* of observed praise statements or critical statements and (b) the *proportion* of praise statements or critical statements to all observed parent verbalizations during the 15-minute free play session.

Praise statements include both labelled and unlabelled praise. Labelled praise is operationalized as any specific statement by a parent expressing their favourable judgment of an activity, product, or attribute of the child, such as "That's a terrific house you made." Unlabelled praise is operationalized as a nonspecific verbal comment by the parent expressing a favourable judgment of an activity or attribute of the child, such as "Great" or "Good job." In this analysis, these two types of praise were summed to form a single estimate of parents' total use of praise.

Critical statements are operationally defined as parent verbalizations that find fault with the activities, products, or attributes of the child. Blame statements and guilt-inducing statements are also considered to be critical statements. Examples include, "You're being naughty" and "I don't like your attitude."

Procedures

After completing the self-report measures, parents were asked to play with their child for 15 minutes while the research assistant video recorded the interaction. Parents were instructed to play with their child as they normally would, and the research assistant would let them know when the 15 minutes was over. Video recordings were then sent electronically to trained DPICS coders who were blinded to study hypotheses. Inter-rater reliability, assessed through intraclass correlation for 10% of DPICS assessments, was 0.98 for praise statements and 0.92 for critical statements.

Data were analyzed using SPSS version 22 (IBM Corp., Armonk, NY). Descriptive statistics were used to summarize parents' self-reports of praise and criticism use and observed use of praise and criticism (as frequencies and as proportions of total verbalizations) in a 15-minute play session. Bivariate correlations between parents' self-reported and observed uses of praise or criticism, as well as correlations between self-reported and observed uses of praise and criticism with parent depression and perceived child behaviour problems, were calculated using Spearman's rho. Multiple regression analyses were conducted to test the effects of parent depressive symptoms or perceived child behaviour problems on parents' self-reports of praise and criticism as predictors of their observed use. To address data skewness, outliers were removed using Mahalanobis distance, Cook's distance, and centred leverage values.

RESULTS

Sample characteristics are summarized in Table 1. A majority of the parents were mothers (75.8%), African American (67.2%), unemployed (64.1%), and economically disadvantaged (95.3% reported a household income less than $20,000 or received Medicaid). The mean parent age was 34 years (SD = 10.3). The mean CESD-R score was 17.8 (SD = 15.6); more than 46% of the parents had depressive symptom scores in the clinical range. The average age of the children was 3.64 years (SD = 1.04). More than half of the children were boys (54.7%). Although all of the children were referred for behaviour problems, only 41.7% of the parents reported child externalizing behaviour problems in the clinical or borderline clinical range.

Parents' Use of Praise and Criticism

A majority of the parents (86.7%) reported using praise "often" or "very often," and using criticism "rarely" or "almost never" (77.3%). During their observed parent-child play interactions, parents verbalized a median of three praise statements (range = 0-48) and eight critical statements (range = 0-38) in 15 minutes. A higher proportion of parents' total verbalizations consisted of critical statements compared with praise statements (13.6% vs. 7.4%). These results are presented in Table 2.

TABLE 1. Sample characteristics

Characteristic	Mean (SD)	n (%)
Parent characteristics (n = 128)		
Age, year	34 (10.3)	
Relationship to child		
Mother		97 (75.8)
Other		31 (24.2)
Race/ethnicity		
African American		86 (67.2)
White		30 (23.4)
Hispanic/Latino		6 (4.7)
Education level		
High school graduate or less		79 (61.7)
Some college		28 (21.9)
College graduate or higher		11 (8.6)
Household income < $20,000 or receive Medicaid		121 (95.3)
Unemployed		82 (64.1)
CESD-R score	17.8 (15.6)	
Score ≥ 16		59 (46.1)
Child characteristics (n = 128)		
Age, year	3.6 (1.0)	
Male		70 (54.7)
Externalizing behaviour ≥ borderline clinical range		53 (41.7)

Note. CESD-R, Center for Epidemiologic Studies Depression Scale–Revised; SD, standard deviation.

Relationships Between Parents' Self-Reported and Observed Use of Praise and Criticism

Tables 3 and 4 summarize bivariate correlations between pertinent variables for parent praise and criticism, respectively. We found a positive correlation between parents' self-reported and observed use of praise based on absolute frequency of praise ($r_s = 0.32, p < .01$) and proportion of praise to total parent verbalizations ($r_s = 0.23, p < .01$). In contrast, a negative association was found between parents' self-reported use of criticism and the observed frequency of critical statements ($r_s = -0.21, p < .05$). No relationship was found between parents' self-reports of their use of criticism with their child and the proportion of observed critical statements to total parent verbalizations ($r_s = -0.05$, not significant).

Moderating Effect of Parent Depressive Symptoms on the Relationship Between Parents' Self-Reported and Observed Behaviours

As shown in Table 3, parent depression scores were not significantly associated with parents' use of praise based on self-report ($r = -0.08$, not significant) or observation ($r = -0.05$, not significant). Also based on regression analysis, parents' depressive symptoms did not moderate the relationship between self-reported and observed use of praise (i.e., no significant interaction between depressive symptoms and self-reported use of praise was found; $\beta = -0.10, p =$ not significant).

TABLE 2. Parents' self-reported and observed use of praise and criticism

Variables	f (%)	Median	Mean (SD)	Range	Proportion, %*
Parent self-reports					
"I praise my child…"					
Almost never	1 (0.8)				
Rarely	0 (0)				
Sometimes	16 (12.5)				
Often	46 (35.9)				
Very often	65 (50.8)				
"I criticize my child…"					
Almost never	69 (53.9)				
Rarely	30 (23.4)				
Sometimes	22 (17.2)				
Often	7 (5.5)				
Very often	0 (0)				
Observed parent behaviours					
Total praise statements		3	5.8 (7.7)	0-48	7.4
Labelled praise		0	0.3 (0.7)	0-4	0.3
Unlabelled praise		3	5.5 (7.3)	0-45	7.1
Critical statements		8	8.5 (6.6)	0-38	13.6
Other parent verbalizations		48.5	55.8 (35.7)	1-155	79.0
Total verbal behaviours		61	70.1 (43.4)	2-201	100

Proportion of praise or critical statements to all parent verbalizations.

As shown in Table 4, parents' depression scores were also unrelated to frequency ($r = -0.05$, not significant) and proportion ($r = 0.07$, not significant) of observed critical statements. However, parents with higher depression scores self-reported using more criticism with their children ($r_s = 0.20$, $p < .05$). Parents' depressive symptoms did not moderate the relationship between parents' self-reported and observed use of critical statements (i.e., depressive symptoms and self-reported use of criticism did not interact significantly; $\beta = -0.12$, $p =$ not significant).

Moderating Effect of Parents' Perceptions of the Severity of Their Child's Behaviour Problems on the Relationship Between Their Self-Reported and Observed Behaviours

As shown in Table 3, parents' self-reports of their use of praise was inversely correlated with their perceptions

of their child's externalizing behaviour problems ($r_s = -0.18$, $p < .05$)—that is, parents who rated their children as having more behaviour problems were less likely to report praising their child. However, moderation analysis did not reveal a significant interaction between the child's externalizing behaviour and parents' self-reported use of praise in predicting their observed use ($\beta = -0.03$, $p =$ not significant). Children's externalizing behaviour problems were also unrelated to parents' use of critical statements based on self-report and observation (see Table 4). Finally, there was no evidence that parents' perceptions of the severity of their children's externalizing behaviour problems moderated the relationships between parents' self-reported and observed use of critical statements (i.e., no significant interaction was found between perceived child externalizing behaviour problems and self-reported criticism use; $\beta = -0.06$, $p =$ not significant).

TABLE 3. Bivariate Spearman's rank correlation coefficients for main variables related to parent praise

Variables	1	2	3	4	5
1 Self-reported praise		0.32†	0.23†	−0.08	−0.18*
2 Observed praise			0.89†	−0.05	−0.003
3 Praise as proportion				−0.001	−0.02
4 Parent's depressive symptoms					0.31†
5 Child's externalizing behaviours					

Correlation coefficient significant at p < .05.
†Correlation significant at p < .01.*

TABLE 4. Bivariate Spearman's rank correlation coefficients for main variables related to parent criticism

Variables	1	2	3	4	5
1 Self-reported criticism		−0.21*	−0.05	0.20*	0.15
2 Observed criticism			0.65†	−0.05	0.13
3 Criticism as proportion				0.07	0.12
4 Parent depressive symptoms					0.31†
5 Child externalizing behaviours					

Correlation coefficient significant at p < .05.
†Correlation significant at p < .01.*

DISCUSSION

Parents' praise and criticism are powerful sources of feedback in shaping their young children's behaviour and development. These parenting behaviours have been a key focus in child development research and serve as important indicators of positive or negative parenting in families of children with mental, emotional, and behaviour disorders. Although many studies use parents' self-reports of praise and criticism, the extent to which we can rely on parent report as reliable indicators of their actual use remains unclear. Data obtained from this clinic sample suggest that parents tend to overestimate their use of praise and underestimate their use of criticism with their preschool children.

> Data obtained from this clinic sample suggest that parents tend to overestimate their use of praise and underestimate their use of criticism with their preschool children.

Although parents who reported praising their child more often were observed to use more praise, the magnitude of the effect was small ($r_s = 0.32$). This modest correlation is consistent with prior literature showing generally small correlations across methods, suggesting that self-report and observation capture different aspects of the same variable (i.e., perceived versus actual parenting behaviour; Gardner, 2000).

Despite the positive correlation between self-reported and observed use of praise, praise was not frequently expressed. Parents verbalized a median of only three praise statements in the 15-minute observed play sessions. On average, only 7% of the parents' statements counted from the parent-child interactions qualified as praise, though these sessions were intended to be a positive one. Yet, nearly 87% of parents reported praising their children "often" or "very often."

Parents' self-reports of their use of criticism was modestly though negatively correlated with their actual use. Specifically, parents who reported using criticisms infrequently were actually *more likely* to criticize their children during the 15-minute play session. There are multiple plausible explanations for this finding. First, parents are aware that being critical is a socially undesirable behaviour and therefore may have reported a more socially acceptable answer. However, it is also possible that parents are truly unaware of how frequently they criticize their children. Indeed, the parents in this sample criticized their children nearly three times more frequently than they praised them (i.e., eight criticisms versus three praise statements) despite their reports to the contrary (77% reported criticizing their children

"rarely" or "almost never"). Another explanation relates to the artificial conditions under which the observed behaviour sample was obtained. Parents with a stronger tendency to criticize their children may have consciously suppressed those comments during the 15-minute play session. Nonetheless, it should be noted that despite the possibility that parents may have modified their behaviour while being observed, the proportion of parents' critical statements were still nearly twice those of their praise statements (i.e., 13.6% vs. 7.6%). We also examined whether two indicators of parents' tendency to hold negative attributions about themselves and their children (i.e., parents' depressive symptoms and parents' ratings of their children's externalizing behaviours) affected concordance between self-report and observed behaviour. Higher depressive symptom scores were associated with more self-reported use of critical statements. However, parents' depression scores did not moderate the relationships between self-reported and observed used of criticism or praise. In addition, parents who rated their children as having more externalizing behaviour problems also reported praising their children less often, but the severity of their child's behaviour problems did not moderate the association between self-reported and observed use of criticism or praise. These data suggest that parents' negative attributions affect how they perceive their children and themselves, but these attributions do not appear to account for the lack of concordance between self-reported and observed behaviour.

Several study limitations should be noted. First, parents' self-reported use of praise and criticism were each measured from a single item extracted from a parent survey. A single item measure may not be an accurate indicator of parents' perceptions of their use of praise or criticism. Second, the behaviour sample used to measure observed parent behaviour was derived from a video-recorded 15-minute play session. Parents' behaviour in this context may not have been representative of their typical behaviour. However, being recorded while playing with one's child would likely elicit more positive behaviour than might be typical. Thus, the number of parent praises observed might have actually been higher and the number of critical statements observed lower than was typical for these participants. Finally, this secondary analysis relied on an existing convenience sample of parents seeking mental health services for their children. As a result, the size of the sample, the study measures used, and the representativeness of the sample were all limited. Additional studies evaluating concordance between parents' self-reports and observed behaviour with their children using larger and more diverse samples in both mental health and community populations are warranted to better understand these discrepancies in measurement and best practices for guiding parents in using more positive parenting strategies with their preschool children.

IMPLICATIONS FOR PRACTICE

Chronic mental health problems in children have now surpassed physical illnesses as one of the five most prevalent disabilities affecting children in the United States (Halfon, Houtrow, Larson, & Newacheck, 2012; Slomski, 2012). Their prevalence points to the importance of screening for behavioural and emotional problems in pediatric primary care and identifying appropriate resources for parents (Weitzman & Wegner, 2015).

Thoughtful discussions with parents in primary care settings about positive strategies for supporting their children's behavioural health, supplemented with written materials on how and when to use these strategies, would be an initial step. For example, Bright Futures includes brief handouts on communicating with children in ways that support their self-esteem (www.brightfutures.org). These handouts, in conjunction with discussions on the importance of parents' positive statements supporting their children's efforts and behaviour, would be an important addition to well-child visits. Referral to parent training programs that are available in many cities across the country would connect parents to interventions that strengthen parents' use of positive skills, such as praise, and teach alternate strategies for discouraging misbehaviour other than criticism. Parent training programs that use brief video-recorded examples of parents using evidence-based parenting strategies to promote positive child behaviour may be useful if parents have not previously been exposed to these strategies (e.g., the Chicago Parent Program, the Incredible Years). The National Registry of Evidence-Base Programs and Practices, sponsored by the Substance Abuse and Mental Health Services Administration, lists more than 70 different parent-training programs. The Web site also provides critical evaluations of each program's evidence and readiness for dissemination along with program contact information for providers and consumers seeking additional information (www.nrepp.samhsa.gov).

It is important to note that although the parents in this sample were seeking help for their children's behaviour, these parents also represent a highly vulnerable population. Most were unemployed and economically disadvantaged, and more than 46% evidenced high levels of depressive symptoms. It is possible that these parents have experienced little praise and a great deal of criticism in their lives. As a result, their perspective on what constitutes "a lot" of praise and "rare" criticism may be skewed. Moreover, parents raising young children in under-resourced communities may feel the need to "toughen" their children to the realities of life. Thus, critical statements may seem to some parents to be a more responsible and realistic way to prepare their children for adulthood than using praise. The challenge for clinicians is to support parents in preparing their children for life's difficulties by building the self-esteem and resilience that their children will need to grow and thrive despite the difficulties.

> The challenge for clinicians is to support parents in preparing their children for life's difficulties by building the self-esteem and resilience that their children will need to grow and thrive despite the difficulties.

We gratefully acknowledge the support of Mirian Ofonedu, Ivonne Begue De Benzo, and Maria Cecelia Lairet-Michelena.

REFERENCES

Achenbach, T. M., & Rescorla, L. A. (2000). *Manual for the ASEBA preschool forms and profiles.* Burlington, VT: University of Vermont, Department of Psychiatry.

Angold, A., Messer, S. C., Stangl, D., Farmer, E. M. Z., Costello, E. J., & Burns, B. J. (1998). Perceived parental burden and service use for child and adolescent psychiatric disorders. *American Journal of Public Health, 88*(1), 75-80.

Barnett, M. A., & Scaramella, L. V. (2013). Mothers' parenting and child sex differences in behavior problems among African American preschoolers. *Journal of Family Psychology, 27*(5), 773-783.

Bohlin, G., Hagekull, B., & Rydell, A. (2000). Attachment and social functioning: A longitudinal study from infancy to middle childhood. *Social Development, 9,* 24-39.

Bowlby, J. (1988). *A secure base: Parent-child attachment and healthy human development.* New York, NY: Basic Books.

Breitenstein, S. M., Gross, D., Fogg, L., Ridge, A., Garvey, C., Julion, W., & Tucker, S. (2012). The Chicago Parent Program: Comparing 1-year outcomes for African American and Latino parents of young children. *Research in Nursing and Health, 35*(5), 475-489.

Brotman, L. M., O'Neal, C. R., Huang, K. Y., Gouley, K. K., Rosenfelt, A., & Shrout, P. E. (2009). An experimental test of parenting practices as a mediator of early childhood physical aggression. *Journal of Child Psychology and Psychiatry, 50*(3), 235-245.

Brummelman, E., Thomaes, S., Orobio de Castro, B., Overbeek, G., & Bushman, B. J. (2014). ''That's not beautiful—that's incredibly beautiful!'': The adverse impact of inflated praise on children with low self-esteem. *Psychological Science, 25*(3), 728-735.

Cassidy, J. (1988). Child-mother attachment and the self in six-year-olds. *Child Development, 59,* 121-134.

Chorpita, B. F., Caleiden, E. L., & Weisz, J. R. (2005). Identifying and selecting the common elements of evidence-based interventions: A distillation and matching model. *Mental Health Services Research, 7*(1), 5-20.

Cimpian, A. (2010). The impact of generic language about ability on children's achievement motivation. *Developmental Psychology, 46*(5), 1333-1340.

Dix, T., Ruble, D. N., Grusec, J. E., & Nixon, S. (1986). Social cognition in parents: Inferential and affective reactions to children of three age levels. *Child Development, 57*(4), 879-894.

Eaton, W., Muntaner, C., Smith, C., Tien, A., & Ybarra, M. (2004). Center for Epidemiologic Studies Depression Scale: Review and revisions (CESD and CESD-R). In M. E. Maruish (Ed.), *The use of psychological testing for treatment planning and outcomes assessment* (3rd ed., pp. 363-377). Mahwah, NJ: Lawrence Erlbaum.

Eyberg, S. M., & Robinson, E. (1992). *Manual for the Dyadic Parent-Child Interaction Coding System*. Seattle, WA: University of Washington Department of Nursing.

Eyberg, S. M., Funderburk, B. W., Hembree-Kigin, T. L., McNeil, C. B., Querido, J. G., & Hood, K. K. (2001). Parent-child interaction therapy with behavior problem children: One and two year maintenance of treatment effects in the family. *Child & Family Behavior Therapy, 23*(4), 1-20.

Fernandez, M. A., & Eyberg, S. M. (2009). Predicting treatment and follow-up attrition in parent-child interaction therapy. *Journal of Abnormal Child Psychology, 37*(3), 431-441.

Furlong, M., McGilloway, S., Bywater, T., Hutchings, J., Smith, S. M., & Donnelly, M. (2013). Cochrane review: Behavioural and cognitive-behavioural group-based parenting programmes for early-onset conduct problems in children aged 3 to 12 years. *Evidence-based Child Health, 8*(2), 318-692.

Gardner, F. (2000). Methodological issues in the direct observation of parent-child interaction: Do observational findings reflect the natural behavior of participants? *Clinical Child and Family Psychology Review, 3*(3), 185-198.

Gross, D. A., Belcher, H. M. E., Ofonedu, M. E., Breitenstein, S., Frick, K. D., & Budhathoki, C. (2014). Study protocol for a comparative effectiveness trial of two parent training programs in a fee-for-service mental health clinic: Can we improve mental health services to low-income families? *Trials, 15*, 70.

Gross, D., Fogg, L., Garvey, C., & Julion, W. (2004). Behavior problems in young children: An analysis of cross-informant agreements and disagreements. *Research in nursing & health, 27*(6), 413-425.

Gross, D., Fogg, L., Young, M., Ridge, A., Cowell, J. M., Richardson, R., & Sivan, A. (2006). The equivalence of the Child Behavior Checklist/1-1/2-5 across parent race/ethnicity, income level, and language. *Psychological Assessment, 18*(3), 313-323.

Gross, D., Fogg, L., Young, M., Ridge, A., Cowell, J. M., Sivan, A., & Richardson, R. (2007). Reliability and validity of the Eyberg Child Behavior Inventory with African American and Latino parents of young children. *Research in Nursing & Health, 30*, 213-223.

Gross, D., Garvey, C., Julion, W., Fogg, L., Tucker, S., & Mokros, H. (2009). Efficacy of the Chicago Parent Program with low-income African American and Latino parents of young children. *Prevention Science, 10*, 54-65.

Halfon, N., Houtrow, A., Larson, K., & Newacheck, P. W. (2012). The changing landscape of disability in childhood. *The Future of Children, 22*(1), 13-42.

Henderlong, J., & Lepper, M. R. (2002). The effects of praise on children's intrinsic motivation: A review and synthesis. *Psychological Bulletin, 128*(5), 774-795.

Leung, D. W., & Slep, A. M. (2006). Predicting inept discipline: The role of parental depressive symptoms, anger, and attributions. *Journal of Consulting and Clinical Psychology, 74*(3), 524-534.

Lorber, M. F., & Egeland, B. (2011). Parenting and infant difficult: testing a mutual exacerbation hypothesis to predict early onset conduct problems. *Child Development, 82*(6), 2006-2020.

McCabe, K. M., Clark, R., & Barnett, D. (1999). Family protective factors among urban African American youth. *Journal of Child Clinical Psychology, 28*, 137-150.

Meltzer, H., Ford, T., Goodman, R., & Vostanis, P. (2011). The burden of caring for children with emotional or conduct disorders. *International Journal of Family Medicine, 2011*, 801203.

Mueller, C. M., & Dweck, C. S. (1998). Praise for intelligence can undermine children's motivation and performance. *Journal of Personality and Social Psychology, 75*(1), 33-52.

Morsbach, S. K., & Prinz, R. J. (2006). Understanding and improving the validity of self-report of parenting. *Clinical Child and Family Psychology Review, 9*(1), 1-21.

Owens, D. J., Slep, A. M., & Heyman, R. E. (2012). The effect of praise, positive nonverbal response, reprimand, and negative nonverbal response on child compliance: A systematic review. *Clinical Child and Family Psychological Review, 15*(4), 364-385.

Scott, S., & Dadds, M. R. (2009). Practitioner review: When parent training doesn't work: Theory-driven clinical strategies. *Journal of Child Psychology and Psychiatry and Applied Disciplines, 50*(12), 1441-1450.

Sivan, A. B., Ridge, A., Gross, D., Richardson, R., & Cowell, J. M. (2008). Analysis of two measures of child behavior problems by African American, Latino, and Non-Hispanic Caucasian parents of young children: A focus group study. *Journal of Pediatric Nursing, 23*(1), 20-27.

Slomski, A. (2012). Chronic mental health issues in children now loom larger than physical problems. *Journal of the American Medical Association, 308*(3), 223-225.

Tung, I., Li, J. J., & Lee, S. S. (2012). Child sex moderates the association between negative parenting and childhood conduct problems. *Aggressive Behavior, 28*(3), 239-251.

Van Dam, N. T., & Earleywine, M. (2011). Validation of the Center for Epidemiologic Studies Depression Scale–Revised (CESD-R): Pragmatic depression assessment in the general population. *Psychiatry Research, 186*(1), 128-132.

Wahler, R. G., & Meginnis, K. L. (1997). Strengthening child compliance through positive parenting practices: What works? *Journal of Clinical Child Psychology, 26*(4), 433-440.

Webster-Stratton, C., & Hammond, M. (1998). Conduct problems and level of social competence in Head Start children: Prevalence, pervasiveness, and associated risk factors. *Clinical Child and Family Psychology Review, 1*(2), 101-124.

Weitzman, C., & Wegner, L. (2015). Promoting optimal development: Screening for behavioral and emotional problems. *Pediatrics, 135*(2), 384-395.

Zentall, S. R., & Morris, B. J. (2010). "Good job, you're so smart": The effects of inconsistency of praise type on young children's motivation. *Journal of Experimental Child Psychology, 107*(2), 155-163.

Nursing Research • July/August 2010 • Vol 59, No 4, 241–249

Subsequent Childbirth After a Previous Traumatic Birth

Cheryl Tatano Beck ▼ Sue Watson

▶ **Background:** Nine percent of new mothers in the United States who participated in the Listening to Mothers II Postpartum Survey screened positive for meeting the *Diagnostic and Statistical Manual of Mental Disorders, Fourth Edition* criteria for posttraumatic stress disorder after childbirth. Women who have had a traumatic birth experience report fewer subsequent children and a longer length of time before their second baby. Childbirth-related posttraumatic stress disorder impacts couples' physical relationship, communication, conflict, emotions, and bonding with their children.

▶ **Objective:** The purpose of this study was to describe the meaning of women's experiences of a subsequent childbirth after a previous traumatic birth.

▶ **Methods:** Phenomenology was the research design used. An international sample of 35 women participated in this Internet study. Women were asked, "Please describe in as much detail as you can remember your subsequent pregnancy, labor, and delivery following your previous traumatic birth." Colaizzi's phenomenological data analysis approach was used to analyze the stories of the 35 women.

▶ **Results:** Data analysis yielded four themes: (a) riding the turbulent wave of panic during pregnancy; (b) strategizing: attempts to reclaim their body and complete the journey to motherhood; (c) bringing reverence to the birthing process and empowering women; and (d) still elusive: the longed-for healing birth experience.

▶ **Discussion:** Subsequent childbirth after a previous birth trauma has the potential to either heal or retraumatize women. During pregnancy, women need permission and encouragement to grieve their prior traumatic births to help remove the burden of their invisible pain.

▶ **Key Words:** phenomenology · posttraumatic stress disorder (PTSD) · subsequent childbirth · traumatic childbirth

I n the United States, 9% of new mothers who participated in the Listening to Mothers II Postpartum Follow-Up Survey screened positive for meeting the *Diagnostic and Statistical Manual of Mental Disorders, Fourth Edition* (American Psychiatric Association, 2000) criteria for posttraumatic stress disorder (PTSD) after childbirth (Declercq, Sakala, Corry, & Applebaum, 2008). In this survey, the mothers' voices revealed a troubling pattern of maternity care.

A large percentage of women giving birth in the United States experienced hospital care that did not reflect the best evidence for practice nor for women's preferences. The Institute of Medicine (2003) identified childbirth as a national healthcare priority for quality improvement. A maternity care quality chasm still exists (Sakala & Corry, 2007).

Researchers and healthcare professionals at an international meeting on current issues regarding PTSD after childbirth recommended the need for research focusing on women's subjective birth experiences (Ayers, Joseph, McKenzie-McHarg, Slade, & Wijma, 2008). Olde, van der Hart, Kleber, and van Son (2006) called for examining the chronic nature of childbirth-related posttraumatic stress lasting longer than 6 months after birth.

The purpose of the current study was to help fill the knowledge gap of one aspect of the chronicity of birth trauma: women's subjective experiences of the subsequent pregnancy, labour, and delivery after a traumatic childbirth.

Review of Literature

Traumatic childbirth is defined as "an event occurring during the labor and delivery process that involves actual or threatened serious injury or death to the mother or her infant. The birthing woman experiences intense fear, helplessness, loss of control, and horror" (Beck, 2004a, p. 28). For some women, a traumatic birth also involves perceiving their birthing experience as dehumanizing and stripping them of their dignity (Beck, 2004a, 2004b, 2006). After a traumatic childbirth, 2% to 21% of women meet the diagnostic criteria for PTSD (Ayers, 2004; Ayers, Harris, Sawyer, Parfitt, & Ford, 2009), involving the development of three characteristic symptoms stemming from the exposure to the trauma: persistent reexperiencing of the traumatic event, persistent avoiding of reminders of the trauma and a numbing of general responsiveness, and persistent increased arousal (American Psychiatric Association, 2000).

Risk Factors

Risk factors contributing to women perceiving their childbirth as traumatic can be divided into three categories: prenatal factors, nature and circumstances of the delivery,

Cheryl Tatano Beck, DNSc, CNM, FAAN, is Distinguished Professor, School of Nursing, University of Connecticut, Storrs.

Sue Watson, is Chairperson, Trauma and Birth Stress, Auckland, New Zealand.

345

and subjective factors during childbirth (van Son, Verkerk, van der Hart, Komproe, & Pop, 2005). Under the prenatal category are factors such as histories of previous traumatic births, prenatal PTSD (Onoye, Goebert, Morland, Matsu, & Wright, 2009), child sexual abuse, and psychiatric counseling. Factors included in the category of nature and circumstances of the delivery include a high level of medical intervention, extremely painful labour and delivery, and delivery type (Ayers et al., 2009). Subjective risk factors during childbirth can include feelings of powerlessness, lack of caring and support from labour and delivery staff, and fear of dying (Thomson & Downe, 2008).

> *A large percentage of women giving birth in the United States experienced hospital care that did not reflect the best evidence for practice nor for women's preferences.*

▼▼▼

Long-Term Impact of Traumatic Childbirth

Researchers are uncovering an unsettling gamut of long-term detrimental effects of traumatic childbirth not only on the mothers themselves but also on their relationships with infants and other family members. Mothers' breastfeeding experiences and the yearly anniversary of their birth trauma can also be negatively impacted.

Impaired mother–infant relationships after traumatic childbirth are being confirmed in the literature. For example, in the study of Ayers, Wright, and Wells (2007) of mothers who experienced birth trauma in the United Kingdom, women described themselves as feeling detached and having feelings of rejection toward their infants. Nicholls and Ayers (2007) reported two different types of mother–infant bonding in couples who shared that PTSD after childbirth affected their relationships with their children; they became anxious/overprotective or avoidant/rejecting. Childbirth-related PTSD also impacted their relationships with their partners, including their physical relationship, communication, conflict, emotions, support, and coping.

Long-term detrimental effects of traumatic childbirth can extend also into women's breastfeeding experiences. In their Internet study, Beck and Watson (2008) explored the impact of birth trauma on the breastfeeding experiences of 52 mothers. For some mothers, their traumatic childbirth led to distressing impediments that curtailed their breastfeeding attempts, such as feeling that their breasts were just one more thing to be violated.

Another aspect of the chronic effect of birth trauma was identified in Beck's (2006) Internet study of the anniversary of traumatic childbirth, an invisible phenomenon that mothers struggled with. Thirty-seven women comprised this international sample of mothers from the United States, New Zealand, Australia, United Kingdom, and Canada. Beck concluded that a failure to rescue occurred for women as the anniversary approached, and all others focused on the celebration of the children's birthdays. This failure to rescue led to unnecessary emotional or physical suffering or both.

Catherall (1998) warned of secondary trauma in families living with trauma survivors. The entire family is vulnerable to becoming secondarily traumatized. The long-term impact of trauma does not result necessarily in PTSD symptoms in family members. Catherall stated that it can have a more insidious effect of a disturbing milieu in the family. The members of the family may be close physically, but their ability to express emotions is limited. True closeness in the family is missing, and their problem solving is impaired. Abrams (1999) identified one of the central clinical characteristics of intergenerational transmission of trauma is the silence that happens in families regarding traumatic experiences. Abrams pleaded that the multigenerational impact of trauma should not be underestimated.

Posttraumatic Growth

Researchers are reporting that traumatic experiences can have positive benefits in a person's life. Posttraumatic growth has been documented in a wide range of people who faced traumatic experiences such as bereaved parents (Engelkemeyer & Marwit, 2008), human immunodeficiency virus caregivers (Cadell, 2007), and homeless women with histories of traumatic experiences (Stump & Smith, 2008). "Posttraumatic growth describes the experience of individuals whose development, at least in some areas, has surpassed what was present before the struggle with the crisis occurred. The individual has not only survived, but has experienced changes that are viewed as important, and that go beyond what was the previous status quo" (Tedeschi & Calhoun, 2004, p. 4). It is not the actual trauma that is responsible for posttraumatic growth but what happens after the trauma. Tedeschi and Calhoun (2004, p. 6) proposed five domains of posttraumatic growth: "greater appreciation of life and changed sense of priorities; warmer, more intimate relationships with others; a greater sense of personal strength; recognition of new possibilities or paths for one's life; and spiritual development."

Childbirth can have an enormous potential to help change how a woman feels about herself and can impact her transition to motherhood (Levy, 2006). Attias and Goodwin (1999, p. 299) noted that a woman who survives a traumatic experience may be able to rebuild her wounded inner self "by having a child, transforming her body from a container of ashes to a container for a new human life." A positive childbirth has the potential to empower a traumatized woman and help her reclaim her life.

One study was located that touched on the positive growth of women after a previous negative birthing experience. In Cheyney's (2008) qualitative study of women in the United States who chose home births after experiencing a negative birth, three integrated conceptual themes emerged from their home birth narratives: knowledge, power, and intimacy. The power of their home births helped heal scars of their past hospital births. Positive growth after birth trauma has yet to be investigated systematically by researchers.

One of the knowledge gaps identified in this literature review focused on an aspect of the long-term effects of birth trauma: mothers' subsequent childbirth. This phenomenological study was designed to answer the research question:

What is the meaning of women's experiences of a subsequent childbirth following a previous traumatic birth?

Methods

Research Design

The term *phenomenology* is derived from the Greek word *phenomenon*, which means "to show itself." The goal of phenomenology is to describe human experiences as they are experienced consciously without theories about their cause and as free as possible from the researchers' unexamined presuppositions about the phenomenon under study. In phenomenology, researchers "borrow" other individuals' experiences to better understand the deeper meaning of the phenomenon (Van Manen, 1984).

The existential phenomenological method developed by Colaizzi (1973, 1978) was used in this Internet study. His method is designed to uncover the fundamental structure of a phenomenon, that is, the essence of an experience. An assumption of phenomenology is that for any phenomenon, there are essential structures that comprise that human experience. Only by examining specific experiences of the phenomenon being studied can their essential structures be uncovered.

Colaizzi's (1973, 1978) method includes features of Husserl's and Heidegger's philosophies. Colaizzi maintains that description is the key to discovering the essence and the meaning of a phenomenon and that phenomenology is presuppositionless (Husserl, 1954). Colaizzi, however, holds a Heideggerian view of reduction, the process of researchers bracketing presuppositions and their natural attitude about the phenomenon being studied. For Colaizzi (1978, p. 58), researchers identify their presuppositions regarding the phenomenon under study not to bracket them off to the side but instead to use them to "interrogate" one's "beliefs, hypotheses, attitudes, and hunches" about the phenomenon to help formulate research questions. Colaizzi agrees with Merleau-Ponty (1956, p. 64) that "the greatest lesson of reduction is the impossibility of a complete reduction." Individual phenomenological reflection about the phenomenon being studied is one approach Colaizzi (1973) offers for assisting researchers to decrease the colouring of their presuppositions and biases on their research activity.

Because the phenomenon of subsequent childbirth after a previous traumatic birth had not been examined systematically before this current study, description of the meaning of women's experiences was the focus of this study. Before the start of the study, the researchers undertook an individual phenomenological reflection. They questioned themselves regarding their presuppositions about the phenomenon of subsequent childbirth after a traumatic birth and how these might influence what and how they conducted their research.

Sample

Thirty-five women participated in the study (Table 1). Saturation of data was achieved easily with this sample size. Their mean age was 33 years (range = 27 to 51 years). All the participants were Caucasian and had two to four children. The length of time since their previous birth trauma to the subsequent birth ranged from 1 to 13 years. Eight of the 35 women (23%) opted for a home birth for their

TABLE 1. Demographic and Obstetric Characteristics

	n	%
Country		
United States	15	43
United Kingdom	8	23
New Zealand	6	17
Australia	5	14
Canada	1	3
Marital status		
Married	34	98
Divorced	1	2
Single	0	0
Education		
High school	3	9
Some college	5	15
College degree	13	38
Graduate	7	19
Missing	7	19
Delivery		
Vaginal	25	72
Cesarean	10	29
Diagnosed PTSD		
Yes	14	40
No	19	55
Missing	2	5
Currently under care of therapist		
Yes	8	23
No	22	63
Missing	5	15

Note. PTSD = posttraumatic stress disorder.

subsequent births. Of these 8 mothers who gave birth at home, 4 lived in Australia, 3 in the United States, and 1 in the United Kingdom. Fourteen mothers (40%) had been diagnosed with PTSD after childbirth.

All the birth traumas were self-defined. Women were not asked if they had experienced other traumas before their birth traumas. Therefore, this was not an exclusionary criterion. The most frequently identified traumatic births focused on emergency cesarean deliveries, postpartum hemorrhage, severe preeclampsia, preterm labour, high level of medical interventions (i.e., forceps, vacuum extraction, induction), infant in the neonatal intensive care unit, feeling violated, lack or respectful treatment, unsympathetic, nonsupportive labour and delivery staff, and "emotional torture."

Procedure

Once institutional review board approval was obtained from the university, recruitment began. Data collection continued for 2 years and 2 months. Women were recruited by means of a notice placed on the Web site of Trauma and Birth Stress (TABS; www.tabs.org.nz), a charitable trust located in New Zealand. The mission of TABS is to support women who have experienced traumatic childbirth and PTSD because of their birth trauma. The sample criteria required that the mother had experienced a traumatic childbirth with a previous labour and delivery, that she was willing to articulate her experience, and that she could read and write English. This international representation of participants was a strength of this recruitment method. A disadvantage, however, was that only women who had access to the Internet and who used TABS for support participated in this study.

Women who were interested in participating in this Internet study contacted the first author at her university e-mail address, which was listed on the recruitment notice. An information sheet and directions for the study were sent by attachment to interested mothers. After reading these two documents, women could e-mail the researcher if they had any questions concerning the study.

Women were asked, "Please describe in as much detail as you can remember your subsequent pregnancy, labor, and delivery following your previous traumatic birth." Women sent their descriptions of their experiences as e-mail attachments to the researcher. The sending of their story implied their informed consent. The length of time varied from when a mother first e-mailed about her interest in the study to when she sent her completed story to the researchers. The shortest turn-around time was 2 days whereas the longest was 9 months. If women did not respond within a certain period, the researchers did not recontact them. The women's wish not to follow through on participation in the study was respected. Throughout this procedure, the first author kept a reflexive journal.

Data Analysis

Colaizzi's (1978) method of data analysis was used. The order of his steps is as follows: written protocols, significant statements, formulated meanings, clusters of themes, exhaustive description, and fundamental structure. It should be noted, however, that these steps do overlap. From each participant's description of the phenomenon, significant statements, which are phrases or sentences that directly describe the phenomenon, are extracted (Table 2). For each significant statement, the researcher formulates its meaning. Here, creative insight is called into play. Colaizzi cautioned that in this step of data analysis, the researcher must take a precarious leap from what the participants said to what they mean. Formulated meanings should never sever all connections from the original transcripts. It is in this step of formulating meanings that Colaizzi's connection to Heidegger can be seen. The next step entails organizing all the formulated meanings into clusters of themes. At this point, all the results to date are combined into an exhaustive description. This step is followed by revising the exhaustive description into a more condensed statement of the identification of the fundamental structure of the phenomenon being studied. The fundamental structure can be shared with the participants to validate how well it captured aspects of their experiences. If any participants share new data, they are integrated into the final description of the phenomenon. Member checking was done with one participant who reviewed the themes and

---

No.	TABLE 2. **Example of Extracting Significant Statements**
	Significant statements
1	One thing that I'd noticed when I was a child was that when my parents got together with other adults, the talk eventually turned to two things: for my father (a Vietnam veteran) and the other men the talk turned to the war and interestingly, to me as a small child, for my mother and the other women the talk always turned to childbirth.
2	It was as if, from a young age, for me, the connections between the two were drawn. A man is tested through war, a women is tested through childbirth.
3	My dad, as abusive as he was, was considered a "good man" because he'd been a good soldier and so, I reasoned forward with a child's intelligence, that all that really mattered for a woman was to be strong and capable in childbirth.
4	And I failed. In the past, with the previous two births (particularly with the one that resulted in PTSD)—that's what it felt like. I failed at being a woman.
5	I don't think that I am alone in feeling. I have a sneaking suspicion that this is pretty universal.
6	Just as a man who "talks" under torture in a POW situation feels as though he's failed, a woman who can't "handle" tortuous situations during childbirth feels like she's failed. It is not true. But it feels true.
7	My dad received two Purple Hearts and a Bronze Star during Vietnam. He, by most standards, would be considered a hero. Where are my Purple Hearts? My Bronze Star? I've fought a war, no less terrifying, no less destroying but there are no accolades. At least that's what it feels like.
8	I am viewed as flawed if not down right strange that I find L & D so terrifying.
9	The medical establishment thinks that I am "mental" and I have no common ground on which to discuss my childbirth experiences with "normal" women.
10	I know, I've tried. And that makes me feel isolated and inferior.

Note. PTSD = posttraumatic stress disorder.

totally agreed with them. In addition, one mother who had not participated in the study but had experienced the phenomenon being studied reviewed the findings and also agreed with them.

Results

The researchers reflected on the written descriptions provided by the 35 women to explicate the phenomenon of their experiences of subsequent childbirth after a previous traumatic birth. These reflections yielded 274 significant statements that were clustered into four themes and finally into the fundamental structure that identified the essence of this phenomenon (Table 3).

Theme 1: Riding the Turbulent Wave of Panic During Pregnancy

Fear, terror, anxiety, panic, dread, and denial were the most frequent terms used to describe the world women lived in during their pregnancy after a previous traumatic birth.

> I remember the exact moment I realized what was happening. I was on my lunch break at work, sitting under a large oak tree, watching cars go by my office, talking with my husband. I suddenly knew... I am pregnant again! I remember the exact angle of the sun, the shading of the objects around me. I remember looking into the sun, at that tree, at the windows to the office thinking, "NO! God PLEASE NO!" I felt my chest at once sink inward on me and take on the weight of a 1000 bricks. I was short of breath, my head seared. All I could think of was "NOOOOOOOOO!"

Another woman described in detail the day she took her pregnancy test.

> I took the test and crumpled over the edge of our bed, sobbing and retching hysterically for hours. I was dizzy. I was nauseous. I was sick. I could not breathe. I thought my chest would implode. I had a terrible migraine. I could not move from the spot where I had crumpled. I could not talk to my husband or see our daughter. I felt torn to pieces, shredded as shards of glass. I spent the next 2 trimesters hanging on for my life with suicidal

thoughts but no real desire to carry them out through. I wanted to see my little girl. It was hell on earth.

Some women went into denial during the first trimester of their pregnancy to cope. Throughout her pregnancy, one woman revealed that she "felt numb to my baby." Some women described how they turned their denial of pregnancy into something positive. One multipara explained that after she was in denial for a few months, she then became determined to make things different this next time, and right at the end of her pregnancy she felt empowered by all that she had learned: "After 3 months of ignoring the fact that I was going to have to go through birth again, I decided I would treat my next labor and delivery as a healing and empowering experience."

Other mothers remained in a heightened state of anxiety throughout their pregnancy, and for some this anxiety escalated to panic and terror. Knowing she may have to go through the same "emotional torture" she endured with her previous traumatic birth, one woman shared, "My 9 months of pregnancy were an anxiety filled abyss which was completely marred as an experience due to the terror that was continually in my mind from my experience 8 years earlier." As the delivery date got closer, some mothers reported having panic attacks.

Theme 2: Strategizing: Attempts to Reclaim Their Body and Complete the Journey to Motherhood

"Well, this time; I told myself *things would be different*. I actually started planning for this birth literally while they were stitching me up from the traumatic first birth." During pregnancy women described a number of different strategies they used to help them survive the 9 months of pregnancy while waiting for what they were dreading: labour and delivery (Table 4). Some women spent time nurturing themselves by swimming, walking, going to yoga classes, and spending time outdoors.

Keeping a journal throughout the pregnancy helped mothers because they had somewhere to write things down, especially if they felt that family and friends did not understand just how difficult this pregnancy, subsequent to their prior traumatic delivery, was. Inspirational quotes were placed around the house to read and motivate women.

TABLE 3. Fundamental Structure of the Phenomenon

Subsequent childbirth after a previous traumatic birth far exceeds the confines of the actual labour and delivery. During the 9 months of pregnancy, women ride turbulent waves of panic, terror, and fear that the looming birth could be a repeat of the emotional and/or physical torture they had endured with their previous labour and delivery. Women strategized during pregnancy how they could reclaim their bodies that had been violated and traumatized by their previous childbirth. Women vowed to themselves that things would be different and that this time they would complete their journey to motherhood. Mothers employed strategies to try to bring a reverence to the birthing process and rectify all that had gone so wrong with their prior childbirth. The array of various strategies entailed such actions as hiring doulas for support during labour and delivery, becoming avid readers of childbirth books, writing a detailed birth plan, learning birth hypnosis, interviewing obstetricians and midwives about their philosophy of birth, doing yoga, and drawing birthing art. All these well-designed strategies did not ensure that all women would experience the healing childbirth they desperately longed for. For the mothers whose subsequent childbirth was a healing experience, they reclaimed their bodies, had a strong sense of control, and their birth became an empowering experience. The role of caring supporters was crucial in their labour and delivery. Women were treated with respect, dignity, and compassion. Although their subsequent birth was positive and empowering, women were quick to note that it could never change the past. Still elusive for some women was their longed-for healing subsequent birth.

TABLE 4. Strategies Used to Cope With Pregnancy and Looming Labour and Delivery

- Writing a detailed birth plan
- Mentally preparing for birth
- Learning birth hypnosis
- Doing birth art
- Writing positive affirmations
- Preparing for birthing at home
- Hiring a doula for labour and delivery
- Celebrating upcoming birth
- Avoiding ultrasounds
- Trying not to think about upcoming birth
- Reading books on healthy pregnancy and birth
- Mapping out your pelvis
- Learning birthing positions to open up the pelvis
- Practicing hypnosis for labour
- Researching birth centers and scheduling tours
- Interviewing obstetricians and midwives
- Exercising to help baby get in the correct position
- Using Internet support group
- Hiring a life coach
- Painting previous birth experience
- Creating "what if" sheet with all possible concerns and then solutions for them
- Creating "Yes, if necessary No" sheet for labor of what the mother wanted to happen
- Determining role of supporters during birth
- Researching homeopathic remedies to prepare body for labour and birth
- Developing a tool kit to help cope in labour
- Developing trust with healthcare provider

Figure 1 is an illustration of one mother's poster that she put up in her home.

Women strategized how to ensure that their looming labour and delivery was not another traumatic one. As one multipara explained, "I need to bring a reverence to the process so I won't feel like a piece of meat lost in the system." Attempts were made to put into place a plan that would attempt to rectify all that had gone wrong with the previous childbirth. Some women turned to doulas in hopes of being supported during their subsequent labour and delivery. Hypnobirthing was a plan used by some women to keep the first traumatic birth from being repeated.

Women reported reading avidly to understand the birth process fully. The most frequently cited books were *Rebounding from Childbirth* (Madsen, 1994), *Birthing from Within* (England & Horowitz, 1998), and *Birth and Beyond* (Gordon, 2002). Mothers often engaged in birth art exercises.

> Toward the end of pregnancy I did the birth art exercises out of the book *Birthing from Within*... I began to trust myself. That will stay with me forever. That is more than

just what I needed to birth the way I wanted to. That is what I needed to become a real woman.

Opening up to their healthcare providers about their previous traumatic births was helpful for some mothers. Once clinicians knew of their history, they would address the mothers' concerns during each prenatal visit. Also sharing with their partners their fears and insecurities around pregnancy and birth helped women's emotional preparedness.

Theme 3: Bringing Reverence to the Birthing Process and Empowering Women

Three quarters of the women who participated in this Internet study reported that their subsequent labour and delivery was either a "healing experience" or at least "a lot better" than their previous traumatic birth. Women became more confident in themselves as women and as mothers in that they really did know what was best for their babies and themselves. The role of supporters throughout labour and delivery was crucial. What was it that made a subsequent birth a healing experience? In the mothers' own words:

> I was treated with respect, my wishes and those of my husband were listened to. I wasn't made to feel like a piece of meat this time but instead like a woman experiencing one of nature's most wonderful events.

> Pain relief was taken seriously. First time around I was ignored. I begged and pleaded for pain relief. Second time it was offered but because I was made to feel in control, I was able to decline.

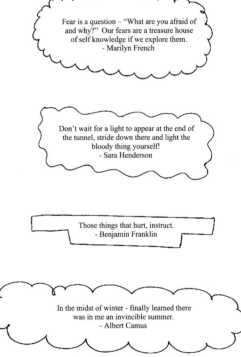

Fear is a question – "What are you afraid of and why?" Our fears are a treasure house of self knowledge if we explore them.
- Marilyn French

Don't wait for a light to appear at the end of the tunnel, stride down there and light the bloody thing yourself!
- Sara Henderson

Those things that hurt, instruct.
- Benjamin Franklin

In the midst of winter - finally learned there was in me an invincible summer.
- Albert Camus

FIGURE 1. A poster of inspirational quotes by one mother.

I wasn't rushed! My baby was allowed to arrive when she was ready. When my first was born, I was told "5 minutes or I get the forceps" by the doctor on call. I pushed so hard that I tore badly.

Communication with labor and delivery staff was so much better the second time. The first time the emergency cord was pulled but no one told me why. I thought my baby was dead and no one would elaborate.

Women reclaimed their bodies, had a strong sense of control, and birth became an empowering experience. Only essential fetal monitoring and minimal medical intervention occurred. Women were allowed to start labour on their own and not be induced. Under gentle supervision of caring and supportive healthcare professionals, women were reassured to just do what their body felt like doing and to follow their body's lead. The number of vaginal examinations was kept at a minimum, and women were permitted to walk around and choose the position they felt best labouring in. One mother described her healing birth:

I pushed my baby into the world and I was shocked. I had never dared to dream for such a perfect delivery. They let me push spontaneously and my baby was delivered into my arms. My husband and I both cried with utter relief that I had given birth exactly how I wanted to and my trauma was healed.

For some women, the birth plan they had prepared during their pregnancy was honoured by the labour and delivery staff, which helped them feel like they had some control and were a part of the birth and not just a witness.

Eight women opted for home births after their previous traumatic births, and for six of them, it did end in fulfilling their dream.

It was as healing and empowering as I had always hoped for. I did not want any high tech management. My home birth was the proudest day of my life and the victory was sweeter because I overcame so very much to come to it.

Another mother who had a successful home birth laboured mostly in her bedroom under candlelight and music playing. She described it as very peaceful being at home surrounded by all her things. Her dog kept vigil by her side. She shared how it was such a gentle way for her baby to be born.

My baby cried for a minute or two as if telling me his birth story and crawled up my body and found my heart and left breast. My heart swelled with so many emotions—love, joy, happiness, pride, relief, and wonderment.

A couple of women explained that their subsequent birth was healing, but at the same time they mourned what they had missed out with their prior birth. The following quote illustrates this.

Even though it was an enormously healing experience, the expectations I had were unrealistic. What I went through during and after my first delivery cannot be erased from memory. If anything with this second birth being so wonderful, it makes dealing with my first birth harder. It makes it sadder and me angrier as before I had nothing to compare it to. I didn't know how different it could be or

how special those first few moments are. I didn't fully understand what I had missed out on. So now 3 years later I find myself grieving again for what we went through, how I was treated and what I missed out on.

Other mothers admitted that although their subsequent births were healing, they could never change the past.

All the positive, empowering births in the world won't ever change what happened with my first baby and me. Our relationship is forever built around his birth experience. The second birth was so wonderful I would go through it all again, but it can never change the past.

Theme 4: Still Elusive: The Longed-for Healing Birth Experience

Sadly, some mothers did not experience the healing subsequent birth they had hoped for. Two women chose to try a home birth after their previous traumatic birth but did not end up with the healing experience they longed for. One mother did deliver at home, but because of postpartum hemorrhage, she was transported by ambulance to the hospital, terrified she would not live to raise her baby. After labouring at home, another multipara who attempted a vaginal birth after cesarean needed to be transported by ambulance for a repeat cesarean birth after she failed to progress.

When the ambulance arrived I felt rescued. I have never been so grateful that hospitals exist. The blue light ambulance journey was terrifying and I was in excruciating pain. By this point I was trying to detach my head from my body, as I had done years earlier when I was being raped.

She went on to vividly describe that as she lay on the operating table:

...with my legs held in the air by 2 strangers while a third mopped the blood between my legs I felt raped all over again. I wanted to die. I had failed as a woman. My privacy had been invaded again. I felt sick.

One multipara shared that although this birth had been a better experience, she would not say it was healing in relation to her first birth that had been so traumatic. "The contrast in the way I was treated just emphasized how bad the first one was. I had no sense of healing until 30 years later when I received counseling for PTSD."

Discussion

Healthcare professionals' failure to rescue women during their previous traumatic childbirth can result in a troubling effect on mothers as they courageously face another pregnancy, labour, and delivery. Subsequent childbirth after a previous birth trauma provides clinicians with not only a golden opportunity but also a professional responsibility to help these traumatized women reclaim their bodies and complete their journey to motherhood.

To help women prepare for a subsequent childbirth after a previous traumatic birth, clinicians first need to identify who these women are. There are instruments available to screen women for posttraumatic stress symptoms due to birth trauma. An essential part of initial prenatal visits should be taking time to discuss with women their previous births. Traumatized women need permission and encouragement to grieve their prior traumatic births to help remove the burden of their invisible pain. Pregnancy is a valuable time for healthcare professionals to help women recognize and deal with unresolved, buried, or traumatic issues. Women should be asked about their hopes and fears for their impending labour and delivery and how they envision this birth. If a woman is exploring the possibility of a home birth, clinicians should question the mother about her previous births. Opting for a home birth may be an indication of a prior traumatic birth (Cheyney, 2008). If women need mental health follow-up during their pregnancy, cognitive behavior therapy and eye movement desensitization reprocessing treatment are two options for PTSD because of birth trauma. Treatment can be given in conjunction with a woman's family members to address secondary effects of PTSD.

Strategies can be employed to help mothers heal and increase their confidence before labour and delivery. Clinicians can share with mothers the Web site for TABS (www.tabs.org.nz), a charitable trust in New Zealand that provides support for women who have suffered through a traumatic birth. Obstetric care providers can suggest to the women some of the numerous strategies that mothers in this study described using during their pregnancies. Women can be encouraged to write down their previous traumatic birth stories. Mothers can share their written stories with their current obstetric care providers so that they understand these women. Some women who participated in this study revealed that birthing artwork definitely helped them prepare for their subsequent labour and delivery after a traumatic childbirth.

Some women in this study touched on one of Tedeschi and Calhoun's (2004) domains of posttraumatic growth, a sense of personal growth. These women revealed feelings of empowerment and of reclaiming their bodies with their subsequent childbirths. Future research needs to be focused specifically on examining the five domains of posttraumatic growth in women who have experienced a subsequent childbirth after a previous birth trauma.

When women are traumatized during childbirth, this can leave a lasting imprint on their lives. If subsequent childbirth has the potential to either heal or retraumatize women, healthcare professionals need to be carefully aware of the consequences their words and actions during labour and delivery can have (Levy, 2006). ▼

Accepted for publication January 27, 2010.

To all the courageous women who shared their most personal and powerful stories of their subsequent childbirth after a previous traumatic birth, the authors are forever indebted.

Corresponding author: Cheryl Tatano Beck, DNSc, CNM, FAAN, School of Nursing, University of Connecticut, 231 Glenbrook Road, Storrs, CT 06269-2026 (e-mail: cheryl.beck@uconn.edu).

References

Abrams, M. S. (1999). Intergenerational transmission of trauma: Recent contributions from the literature of family systems approaches to treatment. *American Journal of Psychotherapy, 53*(2), 225–231.

American Psychiatric Association. (2000). *Diagnostic and Statistical Manual of Mental Disorders—text revision.* Washington, DC: Author.

Attias, R., & Goodwin, J. M. (1999). A place to begin: Images of the body in transformation (pp. 287–303). In J. M. Goodwin & R. Attias (Eds.). *Splintered reflections.* New York: Basic Books.

Ayers, S. (2004). Delivery as a traumatic event: Prevalence, risk factors, and treatment for postnatal posttraumatic stress disorder. *Clinical Obstetrics and Gynecology, 47*(3), 552–567.

Ayers, S., Harris, R., Sawyer, A., Parfitt, Y., & Ford, E. (2009). Posttraumatic stress disorder after childbirth: Analysis of symptom presentation and sampling. *Journal of Affective Disorders, 119*(1–3), 200–204.

Ayers, S., Joseph, S., McKenzie-McHarg, K., Slade, P., & Wijma, K. (2008). Post-traumatic stress disorder following childbirth: Current issues and recommendations for future research. *Journal of Psychosomatic Obstetrics and Gynaecology, 29*(4), 240–250.

Ayers, S., Wright, D. B., & Wells, N. (2007). Symptoms of posttraumatic stress disorder in couples after birth: Association with the couple's relationship and parent-baby bond. *Journal of Reproductive and Infant Psychology, 25*(1), 40–50.

Beck, C. T. (2004a). Birth trauma: In the eye of the beholder. *Nursing Research, 53*(1), 28–35.

Beck, C. T. (2004b). Posttraumatic stress disorder due to childbirth: The aftermath. *Nursing Research, 53*(4), 216–224.

Beck, C. T. (2006). The anniversary of birth trauma: Failure to rescue. *Nursing Research, 55*(6), 381–390.

Beck, C. T., & Watson, S. (2008). Impact of birth trauma on breast-feeding: A tale of two pathways. *Nursing Research, 57*(4), 228–236.

Cadell, S. (2007). The sun always comes out after it rains: Understanding posttraumatic growth in HIV caregivers. *Health & Social Work, 32*(3), 169–176.

Catherall, D. R. (1998). Treating traumatized families. In C. R. Figley (Ed.). *Burnout in families: The systematic costs of caring* (pp. 187–215). Boca Raton, FL: CRC Press.

Cheyney, M. J. (2008). Homebirth as systems-challenging praxis: Knowledge, power, and intimacy in the birthplace. *Qualitative Health Research, 18*(2), 254–267.

Colaizzi, P. F. (1973). *Reflection and research in psychology: A phenomenological study of learning.* Dubuque, IA; Kendall/Hunt Publishing Company.

Colaizzi, P. F. (1978). Psychological research as the phenomenologist views it. In R. Valle & M. King (Eds.). *Existential phenomenological alternatives for psychology* (pp. 48–71). New York: Oxford University Press.

Declercq, E. R., Sakala, C., Corry, M. P., & Applebaum, S. (2008). *New mothers speak out: National survey results highlight women's postpartum experience.* New York: Childbirth Connection.

Engelkemeyer, S. M., & Marwit, S. J. (2008). Posttraumatic growth in bereaved parents. *Journal of Traumatic Stress, 21*(3), 344–346.

England, P., & Horowitz, R. (1998). *Birthing from within.* Alburquerque, NM: Partera Press.

Gordon, Y. (2002). *Birth and beyond.* London: Vermilion.

Husserl, E. (1954). *The crisis of European sciences and transcendental phenomenology.* The Hague: Martinus Nijhoff.

Institute of Medicine. (2003). *Board on Health Care Services Committee on identifying priority areas for quality improvements.* Washington, DC: National Academy Press.

Levy, M. (2006). Maternity in the wake of terrorism: Rebirth or retraumatization? *Journal of Prenatal and Perinatal Psychology and Health, 20*(3), 221–249.

Madsen, L. (1994). *Rebounding from childbirth: Toward emotional recovery.* Westport, CT: Bergin & Garvey.

Merleau-Ponty, M. (1956). What is phenomenology? *Crosscurrents, 6,* 59–70.

Nicholls, K., & Ayers, S. (2007). Childbirth-related post-traumatic stress disorder in couples: A qualitative study. *British Journal of Health Psychology, 12*(Pt. 4), 491–509.

Olde, E., van der Hart, O., Kleber, R., & van Son, M. (2006). Post-traumatic stress following childbirth: A review. *Clinical Psychology Review, 26*(1), 1–16.

Onoye, J. M., Goebert, D., Morland, L., Matsu, C., & Wright, T. (2009). PTSD and postpartum mental health in a sample of Caucasian, Asian, and Pacific Islander women. *Archives of Women's Mental Health, 12*(6), 393–400.

Sakala, C., & Corry, M. P. (2007). Listening to Mothers II reveals maternity care quality chasm. *Journal of Midwifery & Women's Health, 52*(3), 183–185.

Stump, M. J., & Smith, J. E. (2008). The relationship between post-traumatic growth and substance use in homeless women with histories of traumatic experience. *American Journal on Addictions, 17*(6), 478–487.

Tedeschi, R. G., & Calhoun, L. G. (2004). Posttraumatic growth: Conceptual foundations and empirical evidence. *Psychological Inquiry, 15*(1), 1–18.

Thomson, G., & Downe, S. (2008). Widening the trauma discourse: The link between childbirth and experiences of abuse. *Journal of Psychosomatic Obstetrics and Gynaecology, 29*(4), 268–273.

Van Manen, M. (1984). Practicing phenomenological writing. *Phenomenology + Pedagogy, 2*(1), 36–69.

Van Son, M., Verkerk, G., van der Hart, O., Komproe, I., & Pop, V. (2005). Prenatal depression, mode of delivery and perinatal dissociation as predictors of postpartum posttraumatic stress: An empirical study. *Clinical Psychology & Psychotherapy, 12*(4), 297–312.

Orthopedic Nursing. 2016 Jan–Feb; 35(1): 20–9

A Randomized Controlled Trial of an Individualized Preoperative Education Intervention for Symptom Management After Total Knee Arthroplasty

Rosemary A. Wilson ▼ Judith Watt-Watson ▼ Ellen Hodnett ▼ Joan Tranmer

Pain and nausea limit recovery after total knee arthroplasty (TKA) patients. The aim of this study was to determine the effect of a preoperative educational intervention on postsurgical pain-related interference in activities, pain, and nausea. Participants (n = 143) were randomized to intervention or standard care. The standard care group received the usual teaching. The intervention group received the usual teaching, a booklet containing symptom management after TKA, an individual teaching session, and a follow-up support call. Outcome measures assessed pain, pain interference, and nausea. There were no differences between groups in patient outcomes. There were no group differences for pain at any time point. Respondents had severe postoperative pain and nausea and received inadequate doses of analgesia and antiemetics. Individualizing education content was insufficient to produce a change in symptoms for patients. Further research involving the modification of system factors affecting the provision of symptom management interventions is warranted.

Introduction

In Canada, more than 42,000 total knee arthroplasty (TKA) surgeries were performed from 2012 from 2013 (Canadian Institute for Health Information, 2014). TKA is a common, successfully performed joint replacement procedure for pain and immobility associated with knee joint compromise. Arthritis is the most common preoperative diagnosis (95.4% osteoarthritis and 2.2% rheumatoid arthritis). The purpose of joint replacement for these patients is to reduce pain and knee joint stiffness, and thereby increase mobility and function.

Pain and nausea are common symptoms for patients after this procedure. Moderate to severe pain on movement and at rest has been documented during the first 3 postoperative days (Brander et al., 2003; Salmon, Hall, Perrbhoy, Shenkin, & Parker, 2001; Strassels, Chen, & Carr, 2002; Wu et al., 2003). Similarly, nausea has been found to be worse on postoperative day 1, but has the greatest impact on patients on day 2 (Wu et al., 2003).

Previous research (Beaupre, Lier, Davies, & Johnston, 2004; Bondy, Sims, Schroeder, Offord, & Narr, 1999; Lin, Lin, & Lin, 1997; McDonald, Freeland, Thomas, & Moore, 2001; McDonald & Molony, 2004; McDonald, Thomas, Livingston, & Severson, 2005; Roach, Tremblay, & Bowers, 1995; Sjoling, Nordahl, Olofsson, & Asplunf, 2003) has explored education interventions for pain prevention and treatment in the TKA population. These trials used a variety of delivery methods for the intervention including video, pamphlets, and classroom sessions, and the impact on pain outcomes was variable. Three studies reported that the education intervention resulted in moderately lower pain scores (McDonald & Molony, 2004, McDonald et al., 2001, Sjoling et al., 2003). Despite the relationship between pain and nausea and their prevalence after TKA, none of the studies addressed analgesic pain management or antiemetic therapy.

Many factors may impact the effectiveness of the preoperative education intervention, including timing and content. Stern and Lockwood (2005), in a systematic review of 15 randomized controlled trials (RCTs), concluded that preadmission written material combined with verbal instruction was more effective and resulted in better performance of postoperative exercises or skills than information provided postoperatively. A systematic review of 13 studies (Louw, Diener, Butler, & Puentedura, 2013) indicated that preoperative education, which focused on pain communication and

Rosemary A. Wilson, RN(EC), PhD, Assistant Professor, School of Nursing, Queen's University, Kingston, Ontario, Canada.

Judith Watt-Watson, RN, PhD, Professor Emeritus, Lawrence S. Bloomberg Faculty of Nursing, Senior Fellow, Massey College, University of Toronto, Toronto, Ontario, Canada.

Ellen Hodnett, RN, PhD, Professor Emeritus, Lawrence S .Bloomberg Faculty of Nursing, University of Toronto, Toronto, Ontario, Canada.

Joan Tranmer, RN, PhD, Professor, School of Nursing, Queen's University, Kingston, Ontario, Canada.

This original research was partially funded by an award from the Kingston General Hospital Women's Auxiliary Millennium Fund.

The authors declare that there are no conflicts of interest.

DOI: 10.1097/NOR.0000000000000210

management strategies, may result in better patient outcomes than education focused on pathophysiology. Preoperative education for patients with TKA had a significant, positive effect in one study (McDonald et al., 2001). The authors hypothesized that this was due to the difference in educational content of the intervention: a focus on pain management and communication rather than the anatomy and physiology of the surgery. Louw et al. (2013) advised more investigation regarding the content of educational interventions associated with TKA. Further, Wallis and Taylor (2011) conducted a systematic review and meta-analysis of 23 RCTs involving both patients with hip and knee replacement. The meta-analysis ($n = 2$) included 99 participants and provided minimal quality evidence that preoperative exercise combined with education leads to quicker return to mobility and activity after joint replacement, compared with standard preoperative care (standard mean difference = 0.50 [0.10, 0.90]).

Education that includes ways for patients to communicate pain and underlines the use of pain management strategies, including analgesics, has been used in other patient groups. Watt-Watson et al. (2004) addressed common patient concerns with taking analgesics in addition to reviewing the importance of pain relief and pain communication in a study of 406 patients with coronary artery bypass. Patients in the intervention group reported fewer concerns about taking analgesics (22.6 ± 14.7 vs. 18.5 ± 14.1, $p < .05$) and fewer concerns about addiction (3.7 ± 3.6 vs. 4.8 ± 3.8). The finding that most patients would not ask for analgesics, despite having fewer concerns about addiction and taking analgesics because they expected clinicians to know when these were needed, suggested that discussion of these beliefs about postoperative symptom management would be important for TKA patients, as well.

An individualized preoperative education approach has been used successfully to reduce symptoms in patients with cancer (Benor, Delbar, & Krulik, 1998; DeWit et al., 2001; Sherwood et al., 2005; Velji, 2006; Yates

et al., 2004). Further, systematic reviews have recommended individualization of preoperative educational content (Johansson, Nuutila, Virtanen, Katajisto, & Salantera, 2005; McDonald, Page, Beringer, Wasiak, & Sprowson, 2014). However, no studies were found that used an individualized approach to preoperative patient education for patients with TKA.

Therefore, the intervention used in this trial was designed to be an individualized, preoperative approach to patient education and was informed by an adaptation of Wilson and Cleary's (1995) conceptual model of patient outcomes (Figure 1). The intervention focused on patient communication for pain management, analgesic use, and antiemetic use (see Table 1). This study aimed to investigate the impact of an individually delivered preoperative education intervention on pain-related interference, pain, and nausea for patients undergoing unilateral TKA.

Research Questions

- *Primary research question:* What is the effect of an individualized preoperative education intervention for patients with TKA on pain-related interference with usual activities on postoperative day 3?
- *Secondary research question:* What is the effect of an individualized preoperative education intervention for patients with TKA on nausea, pain, and analgesic and antiemetic administration on postoperative days 1, 2, and 3?

Methods

TRIAL DESIGN

An RCT design was used to evaluate outcomes on the first, second, and third days after TKA surgery (see Figure 2). This trial was conducted at an academic health sciences centre in Southeastern Ontario. Ethics approval was obtained from the associated university's Research Ethics Board and the Trial Site Hospital's Research Ethics Board.

TABLE 1. PRE-KNEE SYMPTOM EDUCATION INTERVENTION CONTENT

Topic	Supporting Evidence
Pain, importance of pain management	McDonald et al. (2001); Chang et al. (2005); Johnson, Rice, Fuller, and Endress (1978); Lin et al. (1997); McDonald et al. (2004); Melzack and Wall (1996); Sjoling et al. (2003); Watt-Watson et al. (2004)
Importance of pain management to promote activity	McDonald et al.; Lin et al.; Sjoling et al.; Watt-Watson et al.
Communicating pain to health professionals	McDonald et al.; Johnson et al.; McDonald et al.; Sjoling et al.; Watt-Watson et al.
Asking for analgesics	McDonald et al.; Johnson et al.; Sjoling et al.; Lin et al.; Watt-Watson et al.
Asking for antiemetics	Gan et al. (2003); Melzack and Wall
Preventing dehydration (fluids)	Hodgkinson et al. (2003); Phillips, Johnston, and Gray (1993)
Misbeliefs about taking medication	Chang et al.; Watt-Watson et al.; Wilson, Goldstein, VanDenKerkhof, and Rimmer (2005)
Nonpharmacological measures	Melzack and Wall; Watt-Watson et al.

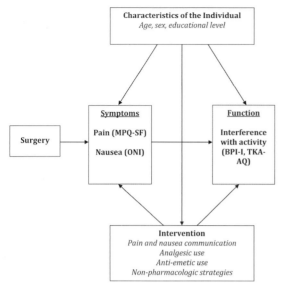

FIGURE 1. Conceptual framework: adaptation of Wilson and Cleary's (1995) model.

STUDY PARTICIPANTS

Patients were included if they were scheduled for elective unilateral primary TKA using planned intrathecal (spinal) anesthetic technique; had grade I–II American Society of Anesthesiologists Physical Status Classification (Larson, 1996); were able to speak and understand English; were able to be reached by telephone; were planned for home discharge; and consented to participate in this trial. Patients were excluded if they were not expected to be discharged home, or were booked for hemi, revision, or bilateral knee arthroplasty.

Recruitment took place at the weekly outpatient orthopaedic preadmission testing clinic at a facility affiliated with the trial centre. Potential participants were identified by clinic staff, and eligible patients were asked for their permission by hospital staff to release their names to the investigator using a standardized script. The trial research assistant gave all willing patients a detailed verbal and written explanation of the trial during their preadmission appointment. Before randomization, written consent was gained by the trial research assistant, who then collected baseline demographic characteristics and clinical information.

Interventions

INTERVENTION: THE PRE-KNEE SYMPTOM EDUCATION INTERVENTION

The Pre-Knee Symptom Education intervention was composed of three components: the booklet, an individual teaching session, and a follow-up support telephone call. Content used in this intervention was drawn from trials of preoperative education programs in surgical patients (McDonald et al., 2001; McDonald & Molony., 2004; Sjoling et al., 2003; Watt-Watson et al., 2004) and supported by focus groups' findings of indi-

vidual areas of concern for patients with TKA (Chang et al., 2005). To ensure concerns, found in the literature, were consistent with those of patients with TKA at the trial site, pilot interviews of 10 patients were conducted on day 2 or 3 post-TKA surgery. The Pre-Knee Symptom Education Booklet was reviewed with each consenting participant in an individualized, private teaching session during the preoperative patient visit to the Pre-Surgical Screening (PSS) Centre. This component was adapted from an educational tool used by Watt-Watson and colleagues (2004) for relevance to TKA postoperative recovery and the result of the pilot interviews done with local patients. The booklet was 12 pages long and included the content provided in Table 1 in addition to diagrams, pictures, and a space for recording questions for the investigator during the telephone follow-up call. The teaching session and booklet review were provided in a quiet examination room. The principal investigator delivered all intervention components during the PSS clinic appointment within 4 weeks of surgery. New concerns identified by trial participants as well as strategies presented were recorded on the Individualized Education Content Tool and reinforced during the follow-up support telephone call along with discussion of any questions raised by participants in the intervening time. The follow-up support telephone call occurred during the week before the scheduled surgical date.

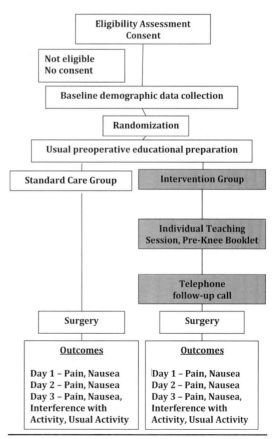

FIGURE 2. Schema of trial design.

Questions asked by participants focused on (a) use of the intravenous patient-controlled analgesia (PCA-IV) pump, (b) concerns about the adverse effects of opioid analgesics, (c) physiotherapy timing, (d) home discharge analgesia, and (e) presurgical fasting guidelines and information regarding oral fluid intake.

Standard Care

Participants in both groups received standard care, including an educational session provided by a physiotherapist outlining physiotherapy activities, a 30-minute video explaining the surgical procedure and postoperative orthopaedic routines, and a brief review of the use of PCA-IV by clinic nursing staff.

Outcomes

Baseline demographic data were collected using the self-reported Baseline Demographic Questionnaire before the intervention.

The primary outcome, pain interference, was measured using the Brief Pain Inventory, Interference (BPI-I) subscale on postoperative day 3 (Cleeland & Ryan, 1994). Pain-related interference, as measured by the BPI-I, refers to the extent to which pain interferes with general activities, sleep, mood, walking, movement from bed to chair, and relationships with others. This measure has well-established construct validity (Mendoza et al., 2004b, 2004a; Tan, Jensen, Thornby, & Shanti, 2004; Watt-Watson et al., 2004). Psychometric testing of postoperative use of the BPI-I demonstrates a consistent subscale structure between acute and chronic pain states (Mendoza et al., 2004a, 2004b; Watt-Watson et al., 2004; Zalon, 1999) as well as sensitivity to change (Mendoza et al., 2004a) and sex differences (Watt-Watson et al., 2004). The use of the BPI-I in the immediate postoperative period (Zalon, 1997) and beyond postoperative day 3 has been demonstrated (Mendoza et al., 2004a; Watt-Watson et al., 2004). Two items were deleted: "normal work" and "enjoyment of life" as these items were not relevant to the early postoperative period. The addition of one item addressing the activity of transferring from bed to chair was added, and the modified tool was pilot tested on the third postoperative day in a group of TKA patients ($n = 14$). The additional item, transferring from bed to chair, was easily answered by all participants and similarly judged to be an appropriate item for the administration time. Similar adaptation of the BPI-I items took place in a study by Watt-Watson et al. (2004) where both "normal work" and "enjoyment of life" were deleted and "deep breathing and coughing" was inserted for use in a postoperative patient population. Cronbach's α for this change was reported as .71.

Secondary outcomes included levels of pain and nausea, and analgesic and antiemetic use. Pain and pain quality were measured using the Short Form McGill Pain Questionnaire (MPQ-SF) (Melzack, 1987; Melzack et al., 1987). Nausea was measured using the Overall Nausea Index (ONI), one component of the Nausea Questionnaire (Melzack, 1989), used previously by Parlow et al. (2004) in a trial of postoperative anti-emetic therapies.

Antiemetic and opioid administration data were recorded from the chart for each of postoperative days 1 to 3.

Sample Size

Sample size for this trial was based on group means from another study ($n = 406$) using the BPI-I as a primary outcome (Watt-Watson et al., 2004). Using a moderate effect size of .5 based on between standard deviation and within standard deviation (Cohen, 1988), the sample size required was 64 per arm (α = .05, power = 80%). A reduction of half the standard deviation of the general population, as reported by Watt-Watson et al. (2004), is a reasonable estimate of the clinically important effect of this intervention. Minimal trial attrition was expected as all measurements were taken during the inpatient hospital stay. A conservative estimate of 10% was used. As a result the sample size required for this trial was 140 in total, with an α level of .05 and power of 80%.

Randomization and Blinding

Participants were randomly assigned to the intervention plus standard care group or the standard care group using a randomization service provided by a research program not connected to this trial. Personnel at the research office used a computer-generated block randomization table provided by statistical services. The research assistant called the research office number, provided the participant number, and received group assignment information. Group assignment was recorded on the Baseline Demographics Questionnaire and was stored in a location separate from all postoperative data collection forms.

The intervention was initiated immediately after randomization for participants in the experimental group in a private room in the presurgical screening area. Although participants could not be unaware of group allocation, the research assistants collecting postoperative outcome data were blinded to group allocation, reducing the potential for cointervention or the introduction of bias by trial personnel during data collection.

Statistical Analysis

Results were analyzed using an intention-to-treat approach. Baseline data were analyzed using descriptive statistics. A two-tailed level of significance of .05 was used for all analyses. Data were analyzed using the SPSS/PASW software package, version 18.

Independent samples t test was used to determine differences in pain-related interference with activity between the intervention and standard care groups on postoperative day 3 on total and component scores. Repeated measures-analysis of covariance was used to determine differences between groups and over the measurement periods in pain scores (MPQ-SF, Numeric Rating Scale [NRS] questions), nausea scores (ONI), and total 24-hour analgesic administration. Differences in antiemetic administration between the two groups were determined using χ^2. Linear-by-linear χ^2 was also used to detect differences in frequency of postoperative activities completed (TKA-AQ). Separate analyses were conducted using participants, rating moderate to severe worst pain and nausea—scores of 4 to 10 (Jones et al., 2005)—in the last 24 hours with antiemetic and analgesic administration.

Results

A total of 337 patients were screened for participation in this trial (see Figure 3). Of these, 162 were eligible and only 19 of these declined to participate.

Therefore, 143 were randomized after baseline demographic data collection in the preadmission phase of surgery preparation. One participant in the standard care group did not meet eligibility criteria at the time of surgery as a result of a change of procedure type (bilateral vs. unilateral TKA), and one participant in each group had the procedure cancelled indefinitely. As a result, the total number for the analysis of baseline characteristics was 143 and 140 for postoperative outcomes. No participants withdrew from the trial during data collection. Baseline demographic data are included in Table 2.

Baseline characteristics were similar between groups with a mean age of 67 ± 8 years in the intervention group and 66 ± 8 years in the standard care group, consistent with many studies of patients with TKA and national TKA data. The primary diagnosis requiring surgery was osteoarthritis in both groups, with approximately one third of participants requiring opioid analgesics for arthritic pain preoperatively.

PRIMARY RESEARCH QUESTION

Day 3 measurements of the BPI-I are presented in Table 3. Total scores for the standard care group (22.4 ± 15.1) and the intervention group (24.4 ± 14.4) were not significantly different ($p = .45$). Independent sample t tests were nonsignificant for all BPI-I items. Highest interference scores for both groups at day 3 were in the moderate range and included general activity (standard care: 5.6 ± 3.2; intervention: 5.8 ± 3.2) and transfer from bed to chair (standard care: 5.0 ± 3.4; intervention: 4.6 ± 2.9). It is important to note that these pain-related interference scores were measured on the third postoperative day, 1 day before the expected discharge date for this group of patients.

SECONDARY RESEARCH QUESTIONS

Pain

Postoperative pain was measured using the MPQ-SF on each of postoperative days 1, 2, and 3 (see Table 4). There were no significant group differences on any of the three postoperative days in either pain right now at rest, pain now with movement, or worst pain in last 24 hours. There was, however, a significant effect for time in pain

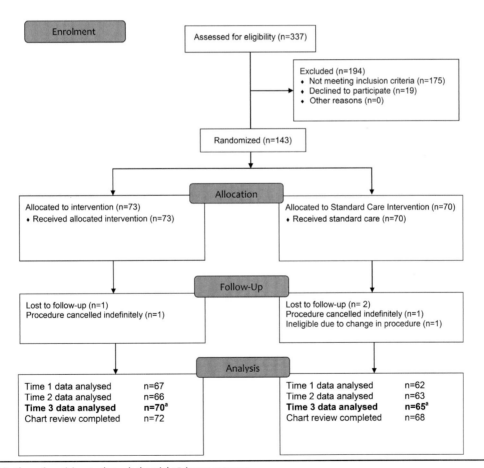

FIGURE 3. Flow of participants through the trial. ªPrimary outcome.

TABLE 2. BASELINE DEMOGRAPHICS OF PARTICIPANTS

Demographics	Intervention (n = 73) n (%)	Standard Care (n = 70) n (%)
Sex		
Female	46 (63)	43 (61)
Home status		
Live alone	13 (18)	15 (21)
Highest education level		
Less than high school	34 (47)	36 (51)
Postsecondary	39 (53)	34 (49)
Home pain medication		
None	13 (18)	18 (26)
Opioid	21 (29)	24 (34)
Nonopioid	39 (53)	28 (40)
Preoperative diagnosis		
Osteoarthritis	70 (96)	67 (96)
Rheumatoid arthritis	3 (4)	3 (4)

TABLE 4. PAIN ON POSTOPERATIVE DAYS 1, 2, AND 3

NRS (0–10)	Intervention (n = 62) M (SD)	Standard Care (n = 55) M (SD)
Pain right now at rest[a]		
Postoperative day 1	4.1 (2.9)	3.7 (2.8)
Postoperative day 2	3.3 (3.0)	2.9 (2.2)
Postoperative day 3	2.8 (2.5)	2.8 (2.7)
Pain right now when moving[b]		
Postoperative day 1	6.4 (2.6)	6.4 (2.7)
Postoperative day 2	6.2 (2.8)	5.9 (2.4)
Postoperative day 3	5.4 (3.0)	6.1 (2.5)
Worst pain last 24 hours[c]		
Postoperative day 1	7.5 (2.5)	7.2 (2.8)
Postoperative day 2	7.7 (2.4)	7.5 (2.1)
Postoperative day 3	7.0 (2.4)	7.0 (2.3)

Note. NRS = Numeric Rating Scale.
[a]$F = 0.36, p = .70.$
[b]$F = 1.61, p = .20.$
[c]$F = 0.14, p = .87.$

right now at rest ($p = .0002$) and worst pain last 24 hours ($p = .013$), with pain decreasing over time but not for the item, pain right now when moving ($p = .06$). Similarly, there was a significant effect for time in the Present Pain Intensity (PPI) global pain rating (0–5) ($p = .001$) but no group difference across time ($p = .70$). As with the NRS and PPI, there was a significant effect of time for both the PRI-S ($p = .02$), the PRI-A ($p = .05$) and the PRI-T ($p = .02$), but there were no significant group differences across the three measurement times. Across both groups, the average rating of worst pain in the last 24 hours was 7 ± 2.4, in the severe range on each of the three postoperative days. Seventy-three percent of the total sample reported moderate to severe pain on movement on day 3, whereas 81% of the sample reported having experienced moderate to severe pain in the last 24 hours.

TABLE 3. PAIN-RELATED INTERFERENCE WITH ACTIVITY ON POSTOPERATIVE DAY 3

Interference Scores BPI-I	Intervention (n = 70) M (SD)	Standard Care (n = 65) M (SD)
Total (scores 0–60)[a]	24.4 (14.4)	22.4 (15.1)
Subscales (scores 0–10)		
General activity	5.6 (3.2)	5.8 (3.2)
Walking	4.8 (3.0)	4.4 (3.5)
Mood	3.3 (3.2)	2.4 (3.2)
Transfer from bed to chair	4.8 (2.9)	5.0 (3.4)
Sleep	3.8 (3.5)	3.3 (3.1)
Relationships with others	1.9 (2.9)	1.6 (2.7)

Note. BPI-I = Brief Pain Inventory, Interference.
[a]$t = -0.76: p = .45.$

NAUSEA

The impact of the intervention on nausea was measured using the six-point ONI. There was no difference between groups in nausea scores (previous 24 hours) over time ($F = 0.02; p = .88$); however, there was a difference within groups in nausea scores (previous 24 hours) over time ($F = 50.9; p < .01$) with nausea decreasing over the 3-day period.

ANALGESIC AND ANTIEMETIC ADMINISTRATION

PCA-IV opioids prescribed for participants postoperatively during the 3-day study period were morphine (82%) and hydromorphone (18%). Oral opioids prescribed on day 3 were morphine, hydromorphone, or oxycodone (67%, 14%, and 18% of participants, respectively) and one participant received oral codeine. Repeated-measures analysis of variance demonstrated no difference between groups in daily 24-hour opioid administration, but for the total sample there was a significant main effect for time as analgesic administration in both groups declined over the 3 postoperative days ($F = 36.1; p = .000$). For patients consistently reporting moderate to severe pain on each day, opioid analgesic administration also declined over their hospital stay (see Table 5). Overall, 7 participants did not receive any opioid analgesic doses on postoperative day 3, two of whom did not receive any doses on postoperative day 2. One participant did not receive any opioid over the 3-day period.

The routine dosing protocol ordered for all patients with TKA reporting even mild nausea was three doses of a prescribed antiemetic (ondansetron). Overall, 79 (56%) participants were administered at least one dose of antiemetic over the 3-day trial period. However, for those reporting moderate to severe nausea on the first postoperative day, 29% in the intervention group and 25% in the standard care group received no antiemetics

TABLE 5. TOTAL OPIOID ANALGESIC ADMINISTRATION FOR ALL PARTICIPANTS IN MILLIGRAMS OF ORAL MORPHINE EQUIVALENTS FOR 24 HOURS ON EACH OF THE 3-DAY TRIAL PERIOD

	Intervention (n = 72) Median (Interquartile Range)	Standard Care (n = 68) Median (Interquartile Range)
Postoperative day 1	78 (69)	78 (87)
Postoperative day 2	62 (65)	56 (55)
Postoperative day 3	40 (45)	40 (42)

in the previous 24-hour period. For those reporting either no or mild nausea in each group, 17% received at least one dose of antiemetic during the same period.

Discussion

There were no significant group differences in any of the outcomes in this trial. However, the results of the total sample are important to highlight. There were no differences in total or component scores for pain-related interference with activity as measured by the BPI-I Interference with general activity, walking, and transfer from bed to chair were in the moderate to severe range and consistent with results reported by Akyol, Karayurt, and Salmond (2009). A major emphasis of the education content within all three components of intervention delivery was the importance of appropriately timed analgesic use to increase opioid administration and improve pain and pain-related interference with activity. In the context of similar opioid use on postoperative day 3 in both groups—median daily oral morphine equivalents: intervention 40 mg (interquartile range = 45 mg), standard care 40 mg (interquartile range = 42 mg)—moderate to severe BPI-I scores in the intervention group illustrate that placing the focus on the patient alone to ensure pre-activity analgesia administration is not sufficient to improve pain-related interference. Watt-Watson and colleagues (2004) reported that only 33% of prescribed analgesics were administered in 53% of patients reporting moderate to severe pain in their study of 406 patients with cardiac surgery. These authors identified a lack of understanding of opioid analgesia among health professionals, and recommended future trials include focus groups with nursing staff in particular to discuss issues affecting pain management in the postoperative setting.

The education provided by all three components of the intervention that focused on strategies to prevent resting pain and pain on movement, including appropriate communication of pain to healthcare providers, failed to produce a difference in pain ratings and qualitative aspects of pain description. Moderate to severe pain, in the context of declining and inadequate opioid analgesic administration, is troubling and raises important questions about the postoperative environment in terms of clinical care. Components of the intervention that reinforced analgesic use before movement in an interval appropriate to the type of analgesic administered

were intended to maximize pain relief and improve mobility to prevent further complications, but the intervention focused on the patients and ignored the roles of the care providers. Additionally, data were not collected that discriminated between surgical pain and other pain. Wittig-Wells, Shapiro, and Higgins (2013) found that other or nonsurgical pain, present in 37% of their sample, interfered with walking, mood, sleep, and relationships with other people. Kearney et al. (2011) reported a similar lack of effect on postoperative pain or activity in a trial of structured preoperative information in joint replacement patients.

Opioid analgesic administration (see Table 5) declined over the 3-day study period ($F = 36.1; p = .000$), whereas pain ratings on movement stayed in the moderate range in both groups across all 3 postoperative days. It is important to note that the median oral morphine equivalent administration was 40 mg for patients in both trial groups, only one third of the opioid doses that were prescribed. This finding is similar to the 33% of prescribed doses administered in the study by Watt-Watson and colleagues (2004).

Unrelieved pain and stress response as a result of acute, surgical injury can have psychological and physiological consequences for patients (Apkarian, Bushnell, Treede, & Zubieta, 2005; Carr & Thomas, 1997; Kehlet, 1997). The phenomenon of central sensitization of dorsal horn neurons by prolonged and repetitive nociceptive input can create the physiology for a longer-term pain problem (Bausbaum & Jessell, 2000) predisposing patients to related comorbidities. Patients with TKA with persistent, unrelieved pain are less likely to do specific physiotherapy activities (i.e., range of motion and weight bearing) that may result in delayed rehabilitation and knee stiffness.

Concomitant moderate to severe nausea rates in this trial may reflect the established interrelationship between pain and nausea. Twenty-eight percent of the intervention and 24% of the standard care groups reported experiencing moderate to severe nausea in the previous 24 hours on postoperative day 3. The attenuation of the pain experience by the presence of nausea and the production of nausea by the pain experience (Fields, 1999; Julius & Bausbaum, 2001; Kandel, Schwartz, & Jessell, 2000) reinforces the need to address both of these symptoms simultaneously.

This trial presents clear evidence that there are significant system issues influencing postoperative symptom management after TKA. Participants in both groups who were reporting moderate to severe nausea or pain frequently did not receive the antiemetic therapy or analgesics ordered. Evidenced-based protocols for nausea management were in place at the trial site, but data show that they were not followed consistently and in some cases, not at all. Antiemetic agents used in these protocols, ondansetron and prochlorperazine, are effective for postoperative nausea when given appropriately (Dzwonczyk, Weaver, Puente, & Bergese, 2012). In this trial, 25% of participants who reported moderate to severe nausea had no antiemetics administered at all. Similarly, participants who reported moderate to severe pain received approximately one third of the prescribed doses of oral analgesic on postoperative day 3 despite hospital-wide programs that support the need for effective pain management (e.g., Pain, the 5th Vital Sign). Other research has suggested that this is not an unusual finding; nursing staff education and attitude may be contributing factors. Gordon and colleagues (2008), in a study of practice-associated pro re nata (PRN) administration of opioids in 602 registered nurses, found that comfort with dose titration was directly and positively related to years of practice experience.

At the trial site, the pain management service is available for consultation by the nursing staff at all times to modify or increase analgesic doses. Although patients reporting scores in the moderate to severe range on pain assessment should, by institutional policy, be reviewed either by the attending service or the pain service, they were not. Although an inadequate explanation for deficiencies in care, staffing resources and patient acuity may have contributed to fewer pain and nausea assessments, placing the onus on the patient to report symptoms requiring treatment.

It appears that the current postoperative environment does not support best practice for nursing staff in terms of symptom management regardless of the measures put in place. This finding is not unique to orthopaedic patient care. In a systematic review of 16 trials of labour support during childbirth in institutional settings, Hodnett, Gates, Hofmeyr, and Sakala (2009) concluded that the effectiveness of labour support interventions was mediated by the environment in which the interventions were provided. Although this clinical group has different requirements than patients with TKA, findings of the review in terms of environmental factors were similar. The ability of interventions with patients to overcome barriers present in the environment is limited if strategies to address these barriers are not also included.

Limitations of this trial are primarily related to support for the implementation of the educational material in the postoperative setting. As the intervention for this trial was directed only at the participants with no component for staff education or protocol development or monitoring, the influence of the healthcare environment on the ability of the participants to engage in the associated behaviours was not reinforcing. Systems issues such as staff lack of adherence to established protocols for symptom management may have resulted in more pain and nausea and greater functional interference.

Institutional accountability reflecting hospital accreditation standards in the clinical environment for the provision of symptom management and early identification and investigation of activity and mobility concerns needs to be established. A consistent approach used by disciplines involved in the care of patients with TKA needs to span from initial assessment for surgery to postoperative care and includes all points of contact between. In the preoperative setting, nursing staff caring for orthopaedic patients must take the lead in ensuring surgical preparation, which includes education that is reinforced by all team members, regardless of their role. Postoperatively, orthopaedic nursing staff must attend to the need for temporally appropriate symptom assessment and pharmacologic and nonpharmacologic interventions for patients. As this trial demonstrates that the delivery of individualized educational content with reinforcement provided by booklet and telephone follow-

up was not sufficient to impact postoperative symptoms after TKA surgery, the nursing role as a symptom management provider and patient advocate is essential to the recovery after TKA. Further trials that also include standardized information provided to patients by preadmission, surgical scheduling and postoperative nursing and medical staff would be beneficial in supporting learned behaviours and knowledge uptake. Consistent with the recommendations of Watt-Watson and colleagues (2004), a qualitative research approach using focus groups of orthopaedic nursing, medical, and physiotherapy staff could be undertaken to determine the environmental and patient-related characteristics, affecting the provision of analgesics and antiemetics and the relationship to postoperative activity.

Conclusion

The numbers of Canadians requiring primary TKA has increased 140% over the last 10 years (CIHI, 2013). The highest rate of TKA surgery is in the 75- to 84-year-age range (65%). There are no published guidelines for the preoperative preparation or postoperative care of these relatively older aged patients. Inadequate management of symptoms such as pain and nausea in the early postoperative period may result in increased morbidity for patients and increased costs for the healthcare system. The purpose of the trial was to examine the impact of individualizing preoperative patient education as a means to address postoperative symptoms affecting recovery from TKA.

Providing information to patients alone was not sufficient to address the need for postoperative symptom prevention and management after TKA. A broader, consistent approach that includes healthcare providers at all levels of patient contact is required to support recovery and rehabilitation after this type of surgery. Further research is required to delineate the barriers in the healthcare environment to appropriate pain and nausea management and to provide more evidence for the relationship between pain and nausea and functional outcomes for patients who have had TKA.

REFERENCES

Akyol, O., Karayurt, O., & Salmomd, S. (2009). Experiences of pain and satisfaction with pain management in patients undergoing total knee replacement. *Orthopedic Nursing, 28,* 79–85.

Apkarian, A., Bushnell, M., Treede, R., & Zubieta, J. (2005). Human brain mechanisms of pain perception and regulation in health and disease. *European Journal of Pain, 9*(4), 463–484.

Bausbaum, A. I., & Jessell, T. M. (2000). The perception of pain. In E. Kandel, J. Schwartz, & Jessell, T. (Eds.), *Principles of neural science* (4th ed., pp. 472–491). New York: McGraw-Hill.

Beaupre, L. A., Lier, D., Davies, D. M., & Johnston, D. B. C. (2004). The effect of a preoperative exercise and education program on functional recovery, health related quality of life, and health service utilization following primary total knee arthroplasty. *Journal of Rheumatology, 31,* 1166–1173.

Benor, D.E., Delbar, V., & Krulik, T. (1998). Measuring the impact of nursing interventions on cancer patients' ability to control symptoms. *Cancer Nursing, 21,* 320–334.

Bondy, L. R., Sims, N., Schroeder, D. R., Offord, K. P., & Narr, B. J. (1999). The effect of anesthetic patient education on preoperative patient's anxiety. *Regional Anesthesia and Pain Medicine, 24*, 158–164.

Brander, V. A., Stulberg, S. D., Adams, A. D., Harden, R. N., Bruehl, S., Stanos, S. P., & Houle, T. (2003). Ranawat Award Paper: Predicting total knee replacement pain: A prospective, observational study. *Clinical Orthopaedics and Related Research, 416*, 27–36.

Canadian Institute for Health Information. (2014). *Hip and knee replacements in Canada 2012–2013 quick stats.* Canadian Institute for Health Information. Retrieved from http://www.cihi.ca

Canadian Institute for Health Information. (2013). *Hip and knee replacements in Canada—Canadian Joint Replacement Registry 2013 Annual Report.* Ottawa: CIHI; 2013.

Carr, E., & Thomas, V. (1997). Anticipating and experiencing post-operative pain: The patient's perspective. *Journal of Clinical Nursing, 6*, 191–201.

Chang, H. J., Mehta, P. S., Rosenberg, A., & Scrimshaw, S. C. (2004). Concerns of patients actively contemplating total knee replacement: Differences by race and gender. *Arthritis and Rheumatism, 51*(1), 117–123.

Cleeland, C., & Ryan, K. (1994). Pain assessment: Global use of the Brief Pain Inventory. *Annals of Academic Medicine Singapore, 23*, 129–138.

Cohen, J. (1988). *Statistical power analysis for the behavioral sciences* (2nd ed.). Hillsdale: Earlbaum Associates.

De Wit, R., & Van Dam, F. (2001). From hospital to home care: A randomized controlled trial of a Pain Education Programme for cancer patients with chronic pain. *Journal of Advanced Nursing, 36*(6), 742–754.

Dzwonczyk, R., Weaver, T., Puente, E., & Bergese, S. (2012). Postoperative nausea and vomiting prophylaxis from an economic point of view. *American Journal of Therapeutics, 19*(1), 11–15.

Fields, H. (1999). Pain: An unpleasant topic. *Pain, Supplement, 6*, S61–S69.

Gan, T. J., Meyer, T., Apfel, C. C., Chung, F., Davis, P. J., Eubanks, S., ... Tramèr, M. R. (2003). Consensus guidelines for managing postoperative nausea and vomiting. *Anesthesia & Analgesia, 97*(1), 62–71.

Gordon, D., Pellino, T., Higgins, G., Pasero, C., & Murphy-Ende, K. (2008). Nurses' opinions of administration of PRN range opioid oral orders for acute pain. *Pain Management Nursing, 9*(3), 131–140.

Hodnett, E., Gates, S., Hofmeyr, G.J., & Sakala, C. (2009). Continuous support for women during childbirth. *Cochrane Database of Systematic Reviews, 3*, CD003766.

Hodgkinson, B., Evans, D., & Wood, J. (2003). Maintaining oral hydration status in older adults: A systematic review. *International Journal of Nursing Practice, 9*, S19–S28.

Johansson, K., Nuutila, L., Virtanen, H., Katajisto, J., & Salantera, S. (2005). Preoperative education for orthopaedic patients: Systematic review. *Journal of Advanced Nursing, 50*, 212–223.

Johnson, J., Rice, V., Fuller, S., & Endress, P. (1978). Sensory information, instruction in a coping strategy, and recovery from surgery. *Research in Nursing and Health, 1*(1), 4–17.

Jones, D., Westby, M., Griedanus, N., Johanson, N., Krebs, D., Robbins, L., Rooks, D., & Brander, V. (2005). Update on hip and knee arthroplasty: Current state of evidence. *Arthritis and Rheumatism, 53*(5), 772–780.

Julius, D., & Bausbaum, A. (2001). Molecular mechanisms of nociception. *Nature, 413*, 203–210.

Kandel, E., Schwartz, J., & Jessell, T. (2000). The perception of pain. *Principles of neural science* (4th ed., pp. 472–491). New York: McGraw-Hill.

Kearney, M., Jennrich, M. K., Lyons, S., Robinson, R., & Berger, B. (2011). Effects of preoperative education on patient outcomes after joint replacement surgery. *Orthopaedic Nursing, 30*(6), 391–6

Kehlet, H. (1997). Multimodal approach to control postoperative pathophysiology and rehabilitation. *British Journal of Anaesthesia, 78*, 606–617.

Larson, C. P. (1996). Evaluating the patient and preoperative preparation. In P. G. Barash, B. F. Cullen, & Stoelting, R. K. (Eds.), *Handbook of clinical anesthesia* (2nd ed., pp. 3–15). Philadelphia: Lippincott-Raven.

Lin, P. C., Lin, L. C., & Lin, J. J. (1997). Comparing the effectiveness of different educational programs for patients with total knee arthroplasty. *Orthopedic Nursing, 16*, 43–49.

Louw, A., Diener, I., Butler, D. S., & Puentedura, E. J. (2013). Preoperative education addressing postoperative pain in total joint arthroplasty: Review of content and educational delivery methods. *Physiotherapy Theory and Practice, 29*(3), 175–194. doi:10.3109/0959 3985.2012.727527

McDonald, D. D., Freeland, M., Thomas, G., & Moore, J. (2001). Testing a preoperative pain management intervention for elders. *Research in Nursing and Health, 24*, 402–409.

McDonald, D. D., & Molony, S. L. (2004). Postoperative pain communication skills for older adults. *Western Journal of Nursing Research, 26*, 836–852.

McDonald, D., Thomas, G., Livingston, K., & Severson, J. (2005). Assisting older adults to communicate their postoperative pain. *Clinical Nursing Research, 14*(2), 109–126. doi:10.1177/1054773804271934

McDonald, S., Page, M. J., Beringer, K., Wasiak, J., & Sprowson, A. (2014). Pre-operative education for hip and knee replacement (Review). *Cochrane Database of Systematic Reviews, 5*, 10.1002/14651858.CD003526. pub3.

Melzack, R. (1989). Measurement of Nausea. *Journal of Pain and Symptom Management, 4*, 157–160.

Melzack, R. (1987). The short form McGill Pain Questionnaire. *Pain, 30*, 191–197.

Melzack, R., Abbott, F., Zackon, W., Mulder, D., & Davis, W. (1987). Pain on a surgical ward: a survey of the duration and intensity of pain and the effectiveness of medication. *Pain, 29*, 67–72.

Melzack, R., & Wall, P. (1996). *The challenge of pain* (2nd ed.). London: Penguin.

Mendoza, T. R., Chen, C., Brugger, A., Hubbard, R., Snabes, M., & Palmer, S. N., ...Cleeland, C. S. (2004a). The utility and validity of the modified brief pain inventory in a multiple-dose postoperative analgesic trial. *The Clinical Journal of Pain, 20*(5), 357–362.

Mendoza, T. R., Chen, C., Brugger, A., Hubbard, R., Snabes, M., & Palmer, S. N., ...Cleeland, C. S. (2004b). Lessons learned from a multiple-dose post-operative analgesic trial. *Pain, 109*(1), 103–109.

Parlow, J., Costache, I., Avery, N., & Turner, K. (2004). Single-does haloperidol for the prophylaxis of postoperative nausea and vomiting after intrathecal morphine. *Anesthesia and Analgesia, 98*, 1072–1076.

Phillips, P. A., Johnston, C. I., & Gray, L. (1993). Disturbed fluid and electrolyte homeostasis following dehydration in elderly people. *Age and Aging, 22*, S26–S33.

Roach, J. A., Tremblay, L. M., & Bowers, D. L. (1995). A preoperative assessment and education program:

implementation and outcomes. *Patient Education and Counseling, 25,* 83–88.

Salmon, P., Hall, G., Perrbhoy, D., Shenkin, A., & Parker, C. (2001). Recovery from hip and knee arthroplasty: Patients' perspective on pain, function, quality of life, and well-being up to 6 months post-operatively. *Archives of Physical Medicine and Rehabilitation, 82,* 360–366.

Sherwood, P., Given, B., Given, C., Champion, V., Doorenbos, A., Azzouz, F., ... Monahan, P. O. (2005). A cognitive behavioural intervention for symptom management in patients with advanced cancer. *Oncology Nursing Forum, 32,* 1190–1198.

Sjoling, M., Nordahl, G., Olofsson, N., & Asplund, K. (2003). The impact of preoperative information on state anxiety, postoeprative pain and satisfaction with pain management. *Patient Education and Counseling, 51,* 169–176.

Stern, C., & Lockwood, C. (2005). Knowledge retention from preoperative patient information. *International Journal of Evidence-Based Healthcare, 3,* 45–63.

Strassels, S. A., Chen, C., & Carr, D. (2002). Postoperative analgesia: Economics, resource use, and patient satisfaction in an urban teaching hospital. *Anesthesia and Analgesia, 94,* 130–137.

Tan, G., Jensen, M. P., Thornby, J. L., & Shanti, B. F. (2004). Validation of the Brief Pain Inventory for chronic non-malignant pain. *Journal of Pain, 5,* 133–137.

Velji, K. (2006). Effect of an individualized symptom education program on the symptom distress of women receiving radiotherapy for gynecological cancer. Available from ProQuest database (AAT NR21992).

Wallis, J., & Taylor, F. (2011). Pre-operative interventions (non-surgical and non-pharmacological) for patients with hip or knee osteoarthritis awaiting joint replacement surgery—a systematic review and meta-analysis. *Osteoarthritis and Cartilage, 19*(12), 1381–1395. doi:10.1016/j.joca.2011.09.001

Watt-Watson, J., Stevens, B., Katz, J., Costello, J., Reid, G., & David, T. (2004). Impact of pre-operative education on pain outcomes after coronary artery bypass graft surgery. *Pain, 109,* 73–85.

Wilson, I. B., & Cleary, P. D. (1995). Linking clinical variables with Health-Related Quality of Life: A conceptual model of patient outcomes. *Journal of the American Medical Association, 273,* 59–65.

Wilson, R., Goldstein, D., VanDenKerkhof, E., & Rimmer, M. (2005). APMS clinical dataset. October 1, 2004, to October 1, 2005. Kingston, Ontario, Unpublished.

Wittig-Wells, D. R., Shapiro, S. E., & Higgins, M. K. (2013). Patients' experiences of pain in the 48 hours following total knee Arthroplasty. *Orthopaedic Nursing, 32*(1), 39–44.

Wu, C., Naqibuddin, M., Rowlingson, A., Lietman, S., Jermyn, R., & Fleisher, L. (2003). The effect of pain on health-related quality of life in the immediate postoperative period. *Anesthesia and Analgesia, 97,* 1078–1085.

Yates, P., Edwards, H., Nash, R., Aranda, S., Purdie, D., & Najman, J., ...Walsh, A. (2004). A randomized controlled trial of a nurse-administered educational intervention for improving cancer pain management in ambulatory settings. *Patient education and counseling, 53*(2), 227–237.

Zalon, M. L. (1997). Pain in frail, elderly women after surgery. *Image: Journal of Nursing Scholarship, 29*(1), 21–26.

Critique of Wilson et al.'s (2016) Study: "A Randomized Controlled Trial of an Individualized Preoperative Education Intervention for Symptom Management After Total Knee Arthroplasty"

OVERALL SUMMARY

This report was a well-written description of a strong quantitative study that used a rigourous randomized controlled design (randomized controlled trial [RCT]), with appropriate randomization and blinding procedures. The preoperative education intervention for patients undergoing total knee arthroplasty (TKA) was designed on the basis of earlier research and a broad conceptual model. The authors provided good information about the intervention's educational components and a rationale for the content. Although the intervention versus control group differences results were not statistically significant, the findings were credible—that is, the results are unlikely to reflect problems with inadequate statistical power or biases in the design. The authors concluded that a patient education approach to pain management for patients undergoing TKA might not be effective without changing the overall systems of pain management in hospitals. Their conclusions could perhaps have been bolstered by the inclusion of a qualitative component to learn more about *why* patients in the intervention group did not get more pain medication than they in fact received.

TITLE

The title of this report effectively communicated the nature of the study design (an RCT), the nature of the intervention (individualized preoperative education), the outcomes (symptom management), and the population (patients undergoing TKA).

ABSTRACT

The abstract for this paper was written as a traditional abstract, without subheadings. The abstract was succinct but conveyed critical information about the study aim, the nature of the intervention, the RCT study design, and the sample size ($N = 143$). Key outcomes were identified (pain, pain interference, and nausea). The abstract also reported the findings, i.e., the absence of significant differences between the intervention and control group on key outcomes. Finally, the authors provided a brief interpretation of their findings and suggestions for future research. The abstract provided information that readers would need in deciding whether to read the full report.

INTRODUCTION

The introduction provided a reasonable rationale for this study. The authors explained the nature and scope of the problem (i.e., pain and nausea as symptoms for patients undergoing TKA, with many such procedures being undertaken). They also noted that several trials to address this problem through educational interventions have been tested, using a variety of delivery methods, and that some had been found to result in lower pain scores. However, the results of these trials were mixed, and no trials had addressed issues relating to nausea following the TKA procedure.

The authors acknowledged that they were guided in the design of their intervention by several systematic reviews. The researchers also were guided by the positive results of individualized preoperative interventions tested with other patient groups (e.g., patients with cancer). Based on earlier studies and using a broad conceptual model (a conceptual map for which was provided in Fig. 1), the researchers developed a multicomponent intervention. The model itself does not appear to have been the foundation for specific intervention components, however. For example, it was not a model that purported to explain the mechanisms through which the intervention would lead to positive effects (e.g., by decreasing anxiety about potential addiction by using opioids, by enhancing patients' self-efficacy, by improving patients' communication skills).

The content for the intervention was derived from several earlier studies; topics and supporting evidence were nicely summarized in their Table 1. The introduction concluded with a statement of the study purpose: "This study aimed to investigate the impact of an individually delivered preoperative education intervention on pain-related interference, pain, and nausea for patients undergoing unilateral TKA."

RESEARCH QUESTIONS

The researchers specified two questions. The primary question asked about the effect of the intervention on pain-related interference on postoperative day 3. The secondary question asked about effects of the intervention on pain, nausea, and analgesic and antiemetic administration on postoperative days 1, 2, and 3. The researchers did not formally state hypotheses, but the implication was that the researchers predicted that the intervention would reduce pain, nausea, and pain interference.

The researchers did not test the effects of the intervention on possible mechanisms through which the intervention might have had positive effects. For example, if the researchers had expected lower pain levels among those in the intervention group because the educational content was expected to decrease fears of addiction, they might have asked study participants about such fears as an additional outcome. Several other factors might be expected to mediate the effect of the intervention on the outcomes, and questions about these mediators could have been addressed.

METHODS

The "Methods" section was well organized into several subsections.

Trial Design

Wilson and colleagues used a strong two-group randomized controlled design to evaluate the effectiveness of the educational intervention. Their Figure 2 nicely summarized schematically the progression of activities and events in the trial, from eligibility assessment to the measurement of outcomes. The design was well-suited to testing the effects of an intervention and was excellent in terms of internal validity. The trial was conducted at a single academic health sciences centre in Ontario, Canada, which could limit the generalizability of the results.

Study Participants

The researchers clearly delineated the inclusion and exclusion criteria for participation in the trial. Participants had to be scheduled for elective TKA using planned intrathecal anesthetics. They also had to be English speakers with telephone access and had to be planned for discharge to home. Patients who were booked for hemi, revision, or bilateral knee arthroplasty were excluded. The report provided adequate information about the recruitment and enrolment process.

Interventions

Wilson and colleagues presented the details about the three components of the intervention (a special booklet, an individualized teaching session, and a follow-up support telephone call). The researchers provided information about who delivered the intervention (the principal investigator in every case) and the timing of the delivery of intervention components (within 4 weeks before surgery for the teaching session and review of the booklet and during the week before the scheduled surgery date for the telephone follow-up). The report did not describe the researchers' rationale for this schedule (e.g., why the follow-up was not within a day or two of the surgery).

The report also presented information about standard care, which is commendable. Patients in both the intervention and control group received an educational session by a physiotherapist, a 30-minute video explaining the surgical procedure, and a brief review of using the intravenous patient-controlled analgesia pump by clinic nursing staff. The timing of providing these supports was not indicated.

Outcomes

In a section labelled "Outcomes," the researchers described the instruments they used to collect baseline and outcome data. They used existing self-report scales to measure pain, nausea, and pain interference. The measure of pain interference was the Brief Pain Inventory, Interference (BPI-I), a scale with items tapping the extent to which pain interferes with general activities, sleep, mood, movements, and relationships with others. The researchers adapted the BPI-I slightly by deleting two items and adding a new item (transferring from bed to chair) to enhance the relevance of the scale to patients in the study. The researchers noted that the original measure has well-established construct validity and sensitivity to change. The researchers did a small pilot test of the adapted scale, but they did not compute its internal consistency. They did note that a similarly adapted scale had an internal consistency reliability of .71, which is modest. The researchers stated that secondary outcomes were measured using the Short Form McGill Pain Questionnaire (MPQ-SF) and the Overall Nausea Index. No information was provided about the reliability and validity of these scales. Ideally, the researchers should have computed and reported a coefficient alpha to indicate the internal consistency of all of their scales, using data from their sample. Also, the authors did not provide readers with information about how the BPI-I scale was scored. Readers cannot be sure if higher scores on the BPI-I are associated with greater or lesser degrees of interference from pain, making it difficult to interpret the results (although it seems likely that higher scores correspond to greater interference). Data regarding the secondary outcomes of analgesic and antiemetic administration were recording from the patients' charts.

Sample Size

The researchers did a power analysis to estimate the sample size they would need in this study. They based their estimate of the effect size ($d = .5$) on a previous study by one of the team members. The power analysis indicated that a sample of 64 patients in each group would be required, but they built in a cushion of 10% for attrition. Thus, the researchers sought a sample size of 140 patients. Commendably, the researchers further justified their effect size estimate by noting that a d of .50 would be a clinically significant amount of improvement.

Randomization and Blinding

The researchers used an excellent randomization method—they relied on a randomization service not connected to the trial. Such a service is preferred to randomization by the team members because it minimizes the risk of bias. Although neither the patients nor the person delivering the intervention could be blinded because of the nature of the intervention, the research assistants who collected the postoperative outcome data were blinded to group assignment.

Statistical Analysis

The researchers provided a good description of the statistical tests and the statistical software they used. For the primary question relating to pain interference, which was measured only once on postoperative day 3, they used an independent groups t-test to compare the two study groups. For the secondary questions relating to pain and nausea, a repeated measures analysis of covariance was used, which was appropriate because these outcomes were measured three times. Finally, for the data on administration of analgesics and antiemetic medication, chi-squared tests were used to compare the intervention and control groups.

RESULTS

The "Results" section began with a description of the study sample. A useful flow chart was included that showed how many patients were screened for eligibility ($N = 337$), how many were excluded for various reasons ($N = 194$), how many were randomized ($N = 143$), and how many actually received the treatment to which they were assigned. A total of 140 were measured for postoperative outcomes, which is the number the power analysis suggested the researchers needed. Background characteristics of the sample were presented in Table 2, which showed that the two groups were similar in terms of sex, education, use of pain medication, and their preoperative diagnosis.

Primary Research Question

The researchers reported that group differences on the pain interference measure (the BPI-I scale) were not statistically significant ($p = .45$). The mean score for those in the intervention group was modestly (but not significantly) *higher* than the mean score for the control group. Table 3 also showed mean scores for six subscale scores on the BPI-I, and group differences were not significant for any of them.

Secondary Research Question

With regard to pain, the researchers stated that there were no group differences in levels of pain on any of the postoperative days. One potentially confusing aspect of the report is that the authors stated in their section labelled "Outcomes" that pain and pain quality were measured using the MPQ-SF. In the "Results" section, the authors mentioned another measure not previously described, the Present Pain Intensity (PPI) global pain rating. They also refer to other pain measures using acronyms without any explanation (PRI-S, PRI-A, and PRI-T). Information about these measures should have been presented in the "Methods" section. Also, Table 4, which summarizes some of the results for pain outcomes, refers to a "Numeric Rating Scale" (NRS) without indicating whether these scores are for the MPQ-SF. In any event, for several of these measures, the researchers reported significantly declines in pain scores over time but not significant differences between the intervention and the control groups.

With regard to nausea, the researchers reported that differences between the intervention and control group on the measure of nausea was not significant ($p = .88$). In both groups, nausea declined over the 3-day period.

Similarly, there were no significant differences between the intervention and control groups with regard to daily opioid administration, but there were significant declines over time in both groups. The "Results" section also presented interesting descriptive information about the use of medications in this sample. For example, the researchers reported that seven participants received no opioid analgesic doses on day 3 and that only 56% of patients were administered at least one dose of antiemetic over the 3-day period.

DISCUSSION

The researchers concluded that their intervention was not effective in reducing pain, nausea, and pain interference in patients undergoing TKA. With nonsignificant results, it is sometimes risky to draw such conclusions because of the possibility of a Type II error, but the authors' conclusions seem appropriate because they used a powerful RCT design, their analysis had adequate power, and the results were consistent across all outcomes.

The researchers' main conclusion was that patient education was ineffective because the problem of appropriately timed and appropriately dosed medication reflected a systems-wide problem. They noted that the trial presented "clear evidence that there are significant systems issues influencing postoperative symptom management after TKA." They pointed out that the patients often did not receive the medications ordered, that evidence-based protocols for nausea management were not followed, and that the pain service in the hospital did not review cases with high levels of pain, as mandated by institutional policy.

Although these conclusions are very likely to be legitimate, the researchers do not appear to have considered alternative or supplementary explanations for the disappointing results, such as deficiencies with the intervention itself or barriers to symptom management stemming from the patient population (in addition to system barriers). It likely would have been useful if this study had been designed as a mixed methods project—that is, if patients had been asked to provide in-depth information about their symptom experiences, their requests for medication, or their reluctance to request analgesics. The researchers did, however, suggest that a future trial should include a qualitative component targeting orthopedic nursing, medical, and physiotherapy staff. The study might also have benefited by including measures of some proximal outcomes of the intervention—such as patients' knowledge of and attitudes toward pain management strategies.

The researchers noted in their discussion that a limitation of this study was that staff education should have been included as a supplementary component. However, this would not have been feasible with the existing research design because staff education would have benefited members of both the intervention and the control group. To test whether a combined patient–staff education effort would result in better symptom management, the trial would have to be conducted in multiple sites, with some sites randomly assigned to either receive or not receive the multipronged intervention.

One final comment is that the researchers did not discuss their findings within the context of earlier research. Prior intervention trials, such as studies by McDonald, were described in the introduction as having positive impacts on pain. The authors did not present an explanation of why their results might be at odds with those of previous studies that helped to guide this research.

OTHER COMMENTS

Presentation

This report was clearly written and well organized. Except for a few areas of confusion regarding pain outcomes, the report provided excellent information about what was done, why it was done, and what was discovered. The report included several excellent figures and tables.

Ethical Aspects

The authors stated that ethical approval for this study was obtained from the Research Ethics Board of both the university where the researchers worked and the hospital where the data were collected. Potential participants were asked for their permission by hospital staff to release their names to the investigator, using a standardized script. Written informed consent was obtained before randomization. Nothing in the description of this study suggested ethical transgressions.

Differences in Perceptions of the Diagnosis and Treatment of Obstructive Sleep Apnea and Continuous Positive Airway Pressure Therapy Among Adherers and Nonadherers

Amy M. Sawyer • Janet A. Deatrick •
Samuel T. Kuna • Terri E. Weaver

▶ **Abstract:** Obstructive sleep apnea (OSA) patients' consistent use of continuous positive airway pressure (CPAP) therapy is critical to realizing improved functional outcomes and reducing untoward health risks associated with OSA. We conducted a mixed methods, concurrent, nested study to explore OSA patients' beliefs and perceptions of the diagnosis and CPAP treatment that differentiate adherent from nonadherent patients prior to and after the first week of treatment, when the pattern of CPAP use is established. Guided by social cognitive theory, themes were derived from 30 interviews conducted postdiagnosis and after 1 week of CPAP use. Directed content analysis, followed by categorization of participants as adherent/nonadherent from objectively measured CPAP use, preceded across-case analysis among 15 participants with severe OSA. Beliefs and perceptions that differed between adherers and nonadherers included OSA risk perception, symptom recognition, self-efficacy, outcome expectations, treatment goals, and treatment facilitators/barriers. Our findings suggest opportunities for developing and testing tailored interventions to promote CPAP use.

▶ **Key Words:** Adherence · compliance · content analysis · decision making · health behaviour · mixed methods · sleep disorders · social cognitive theory

Obstructive sleep apnea (OSA), characterized by repetitive nocturnal upper airway collapse resulting in intermittent oxyhemoglobin desaturation and sleep fragmentation, contributes to significant disabling sequelae, including daytime sleepiness, impaired cognitive and executive function, mood disturbances, and increased cardiovascular and metabolic morbidity (Al Lawati, Patel, & Ayas, 2009; Harsch et al., 2004; Nieto, et al.

Qualitative Health Research, 2010; 20(7):873–892.   Copyright © 2010. Reprinted by permission of SAGE Publications.

2000; Peppard, Young, Palta, & Skatrud, 2000). The prevalence of OSA, based on minimal diagnostic criteria (apnea/hypopnea index [AHI] of 5 events/hour), has been estimated at 2% in women and 4% in men in the United States (Young et al., 1993). More recently, large U.S.-cohort studies have provided additional evidence of the prevalence of OSA, estimating that approximately one in five adults with a mean body mass index (BMI) of at least 25 kg/m^2 has at least mild OSA, defined as an apnea-hypopnea index (AHI) $\geq$ 5 events/hour; and one in 15 adults with a mean BMI of at least 25 kg/m^2 has at least moderate OSA (i.e., AHI $\geq$ 15 events/hour; Young, Peppard, & Gottlieb, 2002). Continuous positive airway pressure (CPAP) therapy is the primary medical treatment for adults with OSA, eliminating repetitive, nocturnal airway closures; normalizing oxygen levels; and effectively improving daytime impairments (Gay, Weaver, Loube, & Iber, 2006; Sullivan, Barthon-Jones, Issa, & Eves, 1981; Weaver & Grunstein, 2008).

Nonadherence to CPAP is recognized as a significant limitation in the effective treatment of OSA, with average adherence rates ranging from 30% to 60% (Engleman, Martin, & Douglas, 1994; Kribbs et al., 1993; Krieger, 1992; Reeves-Hoche, Meck, & Zwillich, 1994; Sanders, Gruendl, & Rogers, 1986; Weaver, Kribbs, et al., 1997). Nonadherent users begin skipping nights of CPAP use during the first week of treatment, and their hourly use of CPAP on days used is significantly shorter than those who apply CPAP consistently (Aloia, Arnedt, Stanchina, & Millman, 2007; Weaver, Kribbs, et al., 1997). Patients who are nonadherent during early treatment generally remain nonadherent over the long term (Aloia, Arnedt, Stanchina, et al., 2007; Krieger, 1992; McArdle et al., 1999; Weaver, Kribbs, et al., 1997). The return of symptoms and other manifestations of OSA with even one night of nonuse underscores the critical nature of adherence to CPAP (Grunstein et al., 1996; Kribbs et al., 1993).

Many studies have explored what factors predict adherence to CPAP (Engleman et al., 1996; Engleman, Martin, et al., 1994; Kribbs et al., 1993; Massie, Hart, Peralez, & Richards, 1999; McArdle et al., 1999; Meurice et al., 1994; Reeves-Hoche et al., 1994; Rosenthal et al., 2000; Schweitzer, Chambers, Birkenmeier, & Walsh, 1997; Sin, Mayers, Man, & Pawluk, 2002). Self-reported side effects of CPAP do not distinguish between adherers and nonadherers to CPAP. Subjective sleepiness, severity of OSA as determined by apnea-hypopnea index, and severity of nocturnal hypoxia are inconsistently identified as correlates, albeit weak, of CPAP adherence (Weaver & Grunstein, 2008). The majority of these studies have focused on physiological variables and patient characteristics as predictors of adherence. Over the past 10 years, studies have identified psychological and social factors and cognitive perceptions, such as self efficacy, risk perception, and outcome expectancies, as determinants of CPAP use (Aloia, Arnedt, Stepnowsky, Hecht, & Borrelli, 2005; Lewis, Seale, Bartle, Watkins, & Ebden, 2004; Russo-Magno, O'Brien, Panciera, & Rounds, 2001; Stepnowsky, Bardwell, Moore, Ancoli-Israel, & Dimsdale, 2002; Stepnowsky, Marler, & Ancoli-Israel, 2002; Wild, Engleman, Douglas, & Espie, 2004). Social and situational variables have also been suggested as influential on CPAP adherence, with those who live alone, who have had a recent life event, and who experienced problems with CPAP on the first night of exposure having lower adherence to CPAP therapy (Lewis et al., 2004). Support group attendance has also been identified as contributing to higher CPAP use in older men (Russo- Magno et al., 2001). Findings of both of these studies suggest that social support is an important factor influencing decisions to use CPAP, yet the sociostructural context of accepting and adhering to CPAP treatment has not been described from the perspective of the patient in the extant literature. Other studies have identified that early experiences with CPAP (i.e., during the first week) are an important influence on patients' perceptions and beliefs about the OSA diagnosis and treatment with CPAP (Aloia, Arnedt, Stepnowsky, et al., 2005; Stepnowsky, Bardwell, et al., 2002).

From the collective published evidence, early experiences with CPAP, combined with patients' perceptions and beliefs about OSA and CPAP and the balance of their sociostructural facilitators/barriers, are critical factors that influence patients' decisions to use CPAP. To date, there are relatively few studies that have systematically examined the influence of disease and treatment perceptions and beliefs on CPAP adherence. Because the first week of CPAP treatment is critically influential on OSA patients' decisions to use CPAP, it is imperative that the contextual experiences and underlying beliefs and perceptions of the diagnosis and treatment be described. There are no published studies that have addressed this significant gap in the scientific literature. Furthermore, no study has directly explored patient perspectives, employing qualitative methodology, both at diagnosis and with treatment, to more fully describe contextual factors that differentiate CPAP adherers and nonadherers. Our study addressed several important questions: (a) What are adult OSA patients' beliefs and perceptions about OSA, the associated risks, and treatment with CPAP prior to treatment use? (b) What are the consequences of these beliefs and perceptions on the use of CPAP? (c) What are the beliefs and perceptions of adults with OSA after 1 week of CPAP use, including perceived benefits of treatment, effect of treatment on health, and perceived ability to adapt to CPAP? and (d) Do differences exist between adherers and nonadherers with regard to their beliefs and perceptions at diagnosis and with treatment use that might, in part, explain differences in CPAP adherence outcomes? To our knowledge, our study findings provide the first published description of beliefs of those who adhere and those who choose not to adhere to CPAP treatment. These findings contribute to understanding patient treatment decisions regarding CPAP use, suggest opportunities for identifying those at risk for nonadherence

to CPAP, and contribute toward developing tailored interventions to promote CPAP use.

■ Conceptual Framework

Acceptance and consistent use of CPAP is influenced by a multitude of factors, as is evidenced in previous studies examining predictors of CPAP adherence (Weaver & Grunstein, 2008). It is therefore important to approach the phenomenon of CPAP adherence from a multifactorial perspective that addresses the complex nature of this particular health behaviour. The application of social cognitive theory has been widely applied in studies of adoption, initiation, and maintenance of health behaviours (Bandura, 1977, 1992; Schwarzer & Fuchs, 1996). The core determinants of the model include knowledge, perceived self-efficacy, outcome expectations, health goals, and facilitators/barriers. The model posits that health promoting behaviours are primarily influenced by patients' self-efficacy, or their belief in their ability to exercise control over personal health habits, which influences other critical determinants: knowledge, outcome expectations, goals, and perceived facilitators and impediments (Bandura, 2004; see Figure 1). Knowledge of health risks and specific benefits relative to health behaviours is a necessary determinant for health behaviours, but rarely does knowledge alone promote change in behaviours. Outcome expectations, or the expectancies one holds for investing in a particular health behaviour, are evaluated by the individual in terms of costs and benefits, including physical, social, and psychological. Individuals who anticipate that the benefits of a health behaviour outweigh the costs are more inclined to perceive the health behaviour as favourable, and more inclined to set short- and long-term personal goals to guide adoption of that health behaviour. This cascade of health behaviour determinants does not occur in isolation, but is influenced by barriers and facilitators that derive from personal, social,

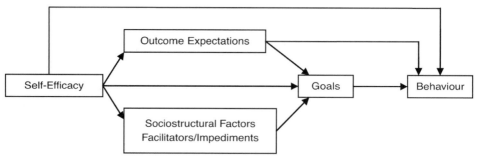

Figure 1. Social cognitive theory health determinants: Pathways of influence of self-efficacy on health behaviours. From Bandura, A. (2004). Health promotion by social cognitive means. *Health Education & Behavior, 31*(2), 146. Copyright 2004 by Sage Publications. Reprinted with permission of the publisher.

and environmental circumstances. As individuals identify facilitators for the health behaviour and overcome barriers, their belief in their ability to successfully change or adopt a health behaviour (i.e., perceived self-efficacy) increases.

Recognizing that individuals exist within a collective agency or community, the construct of self-efficacy is not confined solely to personal capabilities. Although commonalities in the basic concepts of self-efficacy exist across cultures, the "cultivated identities, values, belief structures, and agentic capabilities are the psychosocial systems through which experiences are filtered" (Bandura, 2002, p. 273). Bandura suggested that the application of social cognitive theory must be situated in context, recognizing that "human behavior is socially situated, richly contextualised, and conditionally expressed" (2002, p. 276). From this conceptual perspective and in a predominantly qualitative research paradigm, we examined patients' perceptions, beliefs, and experiences within their own context to permit an explicit description of salient factors that influenced OSA patients' decisions to use or not use CPAP.

■ Method

DESIGN

Using a concurrent nested, mixed method design, we conducted a longitudinal study

extending from initial diagnosis through the first week of home CPAP treatment of newly diagnosed OSA patients. We conducted two individual interviews with participants and collected first-week CPAP adherence data. In contrast to a triangulation design, the concurrent nested study design emphasizes one methodology, and the data are mixed at the analysis phase of the study (Creswell, Plano Clark, Gutmann, & Hanson, 2003). Nesting the less dominant quantitative method within the predominant qualitative method permitted an enriched description of the participants and a more in-depth analysis of the overall phenomenon of interest: CPAP adherence (Creswell et al., 2003).

PARTICIPANTS

Adults with suspected OSA were recruited from a sleep clinic at an urban Veterans Affairs medical centre during a 5-month enrolment period. One sleep specialist referred potential participants who were clinically likely to have OSA to the study. Our purposive sampling strategy was to include patients who (a) provided detailed information during their initial clinical visit and were willing to openly discuss their health and health care; (b) had at least moderate OSA (AHI $\geq$ 15 events/hour; American Academy of Sleep Medicine Task Force, 1999) and were prescribed CPAP treatment; (c) initially accepted CPAP for home

Qualitative Health Research, 2010; 20(7):873–892.   Copyright © 2010. Reprinted by permission of SAGE Publications.

use; and (d) were able to speak and understand English. To ensure that participants would be prescribed CPAP treatment based on Veterans Health Administration CPAP prescribing guidelines in place during study enrolment, patients with mild OSA (AHI < 15 events/hour) were excluded. We also excluded participants who had current or historical treatment with CPAP or any other treatment for OSA, a previous diagnosis of OSA, refusal of CPAP treatment by the participant prior to any CPAP exposure (i.e., in-laboratory CPAP titration sleep study), and those who required supplemental oxygen in addition to CPAP and/or bilevel positive airway pressure therapy for treatment of sleep-disordered breathing during their in-laboratory CPAP titration sleep study.

Previous studies have identified that decisions to adhere to CPAP emerge by the second to fourth day of treatment (Aloia, Arnedt, Stanchina, et al., 2007; Weaver, Kribbs, et al., 1997). Therefore, it is possible that patients' beliefs, perceptions, and experiences during the first several experiences with CPAP might significantly influence short- and long-term CPAP adherence patterns. For this reason, we did not include individuals who refused CPAP treatment prior to any CPAP experience, because we sought to describe salient factors preceding and during initial CPAP exposure. The protocol was approved by the research site and the affiliated university's institutional review boards. All participants provided informed consent prior to participating in any study activities.

PROCEDURE

After study enrolment, each participant had two in-laboratory, full-night sleep studies (i.e., polysomnograms). The first sleep study was a diagnostic study and the second sleep study was to determine the therapeutic CPAP pressure necessary to eliminate obstructive sleep apnea events. All sleep studies were performed and scored using standard criteria (American Academy of Sleep Medicine Task Force, 1999; Rechtschaffen & Kales, 1968). The AHI, a

measure of disease severity in OSA, was computed from the diagnostic polysomnogram as the number of apneas and/or hypopneas per hour of sleep. The therapeutic CPAP pressure, the pressure required to eliminate hypopneas and apneas, was determined on a manual CPAP titration polysomnogram performed about 1 week (7.9 ± 6.9 days) after the diagnostic polysomnogram.

Semistructured Interviews. Semistructured interviews, conducted by one study investigator, were scheduled with participants at two intervals: within 1 week following diagnosis but prior to the CPAP titration sleep study, and after the first week of CPAP treatment at home (see Figure 2). All interviews were conducted in an informal, private room at the medical centre to ensure privacy, participant comfort, and promote open sharing of information (Streubert Speziale & Carpenter, 2003). To minimize attrition, participants were offered the opportunity to participate in interviews at an alternative location or by telephone if transportation difficulties or ambulatory limitations precluded study participation.

Interview guides, consisting of specific questions and probes (i.e., prompts to encourage focus on the particular issue of interest) were used for each interview to ensure that a consistent sequence and set of questions were addressed across participants. A funnel approach was used in the development and execution of the interview guides. This approach begins with broad questions and gradually progresses to focused questions specific to the phenomenon of interest to promote sharing of experiences by the participants (Tashakkori & Teddlie, 1989). The first interview focused on perceptions of the diagnosis, perceived health effects of the diagnosis, pretreatment perceptions of CPAP, and the social and cultural precedents that led to the participant seeking medical care for their sleep problems (see Table 1). The second interview focused on perceived effects of treatment with CPAP, supportive mechanisms or barriers to using CPAP, and how beliefs and perceptions about the diagnosis, associated risks of

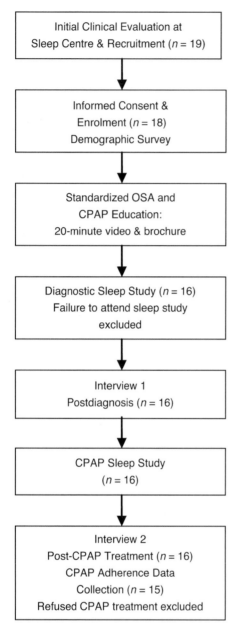

Figure 2. Study design.

the diagnosis, and the treatment experience might have affected CPAP adherence (see Table 2). Interviews were digitally audio-recorded and transcribed to an electronic format by a professional transcriptionist not affiliated with the study. Field notes were maintained by the interviewer before and after each interview to describe the environment of the interview, describe the participant at the time of the interview, and note any aberrations from the planned interview guide that occurred and a description of such aberrations. The field notes not only served as a descriptive context of the interview, but also served as interviewer reflexivity notations (i.e., interviewer biases, suppositions, and presuppositions of the research topic). The purpose of maintaining reflexivity notations was to ensure that interviewer-imposed assumptions did not take precedent over the participant's described experience.

CPAP Adherence. In accordance with the standard of clinical care at the sleep centre, all participants were issued the same model CPAP machine (Respironics Rem- Star Pro®) that records on a data card (SmartCardTM) the time each day that the CPAP circuit is pressurized, an objective measurement of daily CPAP mask-on time. CPAP use was defined as periods when the device was applied for more than 20 minutes at effective pressure. One week of CPAP adherence data were uploaded to a personal computer for software analysis (Respironics EncorePro®) at the time of the second semistructured interview. Graphic adherence data were used as probes to discuss specific occurrences of CPAP nonuse. The objectively measured CPAP adherence data were also used to identify adherent ($\geq$ 6 hours/night CPAP use) and nonadherent participants ($<$ 6 hours/night CPAP use). A cut-off point of 6 hours/night was selected a priori to describe adherers and nonadherers to CPAP treatment, as recent evidence suggests that 6 or more hours of CPAP use per night is necessary to improve both functional and objective sleepiness outcomes (Weaver et al., 2007).

ANALYSIS

A sequential analysis was conducted, with qualitative-directed content analysis of interview data followed by quantitative descriptive

Table 1. Postdiagnosis Interview Guide

Concept	Topic/Question
Perceptions and knowledge of diagnosis	How did you know about sleep disorders and the sleep centre before coming to your first appointment?
	Before being told you have OSA,[a] had you heard of OSA? If so, what did you know about OSA?
	What do you now understand about OSA?
	After having your sleep study, what are your thoughts about OSA and what it means to you?
Perceived effects of diagnosis	How do you believe OSA affects you in your daily life?
Sociocultural precedents and influences on health, illness/disease, and care seeking	Do you know anyone else who has been diagnosed with OSA? If so, how did that impact you and your interest in coming to the sleep center?
	Why did you seek care from the sleep center?
	Is there anyone who influenced you to seek care for this problem?
	Is there anyone who has helped you understand what OSA is? If so, how did that information impact your desire to receive treatment?
	What has you experience with a health care system been to this point?
	Do sleep, sleeping, and/or the sleep environment have any specific meaning(s) to you? To your family? To your spouse/significant other/bed partner?

[a]OSA = Obstructive sleep apnea

analysis of the CPAP adherence data. By sequentially analyzing the data, the priority of the individual as informant was emphasized and the investigators were blinded to CPAP adherence until the final analysis procedure, a mixed methods analysis, was conducted (see Figure 3). By dividing the participants into categories of adherent (i.e., $\geq$ 6 hrs/night CPAP use) and nonadherent (i.e., $<$ 6 hrs/night CPAP use), we examined across-case consistencies in subthemes and themes to describe the contextualized experience of adhering or not adhering to CPAP treatment.

Each transcript was read in its entirety, highlighting, extracting, and condensing text from individual interviews that addressed individual beliefs, perceptions, and/or experiences during diagnosis and early treatment with CPAP. This process of text analysis brought forward the manifest content of the qualitative data (Graneheim & Lundman, 2004). These responses were separated from the interview text, identified by participant identification number, and entered into an analysis table. Abstraction, or the process of taking condensed, manifest data and interpreting the underlying meaning (i.e., latent meaning), followed as participant responses were then described in a condensed format and interpreted for meaning within a thematic coding process. Trustworthiness was enhanced as the likelihood of investigator bias was minimized by first highlighting relevant text for coding, extracting relevant text from complete interviews transcripts, and then coding the meaning units for theory-driven categories or themes and then for subthemes (Hsieh & Shannon, 2005).

Table 2. One Week Post-CPAP Use Interview Guide

Concept	Topic/Question
Perceived effects and knowledge of treatment with CPAP	Have you been using CPAP[a] for the treatment of your OSA[b]? How would you describe your use of CPAP? Are you experiencing any improvement in the way that you feel since you have started using CPAP? When did you first learn about CPAP? Who first described CPAP to you? What did you think when you first learned about CPAP? First saw CPAP? First used CPAP in the sleep laboratory? What do you see as the most important reason for using CPAP in the short term? In the long term?
Supportive mechanisms or barriers to incorporating CPAP into daily life	How was the first week of CPAP treatment? What kinds of problems are you experiencing using CPAP? What has prevented you from regularly using CPAP? What has been helpful to you in regularly using CPAP?
Sociocultural perspectives of health-related decisions to use or not use CPAP	Do you believe CPAP treatment is a treatment you can [continue to] use? Did this belief change since you first learned about your OSA diagnosis? Since starting CPAP? Do you envision yourself using CPAP during the next 3 months? During the next year? During the next 5 years? Do you have any concerns about the CPAP unit? About your sleep [ability or quality]? About your sleep environment that might affect your CPAP use? How does the diagnosis of OSA and treatment with CPAP affect or been affected by those around you?

[a]CPAP = continuous positive airway pressure.
[b]OSA = obstructive sleep apnea.

The overarching, theory-derived themes were initially determined by applying the broad determinants of health as described in the study's conceptual framework, social cognitive theory (Bandura, 2004). These themes included knowledge, perceived barriers and facilitators, perceived self-efficacy, outcome expectations, and goals. This approach permitted the investigators to examine the applicability of the theoretical framework to the phenomenon of CPAP adherence and elaborate on previous findings suggesting the framework's concepts as measurable predictors of CPAP-related health behaviours (Aloia,

Arnedt, Stepnowsky, et al., 2005; Stepnowsky, Bardwell, et al., 2002; Wild et al., 2004). Emergent subthemes were identified as thematic content analysis progressed. The subthemes were then categorized within the overarching conceptual framework themes (see Table 3). We designed the analysis strategy to be consistent with other recent empirical studies of CPAP adherence while permitting a more robust, narrative description of what these theoretically derived variables mean from the perspective of the OSA patient.

Theme definitions were developed by the investigators and reviewed by an expert

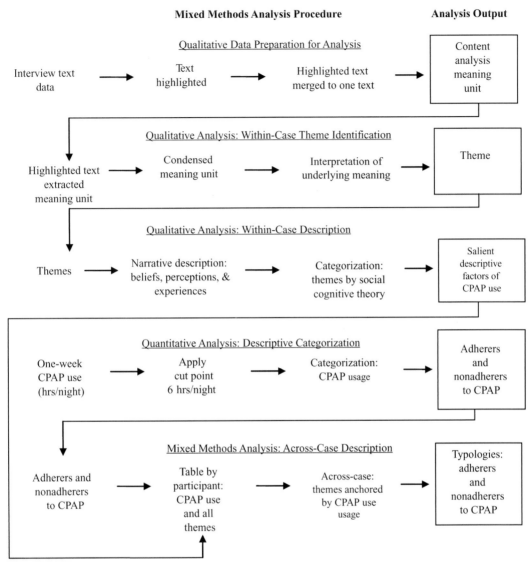

Figure 3. Sequential analysis procedure.

qualitative methodologist and an expert in the research application of theoretical constructs. One study investigator, blinded to CPAP adherence data, coded all interview data for the study. Valid application of the themes was examined by an independent expert coder. Coded interviews were independently recoded by the expert coder to establish validity and reliability of the application of the codes to the interview data. All extracted interview

data were eligible for recoding; approximately 15% of the data from each total interview were randomly selected for expert recoding. Agreement of the study coder and the expert coder was 94%, meeting the established criteria of 80% agreement for acceptance of the coded data. When differences in application of codes were identified, code definitions were reviewed by coders, discussion of specific application of the code(s) was held, and

Qualitative Health Research, 2010; 20(7):873–892. Copyright © 2010. Reprinted by permission of SAGE Publications.

Table 3. Social Cognitive Theory Determinants of Health as Categorizing Framework for Themes From Content Analysis

Determinants of Health Behaviour	Themes[a] Derived From Content Analysis
Knowledge	Fear of death
	Gathering information about OSA/CPAP gives rise to determining the importance of getting to treatment and decisions to accept/reject treatment
	Most immediate impact of OSA on daily life [single symptom] as a motivator to pursue diagnosis and treatment
	Justifying symptoms provides explanation for not pursuing diagnosis and/or treatment
	OSA impacts not only health but also quality of life
	Pervasive effects of OSA on life
	Sleepiness plays a limited role in life and can be accommodated
	Perceived health effects of a disorder are important to valuing diagnosis/treatment
	Associating health risks and functional limitations with OSA contributes to recognizing OSA as a health problem with significant effects on overall well-being
	Perception of seriousness of symptoms influenced by perceived effects symptoms have on individual [health risks] and those around individual [social network]
	Perceived health risks of OSA
	Information provided to individual and applicability of information influences individual's assumptions of responsibility for OSA and CPAP treatment
	Symptoms of OSA have impact on social roles, functions, and relationships
Perceived barriers and facilitators	Social influences as motivators to recognize health problem, seek diagnosis/treatment, and use CPAP
	Objective measures of OSA important to health care decision making
	Differences in perception of urgency of treatment between patient and provider influences valuing of diagnosis and treatment by patient
	Social networks contribute to treatment acceptance but not necessarily to treatment use
	Perceived seriousness of symptoms influenced by perceived effects of symptoms on individual [health risks] and those around individual
	Social networks provide support, help problem solve health concerns, and are sources of health-related information commonality of symptoms of OSA promotes perception of normalcy: Barrier to seeking diagnosis/treatment

(continued)

Qualitative Health Research, 2010; 20(7):873–892. Copyright © 2010. Reprinted by permission of SAGE Publications.

Table 3. *(Continued)*

Determinants of Health Behaviour	Themes[a] Derived From Content Analysis
	Social influences as motivators to recognize health problem, seek diagnosis and treatment, and use treatment
	Silent symptoms: Fear of what it means if symptoms of OSA are undetectable
	Family and social networks contribute to health beliefs about sleep
	Expectations of health delivery vs. the actual delivery of health care services impact on the importance individual's place on their health and the value they place on their relationship with health care providers
Perceived self-efficacy	Knowledge and information provided to individual and applicability of information influences individual's assumption of responsibility for OSA and CPAP treatment
	Early response to CPAP, consistent or inconsistent with outcome expectations, facilitates or is a barrier to treatment use
	Early experience with CPAP is a source of support or a barrier to belief in own ability to use treatment
	Fitting treatment into life
	Problem-solving difficulties/routinization of CPAP responsibilities contribute to disease management
Outcome expectations	Understanding why symptoms exist and associating specific symptoms with a diagnosis provides hope that treatment will address experienced symptoms and improve overall quality of life
	Expectations of treatment outcomes are facilitators of treatment initiation and use
	Early response to CPAP, consistent or inconsistent with outcome expectations, facilitates or is a barrier to using treatment
Goals	Problem-solving difficulties/routinization of CPAP responsibilities contribute to disease management

[a] Themes derived from participant text data were categorized as a determinant of health behaviour from social cognitive theory. Themes are not mutually exclusive. Theme definitions were mutually agreed on by investigators of the study and applied to the directed content analysis procedure by a single investigator acting as the primary coder of text data.

mutual agreement was achieved in all instances of coding differences.

After all interview data were coded for themes, the investigators used the average daily CPAP use during the first week of treatment to separate adherers (≥ 6 hours CPAP use/night) and nonadherers (< 6 hours CPAP use/ night). Descriptive statistics were used in the analysis of 1 week of CPAP adherence data (mean ± standard deviation [SD]).

Across-case analysis of themes and subthemes was then examined from an integrative perspective, using adherent and nonadherent as anchors, or as a unique descriptive qualifier, to identify common perceptions, beliefs, and experiences within the groups of interest. The across-case analysis, including both qualitative and quantitative data sets as complementary within an analysis matrix, gave rise to cases that had common descriptive aspects.

Qualitative Health Research, 2010; 20(7):873–892.   Copyright © 2010. Reprinted by permission of SAGE Publications.

RESULTS

With the recurrence of themes in the content analysis phase, data saturation was reached at 15 participants and the sampling procedure was considered complete. The participants were all veterans, predominantly middleaged (53.9 ± 12.7 years) men (88%; see Table 4). The participants were well educated, with

Table 4. Sample Description

Characteristic	Frequency (%) (*n* = 15)
Gender	
Men	13 (87%)
Women	2 (13%)
Race/ethnicity	
African American	9 (60%)
White	5 (33%)
Other	1 (7%)
Marital status	
Married	7 (47%)
Single	3 (20%)
Divorced	3 (20%)
Widowed	2 (13%)
Highest education	
Middle school	1 (7%)
High school	7 (47%)
2 yr college	4 (27%)
4+ yr college	3 (20%)
Shift work	3 (20%)
Employed	6 (40%)
Retired	6 (40%)
	Mean 6 Standard Deviation
Age, years	53.9 ±12.7
Weight, pounds	248.9 ± 68.7
AHI, events/hour	53.5 ± 26.5
O2 Nadir, %	66.4 ± 13.2
CPAP pressure, cmH$_2$O	10.7 ± 1.6
1 week CPAP adherence, hours	4.98 ± 0.5

93% (*n* = 14) of the sample achieving a high school education or higher. The sample, on average, had severe OSA (AHI 53.5 ± 26.5 events/hr), with an oxygen nadir of 66.4% (± 13.2%). The average CPAP pressure setting was 10.7 ± 1.6 cmH$_2$O. Average CPAP use during the first 7 days of CPAP treatment was 4.98 ± 0.5 hours/night. Sorting on CPAP adherence (i.e. ≥ 6hrs/night CPAP use and < 6 hrs/ night CPAP use), there were six adherers and nine nonadherers. The interview prior to CPAP exposure was conducted after the diagnostic polysomnogram, on average at Day 9 (range 2 to 28 days), and the second interview was conducted following at least 1 week of CPAP treatment (average number of days from Day 1 of CPAP use, 18; range 7 to 47 days).

ADHERERS AND NONADHERERS TO CPAP THERAPY

Knowledge and Perceived Health Risks. Knowledge, or the "knowing" an individual has about the health risks and benefits of health behaviours (Bandura, 2004) was a predominant theme in both interviews for all participants. Saturation on nearly every knowledge theme suggests that participants identified that having an understanding of OSA and CPAP is an important part of the experience of being diagnosed with OSA and treated with CPAP. Adherent participants related their knowledge of risks and benefits of CPAP to their own outcome expectations after being diagnosed with OSA. For some participants, knowledge of OSA being simply more than snoring was a first step in recognizing OSA as a syndrome with health implications. One participant described this, saying, "I knew sleep apnea existed, but it just never dawned on me how serious it was in my case. I just didn't pay any attention to it. I just figured I was going to snore for the rest of my life."

For many participants, "putting the whole picture together" after receiving education about OSA and CPAP treatment helped them

Qualitative Health Research, 2010; 20(7):873–892.   Copyright © 2010. Reprinted by permission of SAGE Publications.

understand that they not only were experiencing symptoms of OSA on a daily basis, but their overall health and quality of life was impacted by OSA. During the first interview, participants were provided with a summary of their diagnostic sleep study results. The combination of education about the OSA diagnosis and treatment with CPAP, and relating their own diagnosis to their daily health and functioning, was important to adherent participants' formulation of accurate beliefs and perceptions of OSA and CPAP. These beliefs served to motivate or facilitate adherent participants' determination to pursue CPAP after diagnosis:

> I didn't know anything really, how the CPAP worked or anything like that. I just knew that there was a disease called sleep apnea and that a lot of people have it and people don't realize it. I really still didn't know anything about it til after I went through the test [diagnostic polysomnogram]. . . . Five [breathing events] is normal and thirty is severe and I'm doing ninety an hour. You know that literally scared the hell right out of me because all I could think of is I'm going to die in my sleep.
>
> [T]hen when you told me about driving, being tired, I remembered that every time we take off on a long trip, the first hour I got to pull over and rest. So it all came together. So I figured maybe I do have it [OSA].

For many adherent participants, knowledge of health risks associated with OSA was limited to "being sluggish" or "having low energy levels." For some, their perception of OSA was only relative to "falling asleep when I sit down." Participants who "put the whole picture together," relating their diagnosis to their own health status, were motivated to accept CPAP treatment from the outset. For example, one participant said, "It's [OSA] got to take a toll in the long run on a lot of things, like high blood pressure. I'm hoping that it helps me to drop my high blood pressure." These perceptions provided hope for adherent participants that expanded beyond the management of their OSA to other disease and health experiences:

> If I have more energy and I'm not so sluggish— because I go to the local high school track and get in five or six laps, walking around the track—I

will have more energy to do those kinds of things that keep you healthy.

Posttreatment, there was less emphasis on knowledge-based themes among adherent participants. This suggested a shift of emphasis among adherers from knowledge of risks and benefits of OSA to perceptions derived from the actual experience of CPAP treatment.

Nonadherent participants' knowledge at diagnosis was not different from adherent participants' knowledge. However, those with knowledge that served as a barrier, rather than a facilitator, to diagnosis were less likely to pursue a diagnostic sleep study in a timely fashion. This was particularly true for those who had inaccurate knowledge and perceptions of OSA, such as OSA being a condition of simple snoring. Even though many acknowledged they probably had OSA, the snoring was the "problem" that defined OSA, not apneic events and resultant untoward health and functional outcomes. As one participant described,

> My brother does it [snores], and he stopped [breathing] all the time in the middle of the night. My father did it, you know, and I do it. I knew I do it so it's been a while, I mean, I don't remember not being a loud snorer. . . . Like I said, my condition is hereditary. I'm sure my oldest son has it and I'm sure my youngest son is going to end up with it. My brother had it and my father had it, you know, my mother probably had it 'cause she's a snorer. I didn't think it was serious of a problem 'cause it's [snoring, stops in breathing] something that I had experienced for so many years.

Furthermore, describing early knowledge of "having to wear a mask" for the treatment of OSA served as a barrier to both seeking diagnosis and treatment for some. This perception was not consistent among only nonadherers though, as many of the participants expressed concerns about the anticipated treatment of their OSA. CPAP adherers and nonadherers described critically important differences in their own ability to reconcile the following: (a) their OSA diagnosis; (b) their experience of symptoms; (c) their goals for treatment use; and (d) their outcome expectations that were met after treatment exposure. These factors,

Qualitative Health Research, 2010; 20(7):873–892. Copyright © 2010. Reprinted by permission of SAGE Publications.

when reconciled by the individual, facilitated overall positive perceptions of the diagnosis and treatment experience.

Goal Setting and Outcome Expectancies.

Outcome expectancies are the expected or anticipated costs and benefits for healthful habits/behaviours that support or deter from an individual's investment in the behaviour (Bandura, 2004). Among the participants, postdiagnosis outcome expectancies that were consistently met were highly influential on participants' decisions to use CPAP. For example, after being diagnosed with OSA, one participant brought all his experienced symptoms into perspective, relating them to his OSA. With treatment, he was hopeful that these symptoms would resolve. He stated, "It seems like sleep apnea basically causes all those problems. So I figure if I can get this taken care of [by wearing CPAP], basically the problems will subside." Making sense of symptoms in terms of treatment outcome expectancies helped adherers commit to trying CPAP and believing that CPAP was going to be a positive experience. One participant summarized his perception of symptoms and outcome expectations like this: "But without me even trying it I know that what I'm experiencing and how it's affected me, and that I want to get better if I can and so there's nothing going to keep me away from getting a CPAP."

A particularly important perception described by participants was their early response to CPAP as influential on future/continued use of CPAP. These early, first experiences were helpful to formulating realistic and personally important outcome expectancies for CPAP use. One participant described his response to CPAP after wearing it for the first time in the sleep laboratory during his second sleep study (i.e., CPAP sleep study):

> But being like I got relief the first night I was at the hospital. I drove home that morning after they woke me up, I went down, I got breakfast, and I'm driving home, I'm saying to myself, gee, I feel great and I only got from one o'clock to six, you know. I feel so much better and I felt so much better that whole day. I felt so good after that five hours of sleep with the machine on that it sold me.

For adherent participants, having a positive response to CPAP during the sleep study night with CPAP was highly motivating for continued CPAP use at home. Furthermore, this early response set the stage for participants to develop an early commitment to the treatment, even when faced with barriers. Persistent, positive responses to CPAP throughout the early treatment period (i.e., 1 week) reinforced participants' outcome expectancies and helped them formulate a perception of the treatment that was conducive to long-term use.

Goals for improved health and for achieving certain health behaviours are an important part of being successful with any health behaviour. According to Bandura (2004), individuals set goals for their personal health, including establishing concrete plans or strategies for achieving those goals. Goal setting among adherent CPAP users focused on "how best to adapt to using CPAP" or identifying "solutions to difficulties with use of CPAP." These goals were established so that adherent CPAP users were able to achieve their outcome expectations. Goal setting was not specifically discussed by adherent participants before using CPAP. With exposure to and experience with CPAP, adherent participants first identified that using CPAP was important and, thereafter, identified "tricks and techniques" to successfully use CPAP. Whether these strategies originated from the participant or were a collaborative effort between participant and a support source, having a plan that addressed how best to adapt to CPAP promoted continued effort directed at using CPAP, as described by one adherent participant:

> I guess the first night I put it on I sort of got a little feeling of claustrophobia, but I pushed it out of my mind, saying to myself, "Don't let this [bother you], this is a machine that is going to help you, you got to wear it," so I just put it in my mind that I was going to wear it.

As this participant described, it was important for him to devise a way that he could use the treatment so that he might realize his overall health goals. Similarly, one participant found that he could not fall asleep with CPAP at full pressure. He emphasized the importance of using CPAP to treat his OSA, but he equated using CPAP to "a tornado blowing through your nose." He recalled being taught about several features on the CPAP machine that might alleviate this sensation. After testing a few tricks on the CPAP machine, he found that he was able to fall asleep on a lower pressure setting while the pressure increased to full pressure setting after he was asleep (i.e., ramp function). By setting an immediate goal to get to sleep while wearing CPAP, he was able to achieve his longer-term goal to wear CPAP each night. The long-term goal of adherent participants was to feel better or sleep better, but the immediate goal was to be able to wear CPAP.

For nonadherers, a negative experience during their CPAP sleep study led them to have an undesirable outlook on CPAP and the overall treatment of OSA. For example, one participant described experiencing no immediate response to CPAP during the CPAP sleep study; therefore, he didn't expect to experience any response to treatment over a more extended period of time:

> I still had the same kind of sleep, I thought. As a matter of fact I thought it took me longer to get to sleep than it did on the first sleep study [without CPAP]. I believe my sleep was still the same type of sleep that I always get, even though, you know, the machine was supposed to make me sleep better. I still woke up in the same condition that I usually wake up in, is what I'm trying to say. I didn't feel any more vigorous or alert or anything after that first night.

Participants' descriptions of their considerations for using CPAP consistently included the question, "What are the down sides of using CPAP?" Combining early negative perceptions of the treatment and early negative experiences with CPAP, nonadherers tended to see the drawbacks of using the treatment as far outweighing any benefits of using the treatment. One participant described both negative perceptions and negative experiences, which caused him to believe that CPAP treatment outcome expectancies were not worth the torment of using the treatment:

> No, I didn't think I couldn't do it from the beginning. I was believing it was gonna do something more than what it did, and it didn't do anything. I'm not getting sleep, I'm still getting up tired. I guess I expected more from it and I didn't get anything, not anything that I could see anyway. No, just a bunch of botheration and I didn't get any sleep.

Among participants who did not adhere, the goal-oriented theme was not present after diagnosis. Nonadherers did not articulate specific goals for attaining treatment and, furthermore, they did not describe strategies to be able to wear CPAP after 1 week of CPAP treatment. For nonadherers, establishing treatment-related goals for use of CPAP was not a priority.

Facilitators of and Barriers to CPAP use.
Perceived facilitators and barriers can be personal, social, and/or structural. Although perceived facilitators and barriers are influential on health behaviours, this process is mediated by self-efficacy (Bandura, 2004). Therefore, the existence of a barrier, in and of itself, might not be particularly influential on an individual's behaviour if their self-efficacy is high. Consistent with this conceptual perspective, some participants identified barriers that were particularly troublesome when using CPAP, but were vigilant users of CPAP despite these barriers. Conversely, those who described numerous facilitators to using CPAP treatment were not necessarily adherent to CPAP.

Adherent participants were less focused on potential or actual facilitators and barriers to using CPAP over time than nonadherers. When adherent participants discussed facilitators and barriers, their overall descriptions were positive, with facilitators being the focus of their experience after using CPAP for 1 week. No adherent participants emphasized barriers to using CPAP after 1 week of treatment. Furthermore, when faced with barriers, adherent participants described perceptions of the treatment as important and identified a belief in their ability to overcome the barrier. For example, one participant experienced a sensation of not being able to breathe during his second night of

Qualitative Health Research, 2010; 20(7):873–892.   Copyright © 2010. Reprinted by permission of SAGE Publications.

CPAP use at home, but his ability to use CPAP was influenced by his commitment to "needing" the treatment:

> Because it was like I couldn't breathe and even though the machine was on, it was like I was paralyzed, and this happened every time when I tried to go back to sleep. How many times? Three more times that very same night until I was getting really anxious because every time I would try to go to sleep, after a while I would get that anxiety again. Finally, I prayed. I got up and I prayed real hard, asked God to really help me with this and I was right to sleep. Ever since then, I pray every night and have no problems.

As this example demonstrates, barriers and facilitators are not independent determinants of health behaviour. Participants described situations and experiences that were labeled as either a facilitator or barrier, but the actual behavioural outcome of getting to diagnosis and using CPAP was not necessarily reflective of such experiences being a barrier or facilitator.

The facilitating experiences described by adherent participants centred on social interactions that provided motivation and facilitation of their CPAP use. Facilitating experiences included descriptions of social support, shared experiences of CPAP use with other CPAP users, and recognition that their own improvement as a result of CPAP treatment was an important influence on social relationships. Social relationships and the ability to be fully engaged in social interactions during their first week of CPAP use was described by several adherent participants as a facilitator to ongoing treatment:

> I see the difference. People see the difference. My wife sees the difference. My kids see the difference. That helps. I think that's 50% of it. People telling you that you have changed and things are getting better and you look a lot better and you a sound a lot better and you act a lot better, because when you have feedback like that you know it's [CPAP] helping.
>
> Our relationship [with spouse] is getting better and better. I think since the sleep machine it's even been more because some things that irritate me, I would speak on and it would cause like a little bit of friction, as it happens in couples. But since I've had the sleep machine, I've been letting the minor things go, things that irritate me or I would complain about before. . . . Communication, our rela-

tionship, so we've been able to talk more and enjoy each other even more since then [starting CPAP]. Yeah, I like the machine, I really do, and I like what it's doing.

Adherent participants clearly emphasized the importance of improved social relationships as a result of their CPAP treatment. Many recognized such improvements after a close friend or family member suggested the improvement was obvious.

Nonadherent participants emphasized barriers rather than facilitators to using CPAP after being diagnosed with OSA. However, after using CPAP for 1 week, nonadherers identified few, if any, actual barriers to treatment. Unlike adherent participants, nonadherers did not discuss social interactions as an important part of their post-CPAP treatment experience. Nonadherent participants also identified themselves as single, divorced, or widowed, with the exception of one participant. Nonadherers did not discuss their social networks (i.e., friends, family outside of their residence, coworkers) as important to their experiences of being diagnosed with OSA and starting CPAP treatment.

Perceived Self-Efficacy. Perceived self-efficacy is the belief that one can exercise control over one's own health habits, producing desired effects by one's own health behaviours (Bandura, 2004). This overarching theme was meaningfully described by participants and represented by several subthemes that were important to both adherers and nonadherers in the study. Within these descriptions, participants offered experiences with being diagnosed with OSA and using CPAP that led to their belief in themselves, or lack thereof, to use or not use the treatment.

Adherers in the sample described generally positive perceived self-efficacy regarding future use of CPAP. Adherers had a positive belief in their ability to use CPAP from the outset, which persisted and became increasingly frequent from diagnosis to early CPAP treatment, even if they first doubted their ability to use the treatment. As one participant described, the first thought of wearing a mask during sleep was not appealing, but with a positive first experience with CPAP, the participant was increasingly confident that CPAP was going to be a part of his life:

> I think I seen the masks sitting there and I thought to myself, I hope I don't have to wear one of those things. Then they came in and said, "Now we're going to put the CPAP on you," and I said, "Okay," and they put the CPAP on me and when they came back into the room I felt great when I woke up at six. They had to wake me up at six o'clock because I was sleeping and you know, I think I felt after that, I didn't care what it was if I got that much sleep from one o'clock to six without getting up. I was going to wear or do whatever I had to do to do it [wear CPAP].

Adherent participants also described that they planned to incorporate CPAP into their daily routine, suggesting an underlying positive belief in their ability to accomplish the health behaviour of using CPAP. Recognizing that using CPAP would necessitate additional daily "work," adherers had well-defined plans of incorporating the added demands to their daily schedule:

> I have to just add some things that I have to do in order to keep the CPAP machine clean and to make sure that it's dry and each week I have to disinfect it, but once I did it, once I decided I was gonna do it, I just went in the bathroom, did the whole thing, it only took about twenty minutes, twenty-five minutes, and I was all done. And getting up in the morning and doing the daily cleaning, you know, that's not a negative but it's just something I have to make an adjustment to.

Nonadherent participants described having largely negative experiences with CPAP during the first exposure (i.e., CPAP sleep study) or during the early phase of home CPAP use. Few nonadherent participants experienced benefits with treatment and nonadherers described unsuccessful or a lack of problem-solving efforts with CPAP difficulties. These negative experiences were important areas of concern with regard to their perceived ability to use CPAP over the long term (perceived self-efficacy). For example, one participant had such an extremely negative experience during the first week he was exposed to CPAP that he firmly doubted his ability to ever use it:

> I couldn't breathe in [the mask]. This thing, I had to suck in to get a breath out of it. Last night I got a good night's sleep but I woke up, then I was claustrophobic. I felt like I was stuck under a bed someplace and couldn't get out and then I woke up. When I wore it the whole night through I wasn't sleeping so that's one of the reasons [I won't use CPAP], like I didn't sleep with it on; it was too aggravating.

Each participant described getting used to CPAP during the first several nights of treatment. With unsuccessful experiences during this period, participants either identified resources to help improve their experience or made decisions to use CPAP less or not at all. For all participants, early experiences with CPAP contributed to their belief in their own abilities to get used to the therapy.

Individuals who had difficulty fitting CPAP into their lives were challenged to be adherent to the treatment. When CPAP was seen as not fitting into a life routine, participants offered doubts as to their ability to continue to use the treatment. One participant described having a routine of falling asleep with television. With CPAP, she had difficulty watching television and therefore she experienced more difficulty getting to sleep. Although she continued to try to use CPAP, she expressed that using CPAP was generally annoying to her. The complexities presented by using CPAP within the constraints of her normal routine were likely to increasingly influence doubt in her ability to use CPAP.

MARRIED AND UNMARRIED CPAP USERS

With the emerging emphasis placed on social support and social networks by adherers in the study, we explored how the social context of daily life impacted on perceptions of OSA and CPAP treatment by examining married ($n = 7$) and unmarried ($n = 8$) participants' responses. Using married and unmarried status from self-reported demographic characteristics as anchors, or as a unique descriptive qualifier, we sorted the subthemes within an analysis matrix to identify common perceptions, beliefs, and experiences within these qualifier groups. We included all participants

Qualitative Health Research, 2010; 20(7):873–892. Copyright © 2010. Reprinted by permission of SAGE Publications.

who identified themselves as married or common-law married as married; all participants who identified themselves as single, divorced, or widowed were included as unmarried.

These groups described different experiences with both diagnosis and CPAP treatment. Married participants offered descriptions of social support resources within immediate proximity that were positive facilitators of seeking diagnosis and starting/staying on treatment. Married participants expressed positive beliefs in their ability to use CPAP with early treatment use, often described in conjunction with a CPAP problem-solving episode that was collaboratively resolved with their partner/spouse. Married participants described overwhelmingly positive early responses and experiences with CPAP treatment. Their outcome expectations were consistent across time. They generally anticipated positive responses to CPAP prior to exposure and experienced positive responses to treatment after 1 week of use. Married participants also identified success in "fitting CPAP into their lives." These participants were able to identify far more benefits from than difficulties with CPAP, benefits that enhanced their ongoing commitment to use of the treatment. Married participants discussed proximate support sources (i.e., spouse, living partner, family members) as important to providing feedback about their response to treatment, trouble-shooting difficulties, and positive reinforcement for persistent use of CPAP.

Unmarried participants commonly identified friends or coworkers as motivating factors (facilitators) to seek diagnosis but less social influence on/facilitation of treatment use after 1 week of CPAP therapy. Without the presence of immediate social support, unmarried participants did not emphasize important social interactions with actual wearing of CPAP. After 1 week of treatment on CPAP, unmarried participants described less confidence in their ability to use CPAP and described less "response" to CPAP than those participants who were married. Unmarried participants described few facilitators of

treatment use during the first week of CPAP therapy. Nearly all unmarried participants identified "self-driven" reasons for pursuing treatment, and there was an absence of social sources of support, or "cheerleaders and helpful problem solvers" while using CPAP during the first week.

TYPOLOGIES OF ADHERENT AND NONADHERENT CPAP USERS

Described differences in beliefs, perceptions, and experiences of being diagnosed with OSA and early treatment with CPAP were explicit between adherers and nonadherers. Adherers perceived health and functional risks of untreated OSA, had positive belief in their ability to use CPAP from early in the diagnostic process, had clearly defined outcome expectations, had more facilitators than barriers as they progressed from diagnosis to treatment, and identified important social influences and support sources for both pursuing diagnosis and persisting with CPAP treatment. Nonadherers described not knowing the risks associated with OSA, perceived fewer symptoms of their diagnosis, did not have clearly defined outcome expectations for treatment, identified fewer improvements with CPAP exposure, placed less emphasis on social support and socially derived feedback with early CPAP treatment, and perceived and experienced more barriers to CPAP treatment. As a result of the across-case analysis in which consistencies and differences emerged among adherers and nonadherers in the described experience of being diagnosed with OSA and treated with CPAP, we suggest typologies, or descriptive profiles, of persons with CPAP-treated OSA (see Table 5). The typologies we propose are consistent with previous empirical studies of CPAP adherence, in that predictive relationships between risk perception, outcome expectancies, perceived self-efficacy, and social support with CPAP use have been identified. Our study findings extend the previous findings by illuminating the importance of contextual meaning persons

Table 5. Typologies of Adherent and Nonadherent CPAP Users

Adherent CPAP Users	Nonadherent CPAP Users
Define risks associated with OSA	Unable to define risks associated with OSA
Identify outcome expectations from outset	Describe few outcomes expectations
Have fewer barriers than facilitators	Do not recognize own symptoms
Facilitators less important later with treatment use	Describe barriers as more influential on CPAP use than facilitators
Develop and define goals and reasons for CPAP use	Facilitators of treatment absent or unrecognized
Describe positive belief in ability to use CPAP even with potential or experienced difficulties	Describe low belief in ability to use CPAP
Proximate social influences prominent in decisions to pursue diagnosis and treatment	Describe early negative experiences with CPAP, reinforcing low belief in ability to use CPAP Unable to identify positive responses to CPAP during early treatment

derive from their experiences, beliefs, and perceptions when progressing from diagnosis with OSA to treatment with CPAP. Moreover, the typologies succinctly describe critical differences between these groups of CPAP-treated OSA persons that support the development of patient-centred or -tailored adherence interventions that recognize individual differences.

■ Discussion

To our knowledge, this is the first study to apply a predominantly qualitative method to describe individuals' beliefs and perceptions of the diagnosis of OSA and treatment with CPAP relative to short-term CPAP adherence. Our findings are consistent with previous, empirical studies with regard to the overall applicability of social cognitive theory to the phenomenon of CPAP adherence. The findings from our study uniquely extend these previous findings by illuminating the importance of the individual experiences, beliefs, and perceptions as influential on decisions to pursue diagnosis and treatment of OSA. The

described differences between adherers and nonadherers in our study suggest critical tailored or patient-centred intervention opportunities that might be developed and tested among patients who are newly diagnosed with OSA and anticipate CPAP treatment. The major findings of the study include the following: (a) adults described and assigned meaning to being diagnosed with OSA and treated with CPAP, which in turn influenced their decisions to accept or reject treatment and the extent of CPAP use; and (b) differences in beliefs and perceptions at diagnosis and with CPAP treatment were identified among CPAP adherers and nonadherers and also described in the social context of married and unmarried CPAP users. The described differences between these groups provide data to support the first published typology, or descriptive profile, of CPAP adherers and nonadherers.

Theoretically derived variables, such as the determinants of health behaviors described in social cognitive theory and applied in our study, are operational concepts that help us understand OSA patients' perceptions and beliefs about OSA and CPAP, and can guide interventions to improve adherence to CPAP.

Framed by Bandura's social cognitive theory (1977), differences among adherers and non-adherers to CPAP can be defined across social cognitive theory determinants of health behaviors: (a) knowledge, (b) perceived self-efficacy, (c) outcome expectancies and goals, and (d) facilitators and barriers. As previous studies have demonstrated, psychosocial constructs, such as those consistent with social cognitive theory, provide possibly the most explained variance, to date, among adherers and nonadherers (Aloia, Arnedt, Stepnowsky, et al., 2005; Engleman & Wild, 2003; Stepnowsky, Bardwell, et al., 2002; Weaver et al., 2003). Furthermore, recent intervention studies to promote CPAP adherence have applied similar theoretical constructs with some positive findings (Aloia, Arnedt, Millman, et al., 2007; Richards, Bartlett, Wong, Malouff, & Grunstein, 2007). As our study findings suggest, decisions to use CPAP are individualized and at least in part dependent on the patient's support environment and early experiences with and beliefs about CPAP. Because early commitments to use or not use CPAP predict long-term use (Aloia, Arnedt, Stanchina, et al., 2007; Weaver, Kribbs, et al., 1997), it is critically important to understand and examine opportunities to intervene on factors that influence early commitments to use CPAP. This insight will potentiate the development of patient-centred and -tailored interventions to improve CPAP adherence at the individual level while collectively promoting the health outcomes of the OSA population.

Our study confirms that social cognitive theory is applicable to the unique health behavior of using CPAP treatment. Indeed, the interacting determinants of health as described by Albert Bandura (1977) in relationship to decisions to accept and use CPAP were clearly described by our study participants. This affirmation suggests that any one measured domain within the model (i.e., barriers, facilitators, outcome expectancies) is not likely to identify persons at risk for nonadherence to CPAP. Rather, our study findings support the complex and reciprocating nature of the theoretical model as it applies to this

health behaviour, and offer clarity to our understanding of CPAP adherence as a multi-factorial, iterative decision-making process. It is therefore important to ascertain an understanding of the context of the individual from the initial diagnosis through early treatment use to address the complex nature of the problem of adherence to CPAP and to prospectively identify those likely to be non-adherent to the treatment.

In our study, the experience and perception of symptoms contributed to the participants' motivation to seek diagnosis and treatment and to adhere to CPAP treatment. Although studies that have examined pre-treatment symptoms, particularly subjective sleepiness, have produced inconsistent results with regard to subsequent CPAP use, these studies have measured symptoms on quantitative scales that define specific scenarios of "impairment" related to the symptom of interest (i.e., Epworth Sleepiness Scale (Johns, 1993), Functional Outcomes of Sleep Questionnaire (Weaver, Laizner, et al., 1997), Stanford Sleepiness Scale (MacLean, Fekken, Saskin, & Knowles, 1992; Engleman et al., 1996; Hui et al., 2001; Janson, Noges, Svedberg-Randt, & Lindberg, 2000; Kribbs et al., 1993; Lewis et al., 2004; McArdle et al., 1999; Sin et al., 2002; Weaver, Laizner, et al., 1997). Yet, as our study highlights, perceptions of need relative to one's experience of symptoms were highly individual and significantly influenced decisions to pursue both diagnosis and treatment. Consistent with perceptions that influence medicine-taking behaviour (Hansen, Holstein, & Hansen, 2009), particular situations necessitated the pursuit of diagnosis and use of the treatment. The experience of symptoms and the impact of symptoms on daily life were highly variable among participants and not readily amenable to discrete categorization. Understanding particular situations is important insight to explaining adherence to CPAP.

Recognizing and acknowledging that perceived symptoms are part of a disease process and logically linked to the diagnosis of OSA was important to the participants of our study,

Qualitative Health Research, 2010; 20(7):873–892.   Copyright © 2010. Reprinted by permission of SAGE Publications.

and to their commitment to move forward from diagnosis to treatment, consistent with Engleman and Wild's findings (2003). A recent intervention study to promote CPAP adherence incorporated specific strategies that address "personalization" of OSA symptoms (Aloia, Arnedt, Riggs, Hecht, & Borrelli, 2004; Aloia, Arnedt, Millman, et al., 2007). Results of this randomized controlled trial showed lower CPAP discontinuation rates among those participants who were in the motivational enhancement and education group when compared with "usual care," suggesting the importance of assisting persons diagnosed with OSA to make the connection between the objectively measured disease/diagnosis and their lived experience of the disease (Aloia, Arnedt, Millman, et al., 2007). Personalizing symptoms, recognizing the impact of symptoms on daily function, and identifying the meaning of disease in terms of the perception of one's own health were clearly described by participants in our study. Adherent and nonadherent participants clearly expressed differences in their experiences of having OSA, including the impact of functional impairment on social relationships. From these differing perspectives, participants defined outcome expectations and health risks associated with OSA in different ways, possibly influencing their eventual decision to use or discontinue CPAP.

The described importance of participants' early experiences with CPAP and their initial response to CPAP treatment, both during the CPAP sleep study and during the first week of CPAP use, were influential on participants' interest in continuing to use CPAP. Our study results are consistent with Van de Mortel, Laird, and Jarrett's (2000) findings in which nonadherent, CPAP-treated OSA patients had complaints about their sleep study experience and described "major" problems on the night of their CPAP titration. Similarly, Lewis et al. (2004) found that problems identified on the first night of CPAP use, albeit on autotitrating CPAP, were consistent with lower CPAP use. Not only has the initial experience in terms of difficulties with CPAP been identified as

important to subsequent CPAP adherence, but also the patient's response to the first night of CPAP (i.e., degree of sleep improvement) has been correlated with subsequent CPAP adherence (Drake et al., 2003). The importance of promoting a positive initial experience with CPAP and providing anticipatory guidance about outcome expectations is highlighted by our findings.

The significance of social support, both proximate and within the broader social network, was an important facilitator of CPAP use among adherers in our study. Differences between the experiences of married and unmarried individuals with OSA revealed the described importance of an immediate, proximate source of support for CPAP use. Our finding is consistent with previous findings that those CPAP users who lived alone were significantly less likely to use their CPAP than those who lived with someone (Lewis et al., 2004). Not only are immediate sources of support important for continued use of CPAP, but also shared experiences with CPAP from less-immediate social sources. Participants in our study described social relationships as motivators to seek diagnosis, providing positive reinforcement for persisting with treatment use, and a source for sharing tips on managing OSA and CPAP. Studies exploring reasons for nonadherence to antituberculosis drugs have similarly identified the importance of social influences on seeking treatment and using treatment (Naidoo, Dick, & Cooper, 2009). Among CPAP-treated OSA patients, intervention studies that included feedback to participants, positive reinforcement, inclusion of a support person, and assistance with trouble-shooting difficulties resulted in higher CPAP adherence among participants in the intervention groups as compared with placebo or usual-care groups (Aloia et al., 2001; Chervin, Theut, Bassetti, & Aldrich, 1997; Hoy, Vennelle, Kingshott, Engleman, & Douglas, 1999). Confirming the applicability of these intervention strategies, the described experiences of participants in our study provide empirical support for adherence interventions that include a support person, provide early feedback and positive reinforcement to patients, and assist with trouble-shooting difficulties in the early treatment period.

Barriers to subsequent CPAP use that were identified by participants of our study included the process of having to put a mask on every night, aesthetic issues with mask/headgear use, inconvenience of having to use a machine to sleep, and daily routines that were disrupted by CPAP. Consistent with previous studies (Engleman et al., 1994; Hui et al., 2001; Massie et al., 1999; Sanders et al., 1986), side effects of CPAP were not emphasized by participants as barriers to CPAP use. Although identified barriers did not necessitate nonadherence to CPAP in our study, it was important for individuals who experienced such barriers to identify positive reasons to use CPAP and successfully mitigate barriers, often with the help of others.

This study had several limitations. First, although the sample size of 15 was adequate for a qualitative study, there was limited power to conduct any exploratory quantitative analyses. Although not the objective of this study, quantitative exploration of commonly used measures of subjective sleepiness, functional impairment, and adherence to CPAP correlated with descriptive, quantified typologies of adherent and nonadherent CPAP users would support the findings of the study. Study participants included predominantly male veterans with severe OSA who had relatively high educational preparation. Examining this typology in a larger, more heterogeneous sample of OSA patients is needed. As the relationship of gender, disease severity, symptom perception, and disease-specific literacy with CPAP adherence has not been clearly defined, replicating this study in a more diverse sample and expanding concurrently measured quantitative outcomes would be informative and supportive of typology refinement or expansion. Finally, to reduce the potential confounding effect of clinically delivered psychoeducation, we enrolled participants referred to the study from a single clinical provider with limited participant–provider interaction at the first prediagnostic evaluation. However, participants may have had telephone contact with the sleep centre staff, or had unscheduled visits at the sleep centre that were not controlled for in any way in our study.

Our mixed methods, exploratory study, employing a predominantly qualitative methodology, achieved saturation of themes regarding the diagnosis of OSA and nightly CPAP use during the first week of treatment. The study results are consistent with previous studies of CPAP, even when adherence, in many previous studies, was defined as four hours/night of use rather than six hours/night of use, as in our study. With recent evidence suggesting better outcomes with longer nightly CPAP use (Stradling & Davies, 2000; Weaver et al., 2007; Zimmerman, Arnedt, Stanchina, Millman, & Aloia, 2006), applying a definition of CPAP adherence of six hours vs. four hours likely contributed to more robust differences in described beliefs and perceptions among adherers and nonadherers. To our knowledge, the results of our study provide the first published, narrative descriptions of CPAP adherers and nonadherers that support an overall composite of characteristics that might be useful in identifying specific subgroups of patients who are most likely to benefit from tailored interventions to lessen the risk for subsequent CPAP nonadherence. To date, studies have provided adherence promotion interventions to unselected groups, possibly minimizing variation of response between intervention and control groups. Future randomized controlled trials testing CPAP adherence interventions delivered to participants who are selected based on their risk for treatment failure because of nonadherence are necessary to evaluate intervention effectiveness.

■ Acknowledgments

We acknowledge the sleep centre staff's commitment to the conduct and completion of the study, and the exemplary transcription services provided by Charlene Hunt at Transcribing4You~Homework4You.

■ Declaration of Conflicting Interests

The authors declared a potential conflict of interest (e.g., a financial relationship with the commercial organizations or products discussed in this article) as follows: Dr. Kuna has received contractural support and equipment from Phillips Respironics, Inc. Dr. Weaver has a licensing agreement with Phillips Respironics, Inc., for the Functional Outcomes of Sleep Questionnaire.

■ Funding

The authors disclosed receipt of the following financial support for the research and/authorship of this article: The study was supported by award number F31NR9315 (Sawyer) from the National Institute of Nursing Research. The content is solely the responsibility of the authors and does not necessarily represent the official views of the National Institute of Nursing Research or the National Institutes of Health.

Bios

Amy M. Sawyer, PhD, RN, is a postdoctoral research fellow at the University of Pennsylvania School of Nursing, Philadelphia, Pennsylvania, and a nurse researcher at the Philadelphia Veterans Affairs Medical Center, Philadelphia, Pennsylvania, USA.

Janet A. Deatrick, PhD, RN, FAAN, is an associate professor and associate director, Center for Health Equities Research, at the University of Pennsylvania School of Nursing, Philadelphia, Pennsylvania, USA.

Samuel T. Kuna, MD, is an associate professor of medicine at the University of Pennsylvania School of Medicine and chief, Pulmonary, Critical Care and Sleep Medicine, at the Philadelphia Veterans Affairs Medical Center, Philadelphia, Pennsylvania, USA.

Terri E. Weaver, PhD, RN, FAAN, is the Ellen and Robert Kapito Professor in Nursing Science, chair, Biobehavioral Health Sciences Division, and associate director, Biobehavioral Research Center, at the University of Pennsylvania School of Nursing, Philadelphia, Pennsylvania, USA.

Corresponding Author
Amy M. Sawyer, University of Pennsylvania School of Nursing, Claire M. Fagin Hall, 307b, 418 Curie Blvd., Philadelphia, PA 19104, USA Email: asawyer@nursing.upenn.edu

REFERENCES

Al Lawati, N. M., Patel, S., & Ayas, N. T. (2009). Epidemiology, risk factors, and consequences of obstructive sleep apnea and short sleep duration. *Progress in Cardiovascular Diseases, 51*, 285–293.

Aloia, M. S., Arndt, J., Riggs, R. L., Hecht, J., & Borrelli, B. (2004). Clinical management of poor adherence to CPAP: Motivational enhancement. *Behavioral Sleep Medicine, 2*(4), 205–222.

Aloia, M. S., Arndt, J. T., Millman, R. P., Stanchina, M., Carlisle, C., Hecht, J., et al. (2007). Brief behavioral therapies reduce early positive airway pressure discontinuation rates in sleep apnea syndrome: Preliminary findings. *Behavioral Sleep Medicine, 5*, 89–104.

Aloia, M. S., Arndt, J. T., Stanchina, M., & Millman, R. P. (2007). How early in treatment is PAP adherence established? Revisiting night-to-night variability. *Behavioral Sleep Medicine, 5*, 229–240.

Aloia, M. S., Arndt, J. T., Stepnowsky, C., Hecht, J., & Borrelli, B. (2005). Predicting treatment adherence in obstructive sleep apnea using principles of behavior change. *Journal of Clinical Sleep Medicine, 1*(4), 346–353.

Aloia, M. S., Di Dio, L., Ilniczky, N., Perlis, M. L., Greenblatt, D. W., & Giles, D. E. (2001). Improving compliance with nasal CPAP and vigilance in older adults with OAHS. *Sleep and Breathing, 5*(1), 13–21.

American Academy of Sleep Medicine Task Force. (1999). Sleep-related breathing disorders in adults: Recommendations for syndrome definitions and measurement techniques in clinical research. *Sleep, 22*, 667–689.

Bandura, A. (1977). Self-efficacy: Toward a unifying theory of behavioral change. *Psychological Reviews, 84*, 191–215.

Bandura, A. (1992). Exercise of personal agency through the self-efficacy mechanism. In R. Schwarzer (Ed.), *Self-efficacy: Thought control of action* (pp. 3–38). Philadelphia: Hemisphere.

Bandura, A. (2002). Social cognitive theory in cultural context. *Applied psychology: An International Review, 51*(2), 269–290.

Bandura, A. (2004). Health promotion by social cognitive means. *Health Education & Behavior, 31*(2), 143–164.

Chervin, R. D., Theut, S., Bassetti, C., & Aldrich, M. S. (1997). Compliance with nasal CPAP can be improved by simple interventions. *Sleep, 20,* 284–289.

Creswell, J. W., Plano Clark, V. L., Gutmann, M. L., & Hanson, W. (2003). Advanced mixed methods research designs. In A. Tashakkori & C. Teddlie (Eds.), *Handbook of mixed methods in social & behavioral research* (pp. 209–240). Thousand Oaks, CA: Sage.

Drake, C. L., Day, R., Hudgel, D., Stefadu, Y., Parks, M., Syron, M. L., et al. (2003). Sleep during titration predicts continuous positive airway pressure compliance. *Sleep, 26,* 308–311.

Engleman, H. M., Asgari-Jirandeh, N., McLeod, A. L., Ramsay, C. F., Deary, I. J., & Douglas, N. J. (1996). Self-reported use of CPAP and benefits of CPAP therapy. *Chest, 109,* 1470–1476.

Engleman, H. M., Martin, S. E., & Douglas, N. J. (1994). Compliance with CPAP therapy in patients with the sleep apnoea/ hypopnoea syndrome. *Thorax, 49,* 263–266.

Engleman, H. M., & Wild, M. (2003). Improving CPAP use by patients with the sleep apnoea/ hypopnoea syndrome (SAHS). *Sleep Medicine Reviews, 7*(1), 81–99.

Gay, P., Weaver, T., Loube, D., & Iber, C. (2006). Evaluation of positive airway pressure treatment for sleep related breathing disorders in adults. *Sleep, 29,* 381–401.

Graneheim, U. H., & Lundman, B. (2004). Qualitative content analysis in nursing research: Concepts, procedures and measures to achieve trustworthiness. *Nursing Education Today, 24,* 105–112.

Grunstein, R. R., Stewart, D. A., Lloyd, H., Akinci, M., Cheng, N., & Sullivan, C. E. (1996). Acute withdrawal of nasal CPAP in obstructive sleep apnea does not cause a rise in stress hormones. *Sleep, 19,* 774–782.

Hansen, D. L., Holstein, B. E., & Hansen, E. H. (2009). "I'd rather not take it, but · · ·": Young women's perceptions of medicines. *Qualitative Health Research, 19,* 829–839.

Harsch, I., Schahin, S., Radespiel-Troger, M., Weintz, O., Jahrei, H., Fuchs, S., et al. (2004). Continuous positive airway pressure treatment rapidly improves insulin sensitivity in patients with obstructive sleep apnea syndrome. *American Journal of Respiratory & Critical Care Medicine, 169,* 156–162.

Hoy, C. J., Vennelle, M., Kingshott, R. N., Engleman, H. M., & Douglas, N. J. (1999). Can intensive support improve continuous positive airway pressure use in patients with the sleep apnea/hypopnea syndrome? *American Journal of Respiratory & Critical Care Medicine, 159,* 1096–1100.

Hsieh, H., & Shannon, S. (2005). Three approaches to qualitative content analysis. *Qualitative Health Research, 15,*1277–1288.

Hui, D., Choy, D., Li, T., Ko, F., Wong, K., Chan, J., et al. (2001). Determinants of continuous positive airway pressure compliance in a group of Chinese patients with obstructive sleep apnea. *Chest, 120,* 170–176.

Janson, C., Noges, E., Svedberg-Randt, S., & Lindberg, E. (2000). What characterizes patients who are unable to tolerate continuous positive airway pressure (CPAP) treatment? *Respiratory Medicine, 94,* 145–149.

Johns, M. (1993). Daytime sleepiness, snoring, and obstructive sleep apnea. The Epworth Sleepiness Scale. *Chest, 103,* 30–36.

Kribbs, N. B., Pack, A. I., Kline, L. R., Smith, P. L., Schwartz, A. R., Schubert, N. M., et al. (1993). Objective measurement of patterns of nasal CPAP use by patients with obstructive sleep apnea. *American Review of Respiratory Diseases, 147,* 887–895.

Krieger, J. (1992). Long-term compliance with nasal continuous positive airway pressure (CPAP) in obstructive sleep apnea patients and nonapneic snorers. *Sleep, 15,* S42–S46.

Lewis, K., Seale, L., Bartle, I. E., Watkins, A. J., & Ebden, P. (2004). Early predictors of CPAP use for the treatment of obstructive sleep apnea. *Sleep, 27,* 134–138.

MacLean, A. W., Fekken, G. C., Saskin, P., & Knowles, J. B. (1992). Psychometric evaluation of the Stanford Sleepiness Scale. *Journal of Sleep Research 1,* 35–39.

Massie, C., Hart, R., Peralez, K., & Richards, G. (1999). Effects of humidification on nasal symptoms and compliance in sleep apnea patients using continuous positive airway pressure. *Chest, 116,* 403–408.

McArdle, N., Devereux, G., Heidarnejad, H., Engleman, H. M., Mackay, T., & Douglas, N. J. (1999). Long-term use of CPAP therapy for sleep apnea/hypopnea syndrome. *American Journal of Respiratory and Critical Care Medicine, 159,* 1108–1114.

Meurice, J. C., Dore, P., Paquereau, J., Neau, J. P., Ingrand, P., Chavagnat, J. J., et al. (1994). Predictive factors of long-term compliance with nasal continuous positive airway pressure treatment in sleep apnea syndrome. *Chest, 105,* 429–434.

Naidoo, P., Dick, J., & Cooper, D. (2009). Exploring tuberculosis patients' adherence to treatment regimens and prevention programs at a public health site. *Qualitative Health Research 19,* 55–70.

Nieto, F., Young, T., Lind, B., Shahar, E., Samet, J., Redline, S., et al. (2000). Association of sleep-disordered breathing, sleep apnea, and hypertension in a large community-based study. *Journal of the American Medical Association, 283,* 1829–1836.

Peppard, P., Young, T., Palta, M., & Skatrud, J. (2000). Prospective study of the association between sleep-disordered breathing and hypertension. *New England Journal of Medicine, 342,* 1378–1384.

Rechtschaffen, A., & Kales, A. (Eds.). (1968). *A manual of standardized terminology, techniques and scoring system for sleep stages in human subjects.* Los Angeles: BIS/BRI. Reeves-Hoche, M. K., Meck, R., & Zwillich, C. W. (1994). Nasal CPAP: An objective evaluation of patient compliance. *American Journal of Respiratory & Critical Care Medicine, 149,* 149–154.

Richards, D., Bartlett, D. J., Wong, K., Malouff, J., & Grunstein, R. R. (2007). Increased adherence to CPAP with a group cognitive behavioral treatment intervention: A randomized trial. *Sleep, 30*, 635–640.

Rosenthal, L., Gerhardstein, R., Lumley, A., Guido, P., Day, R., Syron, M. L., et al. (2000). CPAP therapy in patients with mild OSA: Implementation and treatment outcome. *Sleep Medicine, 1*, 215–220.

Russo-Magno, P., O'Brien, A., Panciera, T., & Rounds, S. (2001). Compliance with CPAP therapy in older men with obstructive sleep apnea. *Journal of American Geriatric Society, 49*, 1205–1211.

Sanders, M. H., Gruendl, C. A., & Rogers, R. M. (1986). Patient compliance with nasal CPAP therapy for sleep apnea. *Chest, 90*, 330–333.

Schwarzer, R., & Fuchs, R. (1996). Self-efficacy and health behaviours. In M. Conner & P. Norman (Eds.), *Predicting health behaviour: Research and practice with social cognition models* (pp. 163–196). Philadelphia: Open Press.

Schweitzer, P., Chambers, G., Birkenmeier, N., & Walsh, J. (1997). Nasal continuous positive airway pressure (CPAP) compliance at six, twelve, and eighteen months. *Sleep Research, 16*, 186.

Sin, D., Mayers, I., Man, G., & Pawluk, L. (2002). Long-term compliance rates to continuous positive airway pressure in obstructive sleep apnea: A population-based study. *Chest, 121*, 430–435.

Stepnowsky, C., Bardwell, W. A., Moore, P. J., Ancoli-Israel, S., & Dimsdale, J. E. (2002). Psychologic correlates of compliance with continuous positive airway pressure. *Sleep, 25*, 758–762.

Stepnowsky, C., Marler, M. R., & Ancoli-Israel, S. (2002). Determinants of nasal CPAP compliance. *Sleep Medicine, 3*, 239–247.

Stradling, J., & Davies, R. (2000). Is more NCPAP better? *Sleep, 23*, S150–S153.

Streubert Speziale, H., & Carpenter, D. (2003). *Qualitative research in nursing* (3rd ed.). Philadelphia: Lippincott Williams & Wilkins.

Sullivan, C., Barthon-Jones, M., Issa, F., & Eves, L. (1981). Reversal of obstructive sleep apnea by continuous positive airway pressure applied through the nares. *Lancet, 1*, 862–865.

Tashakkori, A., & Teddlie, C. (1989). *Mixed methodology: Combining qualitative and quantitative approaches*. London: Sage.

Van de Mortel, T. F., Laird, P., & Jarrett, C. (2000). Client perceptions of the polysomnography experience and compliance with therapy. *Contemporary Nurse, 9*, 161–168.

Weaver, T. E., & Grunstein, R. R. (2008). Adherence to continuous positive airway pressure therapy: The challenges to effective treatment. *Proceedings of the American Thoracic Society, 5*, 173–178.

Weaver, T. E., Kribbs, N. B., Pack, A. I., Kline, L. R., Chugh, D. K., Maislin, G., et al. (1997). Night-to-night variability in CPAP use over first three months of treatment. *Sleep, 20*, 278–283.

Weaver, T. E., Laizner, A. M., Evans, L. K., Maislin, G., Chugh, D. K., Lyon, K., et al. (1997). An instrument to measure functional status outcomes for disorders of excessive sleepiness. *Sleep, 20*, 835–843.

Weaver, T. E., Maislin, G., Dinges, D. F., Bloxham, T., George, C. F. P., Greenberg, H., et al. (2007). Relationship between hours of CPAP use and achieving normal levels of sleepiness and daily functioning. *Sleep, 30*, 711–719.

Weaver, T. E., Maislin, G., Dinges, D. F., Younger, J., Cantor, C., McCloskey, S., et al. (2003). Self-efficacy in sleep apnea: Instrument development and patient perceptions of obstructive sleep apnea risk, treatment benefit, and volition to use continuous positive airway pressure. *Sleep, 26*, 727–732.

Wild, M., Engleman, H. M., Douglas, N. J., & Espie, C. A. (2004). Can psychological factors help us to determine adherence to CPAP? A prospective study. *European Respiratory Journal, 24*, 461–465.

Young, T., Palta, M., Dempsey, J., Skatrud, J., Weber, S., & Badr, S. (1993). The occurrence of sleep-disordered breathing among middle-aged adults. *New England Journal of Medicine, 328*, 1230–1235.

Young, T., Peppard, P., & Gottlieb, D. (2002). Epidemiology of obstructive sleep apnea: A population health perspective. *American Journal of Respiratory & Critical Care Medicine, 165*, 1217–1239.

Zimmerman, M. E., Arnedt, T., Stanchina, M., Millman, R. P., & Aloia, M. S. (2006). Normalization of memory performance and positive airway pressure adherence in memory-impaired patients with obstructive sleep apnea. *Chest, 130*, 1772–1778.

Qualitative Health Research, 2010; 20(7):873–892.   Copyright © 2010. Reprinted by permission of SAGE Publications.

Critique of Sawyer et al.'s (2010) Study: "Differences in Perceptions of Diagnosis and Treatment of Obstructive Sleep Apnea and Continuous Positive Airway Pressure Therapy Among Adherers and Nonadherers"

OVERALL SUMMARY

This was a well-written, interesting report of a study on a significant topic. The mixed methods QUAL + quan approach that was used was ideal for combining rich narrative interview data with objective, quantitative measures of adherence to continuous positive airway pressure (CPAP) treatment. The use of a longitudinal design enabled the researchers to gain insights into changes in patients' perceptions from diagnosis to treatment. The study design and methods were described in detail, and the methods themselves were of high quality. The authors provided considerable information about how the trustworthiness of the study was enhanced. The results were nicely elaborated, and the researchers incorporated numerous excerpts from the interviews. This was, overall, an excellent paper describing a strong study.

TITLE

The title of this report was long; perhaps a few words could have been omitted (e.g., "Differences in" could be removed without affecting readers' understanding of the study). Nevertheless, the title did describe key aspects of the research. The title conveyed the central topic (perceptions about obstructive sleep apnea [OSA] and CPAP therapy). It also communicated the nature of the analysis, which compared perceptions of adherers and nonadherers to CPAP.

ABSTRACT

The abstract was written as a traditional abstract without subheadings. Although brief, the abstract described major aspects of the study. The methods were succinctly presented, covering the overall mixed methods design, the longitudinal nature of the study (two rounds of interviews), the sample (15 OSA patients), the basic type of analysis (content analysis), and the focus on comparing adherent and nonadherent patients using objectively measured CPAP use. Although specific results were not described, the abstract indicated areas in which differences between adherers and nonadherers were observed. Finally, the last sentence suggested some possible applications for the results in terms of developing tailored interventions to promote CPAP use.

INTRODUCTION

The introduction to this study was concise and well organized. It began with a paragraph about OSA as an important chronic health problem, describing its prevalence, effects, and primary medical treatment, i.e., CPAP. This first paragraph conveyed the significance of the topic.

Much of the rest of the introduction discussed adherence to CPAP, which has consistently been found to be low. The researchers set the stage for their study by summarizing evidence about rates of adherence and factors predicting adherence. They also described research that affected design decisions, such as studies that have found that patients' perceptions are influenced by early experiences with CPAP. The studies cited in the introduction included several recent studies, suggesting that the authors were summarizing state-of-the-art knowledge.

The introduction also described knowledge gaps: "To date, there are relatively few studies that have systematically examined the influence of disease and treatment perceptions and beliefs on CPAP adherence." The authors stated their four interrelated research questions, which were well suited to an in-depth qualitative approach.

CONCEPTUAL FRAMEWORK

The article devoted a section to a description of the conceptual framework that underpinned the research. The authors used as their framework Bandura's social cognitive theory, which they summarized and depicted in a useful conceptual map (Fig. 1). They also noted that Bandura's model is relevant within a qualitative inquiry because of explicit recognition of the role of context. One puzzling thing, however, is that both in this section and in the "Results" section, considerable attention was paid to the role of *knowledge* in influencing health behaviours. Yet, knowledge was not a component of the theory depicted in Figure 1.

METHOD

The "Method" section was organized into four subsections and was unusually thorough in providing detail about how the researchers conducted this study.

Design

Sawyer and colleagues used a mixed methods design to study patients' perceptions and beliefs about OSA and CPAP and to explore differences among adherers and nonadherers. The researchers described their design as a concurrent nested mixed methods design and provided a citation to a paper by Creswell and Plano-Clark (2003), the two authors whose more recent work was cited in this textbook. Had Sawyer and colleagues used Morse's notation system, they would have characterized the study as QUAL + quan, which indicates that the data for the two strands were collected concurrently and that the qualitative component was dominant.

The "Design" section also noted that the design was longitudinal, with data collected both at initial OSA diagnosis through the first week of CPAP treatment. Such a longitudinal design was a good way to track patients' perceptions from diagnosis to the early treatment phase. The decision about *when* to collect the two rounds of data was well supported by earlier research. A good graphic (Fig. 2) illustrated the study design and the timing of key events, such as enrolment and collection of demographic data, receipt of treatment education, conduct of the sleep studies, and the two interviews.

Participants

The researchers clearly defined the group of interest and described how participants were recruited. Participants were adults with suspected OSA who were recruited from a Veterans Affairs sleep clinic. To be eligible, patients had to meet various clinical criteria (e.g., had at least moderate OSA, defined as at least 15 apnea or hypopnea events per hour in a sleep study) and practical criteria (had to speak and understand English). Patients were excluded if their responses could be confounded by prior CPAP experiences because the researchers were interested in understanding the perceptions and beliefs early in the diagnosis and CPAP treatment transition.

The researchers also excluded individuals who refused CPAP treatment prior to the actual treatment, and Figure 1 suggests that one such person was dropped from the study. That is, 16 patients were interviewed for the pretreatment interview, but only 15 were interviewed a second time, and the analysis was based on responses from 15 patients.

One comment about this section is that the sampling approach does not appear to be purposive as was described. People were selected if they experienced OSA and use of CPAP, but these were actually eligibility criteria. It appears that the participants were a convenience sample of those meeting the eligibility criteria who were referred by a sleep specialist in one particular clinic. With a small sample, and with a goal of looking at differences between adherers and nonadherers, a purposive strategy of sampling patients on dimensions known to differentiate these groups might have increased the likelihood that both groups would be adequately represented.

Procedures

The section on "Procedures" presented considerable information, focusing primarily on data collection. The section began by describing the two sleep studies that all study participants underwent. In both studies, the patient's apnea/hypopnea index (AHI) was computed via a polysomnogram. The initial AHI helped to determine study eligibility.

Next, the researchers described the major forms of data collection, which included semistructured interviews and instrumentation to assess CPAP adherence objectively. The article specified that the interview data were collected by a single investigator at two points in time: within a week following OSA diagnosis and then after the first week of treatment. The authors noted that participants were given choices about where the interviews would take place in an effort to minimize attrition. And, in fact, there was no attrition in this study.

Table 1 listed questions that guided the initial interview, and Table 2 listed questions for the posttreatment interview. These tables were an excellent way to communicate the nature of the interviews, and the text provided even more detail. Consistency was enhanced by having a single interviewer responsible for conducting all interviews. To maximize data quality, the interviews were digitally recorded and transcribed by a professional transcriptionist.

The interviewer also maintained field notes before and after each interview. Commendably, these field notes were not only descriptive (i.e., describing participants and the interview environments) but also "served as interviewer reflexivity notations (i.e., interviewer biases, suppositions, and presuppositions of the research topic)."

An important feature of this study was that CPAP adherence was not assessed by self-report. Rather, adherence was objectively determined based on quantitative data from the CPAP machine. A standard definition of "CPAP use" was provided, and a criterion of 6 hours or more per night of CPAP use was established for adherence. The researchers provided a convincing rationale for using the 6-hour limit as the cutoff point for adherence versus nonadherence.

The researchers might have considered administering a self-efficacy scale to anchor their discussion of self-efficacy, which is a key construct in their conceptual model. Although many constructs in the model were ones that merited qualitative exploration, self-efficacy is one that perhaps could have been examined from both a qualitative and quantitative perspective, especially in a study that is explicitly mixed methods in design.

Data Analysis

The authors provided a detailed description of their data analysis methods. Not only did they carefully explain data analytic procedures in the text but they also provided a powerful flow chart (Fig. 3) illustrating the sequence of steps they followed.

The qualitative data were content analyzed, an approach that is appropriate for a study that was primarily descriptive. The study purpose was to obtain descriptive information at two points in time about participants' perceptions relevant to OSA and CPAP. The researchers explained the procedures used in the content analysis, and they provided appropriate citations.

The data analysis section explained how theory-driven themes were extracted in a manner consistent with the broad conceptualization of health behaviour articulated in Bandura's theory. The authors offered specific illustrations in Table 3, which listed broad theoretical determinants of health behaviour in the first column and then relevant themes for each determinant as derived from the content analysis. For example, for the broad construct "Perceived self-efficacy," there were five relevant themes, such as "Fitting treatment into life" and "Problem-solving difficulties."

The section on data analysis also included important information about methods the researchers used to enhance trustworthiness. For example, one investigator coded all the interview data. Then, an independent expert recoded a randomly selected 15% of the data from each interview. Overall agreement between the study coder and the expert coder was a high 94%. For any differences of opinion about coding, the discrepancy was resolved by consensus. The theme definitions used in the coding, which were developed by the investigative team, were reviewed by two experts, a qualitative methodologist, and an expert in the application of the theoretical constructs.

Commendably, the qualitative data were coded and content analyzed for themes by an investigator who was blinded to whether the participant was classified as adherent or nonadherent based on the quantitative data. Only after coding was complete was the adherence status of participants revealed. At that point, across-case analysis was examined "from an integrative perspective, using adherent and nonadherent as anchors . . . to identify common perceptions, beliefs, and experiences within the groups of interest."

RESULTS

The "Results" section began with a description of the study sample, all of whom were military veterans. Table 4 showed basic demographic statistics on the 15 participants, including their gender, race/ethnicity, marital and employment status, educational background, and age. Clinical information (e.g., mean weight, AHI events per hour and CPAP adherence in terms of hours per night) was also presented. The text stated that the sample included six adherers and nine nonadherers. The introductory paragraph of the "Results" section also noted that data saturation was reached at 15 participants, and that sampling stopped at that point.

Much of the "Results" section was organized according to differences between adherers and nonadherers to CPAP therapy within major thematic categories, such as "Knowledge and perceived health status," "Facilitators of and barriers to CPAP use," and "Perceived self-efficacy." Key differences between the two groups (and a few areas of overlap) within these major groupings were described and supported with rich excerpts from the interview transcripts.

Social support emerged as an important issue in CPAP adherence, consistent with previous studies. Thus, the researchers performed a useful supplementary analysis in which they examined differences between married and unmarried patients.

The "Analysis" section concluded with a typology (descriptive profiles) of adherent and nonadherent CPAP users based on an integration of the data across themes. Table 5 nicely summarized their typology.

DISCUSSION

Sawyer and colleagues offered a thoughtful discussion of their findings, which highlighted ways in which the findings complement and extend the existing body of evidence on CPAP adherence. The discussion wove together findings from the current study and previous studies and discussed the findings within the context of the theoretical framework.

The authors also noted some study limitations. They pointed out, for example, that study participants were all veterans with fairly high levels of education, and thus exploration with a more diverse population of OSA patients would be desirable. The researchers pointed out that the small sample size of 15 provided limited power for conducting quantitative analyses of numerical data they had at their disposal, such as measures of subjective sleepiness and functional impairment.

Relatively little space was devoted to the implications of the study findings. The researchers noted that "the described differences between adherers and nonadherers in our study suggest critical tailored or patient-centered intervention opportunities . . . " Indeed, they mentioned the opportunity for tailored interventions several times in connection with their discussion of their theoretically derived themes. A bit more elaboration of how the findings could be used in an intervention might have been helpful.

OTHER COMMENTS

Presentation

This report was clearly written, well organized, and offered considerable detail about the research methods. The inclusion of several tables and figures provided explicit and concrete information about various aspects of the study.

Ethical Aspects

The authors briefly stated steps they took to ensure ethical treatment of participants in the subsection labeled "Participants." All participants provided informed consent, and the study protocols were approved by the Research Ethics Board of the affiliated university and the research site.

Note: A few entries in this glossary were not explained in this book, but they are included here because you might come across them in the research literature. These entries are marked with an asterisk (*).

Absolute risk (AR) The proportion of people in a group who experienced an undesirable outcome.

Absolute risk reduction (ARR) The difference between the absolute risk in one group (e.g., those exposed to an intervention) and the absolute risk in another group (e.g., those not exposed).

Abstract A brief description of a study, located at the beginning of a report.

Accessible population The population available for a study; often a nonrandom subset of the target population.

Acquiescence response set A bias in self-report instruments, especially in psychosocial scales, that occurs when participants characteristically agree with statements ("yea-say"), independent of content.

AGREE instrument A widely used instrument (Appraisal of Guidelines Research and Evaluation) for systematically assessing clinical practice guidelines.

Alpha (α) (1) In tests of statistical significance, the significance criterion—the risk the researcher is willing to accept of making a Type I error (false positive); (2) in assessments of the internal consistency of a scale, a reliability coefficient, Cronbach's alpha.

Analysis The organization and synthesis of data to answer research questions and test hypotheses.

Analysis of covariance (ANCOVA) A statistical procedure used to test mean group differences on an outcome variable while controlling for one or more covariates.

Analysis of variance (ANOVA) A statistical procedure for testing mean differences among three or more groups by comparing variability between groups to variability within groups, yielding an F ratio statistic.

Ancestry approach In literature searches, using citations from relevant studies to track down earlier research on which the studies were based (the "ancestors").

Anonymity Protection of participants' confidentiality such that even the researcher cannot link individuals with the data they provided.

Applied research Research designed to find a solution to an immediate practical problem.

*Arm A particular treatment group to which participants are allocated (e.g., the control *arm* or treatment *arm* of a controlled trial).

Assent The affirmative agreement of a vulnerable subject (e.g., a child) to participate in a study, typically to supplement formal consent by a parent or guardian.

Associative relationship An association between two variables that cannot be described as a causal relationship.

403

Assumption A principle that is accepted as being true based on logic or reason, without proof.

Asymmetric distribution A distribution of data values that is skewed, with two halves that are not mirror images of each other.

Attention control group A control group that gets a similar amount of attention as those in the intervention group, without receiving the "active ingredients" of the treatment.

Attrition The loss of participants over the course of a study, which can create bias by changing the characteristics of the sample from those of the sample initially drawn.

Audit trail In a qualitative study, the systematic documentation of decisions, procedures, and data that allows an independent auditor to draw conclusions about trustworthiness.

Authenticity The extent to which qualitative researchers fairly and faithfully show a range of different realities in the collection, analysis, and interpretation of their data.

Autoethnography Ethnographic studies in which researchers study their own culture or group.

Axial coding The second level of coding in a grounded theory study using the Strauss and Corbin approach, involving the process of categorizing, recategorizing, and condensing first-level codes by connecting a category and its subcategories.

Baseline data Data collected at an initial measurement (e.g., prior to an intervention) so that changes can be evaluated.

Basic research Research designed to extend the base of knowledge in a discipline for the sake of knowledge production or theory construction rather than for solving an immediate problem.

Basic social process (BSP) The central social process emerging through analysis of grounded theory data.

Benchmark In measurement, a threshold value on a measure that corresponds to an important value, such as a threshold for interpreting whether a change in scores is meaningful or clinically significant.

Beneficence An ethical principle that involves maximizing benefits for study participants and preventing harm.

*Beta (β) (1) In statistical testing, the probability of a Type II error; (2) in multiple regression, the standardized coefficients indicating the relative weights of the predictor variables in the equation.

Bias Any influence that distorts the results of a study and undermines validity.

Bimodal distribution A distribution of data values with two peaks (high frequencies).

Bivariate statistics Statistical analysis of two variables to assess the empirical relationship between them.

Blind review The review of a manuscript or proposal such that neither the author nor the reviewer is identified to the other party.

Blinding The process of preventing those involved in a study (participants, intervention agents, data collectors, or health care providers) from having information that could lead to a bias, particularly information about which treatment group a participant is in; also called *masking*.

Bracketing In descriptive phenomenological inquiries, the process of identifying and holding in abeyance any preconceived beliefs and opinions about the phenomena under study.

Carryover effect The influence that one treatment can have on subsequent treatments, notably in a crossover design or in test–retest reliability assessments.

Case-control design A nonexperimental design that compares "cases" (people with a specified condition, such as lung cancer) to matched controls (similar people without the condition).

Case study A method involving a thorough, in-depth analysis of an individual, group, or other social unit.

Categorical variable A variable with discrete values (e.g., gender) rather than values along a continuum (e.g., weight).

Category system In studies involving observation, the prespecified plan for recording the behaviours and events under observation; in qualitative studies, a system used to sort, organize, and code the data.

Causal (cause-and-effect) relationship A relationship between two variables wherein the presence or value of one variable (the "cause") determines the presence or value of the other (the "effect").

Cause-probing research Research designed to illuminate the underlying causes of phenomena.

Cell The intersection of a row and column in a table with two dimensions.

Central (core) category The main category or pattern of behaviour in grounded theory analysis using the Strauss and Corbin approach.

Central tendency A statistical index of the "typicalness" of a set of scores, derived from the center of the score distribution; indices of central tendency include the mode, median, and mean.

Certificate of Confidentiality A certificate issued by the National Institutes of Health in the United States to protect researchers against forced disclosure of confidential research information.

Change score A person's score difference between two measurements on the same measure, calculated by subtracting the value at one point in time from the value at the second point.

Chi-squared test A statistical test used in various contexts, most often to assess differences in proportions; symbolized as χ^2.

Clinical practice guidelines Practice guidelines that are evidence-based, combining a synthesis and appraisal of research evidence with specific recommendations for clinical decisions.

Clinical research Research designed to generate knowledge to guide practice in health care fields.

Clinical significance The practical importance of research results in terms of whether they have genuine, palpable effects on the daily lives of patients or on the health care decisions made on their behalf.

Clinical trial A study designed to assess the safety, efficacy, and effectiveness of a new clinical intervention, often involving several phases (e.g., phase III typically is a *randomized controlled trial* using an experimental design).

Closed-ended question A question that offers respondents a set of specified response options.

Cochrane Collaboration An international organization that aims to facilitate well-informed decisions about health care by preparing systematic reviews of the effects of health care interventions.

Code of ethics The fundamental ethical principles established by a discipline or institution to guide researchers' conduct in research with human (or animal) participants.

Coding The process of transforming raw data into standardized form for data processing and analysis; in quantitative research, the process of attaching numbers to categories; in qualitative research, the process of identifying recurring words, themes, or concepts within the data.

Coefficient alpha The most widely used index of internal consistency that indicates the degree to which the items on a multi-item scale are measuring the same underlying construct; also referred to as *Cronbach's alpha*.

Coercion In a research context, the explicit or implicit use of threats (or excessive rewards) to gain people's cooperation in a study.

Cohen's *d* See *d*.

Cohen's kappa See *kappa*.

Cohort design A nonexperimental design in which a defined group of people (a cohort) is followed over time to study outcomes for the cohort; also called a *prospective design*.

Comparison group A group of study participants whose scores on an outcome variable are used to evaluate the outcomes of the group of primary interest (e.g., nonsmokers as a comparison group for smokers); term often used in lieu of *control group* when the study design is not a true experiment.

Complex intervention An intervention in which complexity exists along one or more dimensions, including number of components, number of targeted outcomes, and the time needed for the full intervention to be delivered.

Composite scale A measure of an attribute, involving the aggregation of information from multiple items into a single numerical score that places people on a continuum with respect to the attribute.

Concealment A tactic involving the unobtrusive collection of research data without participants' knowledge or consent, used to obtain an accurate view of naturalistic behaviour when the behaviour would be distorted if participants knew they were being observed.

Concept An abstraction based on observations of behaviours or characteristics (e.g., fatigue, pain).

Concept analysis A systematic process of analyzing a concept or construct, with the aim of identifying the boundaries, definitions, and dimensionality for that concept.

Conceptual definition The abstract or theoretical meaning of a concept being studied.

Conceptual file A manual method of organizing qualitative data, by creating file folders for each category in the coding scheme and inserting relevant excerpts from the data.

Conceptual framework See *framework*.

Conceptual map A schematic representation of a theory or conceptual model that graphically represents key concepts and linkages among them.

Conceptual model Interrelated concepts or abstractions assembled together in a rational scheme by virtue of their relevance to a common theme; sometimes called *conceptual framework*.

Concurrent design A mixed methods study design in which the quantitative and qualitative strands of data collection occur simultaneously; symbolically designated with a plus sign, as in QUAN + QUAL.

Concurrent validity The degree to which scores on an instrument are correlated with scores on an external criterion, measured at the same time.

Confidence interval (CI) The range of values within which a population parameter is estimated to lie, at a specified probability (e.g., 95% CI).

Confidentiality Protection of study participants so that data provided are never publicly divulged.

Confirmability A criterion for trustworthiness in a qualitative inquiry, referring to the objectivity or neutrality of the data and interpretations.

Confounding variable A variable that is extraneous to the research question and that confounds understanding of the relationship between the independent and dependent variables; confounding variables can be controlled in the research design or through statistical procedures.

Consecutive sampling The recruitment of *all* people from an accessible population who meet the eligibility criteria, over a specific time interval or for a specified sample size.

Consent form A written agreement signed by a study participant and a researcher concerning the terms and conditions of voluntary participation in a study.

CONSORT guidelines Widely adopted guidelines (Consolidated Standards of Reporting Trials) for reporting information for a randomized controlled trial, including a checklist and flow chart for tracking participants through the trial, from recruitment through data analysis.

Constant comparison A procedure used in a grounded theory analysis wherein newly collected data are compared in an ongoing fashion with data obtained earlier to refine theoretically relevant categories.

Construct An abstraction or concept that is invented (constructed) by researchers based on inferences from human behaviour or human traits (e.g., health locus of control).

Construct validity The validity of inferences from *observed* persons, settings, and interventions in a study to the constructs that these instances might represent; for a measuring instrument, the degree to which it measures the construct under investigation.

Constructivist grounded theory An approach to grounded theory, developed by Charmaz, in which the grounded theory is constructed from shared experiences and relationships between the researcher and study participants and interpretive aspects are emphasized.

Constructivist paradigm An alternative paradigm to the positivist paradigm that holds that there are multiple interpretations of reality and that the goal of research is to understand how individuals construct reality within their context; associated with qualitative research; also called *naturalistic paradigm*.

***Contamination** The inadvertent, undesirable influence of one treatment condition on another treatment condition, as when members of the control group receive the intervention.

Content analysis The process of organizing and integrating material from documents, often the narrative information from a qualitative study, according to key concepts and themes.

Content validity The degree to which a multi-item measure has an appropriate set of relevant items reflecting the full content of the construct domain being measured.

Content validity index (CVI) An index of the degree to which an instrument is content valid based on ratings of a panel of experts; content validity for individual items and the overall scale can be assessed.

Continuous variable A variable that can take on an infinite range of values along a specified continuum (e.g., height); less strictly, a variable measured on an interval or ratio scale.

Control, research The process of holding constant confounding influences on the dependent variable (the outcome) under study.

Control group Subjects in an experimental study who do not receive the experimental intervention and whose performance provides a counterfactual against which the effects of an intervention can be measured.

Controlled trial A trial of an intervention that includes a control group, with or without randomization.

Convenience sampling Selection of the most readily available persons as participants in a study.

Convergent design A concurrent, equal-priority mixed methods design in which different but complementary data, quantitative and qualitative, are gathered about a central phenomenon under study; symbolized as QUAN + QUAL; sometimes called a *triangulation design*.

Core category (variable) In a grounded theory study, the central phenomenon that is used to integrate all categories of the data.

Correlation A bond or association between variables, with variation in one variable systematically related to variation in another.

Correlation coefficient An index summarizing the degree of relationship between variables, typically ranging from +1.00 (a perfect positive relationship) through 0.0 (no relationship) to −1.00 (a perfect negative relationship).

Correlation matrix A two-dimensional display showing the correlation coefficients between all pairs in a set of several variables.

Correlational research Research that explores the interrelationships among variables of interest, with no researcher intervention.

Cost (economic) analysis An analysis of the relationship between costs and outcomes of alternative nursing or other health care interventions.

*Counterbalancing The process of systematically varying the order of presentation of stimuli or treatments to control for ordering effects, especially in a crossover design.

Counterfactual The condition or group used as a basis of comparison in a study, embodying what would have happened *to the same people* exposed to a causal factor if they *simultaneously* were *not* exposed to the causal factor.

Covariate A variable that is statistically controlled (held constant) in ANCOVA, typically a confounding influence on the outcome variable, or a preintervention measure of the outcome.

Covert data collection The collection of information in a study without participants' knowledge.

Credibility A criterion for evaluating integrity and trustworthiness in qualitative studies, referring to confidence in the truth of the data; analogous to internal validity in quantitative research.

Criterion sampling A purposive sampling approach used by qualitative researchers that involves selecting cases that meet a predetermined criterion of importance.

Criterion validity The extent to which scores on a measure are an adequate reflection of (or predictor of) a criterion—i.e., a "gold standard" measure.

Critical ethnography An ethnography that focuses on raising consciousness in the group or culture under study in the hope of effecting social change.

*Critical incidents technique A method of obtaining data from study participants by in-depth exploration of specific incidents and behaviours related to the topic under study.

Critical theory An approach to viewing the world that involves a critique of society, with the goal of envisioning new possibilities and effecting social change.

Critique A critical appraisal that analyzes both weaknesses and strengths of a research report.

Cronbach's alpha See *coefficient alpha*.

Crossover design An experimental design in which one group of subjects is exposed to more than one condition or treatment in random order.

Cross-sectional design A study design in which data are collected at one point in time; sometimes used to infer change over time when data are collected from different age or developmental groups.

Crosstabs (contingency) table A two-dimensional table in which the frequencies of two categorical variables are crosstabulated.

Crosstabulation A calculation of frequencies for two variables considered simultaneously—e.g., gender (male/female) crosstabulated with smoking status (smoker/nonsmoker).

d statistic A widely used effect size index for comparing two group means, computed by subtracting one mean from the other and dividing by the pooled standard deviation; also called *Cohen's d* or *standardized mean difference*.

Data The pieces of information obtained in a study (singular is *datum*).

Data analysis The systematic organization and synthesis of research data and, in quantitative studies, the testing of hypotheses using those data.

Data collection protocols The formal procedures researchers develop to guide the collection of data in a standardized fashion.

Data saturation See *saturation*.

Data set The total collection of data on all variables for all study participants.

Data triangulation The use of multiple data sources for the purpose of validating conclusions.

Debriefing Communication with study participants after participation is complete regarding aspects of the study (e.g., explaining the study purpose more fully).

Deception The deliberate withholding of information, or the provision of false information, to study participants, usually to reduce potential biases.

Deductive reasoning The process of developing specific predictions from general principles (see also *inductive reasoning*).

Degrees of freedom (*df*) A statistical concept referring to the number of sample values free to vary (e.g., with a given sample mean, all but one value would be free to vary).

Delayed treatment design A design for an intervention study that involves putting control group members on a waiting list to receive the intervention after follow-up data are collected; also called a *wait-list design*.

Delphi survey A technique for obtaining judgments from an expert panel about an issue of concern; experts are questioned individually in several rounds, with a summary of the panel's views circulated between rounds, to achieve some consensus.

Dependability A criterion for evaluating integrity in qualitative studies, referring to the stability of data over time and over conditions; analogous to reliability in quantitative research.

Dependent variable The variable hypothesized to depend on or be caused by another variable (the *independent variable*); the outcome of interest.

Descendancy approach In literature searches, finding a pivotal early study and searching forward in citation indexes to find more recent studies ("descendants") that cited the key study.

Descriptive phenomenology An approach to phenomenology that focuses on the careful description of ordinary conscious experience of everyday life.

Descriptive qualitative study An in-depth study that involves the collection of rich qualitative data but does not have roots in a particular qualitative tradition; data are often analyzed using content analysis.

Descriptive research Research that typically has as its main objective the accurate portrayal of people's characteristics or circumstances and/or the frequency with which certain phenomena occur.

Descriptive statistics Statistics used to describe and summarize data (e.g., means, percentages).

Descriptive theory A broad characterization that thoroughly accounts for a phenomenon.

Determinism The belief that phenomena are not haphazard or random but rather have antecedent causes; an assumption in the positivist paradigm.

Dichotomous question A question with only two response options (e.g., male/female, yes/no).

Directional hypothesis A hypothesis that makes a specific prediction about the direction of the relationship between two variables.

Disconfirming case A concept used in qualitative research that concerns a case that challenges the researchers' conceptualizations; sometimes used in a sampling strategy.

Domain In ethnographic analysis, a unit or broad category of cultural knowledge.

Double-blind A situation (usually in a clinical trial) in which two study groups are blinded with respect to the group that a study participant is in; often a situation in which neither the subjects nor those who administer the treatment know who is in the experimental or control group.

Economic analysis An analysis of the relationship between costs and outcomes of alternative health care interventions.

Effect size (ES) A statistical index expressing the magnitude of the relationship between two variables, or the magnitude of the difference between groups on an attribute of interest (e.g., Cohen's *d*); also used in meta-summaries of qualitative research to characterize the salience of a theme or category.

Effectiveness study A clinical trial designed to test the effectiveness of an intervention under ordinary conditions, usually for an intervention already found to be efficacious in an efficacy study.

Efficacy study A tightly controlled trial designed to establish the efficacy of an intervention under ideal conditions, using a design that stresses internal validity.

Element The most basic unit of a population for sampling purposes, typically a human being.

Eligibility criteria The criteria designating the specific attributes of the target population, by which people are selected for inclusion in a study.

Emergent design A design that unfolds in the course of a qualitative study as the researcher makes ongoing design decisions reflecting what has already been learned.

Emergent fit A concept in grounded theory that involves comparing new data and new categories with previously existing conceptualizations.

Emic perspective An ethnographic term referring to the way members of a culture themselves view their world; the "insider's view."

Empirical evidence Evidence rooted in objective reality and gathered using one's senses as the basis for generating knowledge.

Estimation of parameters Statistical procedures that estimate population parameters based on sample statistics.

Ethical dilemma A situation in which there is a conflict between ethical considerations and the research methods needed to maximize the quality of study evidence.

Ethics A system of moral values that is concerned with the degree to which research procedures adhere to professional, legal, and social obligations to study participants.

Ethnography A branch of human inquiry, associated with anthropology, that focuses on the culture of a group of people, with an effort to understand the worldview and customs of those under study.

Ethnonursing research A term coined by Leininger to denote the study of human cultures, with a focus on a group's beliefs and practices relating to nursing care and related health behaviours.

Etic perspective In ethnography, the "outsider's" view of the experiences of a cultural group.

Evaluation research Research aimed at learning how well a program, practice, or policy is working.

Event sampling A sampling plan that involves the selection of integral behaviours or events to be observed.

Evidence-based practice (EBP) A practice that involves making clinical decisions based on an integration of the best available evidence, most often from disciplined research, with clinical expertise and patient preferences.

Evidence hierarchy A ranked arrangement of the validity and dependability of evidence based on the rigor of the method that produced it; the traditional evidence hierarchy is appropriate primarily for cause-probing research.

Exclusion criteria The criteria specifying characteristics that a population does *not* have.

Expectation bias The bias that can arise when participants (or research staff) have expectations about treatment effectiveness in intervention research; the expectation can result in altered behaviour or altered communication.

Experimental group The study participants who receive the experimental intervention.

Experimental research Research using a design in which the researcher controls (manipulates) the independent variable and randomly assigns people to different treatment conditions; randomized controlled trials use experimental designs.

Explanatory design A sequential mixed methods design in which quantitative data are collected in the first phase and qualitative data are collected in the second phase to build on or explain quantitative findings; symbolized as QUAN → qual or quan → QUAL.

Exploratory design A sequential mixed methods design in which qualitative data are collected in the first phase and quantitative data are collected in the second phase based on the initial in-depth exploration; symbolized as QUAL → quan or qual → QUAN.

External validity The degree to which study results can be generalized to settings or groups other than the one studied.

Extraneous variable A variable that confounds the relationship between the independent and dependent variables and that needs to be controlled either in the research design or through statistical procedures; often called *confounding variable*.

Extreme case sampling A qualitative sampling approach that involves the purposeful selection of the most extreme or unusual cases.

Extreme response set A bias in psychosocial scales created when participants select extreme response options (e.g., "strongly agree"), independent of the item's content.

F **ratio** The statistic obtained in several statistical tests (e.g., ANOVA) in which score variation attributable to different sources (e.g., between groups and within groups) is compared.

Face validity The extent to which an instrument looks as though it is measuring what it purports to measure.

Feminist research Research that seeks to understand, typically through qualitative approaches, how gender and a gendered social order shape women's lives and their consciousness.

Field diary A daily record of events and conversations in the field; also called a log.

Field notes The notes taken by researchers to record the unstructured observations made in the field, and the interpretation of those observations.

Field research Research in which the data are collected "in the field," i.e., in naturalistic settings.

Fieldwork The activities undertaken by qualitative researchers to collect data out in the field, i.e., in natural settings.

Findings The results of the analysis of research data.

Fit An element in Glaserian grounded theory analysis in which the researcher develops categories of a substantive theory that fit the data.

Fixed effects model In meta-analysis, a model in which studies are assumed to be measuring the same overall effect; a pooled effect estimate is calculated under the assumption that observed variation between studies is attributable to chance.

Focus group interview An interview with a small group of individuals assembled to answer questions on a given topic.

Focused interview A loosely structured interview in which an interviewer guides the respondent through a set of questions using a topic guide; also called a *semistructured interview*.

Follow-up study A study undertaken to assess the outcomes of individuals with a specified condition or who have received a specified treatment.

Forest plot A graphic representation of effects in the sample of studies in a meta-analysis, permitting a visual assessment of variation in effects across studies (i.e., heterogeneity).

Framework The conceptual underpinnings of a study—e.g., a *theoretical framework* in theory-based studies or *conceptual framework* in studies based on a specific conceptual model.

Frequency distribution A systematic array of numeric values from the lowest to the highest, together with a count of the number of times each value was obtained.

Frequency effect size In a meta-summary of qualitative studies, the percentage of reports that contain a given thematic finding.

Full disclosure The communication of complete, accurate information to potential study participants.

Functional relationship A relationship between two variables in which it cannot be assumed that one variable caused the other; also called an *associative relationship*.

Gaining entrée The process of gaining access to study participants or data through the cooperation of key gatekeepers in the selected community or site.

Generalizability The degree to which the research methods justify the inference that the findings are true for a broader group than study participants; in particular, the inference that the findings can be generalized from the sample to the population.

Grand theory A broad theory aimed at describing large segments of the physical, social, or behavioural world; also called a *macrotheory*.

Grand tour question A broad question asked in an unstructured interview to gain a general overview of a phenomenon on the basis of which more focused questions are subsequently asked.

Grey literature Unpublished, and thus less readily accessible, research reports.

Grounded theory An approach to collecting and analyzing qualitative data that aims to develop theories about social psychological processes grounded in real-world observations.

Hand searching The planned searching of a journal "by hand" to identify all relevant reports that might be missed by electronic searching.

*Hawthorne effect The effect on the dependent variable resulting from subjects' awareness that they are participants under study.

Health services research The broad interdisciplinary field that studies how organizational structures and processes, health technologies, social factors, and personal behaviours affect access to health care, the cost and quality of health care, and, ultimately, people's health and well-being.

Hermeneutic circle In hermeneutics, the methodologic process in which, to reach understanding, there is continual movement between the parts and the whole of the text that are being analyzed.

Hermeneutics A qualitative research tradition, drawing on interpretive phenomenology, that focuses on the lived experiences of humans and on how they interpret those experiences.

Heterogeneity The degree to which objects are dissimilar (i.e., characterized by variability) on an attribute; heterogeneity of effects in a systematic review can affect whether a meta-analysis is appropriate.

Historical research Systematic studies designed to discover facts and relationships about past events.

History threat The occurrence of events external to an intervention but concurrent with it, which can affect the outcome variable and threaten the study's internal validity.

Homogeneity The degree to which objects are similar (i.e., characterized by low variability); sometimes, a design strategy used to control confounding variables.

Hypothesis A statement of predicted relationships between variables.

Hypothesis testing Statistical procedures for testing whether hypotheses should be accepted or rejected, based on the probability that hypothesized relationships in a sample exist in the population.

Implementation potential The extent to which an innovation is amenable to implementation in a new setting; an assessment of implementation potential is often made in an evidence-based practice project.

Implied consent Consent to participate in a study that a researcher assumes has been given based on participants' actions, such as returning a completed questionnaire.

IMRAD format The organization of a research report into four main sections: the Introduction, Method, Results, and Discussion sections.

*Incidence The rate of new cases with a specified condition, determined by dividing the number of new cases over a given period of time by the number at risk of becoming a new case (i.e., free of the condition at the outset of the time period).

Inclusion criteria The criteria specifying characteristics of a population— characteristics that a prospective participant must have to be considered eligible for a study.

Independent variable The variable that is believed to cause or influence the dependent variable; in experimental research, the manipulated (treatment) variable; the independent variable is both the "I" and the "C" in the PICO framework.

Inductive reasoning The process of reasoning from specific observations to more general rules (see also *deductive reasoning*).

Inference In research, a conclusion drawn from the study evidence, taking into account the methods used to generate that evidence.

Inferential statistics Statistics that are used to make inferences about whether results observed in a sample are likely to be reliable, i.e., found in the population.

Informant An individual who provides information to researchers about a phenomenon under study; a term used mostly in ethnographic studies.

Informed consent A process in the ethical conduct of a study that involves obtaining people's voluntary participation in a study, after informing them of possible risks and benefits.

Inquiry audit An independent scrutiny of qualitative data and relevant supporting documents by an external reviewer to determine the dependability and confirmability of qualitative data.

Insider research Research on a group or culture—usually in an ethnography— by a member of that group or culture; in ethnographic research, an *autoethnography*.

Instrument The device used to collect data (e.g., a questionnaire, test, observation schedule).

Intensity effect size In a meta-summary of qualitative studies, the percentage of all thematic findings that are contained in any given report.

*Intention to treat The gold standard strategy for analyzing data in an intervention study, which involves including participants in the group to which they were assigned, whether or not they received or completed the treatment associated with the group.

Interaction effect The effect of two or more independent variables acting in combination (interactively) on an outcome.

Intercoder reliability The degree to which two coders, working independently, agree on coding decisions.

Internal consistency The degree to which the items on an instrument are interrelated and are measuring the same attribute or dimension, usually as evaluated using coefficient alpha; a measurement property within the reliability domain.

Internal validity The degree to which it can be inferred that the experimental intervention (independent variable), rather than confounding factors, caused the observed effects on the outcome.

Interpretive phenomenology A type of phenomenology that stresses interpreting and understanding, not just describing, human experience; often referred to as *hermeneutics*.

Interrater (interobserver) reliability The degree to which two raters or observers, working independently, assign the same ratings or values for an attribute being measured.

Interval estimation A statistical estimation approach in which the researcher computes a range of values that are likely, within a given level of confidence (e.g., the 95% CI), to contain the true population parameter.

Interval measurement A measurement level in which an attribute of a variable is rank ordered on a scale that has equal distances between points on that scale (e.g., Fahrenheit degrees).

Intervention In experimental research (clinical trials), the treatment being tested; often the "I" in the PICO framework.

Intervention fidelity The extent to which the implementation of a treatment is faithful to its plan.

Intervention protocol The specification of what the intervention and alternative (control) treatment conditions are and how they should be administered.

Intervention research Research involving the development, implementation, and testing of an intervention.

Intervention theory The conceptual underpinning of a health care intervention, which articulates the theoretical basis for what must be done to achieve desired outcomes.

Interview A data collection method in which an interviewer asks questions of a respondent, either face-to-face, by telephone, or over the Internet (e.g., via Skype).

Interview schedule The formal instrument that specifies the wording of all questions to be asked of respondents in structured self-report studies.

Intraclass correlation coefficient (ICC) A statistical index used to estimate the reliability (e.g., test–retest reliability) of a measure.

Intuiting A step in phenomenology, which occurs when researchers remain open to the meaning attributed to the phenomenon by those who experienced it.

Inverse relationship See *negative relationship*.

Investigator triangulation The use of two or more researchers to analyze and interpret a data set, to enhance trustworthiness.

Iowa Model of Evidence-Based Practice A widely used framework that can be used to guide the development and implementation of a project to promote evidence-based practice.

Item A single question or statement on an instrument, such as on a composite scale.

Journal article A report appearing in professional journals such as *Research in Nursing & Health* or *International Journal of Nursing Studies*.

Journal club A group that meets in clinical settings to discuss and critique research articles appearing in journals.

Kappa A statistical index of chance-corrected agreement or consistency between two nominal (or ordinal) measurements, often used to assess interrater reliability.

Key informant A person knowledgeable about the phenomenon of research interest and who is willing to share information and insights with the researcher (e.g., an ethnographer).

Keyword An important term used to search for references on a topic in a bibliographic database.

Knowledge translation (KT) The exchange, synthesis, and application of knowledge by relevant stakeholders within complex systems to accelerate the beneficial effects of research aimed at improving health care.

Known-groups validity A type of construct validity that concerns the degree to which a measure is capable of discriminating between groups known or expected to differ with regard to the construct of interest.

Level of measurement A system of classifying measurements according to the nature of the measurement and the type of permissible mathematical operations; the levels are nominal, ordinal, interval, and ratio.

Level of significance The risk of making a Type I error in a statistical analysis, with the criterion (alpha) established by the researcher beforehand (e.g., $\alpha = .05$).

Likert scale Traditionally, a type of scale to measure attitudes, involving the summation of scores on a set of items that respondents rate for their degree of agreement or disagreement; more loosely, the name attributed to summated rating scales.

Literature review A critical summary of research on a topic, often prepared to put a research problem in context or to summarize existing evidence.

Log In participant observation studies, the observer's daily record of events and conversations.

Logistic regression A multivariate regression procedure that analyzes relationships between one or more independent variables and a categorical dependent variable.

Longitudinal design A study design in which data are collected at more than one point in time, in contrast to a cross-sectional design.

Macrotheory A broad theory aimed at describing large segments of the physical, social, or behavioural world; also called a *grand theory*.

Manifest effect size In meta-summaries, effect sizes calculated from the manifest content represented in the findings of primary qualitative studies; includes *frequency effect sizes* and *intensity effect sizes*.

Manipulation The introduction of an intervention or treatment in an experimental or quasi-experimental study to assess its impact on the dependent (outcome) variable.

*MANOVA See *multivariate analysis of variance*.

Masking See *blinding*.

Matching The pairing of participants in one group with those in a comparison group based on their similarity on one or more characteristic, to enhance group comparability and to control confounding variables.

Maturation threat A threat to the internal validity of a study that results when changes to the outcome (dependent) variable result from the passage of time.

Maximum variation sampling A sampling approach used by qualitative researchers involving the purposeful selection of cases with a wide range of variation.

Mean A measure of central tendency, computed by summing all scores and dividing by the number of cases.

Measure A device whose purpose is to obtain quantitative information to quantify an attribute or construct (e.g., a scale).

Measurement The assignment of numbers to objects according to specified rules to characterize quantities of some attribute.

Measurement error The systematic and random error associated with a person's score on a measure, reflecting factors other than the construct being measured and resulting in an observed score that is different from a hypothetical true score.

Measurement property A characteristic reflecting a distinct aspect of a measure's quality (e.g., reliability, validity).

Median A descriptive statistic that is a measure of central tendency, representing the exact middle value in a score distribution; the value above and below which 50% of the scores lie.

Mediating variable A variable that mediates or acts like a "go-between" in a causal chain linking two other variables.

Member check A method of validating the credibility of qualitative data through debriefings and discussions with informants.

MeSH Medical Subject Headings, used to index articles in MEDLINE.

Meta-analysis A technique for quantitatively integrating the results of multiple studies addressing the same or highly similar research question.

Meta-ethnography A widely used approach to metasynthesis developed by Noblit and Hare.

Metaphor A figurative comparison used by some qualitative analysts to evoke a visual or symbolic analogy.

Meta-summary A process associated with metasyntheses, involving the development of a list of abstracted findings from primary qualitative studies and calculating manifest effect sizes (frequency and intensity effect size).

Metasynthesis The grand narratives or interpretive translations produced from the integration or comparison of findings from qualitative studies.

Method triangulation The use of multiple methods of data collection about the same phenomenon, to enhance trustworthiness.

Methodologic study A study designed to develop or refine methods of obtaining, organizing, or analyzing data.

Methods (research) The steps, procedures, and strategies for gathering and analyzing data in a study.

Middle-range theory A theory that focuses on a limited piece of reality or human experience, involving a selected number of concepts (e.g., a theory of stress).

Minimal important change (MIC) A benchmark for interpreting change scores that represents the smallest change that is important or meaningful to patients or clinicians.

Minimal risk Anticipated risks that are no greater than those ordinarily encountered in daily life or during the performance of routine tests or procedures.

Mixed methods (MM) research Research in which both quantitative and qualitative data are collected and analyzed to address different but related questions.

Mixed studies review A systematic review that integrates and synthesizes findings from quantitative, qualitative, and mixed methods studies on a topic.

Mode A measure of central tendency; the value that occurs most frequently in a distribution of scores.

Model A symbolic representation of concepts or variables and interrelationships among them.

Mortality threat A threat to the internal validity of a study, referring to differential attrition (loss of participants) from different groups.

Multimodal distribution A distribution of values with more than one peak (high frequency).

Multiple comparison procedures Statistical tests, normally applied after an ANOVA indicates statistically significant group differences, that compare different pairs of groups; also called *post hoc tests*.

Multiple correlation coefficient An index that summarizes the degree of relationship between two or more independent variables and a dependent variable; symbolized as *R*.

Multiple regression A statistical procedure for understanding the effects of two or more independent (predictor) variables on a dependent variable.

Multistage sampling A sampling strategy that proceeds through a set of stages from larger to smaller sampling units (e.g., from states, to census tracts, to households).

*****Multivariate analysis of variance (MANOVA)** A statistical procedure used to test the significance of differences between the means of two or more groups on two or more dependent variables, considered simultaneously.

Multivariate statistics Statistical procedures designed to analyze the relationships among three or more variables (e.g., multiple regression, ANCOVA).

N The symbol designating the total number of subjects (e.g., "the total *N* was 500").

n The symbol designating the number of subjects in a subgroup or cell of a study (e.g., "each of the four groups had an *n* of 125, for a total *N* of 500").

Narrative analysis A qualitative approach that focuses on the story as the object of the inquiry.

Naturalistic paradigm See *constructivist paradigm*.

Naturalistic setting A setting for the collection of research data that is natural to those being studied (e.g., homes, places of work).

Nay-sayers bias A bias in self-report scales created when respondents characteristically disagree with statements ("nay-say"), independent of content.

Negative case analysis The refinement of a theory or description in a qualitative study through the inclusion of cases that appear to disconfirm earlier hypotheses.

Negative relationship A relationship between two variables in which there is a tendency for high values on one variable to be associated with low values on the other (e.g., as stress increases, quality of life decreases); also called an *inverse relationship*.

Negative skew An asymmetric distribution of data values with a disproportionately high number of cases at the upper end; when displayed graphically, the tail points to the left.

Nested sampling An approach to sampling in mixed methods studies in which some, but not all, of the participants from one strand are included in the sample for the other strand.

Network sampling See *snowball sampling*.

Nominal measurement The lowest level of measurement involving the assignment of characteristics into categories (e.g., males = 1; females = 2; other = 3).

Nondirectional hypothesis A research hypothesis that does not stipulate the expected direction of the relationship between variables.

Nonequivalent control group design A quasi-experimental design involving a comparison group that was not created through random assignment.

Nonexperimental research Studies in which the researcher collects data without introducing an intervention; also called *observational research*.

Nonparametric tests A class of statistical tests that do not involve stringent assumptions about the distribution of variables in the analysis.

Nonprobability sampling The selection of sampling units (e.g., people) from a population using nonrandom procedures (e.g., convenience and quota sampling).

Nonresponse bias A bias that can result when a nonrandom subset of people invited to participate in a study decline to participate.

Nonsignificant result The result of a statistical test indicating that group differences or an observed relationship could have occurred by chance, at a given level of significance; sometimes abbreviated as NS; sometimes called *negative results*.

Normal distribution A theoretical distribution that is bell-shaped, symmetrical, and not too peaked.

Null hypothesis A hypothesis stating the absence of a relationship between the variables under study; used primarily in statistical testing as the hypothesis to be rejected.

Number needed to treat (NNT) An estimate of how many people would need to receive an intervention to prevent one undesirable outcome, computed by dividing 1 by the value of the absolute risk reduction.

Nursing research Systematic inquiry designed to develop knowledge about issues of importance to the nursing profession.

Nursing sensitive outcome A patient outcome that improves if there is greater quantity or quality of nursing care.

Objectivity The extent to which two independent researchers would arrive at similar judgments or conclusions (i.e., judgments not biased by personal values or beliefs).

Observation A method of collecting information and measuring constructs by directly watching and recording behaviours and characteristics.

Observational research Studies that do not involve an experimental intervention—i.e., nonexperimental research in which phenomena are merely observed; also, research in which data are collected through direct observation.

Odds A way of expressing the chance of an event—the probability of an event occurring to the probability that it will not occur, calculated by dividing the number of people who experienced an event by the number for whom it did not occur.

Odds ratio (OR) The ratio of one odds to another odds, e.g., the ratio of the odds of an event in one group to the odds of an event in another group; an odds ratio of 1.0 indicates no difference between groups.

Open-ended question A question in an interview or questionnaire that does not restrict respondents' answers to preestablished response options.

Open coding The first level of coding in a grounded theory study, referring to the basic descriptive coding of the content of narrative materials.

Operational definition The definition of a concept or variable in terms of the procedures by which it is to be measured.

Operationalization The translation of research concepts into measurable phenomena.

Ordinal measurement A measurement level that rank orders phenomena along some dimension.

Outcome A term often used to refer to the dependent variable, i.e., a measure that captures the outcome (endpoint) of interest; the "O" in the PICO framework.

Outcomes research Research designed to document the effectiveness of health care services and the end results of patient care.

p **value** In statistical testing, the probability that the obtained results are due to chance alone; the probability of a Type I error.

Paradigm A way of looking at natural phenomena that encompasses a set of philosophical assumptions and that guides one's approach to inquiry.

Paradigm case In a hermeneutic analysis following the precepts of Benner, a strong exemplar of the phenomenon under study, often used early in the analysis to gain understanding of the phenomenon.

Parameter A characteristic of a population (e.g., the mean age of all Canadian citizens).

Parametric tests A class of statistical tests that involve assumptions about the distribution of the variables and the estimation of a parameter.

Participant See *study participant*.

Participant observation A method of collecting data through the participation in and observation of a group or culture.

Participatory action research (PAR) A research approach in which researchers and study participants collaborate in all steps of the research process; the approach is based on the premise that the use and production of knowledge can be political and used to exert power.

*****Path analysis** A regression-based procedure for testing causal models, typically using correlational data.

Patient-reported outcome (PRO) A health outcome that is measured by directly asking patients for information.

Pearson's *r* A correlation coefficient designating the magnitude of relationship between two interval- or ratio-level variables; also called *the product–moment correlation*.

Peer debriefing A session with peers of the researcher, to review and explore various aspects of a qualitative study, often used to enhance trustworthiness.

Peer reviewer A researcher who reviews and critiques a research report or proposal and who makes a recommendation about publishing or funding the research.

Perfect relationship A correlation between two variables such that the values of one variable can perfectly predict the values of the other; designated as 1.00 or −1.00.

*****Per protocol analysis** Analysis of data from a randomized controlled trial that excludes participants who did not receive the protocol to which they were assigned.

Persistent observation A qualitative researcher's intense focus on the aspects of a situation that are relevant to the phenomena being studied.

Person triangulation The collection of data from different levels or types of persons, with the aim of validating data through multiple perspectives on the phenomenon.

Personal interview An in-person, face-to-face interview between an interviewer and a respondent.

Phenomenology A qualitative research tradition, with roots in philosophy and psychology, that focuses on the lived experience of humans.

Phenomenon The abstract concept under study, often used by qualitative researchers in lieu of the term *variable*.

Photo elicitation An interview stimulated and guided by photographic images.

Photovoice A technique used in some qualitative studies that involves asking participants to take photographs relating to a topic under study and then interpret them.

PICO framework A framework for asking well-worded questions, and for searching for evidence, where P = population, I = intervention of influence, C = comparison, and O = outcome.

Pilot test A small-scale study, or trial run, done in preparation for a major study, often to assess feasibility.

Placebo A sham or pseudointervention sometimes used as a control group condition.

*Placebo effect Changes in the dependent variable attributable to the placebo.

Plan-Do-Study-Act A framework often used to guide quality improvement projects.

Point estimation A statistical procedure that uses information from a sample (a statistic) to estimate the single value that best represents the population parameter.

Population The entire set of individuals or objects having some common characteristics (e.g., all registered nurses [RNs] in California); the "P" in the PICO framework.

Positive relationship A relationship between two variables in which high values on one variable tend to be associated with high values on the other (e.g., as physical activity increases, pulse rate increases).

Positive results In statistical testing, research results that are consistent with the researcher's hypotheses; negative results are ones that are not statistically significant.

Positive skew An asymmetric distribution of values with a disproportionately high number of cases at the lower end; when displayed graphically, the tail points to the right.

Positivist paradigm The paradigm underlying the traditional scientific approach, which assumes that there is an orderly reality that can be objectively studied; often associated with quantitative research.

***Post hoc* test** A test for comparing all possible pairs of groups following a significant test of overall group differences (e.g., in an ANOVA).

Poster session A session at a professional conference in which several researchers simultaneously present visual displays summarizing their studies while conference attendees circulate around the room perusing the displays.

Posttest data Data collected after introducing an intervention.

Posttest-only design An experimental design in which data are collected from participants only after the intervention has been introduced.

Power The ability of a design or analysis strategy to detect true relationships that exist among variables.

Power analysis A procedure for estimating either the needed sample size for a study or the likelihood of committing a Type II error.

Pragmatism A paradigm on which mixed methods research is often said to be based, in that it acknowledges the practical imperative of the "dictatorship of the research question."

Precision The degree to which an estimated population value (a statistic) clusters closely around the estimate, usually expressed in terms of the width of the confidence interval.

Prediction The use of empirical evidence to make forecasts about how variables will behave with a new group of people.

Predictive validity A type of criterion validity that concerns the degree to which a measure is correlated with a criterion measured at a future point in time.

Predictor variable In regression analyses, a term often used in lieu of independent variable; predictor variables are used to predict the value of the dependent (outcome) variable.

Pretest (1) Data collected prior to an intervention; often called baseline data. (2) The trial administration of a newly developed instrument to identify potential weaknesses.

Pretest–posttest design An experimental design in which data are collected from research subjects both before and after introducing an intervention.

Prevalence The proportion of a population having a particular condition (e.g., fibromyalgia) at a given point in time.

Primary source Firsthand reports of facts or findings; in research, the original report prepared by the investigator who conducted the study.

Primary study In a systematic review, an original study whose findings are used as the data in the review.

Priority A key design feature in mixed methods research, concerning which strand (qualitative or quantitative) will be given more emphasis; in notation, the dominant strand is in all capital letters, as QUAL or QUAN, and the nondominant strand is in lower case, as qual or quan.

Probability sampling The selection of sampling units (e.g., participants) from a population using random procedures (e.g., simple random sampling).

Probing Eliciting more useful or detailed information from a respondent in an interview than was volunteered in the first reply.

Problem statement An expression of a dilemma or disturbing situation that needs investigation.

Process analysis A descriptive analysis of the process by which a program or intervention gets implemented and used in practice.

Process consent In a qualitative study, an ongoing, transactional process of negotiating consent with participants, allowing them to collaborate in the decision making about their continued participation.

Product–moment correlation coefficient (*r*) A correlation coefficient designating the magnitude and direction of relationship between two variables measured on at least an interval scale; also called *Pearson's r*.

Prolonged engagement In qualitative research, the investment of sufficient time during data collection to have an in-depth understanding of the phenomenon under study, thereby enhancing credibility.

Proposal A document communicating a research problem, proposed methods for addressing the problem, and, when funding is sought, how much the study will cost.

Prospective design A study design that begins with an examination of a presumed cause (e.g., cigarette smoking) and then goes forward in time to observe presumed effects (e.g., lung cancer); also called a *cohort design*.

Psychometric assessment An evaluation of the measurement properties of a measure, such as its reliability and validity.

Psychometrics The theory underlying principles of measurement and the application of the theory in the development and testing of measures.

Publication bias The bias resulting from the fact that published studies overrepresent statistically significant findings, reflecting the tendency of researchers, reviewers, and editors to not publish nonsignificant results.

Purposive (purposeful) sampling A nonprobability sampling method in which the researcher selects participants based on personal judgment about who will be most informative.

Q-sort A data collection method in which participants sort statements into piles (usually 9 or 11) according to some bipolar dimension (e.g., most helpful/least helpful).

Qualitative analysis The organization and interpretation of narrative data for the purpose of discovering important underlying themes, categories, and patterns.

Qualitative content analysis See *content analysis*.

Qualitative data Information collected in narrative (nonnumeric) form, such as the information provided in an unstructured interview.

Qualitative research The investigation of phenomena, typically in an in-depth and holistic fashion, through the collection of rich narrative materials using a flexible research design.

Quality improvement (QI) Systematic efforts to improve practices and processes within a specific organization or patient group.

Quantitative analysis The organization and testing of numeric data through statistical procedures for the purpose of describing phenomena or assessing the magnitude and reliability of relationships among them.

Quantitative data Information collected in a quantified (numeric) form.

Quantitative research The investigation of phenomena that lend themselves to precise measurement and quantification, often involving a rigorous and controlled design.

Quasi-experiment A type of design for testing an intervention in which participants are not randomly assigned to treatment conditions; also called a *nonrandomized trial* or a *controlled trial without randomization*.

Questionnaire A document used to gather self-report data via self-administration of questions.

Quota sampling A nonrandom sampling method in which "quotas" for certain subgroups, based on sample characteristics, are established to increase the representativeness of the sample.

r The symbol for a bivariate correlation coefficient, summarizing the magnitude and direction of a relationship between two variables measured on an interval or ratio scale.

R The symbol for the multiple correlation coefficient, indicating the magnitude (but not direction) of the relationship between a dependent variable and multiple independent (predictor) variables, taken together.

R^2 The squared multiple correlation coefficient, indicating the proportion of variance in the dependent variable explained by a set of independent variables.

Random assignment The assignment of participants to treatment conditions in a random manner (i.e., in a manner determined by chance alone); also called *randomization*.

Random effects model In meta-analysis, a model in which studies are not assumed to be measuring the same overall effect but rather reflect a distribution of effects; often preferred to a fixed effect model when there is extensive variation of effects across studies.

Random number table A table displaying hundreds of digits (from 0 to 9) in random order; each number is equally likely to follow any other.

Random sampling The selection of a sample such that each member of a population has an equal probability of being included.

Randomization The assignment of subjects to treatment conditions in a random manner (i.e., in a manner determined by chance alone); also called *random assignment*.

Randomized controlled trial (RCT) A full experimental test of an intervention, involving random assignment to treatment groups; sometimes, an RCT is phase III of a full clinical trial.

Randomness An important concept in quantitative research, involving having certain features of the study established by chance rather than by design or personal preference.

Range A measure of variability, computed by subtracting the lowest value from the highest value in a distribution of scores.

Rating scale A scale that requires ratings of an object or concept along a continuum.

Ratio measurement A measurement level with equal distances between scores and a true meaningful zero point (e.g., weight).

Raw data Data in the form in which they were collected, without being coded or analyzed.

Reactivity A measurement distortion arising from the study participant's awareness of being observed, or, more generally, from the effect of the measurement procedure itself.

Readability The ease with which materials (e.g., a questionnaire) can be read by people with varying reading skills, often determined through readability formulas.

Receiver-operating characteristic (ROC) curve A method used in developing and refining a screening instrument to determine the best cutoff point for "caseness."

Reflexive notes Notes that document a qualitative researcher's personal experiences, self-reflections, and progress in the field.

Reflexivity In qualitative studies, the researcher's critical self-reflection about his or her own biases, preferences, and preconceptions.

Regression analysis A statistical procedure for predicting values of a dependent variable based on one or more independent variables.

Relationship A bond or a connection between two or more variables.

Relative risk (RR) An estimate of risk of "caseness" in one group compared to another, computed by dividing the absolute risk for one group (e.g., an exposed group) by the absolute risk for another (e.g., the nonexposed); also called the *risk ratio*.

Reliability The extent to which a measurement is free from measurement error; more broadly, the extent to which scores for people who have not changed are the same for repeated measurements.

Reliability coefficient A quantitative index, usually ranging in value from .00 to 1.00, that provides an estimate of how reliable an instrument is (e.g., the intraclass correlation coefficient).

Repeated measures ANOVA An analysis of variance used when there are multiple measurements of the dependent variable over time (e.g., in an experimental crossover design).

Replication The deliberate repetition of research procedures in a second investigation for the purpose of assessing whether earlier results can be confirmed.

Representative sample A sample whose characteristics are comparable to those of the population from which it is drawn.

Representativeness A key criterion for assessing the adequacy of a sample in quantitative studies, indicating the extent to which findings from the study can be generalized to the population.

Research Systematic inquiry that uses orderly methods to answer questions or solve problems.

Research control See *control, research*.

Research design The overall plan for addressing a research question, including strategies for enhancing the study's integrity.

Research ethics board (REB) The institutional group that convenes to review proposed and ongoing studies with respect to ethical considerations.

Research hypothesis The actual hypothesis a researcher wishes to test (as opposed to the *null hypothesis*), stating the anticipated relationship between two or more variables.

Research methods The techniques used to structure a study and to gather and analyze information in a systematic fashion.

Research problem A disturbing or perplexing condition that can be investigated through disciplined inquiry.

Research question A specific query the researcher wants to answer to address a research problem.

Research report A document (often a journal article) summarizing the main features of a study, including the research question, the methods used to address it, the findings, and the interpretation of the findings.

Research utilization The use of some aspect of a study in an application unrelated to the original research.

Researcher credibility The faith that can be put in a researcher based on his or her training, qualifications, and experience.

Respondent In a self-report study, the participant responding to questions posed by the researcher.

Responder analysis An analysis that compares people who are *responders* to an intervention, based on their having reached a benchmark on a change score (e.g., the minimal important change), compared to people who are nonresponders (have not reached the benchmark).

Response options The prespecified set of possible answers to a closed-ended question or item.

Response rate The rate of participation in a study, calculated by dividing the number of persons participating by the number of persons sampled.

Response set bias The measurement error resulting from the tendency of some individuals to respond to items in characteristic ways (e.g., always agreeing), independently of item content.

Results The answers to research questions, obtained through an analysis of the collected data.

Retrospective design A study design that begins with the manifestation of the outcome variable in the present (e.g., lung cancer), and a search for a presumed cause occurring in the past (e.g., cigarette smoking).

Risk/benefit assessment An assessment of the relative costs and benefits, to an individual study participant and to society at large, of participation in a study; also, the relative costs and benefits of implementing an innovation.

Risk ratio See *relative risk*.

Rival hypothesis An alternative explanation, competing with the researcher's hypothesis, for interpreting the results of a study.

ROC curve See *receiver-operating characteristic curve*.

Sample A subset of a population comprising those selected to participate in a study.

Sample size The number of people who participate in a study; an important factor in the *power* of the analysis and in statistical conclusion validity in quantitative research.

Sampling The process of selecting a portion of the population to represent the entire population.

Sampling bias Distortions that arise when a sample is not representative of the population from which it was drawn.

Sampling distribution A theoretical distribution of a statistic, using the values of the statistic (e.g., the mean) from an infinite number of samples as the data points in the distribution.

Sampling error The fluctuation of the value of a statistic from one sample to another drawn from the same population.

Sampling frame A list of all the elements in the population, from which a sample is drawn.

Sampling plan The formal plan specifying a sampling method, a sample size, and procedures for recruiting subjects.

Saturation The collection of qualitative data to the point where a sense of closure is attained because new data yield redundant information.

Scale A composite measure of an attribute, involving the adding together of several items that have a logical and empirical relationship to each other, resulting in the assignment of a score to place people on a continuum with respect to the attribute.

Schematic model A graphic representation depicting concepts and relationships between them; also called a *conceptual map*.

Scientific merit The degree to which a study is methodologically and conceptually sound.

Scientific method A set of orderly, systematic, controlled procedures for acquiring dependable, empirical—and typically quantitative—information; the methodologic approach associated with the positivist paradigm.

Scoping review A preliminary review of research findings designed to refine the questions and protocols for a systematic review.

Screening instrument An instrument used to assess whether potential subjects for a study meet eligibility criteria, or for determining whether a person tests positive for a specified condition.

Secondary analysis A form of research in which the data collected in one study are reanalyzed in another investigation to answer new questions.

Secondary source Secondhand accounts of events or facts; in research, a description of a study prepared by someone other than the original researcher.

Selection threat (self-selection) A threat to a study's internal validity resulting from preexisting differences between groups under study; the differences affect the outcome in ways extraneous to the effect of the independent variable.

Selective coding A level of coding in a grounded theory study that begins once the core category has been discovered and involves limiting coding to only those categories related to the core category.

Self-determination A person's ability to voluntarily decide whether or not to participate in a study.

Self-report A data collection method that involves a direct verbal report by study participants (e.g., by interview or questionnaire).

Semistructured interview An open-ended interview in which the researcher is guided by a list of specific topics to cover.

Sensitivity The ability of a screening instrument to correctly identify a "case," e.g., to correctly diagnose a condition.

Sensitivity analysis An effort to test how sensitive the results of a statistical analysis are to changes in assumptions or in the way the analysis was done (e.g., in a meta-analysis, used to assess whether conclusions are sensitive to the quality of the studies included or to the model used).

Sequential design A mixed methods design in which one strand of data collection (qualitative or quantitative) occurs prior to the other, informing the second strand; symbolically shown with an arrow, as QUAL → QUAN.

Setting The physical location and conditions in which data collection takes place in a study.

Significance, clinical See *clinical significance*.

Significance, statistical See *statistical significance*.

Significance level The probability that an observed relationship could be caused by chance; significance at the .05 level indicates the probability that a relationship of the observed magnitude would be found by chance only 5 times out of 100.

Simple random sampling Basic probability sampling involving the selection of sample members from a sampling frame at random.

Site The overall location where a study is undertaken.

Skewed distribution The asymmetric distribution of a set of data values around a central point.

Snowball sampling The selection of participants through referrals from earlier participants; also called *network sampling*.

Social desirability response set A bias in self-report instruments created when participants have a tendency to misrepresent their opinions in the direction of answers consistent with prevailing social norms.

Space triangulation The collection of data on the same phenomenon in multiple sites to enhance the validity of the findings.

Spearman's rho A correlation coefficient indicating the magnitude of a relationship between variables measured on the ordinal scale.

Specificity The ability of a screening instrument to correctly identify noncases.

Standard deviation The most frequently used statistic for designating the degree of variability in a set of scores.

Standard error The standard deviation of a sampling distribution, such as the sampling distribution of the mean.

Standardized mean difference (SMD) In meta-analysis, the effect size for comparing two group means, computed by subtracting one mean from the other and dividing by the pooled standard deviation; also called Cohen's *d*.

Statement of purpose A declarative statement of the overall goals of a study.

Statistic An estimate of a parameter, calculated from sample data.

Statistical analysis The organization and analysis of quantitative data using statistical procedures, including both descriptive and inferential statistics.

Statistical conclusion validity The degree to which inferences about relationships from a statistical analysis of the data are correct.

Statistical control The use of statistical procedures to control confounding influences on the dependent variable.

Statistical inference An inference about the population based on information from a sample, using laws of probability.

Statistical power The ability of a research design and analytic strategy to detect true relationships among variables.

Statistical significance A term indicating that the results from an analysis of sample data are unlikely to have been caused by chance, at a specified level of probability.

Statistical test An analytic tool that estimates the probability that obtained results from a sample reflect true population values.

Stipend A monetary or other payment to individuals participating in a study, as an incentive for participation and/or to compensate for time and expenses.

Strata Subdivisions of the population according to some characteristic (e.g., males and females); singular is *stratum*.

Stratification The division of a sample or a population into smaller units (e.g., males and females), typically to enhance representativeness or to explore results for subgroups of people; used in both sampling and in allocation to treatment groups.

Stratified random sampling The random selection of study participants from two or more strata of the population independently.

Structured data collection An approach to collecting data from participants, either through self-report or observations, in which categories of information (e.g., response options) are specified in advance.

Study participant An individual who participates and provides information in a study.

Subgroup analysis An analysis that examines whether statistical results are consistent for different subsets of the sample (e.g., for males and females).

Subject An individual who participates and provides data in a study; term used primarily in quantitative research.

Subscale A subset of items that measures one aspect or dimension of a multidimensional construct.

Summated rating scale A scale consisting of multiple items that are added together to yield an overall, continuous score for an attribute (e.g., a Likert scale).

Survey research Nonexperimental research that involves gathering information about people's activities, beliefs, preferences, and attitudes via direct questioning.

Symmetric distribution A distribution of values with two halves that are mirror images of the each other.

Systematic review A rigorous synthesis of research findings on a particular research question, using systematic sampling and data collection procedures and a formal protocol.

Systematic sampling The selection of sample members such that every kth (e.g., every 10th) person or element in a sampling frame is chosen.

Tacit knowledge Information about a culture that is so deeply embedded that members do not talk about it or may not even be consciously aware of it.

Target population The entire population in which a researcher is interested and to which he or she would like to generalize the study results.

Taxonomy In an ethnographic analysis, a system of classifying and organizing terms and concepts, developed to illuminate a domain's organization and the relationship among the domain's categories.

Test statistic A statistic used to test for the reliability of relationships between variables (e.g., chi-squared, *t*); sampling distributions of test statistics are known for circumstances in which the null hypothesis is true.

Test–retest reliability The type of reliability that concerns the extent to which scores for people who have not changed are the same when a measure is administered twice; an assessment of a measure's stability.

The canadian nurses association (CNA) The CNA is also known in French as the Association des infirmières et infirmiers du Canada (AIIC), is the national professional association representing Canadian registered nurses (RNs) to other organizations and to governments nationally and internationally.

Theme A recurring regularity emerging from an analysis of qualitative data.

Theoretical framework See *framework*.

Theoretical sampling In qualitative studies, especially in a grounded theory studies, the selection of sample members based on emerging findings to ensure adequate representation of important theoretical categories.

Theory An abstract generalization that presents a systematic explanation about relationships among phenomena.

Thick description A rich, thorough description of the context and participants in a qualitative study.

Threats to validity In research design, reasons that an inference about the effect of an independent variable (e.g., an intervention) on an outcome could be wrong.

Time sampling In structured observations, the sampling of time periods during which observations will take place.

Time triangulation The collection of data on the same phenomenon or about the same people at different points in time, to enhance trustworthiness.

Time-series design A quasi-experimental design involving the collection of data over an extended time period, with multiple data collection points both prior to and after introducing an intervention.

Topic guide A list of broad question areas to be covered in a semistructured interview or focus group interview.

Transferability The extent to which qualitative findings can be transferred to other settings or groups; analogous to generalizability.

Treatment The experimental intervention under study; the condition being manipulated by the researcher.

Tri council policy statement (TCPS) The Tri-Council Policy Statement: Ethical Conduct for Research Involving Humans (TCPS or the Policy) is a joint policy of Canada's three federal research agencies – the Canadian Institutes of Health Research (CIHR), the Natural Sciences and Engineering Research Council of Canada (NSERC), and the Social Sciences and Humanities Research Council of Canada (SSHRC).

Triangulation The use of multiple methods to collect and interpret data about a phenomenon to converge on an accurate representation of reality.

Trustworthiness The degree of confidence qualitative researchers have in their data and analyses, most often assessed using the criteria of credibility, transferability, dependability, confirmability, and authenticity.

***t*-test** A parametric statistical test for analyzing the difference between two means.

Type I error An error created by rejecting the null hypothesis when it is true (i.e., the researcher concludes that a relationship exists when in fact it does not—a false positive).

Type II error An error created by accepting the null hypothesis when it is false (i.e., the researcher concludes that *no* relationship exists when in fact it does—a false negative).

Unimodal distribution A distribution of values with one peak (high frequency).

Unit of analysis The basic unit or focus of a researcher's analysis—typically individual study participants.

Univariate statistics Statistical analysis of a single variable for descriptive purposes (e.g., computing a mean).

Unstructured interview An interview in which the researcher asks respondents questions without having a predetermined plan regarding the content or flow of information to be gathered.

Unstructured observation The collection of descriptive data through direct observation that is not guided by a formal, prespecified plan for observing, enumerating, or recording the information.

Validity A quality criterion referring to the degree to which inferences made in a study are accurate and well-founded; in measurement, the degree to which an instrument measures what it is intended to measure.

Variability The degree to which values on a set of scores are dispersed over a range of values.

Variable An attribute that varies, that is, takes on different values (e.g., body temperature, heart rate).

*Variance A measure of variability or dispersion, equal to the standard deviation squared.

Vignette A brief description of an event, person, or situation to which respondents are asked to express their reactions.

Visual analog scale (VAS) A scaling procedure used to measure certain clinical symptoms (e.g., pain, fatigue) by having people indicate on a straight line the intensity of the symptom; usually measured on a 100-mm scale with values from 0 to 100.

Vulnerable groups Special groups of people whose rights in studies need special protection because of their inability to provide meaningful informed consent or because their circumstances place them at higher-than-average-risk of adverse effects (e.g., children, unconscious patients).

Wait-list design See *delayed treatment design*.

Yea-sayers bias A bias in self-report scales created when respondents characteristically agree with statements ("yea-say"), independent of content.

Page numbers in bold indicate glossary entries.